Physical Activity Instruction of Older Adults

Second Edition

Debra J. Rose, PhD

California State University at Fullerton

Editor

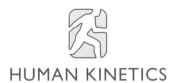

HUMAN KINETICS

Library of Congress Cataloging-in-Publication Data

Names: Rose, Debra J., editor.
Title: Physical activity instruction of older adults / Debra J. Rose, PhD,
 editor.
Description: Second edition. | Champaign, IL : Human Kinetics, 2019. |
 Includes bibliographical references and index.
Identifiers: LCCN 2018000298 | ISBN 9781450431064 (print) | ISBN 9781492570035
 (ebook)
Subjects: LCSH: Physical education for older people. | Aging--Physiological
 aspects.
Classification: LCC GV447 .P575 2019 | DDC 613.7/0446--dc23 LC record available at https://lccn.loc.gov/2018000298

ISBN: 978-1-4504-3106-4 (print)

The web addresses cited in this text were current as of June 2018, unless otherwise noted.

Senior Acquisitions Editor: Amy N. Tocco
Developmental and Managing Editor: Carly S. O'Connor
Copyeditor: Pamela S. Johnson
Indexer: Beth Nauman-Montana
Permissions Manager: Dalene Reeder
Graphic Designer: Denise Lowry
Cover Designer: Keri Evans
Cover Design Associate: Susan Rothermel Allen
Photograph (cover): Ariel Skelley/DigitalVision/Getty Images
Photographs (interior): © Human Kinetics, unless otherwise noted
Photo Asset Manager: Laura Fitch
Photo Production Coordinator: Amy M. Rose
Photo Production Manager: Jason Allen
Senior Art Manager: Kelly Hendren
Illustrations: © Human Kinetics, unless otherwise noted
Printer: Sheridan Books

We thank the Center for Successful Aging at California State University, Fullerton, for assistance in providing the location for the photo shoot for this book.

Printed in the United States of America   10 9 8 7 6 5 4 3 2 1

The paper in this book is certified under a sustainable forestry program.

Human Kinetics
P.O. Box 5076
Champaign, IL 61825-5076
Website: www.HumanKinetics.com

In the United States, email info@hkusa.com or call 800-747-4457.
In Canada, email info@hkcanada.com.
In the United Kingdom/Europe, email hk@hkeurope.com.

For information about Human Kinetics' coverage in other areas of the world,
please visit our website: **www.HumanKinetics.com**

E5724

Contents

Preface

Identifying ways to promote active life expectancy and reduce the onset of physical frailty has become a major focus for gerontology researchers and physical activity instructors throughout the world. People are now living longer, and the population aged 65 years and older is rapidly increasing. Average life expectancy at birth in most developed countries now is approximately 80 years, an average increase of about 25 to 30 years since 1900, with women living between 6 and 8 years longer on average than men. Globally, the 65 and older population is projected to increase to about 1.6 billion by 2050, representing 16.7 percent of the total population of 9.4 billion. This equates to a growth rate of 27.1 million older adults annually between 2015 and 2050 (He, Goodkind, & Kowal, 2016). This surge in the older adult population brings with it many serious challenges, but it also presents numerous opportunities for professionals working in the field of fitness and health promotion.

The recognized value of physical activity in preserving functional capacity and reducing physical frailty in later years has resulted in the proliferation of physical activity programs specifically designed for older adults in communities around the world. Providing safe and effective exercise programs for this population, however, requires specialized knowledge and practical training, particularly because chronic medical conditions will alter older adults' need for and response to exercise. The need for evidence-based curriculum materials to train physical activity instructors of older adults at the international level led to the formation of a coalition of members from 13 countries and a committee of experts from the United States. These members reviewed and critiqued a set of curriculum standards for preparing physical activity instructors of older adults, first published in the *Journal of Aging and Physical Activity* (Jones & Clark, 1998), and a similar set of international curriculum guidelines was published in the form of a final consensus document, *International Curriculum Guidelines for Preparing Physical Activity Instructors of Older Adults* (Ecclestone & Jones, 2004). The training modules based on the agreed-upon guidelines are shown in the figure on page x. The nine training modules cover the essential knowledge and skills that should be included in training programs for entry-level physical activity instructors of older adults. The final consensus document, *International Curriculum Guidelines for Preparing Physical Activity Instructors of Older Adults,* was published in the *Journal of Aging and Physical Activity* in October of 2004 (Ecclestone & Jones, 2004). See appendix A for a more detailed description of each training module.

The Purpose of This Book

The first edition of *Physical Activity Instruction of Older Adults* represented the first collaborative effort to provide a comprehensive textbook that addressed each of the nine international curriculum guideline training modules. This second edition builds upon the content presented in the first edition and provides both an updated review of the literature and a contemporary approach to designing and implementing effective, safe, and fun physical activity programs for older adults. Written for entry-level instructors, undergraduate students, and instructors preparing for certification as well as for personal trainers, activity directors and assistants, therapeutic recreation specialists, and group exercise leaders already working with older adults, this book provides the fundamental knowledge and skills recommended in each of the nine training modules. According to training module 3, for example, it is recommended that instructor training programs include information about how to use results obtained from screening, assessment, and client goal-setting activities to make appropriate decisions regarding individual and group physical

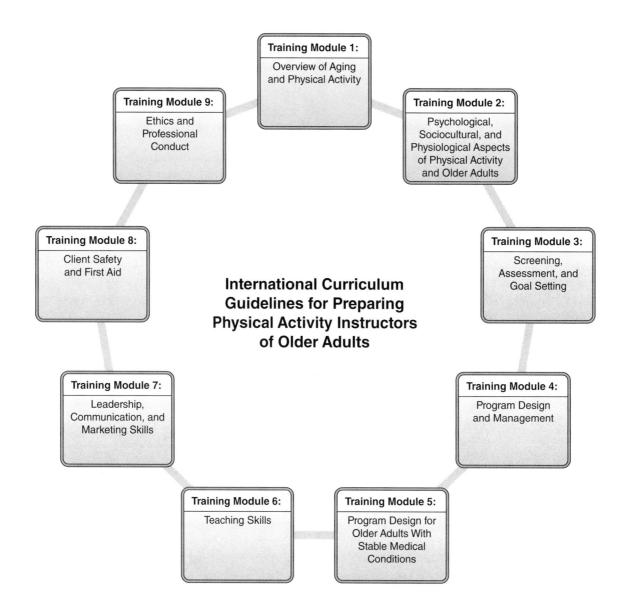

activity program design and management. Training module 5 provides both scientific and practical information on a range of health and fitness considerations—common medical conditions experienced by older adults, signs and symptoms associated with medication-related negative interactions during activity, how to adapt and tailor exercise for clients with different fitness levels, and stable medical conditions—to help prevent injury and other emergency situations.

This edition of the book continues to provide unique features aimed at enhancing understanding of the material and retention of what is learned. Each chapter begins with a list of objectives that familiarize readers with the key concepts they will learn and concludes with a summary and recommended

readings. Terms that are key to learning are highlighted throughout each chapter, as are key points that summarize important content. Students, instructors, and professionals in training will also find the study questions and practical application activities at the end of each chapter particularly useful for reviewing important topics and applying knowledge to practice. A new chapter is also introduced in this edition. Chapter 9, Whole-Person Wellness for Successful Aging, introduces the reader to the multiple dimensions of whole-person wellness and how to integrate each of the six dimensions and associated beliefs into physical activity programs designed for older adults.

Also included for instructors is an image bank containing most of the illustrations, photos, and tables from the text, which can be used to create handouts, PowerPoint presentations, or other learning aids for their students. This resource can be accessed by visiting www.HumanKinetics.com/PhysicalActivityInstructionOfOlderAdults.

All of the continued and expanded features of this edition of *Physical Activity Instruction of Older Adults* are intended to meet the overarching goal of this book—namely, to provide the fundamental knowledge and skills needed to lead safe and effective exercise classes or personal training sessions for older adults with diverse functional capabilities. This book should also prepare the reader to pursue advanced certifications now offered by a number of national and international organizations, including the American College of Sports Medicine (ACSM), American Council on Exercise (ACE), and the United Kingdom–based Later Life Training (LLT).

How This Book Is Organized

This edition is divided into four parts, each of which addresses one or more of the training modules that comprise the international curriculum guidelines. To present the information needed to develop safe and effective physical activity programs for older adults in the most logical and understandable way, the training modules are not addressed in numerical order, and some chapters address more than one module. The best way to read this book is sequentially, in the order that the chapters are presented.

Part I, Overview of Aging and Physical Activity, begins with the overview by Rose and Skelton in chapter 1 of the demographics and definitions of aging, followed by an introduction to a new field of study, *gerokinesiology.* In chapter 2, Rose describes successful aging and summarizes its predictors. In chapter 3, Wilson describes the role of physical activity in the aging process and highlights the psychosocial and cognitive benefits derived from regular physical activity. In chapter 4, MacRae describes the physiological aspects of aging and the functional implications of these changes.

Part II, Screening, Assessment, and Goal Setting, provides the knowledge and skills needed to conduct thorough preexercise and health screenings

and assessments, provide meaningful feedback to clients, evaluate program outcomes, and help clients develop short- and long-term behavioral goals. In chapter 5, Rose describes preexercise screening tools for determining the general health, physical activity level, and disabilities of older adult participants. Rose also explains how to administer and interpret the screening tools and share the results with the participant. In chapter 6, Jones and Rikli describe field-based assessment tools used to measure physical impairments and functional limitations in the older adult population. Finally, in chapter 7, Wilcox and King explain the major personal, environmental, and program-related factors that influence the initiation and maintenance of physical activity by older adults. They also address important theories of behavioral change and cognitive and behavioral strategies that can be used to motivate older adults in group-based and individual settings.

Part III, Core Program Principles and Training Methods, delves further into programming, focusing on the core principles and training methods for exercise programs for older adults. Chapter 8, by Rose, discusses the potential functional benefits of the different types of physical activities that should be included in all well-rounded physical activity programs for older adults. This chapter also addresses how to apply several exercise principles for effective program design. In chapter 9, Montague, Rose, and Aprile introduce the multiple dimensions of whole-person wellness and how to integrate each of the six dimensions into a physical activity program. Kluge describes the warm-up and cool-down components of an exercise program in chapter 10, including specific activities to engage older adults mentally, emotionally, socially, and spiritually. In chapter 11, Rose describes age-associated changes in joint and muscle flexibility, including the effects of these changes on the basic activities of daily living. She describes a number of different dynamic and static flexibility exercises that address every major muscle group and joint in the body. In chapter 12, Signorile describes the resistance-training variables that improve muscle strength, endurance, and power (e.g., resistance, exercise order, repetitions) and provides readers with the skills needed to design a safe and effective resistance-training component for older adults. In chapter 13, Dinan-Young and Skelton provide an overview of the critical principles and variables for designing aerobic endurance programs for older adults, including accommodating different fitness levels and functional abilities. In the last chapter of part III, Rose explains how age-associated physiological changes can affect balance and mobility and provides progressive balance and mobility exercises.

Part IV, Program Design, Leadership, and Risk Management, completes this edition of this book by focusing on the essential skills and knowledge necessary for creating an effective and safe physical activity program for older adults. In chapter 15, Rose presents the key motor learning principles that guide effective skill teaching, including demonstrations and verbal cues, structuring the practice environment, introducing new skills, and providing feedback. In chapter 16, Hawley-Hague and Dinan-Young discuss leadership skills to enhance teaching effectiveness, including motivation and communication strategies. Chapter 17, by Peterson, describes the major disabling conditions that affect older adults and how to modify exercises to enhance safe participation and reduce injury among older adults with specific medical conditions. In the final chapter of the book, Rose discusses several pertinent legal issues and offers guidelines for developing a risk management plan. She ends the chapter with a discussion of professional ethics.

Putting Knowledge Into Practice

The authors who contributed to the first and second editions of *Physical Activity Instruction of Older Adults* are all highly respected experts in their disciplines. They have repeatedly demonstrated their ability to translate cutting-edge theoretical concepts into meaningful guidelines for effective practice. After you read this book and complete the thought-provoking study questions and practical application activities at the end of each chapter, you will have a solid grasp of the essential knowledge and skills for designing and implementing an effective physical activity program that addresses the needs and interests of *all* older adults. As a result of acquiring the skills needed to appropriately select, administer, and interpret preexercise health and activity screening tests, you will also be able to demonstrate the effectiveness of your program and thereby foster higher participation and retention rates among the older adult community.

Together, we will continue to raise the professional standards for all physical activity instructors of older adults and also address one of the most critical worldwide health issues: how to improve the quality of life for all people in their later years.

Acknowledgments

First, I would like to express my deepest appreciation to each of the contributing authors who wrote the chapters in the first edition of *Physical Activity Instruction of Older Adults*. Creating the first-ever edited textbook in the field of gerokinesiology was not an easy task and required considerable time and dedication. I also wish to thank C. Jessie Jones, who co-edited the first edition with me. I realized, after serving as the sole editor of the second edition, how much I missed her wonderful leadership and managerial skills. Finally, I wish to extend my sincere appreciation to each of the new and returning contributing authors who revised the original chapters or contributed a new chapter and then waited *very* patiently for the second edition of the textbook to become a reality. It has been a very long journey for all of us, including the multiple editors at Human Kinetics, but I hope you'll agree that the end product is worth the wait!

My sincere gratitude is also extended to the numerous professionals throughout the world who participated in the development of the 2004 *International Curriculum Guidelines for Preparing Physical Activity Instructors of Older Adults*. The guidelines continue to form the basis of the content in this edition and serve as an important foundation for the preparation of future professionals in gerokinesiology.

To all the staff at Human Kinetics who contributed in any capacity to the production of this edition, I am appreciative of your expertise and publishing skills and for your consistent support and enduring patience with me throughout this unexpectedly long journey.

Finally, to the thousands of older adults who have participated in our research and training programs over the course of the last 23 years at the Center for Successful Aging at California State University at Fullerton, I thank you for your support, wisdom, and mentorship—the faculty and students in the gerokinesiology concentration have learned so much from each and every one of you!

PART

I

Overview of Aging and Physical Activity

Training Module 1:
Overview of Aging and Physical Activity

Training Module 9:
Ethics and Professional Conduct

Training Module 2:
Psychological, Sociocultural, and Physiological Aspects of Physical Activity and Older Adults

Training Module 8:
Client Safety and First Aid

International Curriculum Guidelines for Preparing Physical Activity Instructors of Older Adults

Training Module 3:
Screening, Assessment, and Goal Setting

Training Module 7:
Leadership, Communication, and Marketing Skills

Training Module 4:
Program Design and Management

Training Module 6:
Teaching Skills

Training Module 5:
Program Design for Older Adults With Stable Medical Conditions

Training to become a physical activity instructor of older adults begins with an introduction to the field of gerontology (the science of aging) and knowledge about the physiological and psychological dimensions of the aging process and the role of physical activity. Part I of this text addresses the first two training modules included in the *International Curriculum Guidelines for Preparing Physical Activity Instructors of Older Adults*. Module 1 recommends areas of study that include general background information about the aging process and the benefits of an active lifestyle. These are the topics of chapters 1 and 2. Module 2 recommends areas of study that include psychological, sociocultural, and physiological aspects of physical activity in order to develop safe and effective physical activity and exercise programs for older adults. Chapters 3 and 4 address areas of study contained in both modules 1 and 2.

- Chapter 1 provides an overview of the demographics of aging, compares various definitions of aging, and introduces the reader to an expanding field of study: gerokinesiology.

- Chapter 2 describes the predictors of successful aging. It discusses biological, psychological, and sociological theories of aging and how physical activity promotes successful aging. This information will help you communicate to your clients that successful aging depends on the interplay of many factors, especially staying physically active.

- Chapter 3 debunks common myths and misperceptions about the aging process. It then describes the psychological, cognitive, and social benefits of regular physical activity and ways to promote more physical activity among older adults at both local and national levels.

- Chapter 4 describes the major age-associated changes in physiological systems, the functional implications of these changes, and the types of physical activity that have the potential to counteract or delay these age-related changes. With this knowledge base you will better understand the factors to consider when designing programs to meet the specific goals and preferences of older adults. You will also be able to better articulate and promote the benefits of an active lifestyle to older adults once you have finished reviewing the chapters in part I and completing the questions and application activities at the end of each chapter.

The Field of Gerokinesiology

Debra J. Rose
Dawn A. Skelton

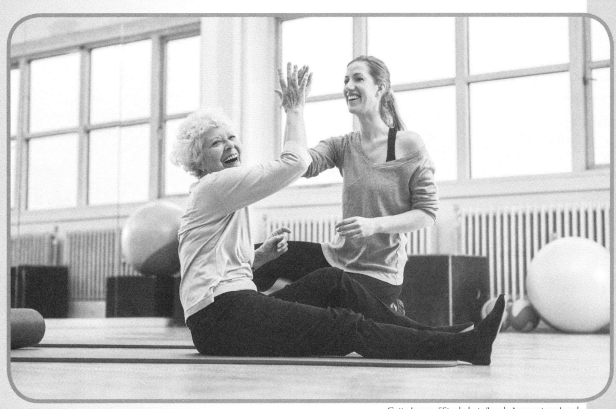

Objectives

After completing this chapter, you will be able to

1. describe the general demographics of aging throughout the world;

2. explain the difference between the terms *chronological*, *biological*, and *functional aging*;

3. differentiate the terms *usual*, *pathological*, and *successful aging*;

4. understand the general benefits of physical activity for promoting health and reducing disease and disability;

5. understand the rationale for the development of the subdiscipline of kinesiology called *gerokinesiology*; and

6. describe the different types of training programs that have been developed to prepare physical activity instructors of older adults.

The academic disciplines of exercise science, kinesiology, and physical education have traditionally focused on children, adolescents, and younger adults. However, as the value of physical activity throughout the life span is recognized and supported by a growing body of research evidence, more attention is being directed to the training of instructors who specialize in leading physical activity programs for older adults. The purposes of this chapter are to describe the demographics of aging throughout the world, summarize the benefits of physical activity for older adults, present the various definitions of aging, and introduce the rapidly expanding field of gerokinesiology.

Demographics of Older Adults

Advancements in medical technology, health care, nutrition, and sanitation have resulted in lower birth and death rates throughout the world. People are living longer, and the population aged 65 years and older is rapidly increasing. Average life expectancy at birth in most developed countries now is approximately 80 years, an average increase of about 25 to 30 years since 1900, with women living between 6 and 8 years longer on average than men. A national report by the U.S. Census Bureau, *An Aging World: 2015* (He, Goodkind, & Kowal, 2016), emphasized that global aging is occurring at

an unprecedented rate. Globally, the 65 and older population is projected to increase to about 1.6 billion by 2050, representing 16.7 percent of the total population of 9.4 billion. This equates to a growth rate of 27.1 million older adults annually between 2015 and 2050 (He et al., 2016). In contrast to this rapid expansion of the older adult population, the under-20 age group is projected to remain almost the same over the next 35 years (2.5 billion in 2015 and 2.6 billion in 2050). A statistic of even perhaps greater significance is that by 2050, the proportion of the population aged 65 and older (15.6%) will be more than double that of children under the age of 5 years (7.2%).

International comparisons in the year 2015 continue to show that Europe remains the oldest region in the world, with 17.4 percent of the total population 65 years and older. North America follows closely with 15.1 percent, and Oceania is third with 12.5 percent of the total regional population (see figure 1.1). Although these regions will remain the oldest through 2050, the percentage of older adults in the regions of Asia and Latin America and the Caribbean will more than double in the same time period. Given the overall size of the population in Asia, which includes China and India, it is projected that this region will account for nearly two-thirds (62.3%) of the world's total older adult population by 2050 (U.S. Census Bureau, 2015).

The rapid acceleration in the aging population, especially people over the age of 85, presents a number of health, social, and economic challenges

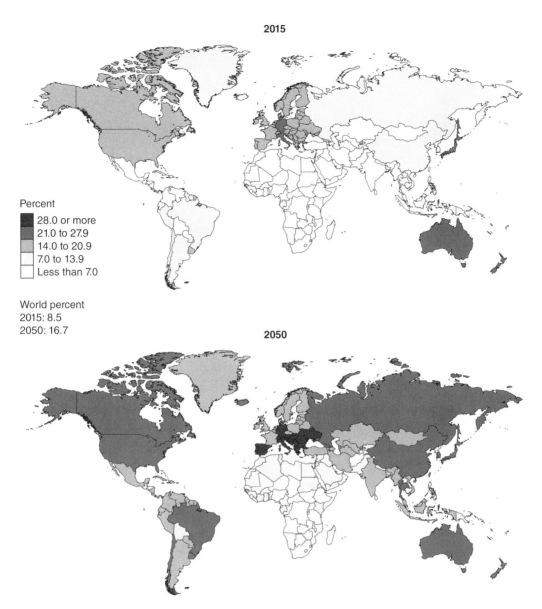

FIGURE 1.1　Percentage of population aged 65 and over: 2015 and 2050.

Reprinted from He, Goodkind and Kowal (2016).

for individuals, families, and governments throughout the world. Two of the greatest challenges will be the fiscal shortfall in health and social security programs for older adults and the rising medical costs associated with chronic disability. In response to these imminent challenges, a worldwide movement is under way to find effective ways to promote *active* life expectancy and reduce the number of years people live with chronic disabilities. Fries and Crapo (1981) defined **active life expectancy** as the number of years of life spent without significant disease or disability, while Katz and colleagues (1983) adopted a more positive tone by defining it as the number of expected years of physical, emotional, and intellectual vigor or functional well-being.

Benefits of Physical Activity

Professionals who have worked in the health and fitness field for many years are well aware of the importance of integrating physical activity into every individual's daily life. Numerous research studies have also reported many health- and performance-related benefits of engaging in regular physical activity, particularly for older adults. It has been shown that a certain level of fitness not only protects the individual from a number of chronic diseases (e.g., heart disease, diabetes, cancer) but also makes performing the many tasks of daily life, as well as participating in a variety of sports and recreational activities, considerably easier. A number of psychological benefits can also be derived from regular participation in physical activity, including emotional well-being, enhanced cognitive function, and a higher perceived quality of life (see chapter 3).

Despite this large body of research evidence, a very low percentage of older adults engage in physical activity on a regular basis. Current estimates based on the National Health Interview Survey conducted in 2015 are that only 49 percent of adults aged over 18 years currently meet the 2008 national physical activity guidelines (U.S. Department of Health and Human Services, 2008) for aerobic activity (based on leisure-time activity); the percentage is even lower for meeting the amount of aerobic and muscle-strengthening activities (20.9%) recommended in the same set of guidelines. Moreover, with increasing age, the percentages decline even further. For example, only 27.1 percent of adults aged 75 and older meet the recommended amount of aerobic activity and only 8.7 percent report engaging in the recommended amount of aerobic and muscle-strengthening activities. A more detailed discussion of the recommendations outlined in the most recently published version of the *Physical Activity Guidelines for Americans* (PAGAC, 2018) will be presented in chapter 8. Unless the current trend is reversed, the costs of physical inactivity among the older adult population will place increasing demands on medical and social services and the public health system in general. It is already the case that approximately one-third of total health care expenditures in the United States are for older adults (over 65 years), a proportion that is expected to rise substantially in the next 25 years. According to Carlson, Fulton, Pratt, Yang, & Adams (2015), this alarming trend "could potentially be reduced by increasing adults' physical activity levels consistent with current guidelines and *Healthy People 2020* objectives" (p. 319). In a review in which the authors merged leisure-time physical activity data from the National Health Interview Survey (2004-2010) with health care expenditure data from the Medi-cal Expenditure Panel Survey (2006-2011), it was estimated that as much as 11 percent ($117 billion per year) of annual total health care expenditures were associated with inadequate levels (classified as inactive or insufficiently active) of physical activity.

Defining Old Age

Defining the term *old age* sounds simple, but it is actually very complex. For example, with the increase in antiaging treatments (e.g., antiaging products and cosmetic surgical procedures) available today, individuals may look much younger than their chronological age. To help you understand the complexity of defining *old age*, the following is a brief description of three main definitions: chronological, biological, and functional aging.

Unfortunately, the most common indicator used to define *old age* is **chronological age**—that is, the passage of time from birth in years. People are often lumped together in a particular age category by chronological age and then provided a label such as "young-old" (aged 65-74 years), "middle-old" (aged 75-84 years), "old-old" (aged 85-99 years), and "oldest-old" (aged 100 or more years). According to the United Nations, in 2015, there were nearly half a million centenarians (100 or more years old) worldwide, with the highest number residing in the United States (72,197 based on 2014 CDC data). Current projections suggest that there will be 3.7 million centenarians across the globe in 2050 (see figure 1.2).

Biological aging, also known as primary aging, refers to a group of processes within the body that eventually lead to loss of adaptability, disease, physical impairments, functional limitations, disability, and eventual death. There are several biological theories of aging, and a number of factors have been proposed that affect the rate of biological aging. The major theories of biological aging are discussed in chapter 2.

Functional age has to do with one's functional fitness in comparison with others the same age and gender. For example, an 80-year-old woman may have the aerobic endurance of a woman in the 60-64 age category (as measured by the six-minute walk; see chapter 6 for Senior Fitness Test items and national performance norms). Therefore her functional age relative to aerobic endurance is between

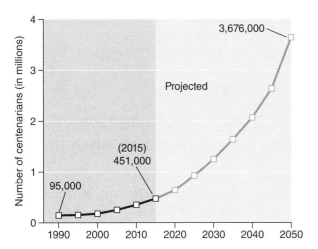

FIGURE 1.2 The worldwide centenarian population is increasing rapidly.

United Nations, Department of Economic and Social Affairs, Population Division (2015). *World Population Prospects: The 2015 Revision: Key Findings and Advance Tables.* Working Paper No. ESA/P/WP.241.

60 and 64 years of age. Impairments in physical fitness parameters (e.g., aerobic endurance, musculoskeletal integrity, flexibility, body composition, and the sensorimotor system) have a direct impact on a person's functional abilities (e.g., walking, stair climbing, rising from a chair), and functional limitations eventually lead to physical disabilities (refer to the Functional Fitness Framework in chapter 6). Spirduso, Francis, and MacRae (2005) hierarchically divided physical function into five levels: physically elite, physically fit, physically independent, physically frail, and physically dependent (see figure 1.3). This hierarchy of physical function in later life may be an effective way to categorize your clients once you have completed the preexercise screening and functional assessments described in chapters 5 and 6, respectively.

It is extremely important to recognize that as people age they become increasingly more diverse in their medical, psychological, and physical status. Differentiating between usual (or normal), pathological (or abnormal), and successful aging is another way of categorizing the way people age. **Usual aging** refers to the way the majority of people age and is characterized by a gradual decline in body function, leading to physical impairments, disease, functional limitations, and eventually the onset of disability and death. **Pathological aging** generally refers to the way individuals age when they are genetically predisposed to certain diseases or have high-risk negative lifestyles (e.g., poor eating habits, smoking, excessive alcohol use) that lead to premature disability and death. **Successful aging**, on

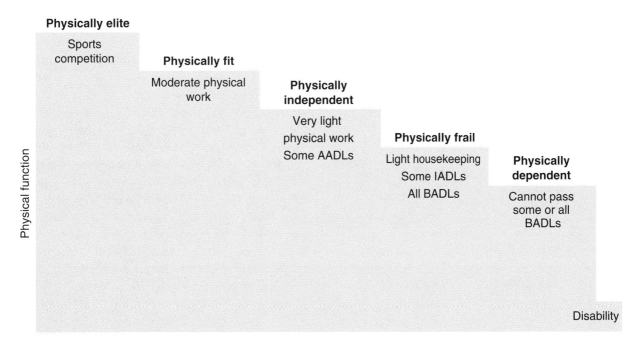

FIGURE 1.3 Hierarchy of physical function. BADL: basic activity of daily living; IADL: instrumental activity of daily living; AADL: advanced activity of daily living.

Reprinted by permission from W. Spirduso, K. Francis, and P. MacRae, *Physical Dimensions of Aging,* 2nd ed. (Champaign, IL: Human Kinetics, 2005), 264.

the other hand, is more difficult to define because the term *success* itself is quite ambiguous. Successful aging is a qualitative description of aging rather than one that refers to longevity or survival. Rowe and Kahn (1987) referred to successful agers as people with better than average physiological and psychosocial characteristics in late life and healthy genes. Successful agers are also more satisfied with life in general. Chapter 2 provides a more in-depth discussion of the major theories and predictors of successful aging.

Physical activity has great value in preserving functional capacity and reducing disease and physical frailty in later years, making physical activity programs for older adults especially important. However, most experts agree that specialized training is needed for activity professionals who develop and implement physical activity programs for older adults.

Gerokinesiology: An Expanding Field of Study

Recognition of the importance of physical activity for older adults and the growing support of the medical community (Kerse, Elley, Robinson, & Arroll, 2005; Noordman, Verhaak, & van Dulmen, 2010) have resulted in more facilities and organizations (e.g., senior centers, hospitals, recreation departments, fitness clubs, churches, YMCAs, retirement communities) offering physical activity programs for this segment of the population. However, many experts, including the authors of this chapter, have argued that because of the large range of medical conditions and functional abilities in the 65 and over population, preparing to be a physical activity instructor for older adults requires more knowledge, skills, and experience than to be an instructor of younger adults. In an effort to promote curriculum development and elevate the quality of professional training programs offered in this area, several experts representing numerous organizations throughout the world convened and developed international curriculum guidelines for preparing physical activity instructors of older adults (Ecclestone & Jones, 2004). The guidelines comprise nine curriculum-training modules and will be detailed later in the

chapter. This text uses the term **gerokinesiology** to describe this rapidly growing field of study, a term based on the input of several expert physical activity instructors of older adults and many university professors throughout the world who currently prepare undergraduate and graduate students to work with older adults in a variety of physical activity settings.

Because of the growing job opportunities for physical activity instructors of older adults and the recognized need for specialized training, more and more universities now offer individual courses addressing physical activity and aging, experiential learning opportunities in real-world contexts, or more comprehensive areas of concentration in gerokinesiology. The increased availability of textbooks that focus on the aging process and the role of physical activity have made it easier to offer stand-alone courses as electives within a broader kinesiology curriculum or even to create a series of courses on which to base an academic concentration (Spirduso et al., 2005; Taylor & Johnson, 2008; Watson, 2017). For example, California State University at Fullerton currently offers an academic concentration in gerokinesiology at both the undergraduate and graduate level. In addition to completing the core academic requirements in kinesiology (i.e., the courses Biomechanics; Exercise Physiology; Motor Control and Learning; Psychology of Sport and Physical Activity; Sociocultural, Philosophical, and Historical Perspectives of Human Movement) students in the gerokinesiology concentration area complete additional coursework specific to the concentration (i.e., Physical Dimensions of Aging, Functional Performance Assessment and Programming for Older Adults, Principles of Teaching Group Fitness, Physical Activity and Behavior Change). Students in the gerokinesiology concentration also complete an internship within the Center for Successful Aging, where they receive hands-on training working with older adults who attend the center's weekly wellness programs. A number of other universities within North America have developed similar academic concentrations, some with supporting centers offering similar opportunities for hands-on training and instructor certifications (e.g., Canadian Centre for Activity and Aging, Western Ontario University). Within the United Kingdom, while there are no specific academic concentrations in gerokinesiology, programs offering degrees in sport and health or physical activity and health are starting to work in collaboration with external training providers to offer the qualifications of the exercise-training framework for their master of science students (e.g., Portsmouth University). Certainly, from a practical perspective, degree content for a master of sport science does not currently provide students with the necessary practical skills to deliver evidence-based programs for frail older people.

> Gerokinesiology is a specialized area of study within the larger discipline of kinesiology that focuses on understanding how physical activity influences all aspects of health and well-being in the older adult population and the aging process in general.

Historically, the academic discipline of kinesiology and physical education focused on preparing students for careers in the areas of teaching and coaching children and young adults. In more recent years, however, the discipline has expanded to include specialized areas of study designed to prepare students for careers in such areas as fitness and health promotion, therapeutic exercise, and sport management (Hoffman & Knudson, 2017). As with a number of other subdisciplines in kinesiology—such as motor control and learning, biomechanics, exercise physiology, sport and exercise psychology, and pedagogy—the emerging new subdiscipline of gerokinesiology was preceded by scientific research and the development of unique curriculum offerings.

Gero- is the root of the word *gerontology.* As a field of study, gerontology adopts a multidisciplinary approach to examining the biological, economic, psychological, social, and health and fitness aspects of the aging process. The National Academy of Kinesiology uses the term *kinesiology* to describe a multifaceted field of study in which movement or physical activity is the intellectual focus. According to this definition, physical activity encompasses exercise performed for the improvement of health and fitness, activities of daily living, sport, dance, work, and play. Moreover, a variety of special populations are studied, including people with injuries, diseases, or disabilities; athletes; children; and the

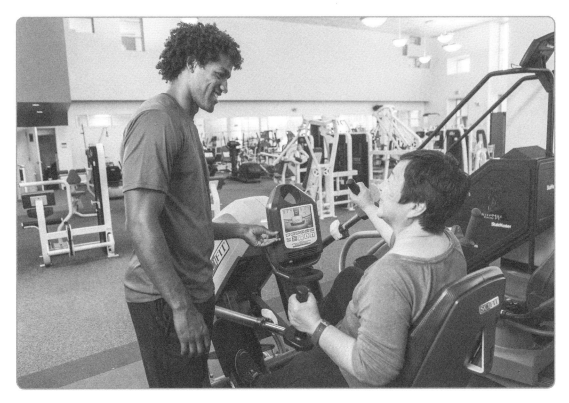

The gerokinesiology curriculum prepares undergraduate and graduate students to work with older adults in a variety of physical activity settings.

elderly. Elements of the two terms *gerontology* and *kinesiology* have been combined to describe a specialized area of study within the larger discipline of kinesiology that focuses on understanding how physical activity influences all aspects of health and well-being in the older adult population and the aging process in general.

Curriculum Development

Curriculum development to prepare physical activity instructors of older adults was minimal prior to the 1990s (Jones & Rikli, 1994). Until recently, instructors and personal trainers who led physical activity programs for older adults reported that they had to rely primarily on self-study, on-the-job training, or workshops and conferences to develop the specific knowledge and skills needed to work with older adults (Jones & Rose, 2005). The slow response by academic institutions to develop curricula aimed at preparing physical activity instructors for older adults has resulted in a number of professional organizations and individual entrepreneurs offering training that culminates in some type of certification. Unfortunately, lacking curriculum guidelines to assist their development, some of these training programs have failed to provide the essential knowledge and practical skills that are essential for safe and effective physical activity programs for older adults.

The *International Curriculum Guidelines for Preparing Physical Activity Instructors of Older Adults,* published by Ecclestone and Jones (2004) in the *Journal of Aging and Physical Activity,* recommend that the following nine curriculum training modules form the basis of any professional training program or academic curriculum subsequently developed:

1. Overview of Aging and Physical Activity
2. Psychological, Sociocultural, and Physiological Aspects of Physical Activity and Older Adults
3. Screening, Assessment, and Goal Setting
4. Program Design and Management
5. Program Design for Older Adults With Stable Medical Conditions
6. Teaching Skills
7. Leadership, Communication, and Marketing Skills
8. Client Safety and First Aid
9. Ethics and Professional Conduct

The content presented in this text is based on these training modules recommended by the international guidelines. Refer to appendix A for a detailed description of the training modules.

Later Life Training Curricula: The Gold Standard for Instructor Training?

The founders of Later Life Training (LLT) are internationally recognized experts in exercise and aging. Indeed, one of the founding directors, Susie Dinan-Young, was part of the International Coalition Membership involved in the development of the *International Curriculum.* At the cutting edge of research and service development, LLT has a proven track record in translating evidence and best practice guidance into progressive, effective, and safe exercise programs in clinical and community exercise settings within National Health Service (NHS) Health and Wellbeing pathways across the United Kingdom. LLT took up the challenge to ensure a continuum of instructor training in order to fill the gap in physical activity provision between the hospital-based rehabilitation setting and the much more active senior exercise classes that can be found in community settings. LLT has been delivering a range of training programs since 2003 (see figure 1.4) and has had a strong influence in the development of national standards of instruction. The United Kingdom is unique in that it has established national standards that all training providers must meet in order to be accredited to provide general physical activity programs for older adults as well as more specialized programs (e.g., exercise referral, fall risk reduction, stroke, frailty). Further information can be found at http://www.skillsactive.com/standards-quals/national-occupational-standards (although these national standards are under review).

Later Life Training's uniqueness within a large training-provider market in the United Kingdom lies

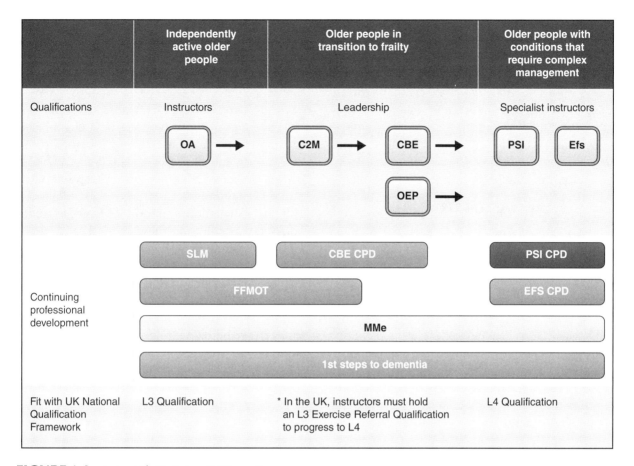

FIGURE 1.4 Later Life Training (LLT) continuum.

Reprinted by permission from D. Skelton et al., *Postural Stability Instructor Manual 2017* (Later Life Training Ltd., Killin, Scotland, UK, 2007), 3. Copyright Later Life Training Ltd.

in the fact that all of its courses are based on the *International Curriculum Guidelines for Preparing Physical Activity Instructors of Older Adults* as well as published evidence in peer-reviewed journals, with proven outcomes for older adults and with a strong emphasis on implementation. The directors and some of the tutors are also academics and ensure that the latest evidence-based information is quickly assimilated into their training. What sets LLT courses apart is the focus on practical skills: Sport and exercise science are integrated with therapy-based approaches to provide exercise tailored to each individual's clinical and functional needs. This facilitates effective transition from primary and secondary care services to voluntary and nongovernmental providers to ensure effective dose and progression of exercise and a seamless exercise pathway for older adults. LLT is a nonprofit organization, with its revenues reinvested back into updating existing courses or developing new

courses as well as continuing professional development for its staff.

In the early days of LLT, a continuum of evidence-based, exercise-training qualifications for health, exercise, and fitness professionals working with frailer older adults was supported by a national expert advisory group and funded by the United Kingdom's Department of Health (Skelton, Dinan, & Laventure, 2004). These three qualifications—the Postural Stability Instructor (PSI) (Skelton, 2004; Skelton, Dinan, Campbell, & Rutherford, 2005), the Chair Based Exercise (CBE) Leader (Skelton et al., 2005; Skelton & Townley, 2008), and the Senior Peer Mentor Physical Activity Motivator (Someone Like Me; SLM) (Laventure, Dinan, & Skelton, 2008)—were developed to ensure effective planning, teaching, and implementation of physical activity programs for older adults. A team of people with extensive expertise in the fields of research, exercise, medicine and general practice, falls and injury prevention, rehabilitation, education, social services, and public health developed each program. Responding to consumers (instructors and commissioners of services), they have gone on to develop a large range of products that address strategies to increase uptake and adherence in a frailer older adult population. Later Life Training has now trained nearly 3,000 PSIs across the United Kingdom, and over 50 percent of falls services in the United Kingdom employ PSIs (Royal College of Physicians, 2012), as recommended by the Department of Health (2009) and as cost-effective commissioning (Public Health England, 2018). PSIs are now considered key to the fidelity of intervention delivery in fall prevention research within the United Kingdom (Gawler et al., 2016; Iliffe et al., 2014; Public Health England, 2018).

Later Life Training also delivers instruction in the well-known New Zealand–based fall prevention program, the Otago Exercise Program (OEP) Leader (Campbell, Robertson, Gardner, Norton, Tilyard, & Buchner, 1997; Skelton & Gawler, 2008; Skelton, Townley, & Gawler, 2015), having trained over 2,500 OEP Leaders in the United Kingdom in the last 10 years. Beginning in 2014, LLT implemented the OEP Cascade Trainer program in 11 different European countries within the ProFouND (Prevention of Falls Network for Dissemination) project. The prerequisite for participating in this higher-level train-the-trainer program is completion of the OEP leader program and experience in delivering training (in-house or external). A total of 151 OEP Cascade Trainers have been certified since 2014, and they have subsequently trained over 3,000 new OEP leaders in the 14 countries, including Singapore.

Two other national qualifications delivered are the Exercise and Fitness after Stroke (EfS) Instructor (based on Mead et al., 2007) and the Adapting Exercise for Independently Active, Older People (OA) (Nelson et al., 2007). In order to provide continuing professional development for instructors, LLT has also developed one-day training updates. One such training day is the Functional Fitness MOT (FFMOT), based on the research of Rikli and Jones (de Jong et al., 2016; Laventure & Skelton, 2016; Rikli & Jones, 1999, 2013), which aims to raise awareness among older people of the need to remain active by comparing their fitness levels to the Senior Fitness Test (SFT) normative standards

developed by Rikli and Jones. (The SFT is described in greater detail in chapter 6.) The course addresses strategies that instructors and health professionals can use to motivate older people to do activities that will improve any areas of functional fitness in need of improvement. They also offer 1st Steps in Dementia for those working with clients with impaired cognition (Laventure & Aherne, 2009, 2010). The Motivate Me (MMe) training day integrates research and learning in behavioral motivation strategies for increasing uptake and adherence and providing tailored support strategies for older adults (Hawley-Hague, Horne, Skelton, & Todd, 2016; King, Rejeski, & Buchner, 1998; Laventure, Hetherington, Street, & Penington, 2016; National Institute for Health and Clinical Excellence, 2007; Yardley et al., 2007). Research has shown that instructors who have undertaken MMe training foster better participant adherence to their group sessions than instructors without this training (Hawley-Hague et al., 2014). All program-related products are nationally accredited by Skills Active and the Register of Exercise Professionals and certain products are also endorsed by the United Kingdom's AGILE (older adults section of the Chartered Society of Physiotherapy), Stroke Association, and relevant universities. Finally, LLT identified a gap in training provision for those older adults transitioning to frailty who were receiving home care. Specifically, an increasing number of frailer older adults were being referred to exercise, but there was a need for care providers to encourage activity and provide consistent messaging for the journey between care and the health and leisure setting, particularly in terms of strength and balance. In 2017, LLT developed a bespoke training approach to support the care sector workforce. The Care To Move (CTM) approach aims to enable health care professionals not qualified in exercise delivery to play a proactive part in the movement continuum. CTM training is informed by behavioral change strategies, communication, and a series of movement prompts embedded within usual packages of care (i.e., outside of exercise programs).

Since 2003, LLT has trained over 9,000 professionals in the United Kingdom and has built a strong network of instructors, leaders, and commissioners of services. It also hosts service evaluations and an instructor locator on its website. LLT maintains a vibrant Facebook page and Twitter account and also provides member forums and newsletters and hosts an annual conference.

Despite international recognition by medical and exercise science professionals and the ever-increasing numbers of older adults wishing, or needing, to become more physically active, in all parts of the world an insufficient number of instructors are training to specialize in teaching older adults. This is likely due to the increasing number of potential instructors choosing to train to work with patient populations; although exciting on many levels, this appears to have resulted in the teaching of healthier, independent older adults being relegated to the backwater of instructor training. Of deeper concern is that many of the qualifications and instructor training courses have been reduced to theoretical and written case-study assessments or multiple-choice exams. The authors of this chapter argue strongly that in addition to knowledge-based training, there must be practical training and assessment of competency in the teaching and leadership skills to ensure effective and progressive programs, underpinned by group management to reduce risks for older adults. LLT, for example, is the only training provider in the United Kingdom to still require a practical assessment with their older adult and specialist qualifications. Furthermore, the delivery of these courses by tutors who are experts and experienced with the full functional range of older participants is crucial to the development of specialized older adult teaching skills.

Career Opportunities

In addition to the many opportunities that now exist for graduates of kinesiology programs to instruct physical activity programs in community settings, expanded opportunities now exist for employment in senior living communities. A 2017 survey conducted by the International Council on Active Aging (ICAA) revealed that 74 percent of retirement communities offered formal structured wellness programs (that probably include physical activity [PA] but are not exclusive to PA) while 24 percent offered a few wellness activities but no formal program. Given that the primary reason a growing number of older adults are choosing to live in retirement communities is so they can maintain an active lifestyle, consumer demand for on-site

wellness centers or physical activity programs led by qualified staff is increasing (ICAA, 2017b). A survey of 3,406 residents living in continuing care retirement communities (CCRCs) or in independent living or assisted living communities found that the availability of a comprehensive wellness program (with appropriate staffing) was a primary reason for choosing a particular retirement community (ICAA, 2017a).

Senior living communities are particularly desirable locations in which to work because they offer the opportunity for full-time employment in one location, competitive salaries, the opportunity for career advancement, and health benefits. Outside of community settings, entrepreneurial opportunities for kinesiology graduates with specialized training in gerokinesiology are also increasing. Older adults in the baby boomer generation with more financial resources available to them are engaging personal trainers who have the necessary knowledge and practical skills to create tailored exercise programs for this segment of the population.

Summary

The increase in the number of people living beyond the age of 65 and the recognized value of physical activity for preventive medicine and health promotion have resulted in the proliferation of physical activity programs especially designed for older adults. Gerokinesiology is a rapidly expanding and specialized area of study that focuses on professional training in and research on physical activity and aging. An increasing number of universities are offering courses that address the role of physical activity in the aging process, with some even developing concentrations in the relatively new subdiscipline of gerokinesiology. Opportunities to become certified fitness or physical activity instructors of older adults are also rapidly increasing, particularly in the United States, although concern persists among experts as to whether sufficient academic rigor is provided to truly prepare professionals to work with an extremely heterogeneous segment of the population. At present, the Later Life Training continuum described earlier in this chapter is clearly the gold standard for preparing instructors to work with older adults across the functional continuum. The model not only provides a hierarchy of training programs that are designed to continually build upon the theoretical knowledge of instructors as they progress through the various training levels, but it also develops and evaluates their instructional and leadership skills as a core component of every training program.

Key Terms

active life expectancy

biological aging

chronological age

functional age

gerokinesiology

pathological aging

successful aging

usual aging

Recommended Readings

Jones, C.J., & Clark, J. (1998). National standards for preparing senior fitness instructors. *Journal of Aging and Physical Activity, 6,* 207-221.

Sullivan, G.M., & Pomidor, A.K. (Eds.). (2015). *Exercise for aging adults. A guide for practitioners.* Springer International Publishing Switzerland.

Study Questions

1. The average life expectancy at birth in most developed countries now is approximately
   a. 68 years
   b. 72 years
   c. 75 years
   d. 80 years

2. The region with the greatest percentage of its total population aged 65 and over is currently
   a. Oceania
   b. United States
   c. Europe
   d. Asia and Latin America

3. What percentage of people in the United States aged 75 years and older currently meet the 2008 Physical Activity Guidelines for Americans (PAGA) for aerobic exercise?
   a. 49 percent
   b. 27.1 percent
   c. 20.9 percent
   d. 8.7 percent

4. *Usual aging* refers to
   a. the process of aging with above-average physiological and psychosocial characteristics
   b. a group of processes in the body that eventually lead to loss of adaptability, disease, physical impairments, functional limitations, disability, and eventual death
   c. the way the majority of people age and is characterized by a gradual decline in body function, leading to physical impairments, disease, functional limitations, and eventually the onset of disability and death
   d. the way individuals age who are genetically predisposed to certain diseases or have high-risk negative lifestyles

5. *Gerokinesiology* is defined as a
   a. specialized area of study within the larger discipline of kinesiology that focuses on understanding how physical activity influences all aspects of health and well-being in the older adult population and the aging process in general
   b. subdiscipline within gerontology that focuses on understanding how physical activity influences all aspects of health and well-being across the life span
   c. new discipline that focuses on understanding how physical activity influences all aspects of health and well-being in the older adult population and the aging process in general
   d. specialized area of study within kinesiology that focuses on physical activity across the life span

6. *International Curriculum Guidelines for Preparing Physical Activity Instructors of Older Adults* was published in
   a. 1998
   b. 2004
   c. 2010
   d. 2016

Application Activities

1. Interview two or three physical activity instructors of older adults and ask them to describe what they consider to be the important knowledge and skills needed to provide safe and effective physical activity programs for older adults.

2. Go online and review the certification programs offered by different professional organizations (e.g., World Instructor Training School, American Senior Fitness Association, National Strength and Conditioning Association, Later Life Training) for physical activity instructors of older adults. Which one would you recommend and why?

Predictors of Successful Aging

Debra J. Rose

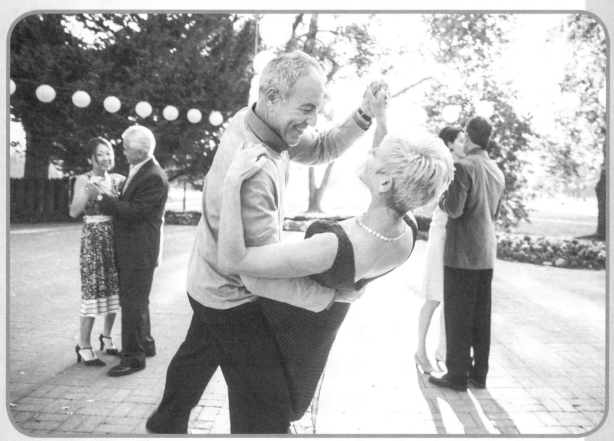

Objectives

After completing this chapter, you will be able to

1. define the term *successful aging*;
2. describe and differentiate the biological, psychological, and sociological theories of aging;
3. describe and differentiate the different models of successful aging; and
4. explain the benefits of physical activity in promoting successful aging.

There is growing consensus among experts who study demographic trends that the United States is on the "brink of a longevity revolution." This prediction is supported by statistics from the Centers for Disease Control and Prevention (2007) showing that by 2030, one in every five Americans will be 65 years or older. Mortality rates and longevity are also expected to improve globally, with life expectancy at birth projected to increase by at least 10 years, reaching approximately 76 years by 2050. As a consequence of this disproportionate growth in the older adult segment of the population, health care spending is also projected to increase by as much as 25 percent unless the health of the older adult population can be maintained or improved substantially (CDC, 2013). Unfortunately, current estimates of the number of older adults (65 years and older) in the U.S. who are considered to be aging "successfully" are alarmingly low. Based on findings from the Health and Retirement Study, only 11.9 percent of older adults were categorized as aging "successfully" in any one year (McLaughlin, Connell, Heeringa, Li, & Roberts, 2009). Moreover, the odds of aging successfully declined by as much as 25 percent over the six-year measurement period (1998-2004) with the adjusted odds being lower for adults 75 years and older, males, and those at a lower socioeconomic level (McLaughlin et al., 2009).

The concept of successful aging (SA) dates back several decades (Baltes & Baltes, 1980; Havighurst, 1961; Palmore, 1979; Rowe & Kahn, 1987). Havighurst (1961) coined the term *successful aging*, referring to it as "adding life to the years" and "getting satisfaction from life." Palmore (1979) defined successful aging as including longevity, lack of disability, and life satisfaction. Rowe and Kahn

(1987) further defined successful agers as people with better than average physiological and psychosocial characteristics in late life and healthy genes. Furthermore, they considered successful agers as having two additional traits: low risk for physical and cognitive diseases and disabilities until the age of 80 or more, and life satisfaction with their physical, mental, social, emotional, and spiritual well-being. Although it is clear that the concept of successful aging and the term itself is not universally accepted, the most often included component of successful aging is physical functioning/disability (Depp & Jeste, 2006). Other components identified in other definitions include cognitive ability, social functioning, life satisfaction, and absence of disease.

As a result of the many different ways in which SA was defined, vastly different proportions of study participants were categorized as aging successfully. Using the objective criteria set forth by Rowe and Kahn (1987) in their model of SA, Strawbridge, Wallhagen, and Cohen (2002) found that only 18.8 percent of the 867 older adults (65-99 years) they studied would be categorized as successfully aging. In contrast, 50.3 percent of the same group of older adults was categorized as successfully aging on the basis of a single question that asked them to rate the extent to which they thought they were aging successfully. On the basis of these divergent findings, a number of researchers have argued that the perceptions of older adults need to be included in any definition of SA (Ferri & James, 2009; Phelan, Anderson, Lacroix, & Larson, 2004; Reichstadt, Sengupta, Depp, Palinkas, & Jeste, 2010). McLaughlin et al. (2009) have also called for a broader definition of SA, particularly if the concept is to be used as a benchmark for assessing the health and functional status of the older adult population. The authors argue that if the term continues to be narrowly defined, "we are likely to classify many older adults with good health and functioning as being in an unhealthy state for what might be relatively minor reasons" (p. 225).

Successful aging should not be limited to one-dimensional stories about older adults who exhibit above average performance speed, intellectual function, and physical health. Gerokinesiologists also need to be careful not to make people feel that they have aged unsuccessfully because they have a disease or are unable to walk without difficulty. However a person defines successful aging, it is certainly not determined by longevity (survival) alone but also by the quality of those years. Although physiological aging is inevitable, the way in which a person ages depends, for the most part, on his or her lifestyle. Successful aging is not something that begins in later life; rather, it is an accumulation of where and how we have lived our lives, experiences we have encountered, people in our lives, how we feel about ourselves, and choices we make regarding how we care for ourselves and manage our lives. This chapter discusses various predictors (determinants) of successful aging addressed by biological, psychological, and sociological theories of aging. Why study theories of aging? Theories provide the basis for addressing basic and applied research questions, developing effective intervention strategies, and creating or changing public policies. At a practical level, this knowledge can help you as a physical activity instructor to create effective exercise programs and physical activity environments that help to promote the successful aging of your clients.

Biological Theories of Aging

The maximum life span (110-120 years) has not changed since prehistoric times, yet very few people live that long. Why? What are the underlying mechanisms that alter our physiology and determine our deterioration and eventual death? Why do people age at different rates? Several biological theories of aging attempt to answer these questions. However, one of the major problems in developing a coherent aging theory is separating causes from effects.

Many theories have been and are still being tested. It is important to remember that theories should not be considered fact and that no single theory can explain the phenomenon of **senescence**, which is defined as the aging of the body, the gradual decline in cell and body functions that eventually leads to death. Although many individual biological theories of aging have been developed over the years, for the purpose of this discussion, they are divided into three main categories: genetic theories, damage theories, and gradual imbalance theories.

Genetic Theories

Genetic theories focus on the role of heredity in determining the rate of aging within the body. Few genes actually control the rate of aging; however, thousands of genes have a significant role in development of pathologies (diseases). According to Medvedev (1981), aging of the body occurs as a result of the gradual breakdown of **deoxyribonucleic acid (DNA**, the chemical makeup of genes) sequences within the cells, causing incomplete cell reproduction. Genetic theories also suggest that the aging process is controlled by a biological clock that is programmed into each cell of the body. This process prevents human cells from growing and dividing forever. One of the oldest and most prominent theories of aging is the Hayflick limit, which states that a human cell can divide only a limited number of times, approximately 50, and then it suddenly stops dividing and dies (Hayflick, 1961). Hayflick's theory has since been challenged because it is now known that not all cells age or divide at the same rate. For example, cells of the immune and endocrine systems divide very few times, while neurons and muscle cells do not divide at all. Even Hayflick conceded that most people die of diseases before they reach the limit of possible cell life.

Damage Theories

The damage theories emphasize the accumulation of cell damage as a key determinant of cellular dysfunction and death. According to these theories, the cells are damaged by an accumulation of DNA errors or cross-linkages, waste products, glucose, or free radicals within the cells. One of the most accepted theories of cell damage is the free-radical theory (Harman, 1956). **Free radicals** are atoms or groups of atoms that have at least one unpaired electron, making them highly reactive. Although free-radical production provides the energy needed for daily living and kills bacterial invaders, excessive free radicals cause harmful oxidation that damages cell membranes, cell components of DNA and **ribonucleic acid (RNA)** synthesis, and enzymes needed for cell metabolism and correct cell division. Free radicals are especially damaging to the cardiovascular, neuromuscular, immune, and endocrine systems. Eventually the accumulation of cellular damage increases a person's risk for a host of diseases, such as cardiovascular disease, diabetes mellitus, neurodegenerative diseases, cancer, and macular degeneration. In addition to the free radicals produced by the body during metabolism (breakdown of food to make energy), cells are exposed to free radicals from radiation and environmental chemicals (especially tobacco smoke) and those formed when the ultraviolet rays of the sun touch the skin.

Another highly supported damage theory relates to **cross-linkage**. As we age, important large molecules (called macromolecules) of connective tissue (elastin and protein collagen) become intertwined or cross-linked, leading to cellular dysfunction. These cross-links are associated with reduced elasticity in skin and muscle tissue, changes in the lens of the eye, stiffening of blood vessel walls, and reduced joint mobility in older adults (Diggs, 2008a). Cross-linkage of molecules also causes large tangles that interfere with intracellular transport of nutrients and chemical messengers. The cross-linkage of fibers is believed to occur due to increases in free-radical oxidation. Interestingly, leading a more active lifestyle and consuming a healthy diet seem to inhibit or delay cross-linking.

Gradual Imbalance Theories

Collectively, the gradual imbalance theories hypothesize that body systems age at different rates, causing imbalances in biological functions, especially within the central nervous (brain and spinal cord), immune, and endocrine systems (Haywood & Getchell, 2014; Spirduso, Francis, & MacRae, 2005). The central nervous system and the endocrine system, often together referred to as the neuroendocrine system, involve a complicated network of biochemicals that regulate the release of hormones to help the body adapt to real or perceived stress or environmental challenges. The ability of the immune system to produce important antibodies and certain types of T cells also declines with age, leading to dysfunction within the thymus, an important structure within the immune system. Malfunctions of these systems result in hormonal imbalances and deficiencies, causing other physiological and metabolic imbalances that negatively affect a number of body functions and increase the risk of disease among older adults.

Each of the biological theories described in this section attempts to explain the deterioration of body systems (senescence) and eventual death. Although there is a lack of agreement on just how much genetics determines the aging process, family studies have demonstrated that approximately 25 percent of the variation in human longevity is the result of genetic factors (Passarino, De Rango, & Montesanto, 2016). With some understanding of the biological theories of aging, you can confidently convey to your clients that much of how they age is within their control. The next section discusses various psychological theories of aging.

> An understanding of the genetic, damage, and gradual imbalance theories of aging will enable you to confidently convey to your clients that much of their aging process is within their control.

Psychological Theories of Aging

Psychological theories of aging attempt to explain the psychological development of a person and the psychological traits associated with successful aging. Three prominent psychosocial theories discussed here are Maslow's (1943) hierarchy of needs, Erikson's psychosocial stages of development (Erikson, Erikson, & Kivnick, 1986), and the theory of selective optimization with compensation developed by Baltes and Baltes (1990).

One of the most popular theories of successful aging is Maslow's (1943) hierarchy of needs. Maslow described a hierarchy of human needs in which lower-level needs must be satisfied before addressing needs at the next higher level (Maslow & Lowery, 1998). According to Maslow, the more self-actualized and transcendent an individual becomes, the wiser he or she also becomes. **Self-actualization** is defined as finding self-fulfillment and realizing one's potential. **Transcendence** is defined as helping others find self-fulfillment and realize their potential. Is there research evidence to support Maslow's theoretical assumptions? The answer is *yes* based on a Gallup World Poll conducted in 155 countries between 2005 and 2010 (Tay & Diener, 2011). While the authors of the study found that fulfillment of the needs described by Maslow appeared to be universal and important to a person's individual happiness, the order in which higher or lower needs were met did not seem to matter. Perhaps even more important was the finding that individual ratings of

well-being were influenced by the ratings of their fellow citizens; that is, individuals rated their subjective well-being more highly when others in their society also had their needs fulfilled.

One of the early theories of personality development is Erikson's psychosocial stages of development (Erikson et al., 1986). According to Erik Erikson, personality development proceeds through eight stages, each characterized by some type of psychosocial crisis, which must be resolved for successful aging to occur (see table 2.1). The last three stages (between young and late adulthood) describe positive personality development leading to successful aging as the ability to (1) form close relationships with friends and lovers, (2) be productive by raising a family or through some form of work, and (3) look back on one's life with pride and satisfaction.

Table 2.1 Erikson's Psychosocial Stages

Stage	Approximate age	Positive outcome	Negative outcome
Trust vs. mistrust	0-1 year	Child develops faith in people, believes that his or her needs will be taken care of.	Child comes to believe that other people cannot be counted on, believes that his or her needs will not be met.
Autonomy vs. shame and doubt	1-3 years	Child develops confidence in his or her ability to do basic tasks independently.	Child lacks self-confidence.
Initiative vs. guilt	3-5 years	Child feels OK about trying new things.	Child is afraid to try new things, afraid of failure or disapproval if he or she does try new things.
Competence vs. inferiority	6-12 years	Child takes pride in being able to accomplish normally expected tasks.	Child feels inferior because he or she cannot do things that other children appear to do with ease.
Identity vs. role confusion	13-18 years	Child develops a sense of who he or she is and how he or she wants to live life.	Child may be unable to settle on an identity (role confusion) or may adopt a negative identity.
Intimacy vs. isolation	Young adulthood	Person is able to form close relationships with friends and lovers.	Person has difficulty forming or sustaining close relationships.
Generativity vs. stagnation	Middle adulthood	Person is productive through raising a family or through some form of work.	Person is unable to be productive.
Ego integrity vs. despair	Late adulthood	Person is able to look back on his or her life with pride and satisfaction and approach death with dignity and acceptance.	Person feels that he or she has not accomplished what he or she set out to accomplish in life and is frustrated by the approaching end of life.

Based on E.H. Erikson, *Childhood and Society,* 2nd ed. (New York, NY: W.W. Norton and Company, 1963), 272-273.

Sociological Theories of Aging

The most widely accepted sociological theory of aging currently is activity theory. This theory simply states that a positive relationship exists between an individual's level of activity and life satisfaction (Diggs, 2008b). Another theory that has gained considerable support over the years is continuity theory (Atchley, 1971, 1999). This theory states that the people who age most successfully carry forward positive health habits, preferences, lifestyles, and relationships from midlife into later life.

A large body of literature provides consistent evidence that a person's social and physical environments influence the aging process (Charles & Carstensen, 2010; Frost et al., 2010). Conversely, inadequate social and physical environments have been found to be associated with an increase in mortality and morbidity and a decrease in overall health and well-being (Umberson & Montez, 2010). A number of studies have shown that the effects of social relationships begin early in childhood and continue throughout life, cumulatively affecting overall health in either a positive or negative manner (Umberson & Montez, 2010). As a physical activity instructor, you can do much to promote the successful aging of your clients by creating fun and social physical activity environments.

Models of Successful Aging

In addition to the more general theories of aging that have been proposed, specific models of successful aging have also been developed and tested over the past 40 years. Perhaps the most popular model of successful aging that has been used to guide gerontology research is one first conceptualized and collaboratively investigated by an interdisciplinary team of scholars assembled by the MacArthur Foundation and chaired by Dr. John Rowe, a geriatrician and physiologist at Mt. Sinai Medical Center (Rowe & Kahn, 1987, 1998). The development of this model was to herald a dramatic paradigm shift in aging research from one that focused on the negative aspects of aging such as disease and disability to one that emphasized the positive aspects of aging and the important role that lifestyle and other psychosocial factors play in helping older adults retain or enhance their ability to function well into their later years.

The ability to maintain three key characteristics formed the basis of Rowe and Kahn's SA model: a low risk of disease and disease-related disability, high mental and physical function, and active engagement with life. In order to be categorized as aging successfully, however, older adults needed to display high levels of all three of the above characteristics. A sample of 1,189 older adults aged between 70 and 79 years who met the objective criteria established for SA (i.e., top 33rd percentile across all three domains) were subsequently followed for the next eight years (Rowe & Kahn, 1987, 1998). In all, the many related studies that followed produced close to 100 scientific publications and a best-selling lay publication titled *Successful Aging* (Rowe & Kahn, 1998), in which a number of myths previously associated with the aging process were successfully debunked.

Baltes and Baltes (1990) subsequently developed a complimentary model of SA known as the Selective Optimization with Compensation (SOC) model. The SOC model was based on findings emerging from the original Berlin Aging Study that followed a sample of 516 persons aged between 70 and 100 years between 1993 and 1998 (Baltes & Mayer, 1999). In contrast to the Rowe and Kahn model of SA, the SOC model focuses more on describing the behavioral and psychological processes involved in adapting to age-associated reductions in physiological reserve and breadth of neural plasticity. The basic assumption of the SOC model is that individuals engage in behaviors that are aimed at optimizing their general reserves as they age, while also compensating for restricted plasticity or adaptive potential. Subsequent research demonstrated that different combinations of the SOC mechanisms are used by adults of different ages to regulate their lives and that higher engagement in SOC-relevant strategies is associated with indicators of SA such as positive psychological functioning, life satisfaction, and emotional well-being, irrespective of age (Freund & Baltes, 2007; Jopp & Smith, 2006).

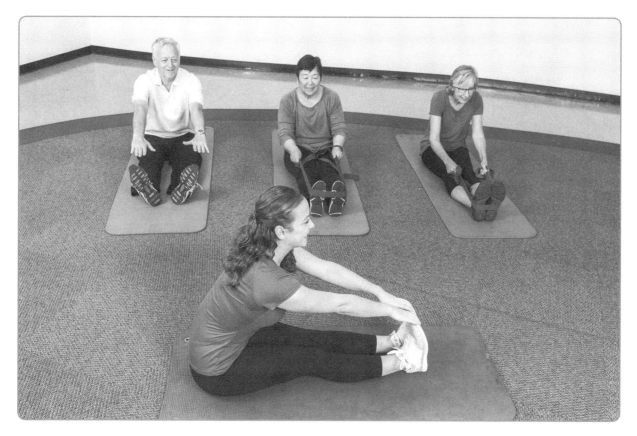

Participating in group-based exercise classes can assist older adults in achieving each of the key characteristics of successful aging identified in the Rowe and Kahn model of successful aging.

Pruchno, Wilson-Genderson, and Cartwright (2010) have begun testing a two-factor model of successful aging. Central to their model of SA is the idea that adults can experience chronic disease and disability and still believe that they are aging successfully and that SA is a characteristic that should not be delimited by age. Unlike the two models of SA described previously, the assumptions of the two-factor model proposed by Pruchno et al. (2010) were tested in a large sample of middle-aged adults (50-74 years). Pruchno and colleagues wanted to understand how and to what extent the objective and subjective aspects of SA were related to each other, as well as the role of age and gender. Their preliminary results provide support for a model of SA that includes both objective and subjective criteria. Moreover, their findings further suggest that certain factors such as cognitive function, social engagement, and psychological well-being, previously identified as components of SA, might be better viewed as predictors or antecedents of SA.

Physical Activity as a Determinant of Successful Aging

A mounting body of empirical evidence has demonstrated that exercise or physical activity provides a number of important physiological, psychological, and social benefits for older adults. Certainly, structured exercise or physical activity is at the core of most, if not all, attempts to prevent the onset of disability, slow the progression of disease or system impairments, or restore function to a level that optimizes independence following a traumatic event. Pope and Tarlov (1999) refer to these as the primary, secondary, and tertiary roles played by physical activity in promoting health.

For each of the components identified in the SA model developed by Rowe and Kahn, physical activity has the potential to serve as the primary vehicle for enhancing or maintaining each of the three key characteristics identified. Indeed, a substantial amount of research has demonstrated an important primary role for physical activity in the prevention of a number of chronic diseases (Nelson et al., 2007) (e.g., cardiovascular disease, type II diabetes, osteoporosis, certain types of cancer), functional limitations (Paterson & Warburton, 2010), and premature disability (Nelson et al., 2007). Moreover, regular engagement in physical activity is associated with the retention of substantially higher levels of cognitive health as characterized by preserved executive control function well into later adulthood (Baker, Meisner, Logan, Kungl, & Weir, 2009; Rejeski, Brawley, & Haskell, 2003; Warburton, Nicol, & Bredin, 2006). Finally, regular engagement in physical activity, particularly in socially supportive group environments, facilitates active engagement in life (Liffiton, Horton, Baker, & Weir, 2012; Meisner, Dogra, Logan, Baker, & Weir, 2010). This is particularly true for older women who are just beginning an exercise program (Hillman, Belopolsky, Snook, Kramer, & McAuley, 2004). Even acute bouts of exercise (as little as 20 minutes) performed at different intensities (moderate or vigorous) have resulted in improved executive function in older women (Peiffer, Darby, Fullenkamp, & Morgan, 2015). The individual benefits of physical activity for older adults are summarized in figure 2.1.

A review of the research investigating how different types of physical activities influence health in the older adult population suggests that a one-type-suits-all physical activity program is not effective (Marcus et al., 2006). As the different roles for physical activity identified earlier in this chapter suggest, relatively healthy older adults can derive

---

Physiological Benefits

Immediate Benefits

- *Glucose levels:* Physical activity helps regulate blood glucose levels.
- *Catecholamine activity:* Both adrenalin and noradrenaline levels are stimulated by physical activity.
- *Improved sleep:* Physical activity has been shown to enhance sleep quality and quantity in individuals of all ages.

Long-Term Effects

- *Aerobic (cardiovascular) endurance:* Substantial improvements in almost all aspects of cardiovascular functioning have been observed following appropriate physical training.
- *Resistance training (muscle strengthening):* Individuals of all ages can benefit from muscle strengthening exercises. Resistance training can have a significant impact on the maintenance of independence in old age.
- *Flexibility:* Exercise that stimulates movement throughout the range of motion assists in the preservation and restoration of flexibility.
- *Balance and coordination:* Regular activity helps prevent or postpone the age-associated declines in balance and coordination that are a major risk factor for falls.
- *Velocity of movement:* Behavioral slowing is a characteristic of advancing age. Individuals who are regularly active can often postpone these age-related declines.

(continued)

FIGURE 2.1   The physiological, psychological, and social benefits of physical activity for older adults.

Psychological Benefits

Immediate Benefits

- *Relaxation:* Appropriate physical activity enhances relaxation.
- *Reduced stress and anxiety:* There is evidence that regular physical activity can reduce stress and anxiety.
- *Enhanced mood state*: Numerous people report elevations in mood state following appropriate physical activity.

Long Term Effects

- *General well-being:* Improvements in almost all aspects of psychological functioning have been observed following periods of extended physical activity.
- *Improved mental health:* Regular exercise can make an important contribution in the treatment of several mental illnesses, including depression and anxiety neuroses.
- *Cognitive improvements:* Regular physical activity may help postpone age-related declines in central nervous system processing speed and improve reaction time.
- *Motor control and performance:* Regular activity helps prevent or postpone the age-associated declines in both fine and gross motor performance.
- *Skill acquisition:* New skills can be learned and existing skills refined by all individuals regardless of age.

Social Benefits

Immediate Benefits

- *Empowered older individuals:* A large proportion of the older adult population voluntarily adopts a sedentary lifestyle, which eventually threatens to reduce independence and self-sufficiency. Participation in appropriate physical activity can help empower older individuals and assist them in playing a more active role in society.
- *Enhanced social and cultural integration:* Physical activity programs, particularly when carried out in small groups or other social environments, enhance social and intercultural interactions for many older adults.

Long-Term Effects

- *Enhanced integration:* Individuals who are regularly active are less likely to withdraw from society and more likely to actively contribute to the social milieu.
- *Formation of new friendships:* Participation in physical activity, particularly in small groups or other social environments, stimulates new friendships and acquaintances.
- *Widened social and cultural networks:* Physical activity frequently provides individuals with an opportunity to widen their available social networks.
- *Role maintenance and role acquisition:* A physically active lifestyle helps foster the stimulating environments necessary for maintaining an active role in society, as well as for acquiring positive new roles.
- *Enhanced intergenerational activity:* In many societies, physical activity is a shared activity. It provides opportunities for intergenerational contact, thereby diminishing stereotypical perceptions about aging and the elderly.

FIGURE 2.1   *(continued)*

significant health benefits or a reduced risk for disability by participating in many different types of physical activity interventions (e.g., walking, cycling, structured exercise classes). On the other hand, older adults living with one or more chronic diseases or system impairments that adversely affect their health and restrict their mobility appear to benefit more from an individually tailored physical activity program that specifically addresses the impairments that are contributing to a more rapid decline in their health. While the overall intensity of the designed program may not differ between these two groups, how the major exercise principles (i.e., overload and specificity) and related exercise variables (i.e., frequency, intensity, time, and type) are manipulated may be very different. (More will be said about each of these exercise principles in chapters 8 and 13.) Finally, for older adults who are frail or transitioning into frailty, individualized physical activity programs that manipulate the major exercise principles and variables in yet another way, and are delivered in combination with other strategies (e.g., medication management, modifications to the living environment) appear to be more effective (Faber, Bosscher, Chin A Paw, & van Wieringen, 2006). Growing evidence also suggests the need for including a behavioral counseling or social-cognitive component within a physical activity program as a means of developing self-regulation skills and better long-term adherence to engaging in physical activity (Brawley, Flora, Locke, & Gierc, 2016; Marcus et al., 2006).

The benefits of exercise on cognitive function among older adults, considered as important as maintaining physical capacity by Rowe and Kahn, have also been explored in a number of studies over the past two decades (Angevaren, Aufdemkampe, Verhaar, Aleman, & Vanhees, 2008; Colcombe & Kramer, 2003; Young, Angevaren, Rusted, & Tabet, 2015). In one of the earliest reviews to systematically investigate the benefits of exercise on cognitive function, Colcombe and Kramer (2003) evaluated the effects of 18 research studies that investigated the impact of different fitness interventions on cognitive function in healthy older adults ranging in age from 55 to 80 years. The benefits of exercise were most apparent for higher-order executive functions such as planning, abstraction, and the selection of relevant sensory information. Larger and more reliable improvements in cognitive function were noted for those fitness interventions that combined aerobic exercise with resistance training and were longer in duration (6+ months). Of further note was the finding that clinical populations showed similar improvements with exercise as did the nonclinical populations studied.

In contrast to these positive findings, subsequent systematic reviews published in 2008 and 2015 that specifically explored the role of aerobic exercise on cognitive function in healthy adults aged over 55 years have yielded mixed findings. While the findings of the 2008 review (Angevaren et al., 2008) demonstrated significant benefits of aerobic exercise on certain cognitive functions in healthy older adults based on a review of 11 research studies, a later review of 12 randomized clinical controlled trials showed no cognitive benefits at all, even in those adults who demonstrated improved cardiorespiratory fitness (Young et al., 2015). Differences in study design quality, the types of cognitive measures used to evaluate intervention efficacy, and the exercise interventions themselves have been identified as possible reasons for the incongruent findings. Clearly, more and better research is needed to determine the nature of the relationship between exercise and cognitive function.

Summary

Successful aging is a difficult concept to define because it is multifaceted. The indicators of successful aging include such factors as length of life, physical and mental health, social competence and productivity, personal control, and life satisfaction. Biological theories of aging—including genetic, damage, and gradual imbalance theories—focus on the factors that cause senescence of the body and increase the risk of morbidity and mortality with age.

Psychosocial theories of aging emphasize how much control people have over how they age. Psychological theories (e.g., Maslow's hierarchy of needs, Erikson's psychosocial stages of development, and the Baltes' theory of selective optimization with compensation) focus on the influence of psychological processes and personality characteristics on the aging process. Research has identified the following psychological factors as being important determinants of successful aging: **intelligence, cognitive capacity, self-efficacy, self-esteem, personal control, coping style**, and **resilience**.

Sociological theories focus on the influence of the social and physical environments on aging. Such theories include the activity theory and the continuity theory. Theories of aging are the basis for research, program development, and public policies. This theoretical knowledge can also help you as a physical activity instructor to create effective exercise programs and physical activity environments that promote the successful aging of your clients.

The final section of the chapter discussed the benefits of physical activity in promoting successful aging, including its physiological, psychological, and social benefits. Successful aging depends on the interplay of such factors as genetics, personal and social environment, lifestyle behaviors, attitudes, adaptability, social supports, and certain personality characteristics. The task of creating a physical activity environment that promotes the successful aging of your clients is not an easy one. Several chapters in this book are designed to prepare you with the knowledge and skills necessary to accomplish this task in a way that meets the needs, desires, and interests of your clients. The quality of life of every older adult you work with will be enhanced through your efforts.

Key Terms

cognitive capacity

coping style

cross-linkage

deoxyribonucleic acid (DNA)

free radicals

intelligence

personal control

resilience

ribonucleic acid (RNA)

self-actualization

self-efficacy

self-esteem

senescence

transcendence

Recommended Readings

Friedman, H.S., & Martin, L.R. (2011). *The longevity project.* New York: Hudson Street Press.

Rowe, J.W., & Kahn, R.L. (1998). *Successful aging.* New York: Pantheon Books.

Study Questions

1. The role of heredity in determining the rate of aging within the body is addressed by a

   a. damage theory of aging

   b. genetic theory of aging

   c. free-radical theory of aging

   d. gradual imbalance theory of aging

2. Maslow's hierarchy-of-needs theory is an example of a

   a. psychological theory of aging

   b. genetic theory of aging

   c. sociological theory of aging

   d. theory of selective optimization with compensation

3. The final stage of Erikson's psychosocial stages of personality development is

   a. generativity versus stagnation

   b. ego integrity versus despair

   c. competence versus inferiority

   d. autonomy versus shame and doubt

4. According to Rowe and Kahn, which of the following characteristic(s) must be maintained in order to age successfully?

   a. low risk of disease and disability

   b. high mental and physical function

   c. active engagement with life

   d. all of the above

5. The theory of selective optimization with compensation states that successful aging has a lot to do with the ability of the older adult to

   a. focus on high-priority areas of life

   b. optimize personal skills and talents

   c. compensate for losses of physical function

   d. all of the above

Application Activities

1. Based on the psychological and sociological theories of aging discussed in this chapter, describe three ways you can promote the successful aging of your clients.

2. Develop a short presentation describing the physical, psychological, and social benefits of physical activity that can be delivered to a group of older adults.

Psychological and Sociocultural Aspects of Physical Activity for Older Adults

Kathleen S. Wilson

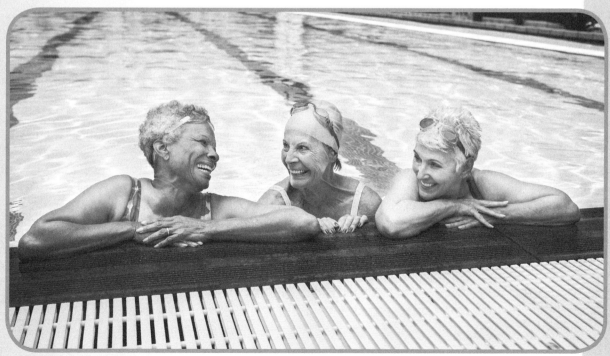

Objectives

After completing this chapter, you will be able to

1. identify the myths and stereotypes associated with aging and participation in physical activity in later life;
2. discuss how physical activity affects older adults' quality of life;
3. explain how physical activity affects psychological well-being in later years, including perceptions of self-esteem, physical self-worth, and self-efficacy;
4. elucidate the relationship between physical activity and cognitive function;
5. describe how physical activity is related to social interactions of older adults; and
6. discuss strategies and national initiatives to promote physical activity among older adults.

There is wide acceptance throughout the industrialized world of the importance of regular physical activity for successful aging. The U.S. Department of Health & Human Services (2008; PAGAC, 2018) published physical activity guidelines for Americans that included a section specifically for older adults. The recommendations for healthy older adults are essentially the same as for adults, which include 150 minutes of aerobic activity and two days of resistance training per week. For those older adults who cannot achieve the goal of 150 minutes, the recommendations are that they should be as active as their abilities and conditions allow. One additional recommendation is that older adults at risk for falls engage in balance training. Recommendations from the American Heart Association and American College of Sports Medicine (Nelson et al., 2007) not only recommend participating in aerobic activity and muscle strengthening activity but also note the importance of participating in flexibility activity at least two days a week. The addition of balance exercises was further recommended if the older adult was experiencing mobility impairments and was at risk for falls (Chodzko-Zajko et al., 2009). These guidelines were further updated in 2011 to include the performance of neuromotor fitness exercises involving balance, agility, and coordination at least two to three days per week for all older adults (Garber et al., 2011). Further discussion of the current Physical Activity Guidelines for Americans

(PAGA) is provided in chapter 8. Unfortunately, the overwhelming majority of older adults (above 60 years of age) are not physically active, with only 24 percent actually meeting the public health recommendations (Troiano et al., 2008; PAGAC, 2018). In adults over the age of 70 years, males, on average, participate in as little as 8.7 minutes per day of moderate to vigorous activity while females average only 5.4 minutes per day (Troiano et al., 2008).

The physical benefits associated with physical activity participation are well known and include reduction in risk factors for many chronic diseases and preservation of numerous aspects of physiological functioning, including cardiovascular function, muscle strength and endurance, balance, and flexibility (Powell, Paluch, & Blair, 2011; U.S. Surgeon General, 1996; Warburton, Nicol, & Bredin, 2006; World Health Organization, 2018). However, despite the wealth of research in this area, the general population is less familiar with the psychological benefits of physical activity including quality of life, psychological well-being, perceptions of ones' self, and cognitive function (Gillison, Skevington, Sato, Standage, & Evangelidou, 2009). In this chapter, we will discuss the various psychosocial benefits that older adults gain from participating in regular physical activity. First, though, we discuss the myths and stereotypes facing older adults.

Aging Stereotypes

One of the most persistent fallacies about aging is the widespread perception that aging is associated with nothing but loss and decline, doom and gloom (Chodzko-Zajko, 1995; Levy, 2009; Lindland, Fond, Haydon, & Kendall-Taylor, 2015). Myths about aging lead to perceptions or stereotypes that associate being old with such conditions as poor health, senility, depression, being boring, declining vitality, and an inability to learn new skills and be productive (Thornton, 2002). One especially prevalent stereotype is the idea of dependency in old age (Levy, 2009). We are exposed to these stereotypes throughout our lives, so internalization begins in childhoods and continues through adulthood and old age (Levy, 2009). These myths and stereotypes contribute to the perception of aging as a negative condition, which can adversely affect the health of older individuals and lead to problems such as higher levels of blood pressure (Levy, 2009) and poorer memory (Levy, 1996).

Robert Butler, the first director of the National Institute on Aging, suggested that there is a widespread tendency throughout society to focus disproportionately on the negative consequences of aging (Butler & Lewis, 1982). Butler referred to this tendency as **ageism**, which he defined as the practice of discriminating against an individual or group of individuals on the basis of their chronological age. According to Butler, ageism has three constituent elements:

- Prejudicial attitudes toward the aged, toward old age, and toward the aging process

- Discriminatory practices against older adults, particularly in employment, but in other social roles as well

- Institutional policies and procedures that perpetuate stereotypical beliefs about older adults, reduce their opportunities for a satisfactory life, and undermine their personal dignity

Butler further concluded that these prejudicial attitudes, discriminatory behaviors, and unjust institutional policies have contributed to the transformation of aging from a natural process into a social problem.

This type of discrimination is generally accepted by society, leading to a widespread prevalence (Angus & Reeve, 2006, Lindland et al., 2015). In a survey of adults older than 50 years of age, 84 percent of Americans reported experiencing at least one of the incidents of ageism identified (Palmore, 2004). Frequently identified instances of ageism included minor events (e.g., jokes that poke fun at old people), experiencing disrespect (e.g., being talked down to because of age), and erroneous assumptions about ailments or frailty (i.e., being told you are too old for that). The prevalence of ageist views suggests that the negative perceptions of aging permeate society and contribute to the view of the aging society as an increasing burden (Angus & Reeve, 2006; Lindland et al., 2015; Thornton, 2002).

These negative perceptions of aging not only are perpetuated by younger adults but also are prevalent among older adults themselves. Older adults may have a positive or negative view of aging stereotypes and these can have a positive or negative effect on a variety of outcomes, both physical and cognitive (Levy, 2009). Based on interviews with older adults, researchers grouped older adults' perceptions of the typical older adult into two types (Horton, Baker, Cote & Deakin, 2008). Some older adults viewed the typical older adult in line with the myths and stereotypes of aging, but viewed themselves as not typical. In contrast, other older adults held a more positive perception of aging and viewed the typical older adult as active and healthy, in which case they described themselves as the typical older adult (Horton, et al., 2008). Positive and negative self-perceptions of older adults such as the ones just mentioned can have a profound impact on their health. Those older adults who held more positive attitudes toward their own aging survived on average 7.5 years longer than those who had a negative attitude toward their own aging (Levy, Slade, Kunkel, & Kasl, 2002). These positive self-perceptions also have been related to functional health status (Levy, Slade, & Kasl, 2002), fewer physical illnesses (Wurm, Tesch-Römer, & Tomasik, 2007), and more preventive health behaviors (Levy & Myers, 2004) including exercise (Wurm, Tomasik, & Tesch-Römer, 2010).

Not only does one's own perceptions of one's own aging influence health and behaviors, but being exposed to either positive or negative stereotypes on a daily basis in the environment also can impact one's own behavior and health. For example, in an experimental study, healthy older adults were subconsciously presented with either a positive or a negative stereotype of aging (Hausdorff, Levy, & Wei, 1999). Those participants who received the positive stereotype of aging showed improved walking performance when compared to those who received the negative stereotypes. These changes in response based on exposure to positive or negative stereotypes of aging highlight the importance of addressing the stereotypes and ageism that are prevalent in society and the broader media.

Given the impact of positive self-perceptions on the health of older adults, physical activity and health professionals can work to promote positive self-perceptions and correct false beliefs about aging. Several strategies have been suggested to help counteract these aging stereotypes and promote positive self-perceptions. First, it is safe to assume that the target audience is aware of the benefits of physical activity. An American Association of Retired Persons (AARP) survey reported that 94 percent of adults older than 50 years reported exercising as a means to improve their overall health while 92 percent reported exercising to feel good about themselves (AARP, 2006). In another study, 95 percent of older adults viewed physical activity as beneficial (Crombie et al., 2004). Several types of messages have also been suggested to help motivate older adults to engage in physical activity. First, it is recommended that promotional messages targeting older adults should feature ordinary people (Ory, Kinney Hoffman, Hawkins, Sanner, & Mockenhaupt, 2003). Older adults find others like them who are physically active and successfully aging to be inspirational, but may find super-fit individuals to be unrealistic and discouraging (Horton et al., 2008). A second recommendation is to provide concrete information such as providing specific directions and guidance for performing physical activities. Guidance may be provided in the form of detailed descriptions of how to perform specific resistance-training exercises, directions to where classes are being offered in the community, or links to websites for more information on programs and classes. Further, it is important that the content of any message be specific, such as including the minimum number of days (e.g., at least five days a week) as opposed to just saying most days of the week. As with other populations, it is important to recognize the challenges that people may face with being active (Ory et al., 2003). By highlighting individuals overcoming these obstacles, older adults may be inspired to be more active. Finally, a key motivator for older adults is their family (Ory et al., 2003). Ageism, which involves the negative perceptions of aging, is pervasive in society from childhood to older adulthood. Such negative perceptions have the potential to impact the health, behavior, and mortality of older adults.

In efforts to motivate older adults to be physically active, instructors can help foster positive attitudes toward physical activity among older adults by actively discussing some of the common myths about physical activity with clients and potential clients (see the sidebar). Providing materials such as books, brochures, or websites that are written for older adults also may help them view physical activity more positively. For example, the *National Blueprint* initiative coordinates a public information campaign designed to dispel common myths and misunderstandings about physical activity. Several other websites provide material that a physical activity instructor could download or share with older adults including the National Institute on Aging (go4life.nia.nih.gov), the National Council on Aging (www.ncoa.org), and the Centers for Disease Control and Prevention (www.cdc.gov/physicalactivity/basics/older_adults/).

Psychosocial Benefits of Physical Activity

Many people associate exercise only with changes in physical fitness. They fail to realize that there are many psychosocial benefits to be gained from regular physical activity. For example, participating in a group exercise program may help to improve ones' satisfaction with their own aging as participants in

> Individuals who are regularly active receive not only physical benefits but also psychological benefits such as improved quality of life, life satisfaction, psychological well-being, and cognitive functioning.

Common Myths About Exercise

Seven general themes about exercise and old age (health status, age, ability, access, intensity, time, and enjoyment) lead to the following common myths and perceived barriers.

- *Myth 1: I'm sick, so I shouldn't exercise; since I'm older, I need to check with my doctor before I exercise.* Many older adults believe that you have to be healthy to exercise. Physical activity can improve quality of life for the vast majority of older adults and may be most effective for people with chronic health conditions and diseases. Instructors can help dispel this myth by pointing out role models in the community who are regularly active despite having health concerns. For some older adults, having a doctor's approval for exercise may give them confidence to be active. Older adults who have no medical conditions and have been physically active recently may not need to check with a doctor. Instructors can also encourage older adults to have regular conversations with their doctors about being physically active.

- *Myth 2: I'm too old to start exercising; it's too late to make a difference in my health; it isn't safe; I don't want to fall and break a hip.* Many older adults do not realize that physical activity has been shown to benefit individuals of all ages, including people as old as 90 or 100 years of age. Instructors can strategically display images of active older adults to help reinforce the notion that age need not be a barrier to activity. Furthermore, many of the typical signs of being "too old" are actually associated with inactivity. Instructors can talk about how specific exercises can help older adults perform activities of daily living. With some older adults being fearful of falling, instructors should address these worries by discussing the ways exercise can improve balance, strength and agility, thereby increasing older adults' mobility and potentially reducing their risk for falling. Instructors can also discuss ways to make exercises safer, such as having a spotter when appropriate and holding on to a support to minimize instability.

- *Myth 3: I'm too weak to start exercising; I'm disabled so I can't exercise.* Exercise can take many different forms and can be modified to your starting point. Someone who is weak from an illness or surgery can build strength by starting slowly and gradually increasing the activity level. For instance, a goal might be to walk across the room four times in a day. Once that becomes manageable, the goal can be increased to walking down the hall. A similar approach works for someone with a disability: identify what activities are appropriate and modify other activities so that they can be performed successfully. Instructors can work with older adults to help them set goals that are appropriate for their current level of functioning. Being flexible and knowing how to modify exercises are important skills for a physical activity instructor.

- *Myth 4: No pain, no gain; exercise will hurt my joints.* Many older adults learned about physical activity at a time when it was thought that exercise had to be of high intensity to be beneficial. It is now recognized that physical activity does not need to be strenuous or exhausting to provide significant health benefits. Physical activity instructors may need to reinforce the notion that light to moderate physical activities, such as social dancing, walking, or gardening, are appropriate and effective ways to include more physical activity in daily life. For those older adults with arthritis, participating in physical activity has been linked to less pain and improved joint function.

(continued)

Common Myths About Exercise *(continued)*

- *Myth 5: You need special clothing, equipment, and access to a gym; I can't afford to join.* No special clothing or equipment is needed. Safe and effective exercise can be performed while wearing comfortable street shoes and loose-fitting everyday clothes. Moreover, effective strength training can be undertaken with inexpensive equipment such as elastic bands and water-filled jugs. These activities can be done in the comfort of home or at a community center and don't require gym access. Also, being active can be achieved without having to spend any money. Instructors can provide older adults with options for exercises that they can do by lifting common household items or nothing but their own body weight. For many older adults, cultural factors influence clothing and exercise choices. It is important that instructors take cultural and generational factors into consideration when choosing physical activity offerings.

- *Myth 6: I'm too busy to exercise; I don't have time.* Few older adults realize that physical activity does not have to occur at a particular time and place but often can be built into daily activities such as shopping, gardening, and household chores. It can also be performed in shorter bouts of 10 to 15 minutes multiple times per day instead of a single 30-minute bout (Murphy, Neville, Neville, Biddle, & Hardman, 2002). Physical activity instructors can help older adults review their busy schedules and identify opportunities for increasing their level of physical activity. Instructors can also provide strengthening exercises that can be done in a short period of time, such as performing leg exercises during commercials. Sometimes, simple exercises can be fit into a daily routine by linking the physical activity to a specific part of the routine. For instance, clients can stretch right after brushing their teeth or do leg raises while waiting for the kettle to boil. Activity becomes easier once it is part of a routine.

- *Myth 7: Exercise is boring; exercise is not enjoyable.* For many, when they think of exercise they think of the repetitive motion of a treadmill or other exercise machine. Repetitiveness exercise can be viewed by some as boring. Exercise doesn't have to be boring. It can take a variety of forms such as playing a game, walking with a friend, playing with grandchildren, gardening, or taking a dance class. As long as the body is moving, it counts as exercise. Instructors can encourage older adults to explore options that they haven't thought about before but are likely to find enjoyable. By introducing a variety of activities into classes, instructors can help make exercise fun and not boring. Another way to help make exercise less boring and more enjoyable is to foster a social atmosphere within the class. Encourage older adults to interact and support each other; by making friends with others, older adults may find the class more enjoyable.

From WebMD. www.webmd.com/healthy-aging/nutrition-world-2/exercise-older-adults

---

the exercise program showed less dissatisfaction with their age than control groups (Klusmann, Evers, Schwarzer, & Heuser, 2012). Numerous research studies with older adults have focused on the relationship of physical activity and overall life satisfaction, quality of life, psychological health and well-being, and cognitive function. The following sections provide an overview of research in these areas.

Physical Activity and Quality of Life

One psychosocial benefit that has received increasing attention is **quality of life** (Bowling, 2007; Bowling & Iliffe, 2011; Depp & Jeste, 2009). Quality of life has been defined as the conscious judgment of the satisfaction an individual has with respect to his or her life (ACSM, 1998). However, it is a broader construct that includes physical, mental, and social indicators of health status (White, Wojcicki, & McAuley, 2009). According to the World Health Organization (1998), quality of life involves six domains: physical health, psychological state, level of independence, social relationships, environment, and spirituality, religiousness, and personal beliefs. In a position stand published by the American College of Sports Medicine (Chodzko-Zajko et al., 2009), physical activity appears to have a positive effect on quality of life; however, this effect may not be the same for all domains of quality of life. These different outcomes are further described later in this chapter.

In a survey of healthy older adults (>60 years of age), Acree et al. (2006) found that those adults who were more physically active demonstrated better physical functioning, fewer role limitations due to physical and emotional health, greater vitality, more positive mental health, greater social function, and better general health than those who were less physically active. Gillison et al. (2009) performed a meta-analysis, which revealed that there were small but significant improvements in psychological and physical domains of quality of life in response to exercise interventions in healthy older adults. Often a life satisfaction scale is used to reflect quality of life (McAuley et al., 2006). Using this global measure of quality of life, links have been seen with participation in light physical activities when based on self-reports of physical activity (Rennemark, Lindwall, Halling, & Berglund, 2009). Given that individuals often over-report their physical activity levels, assessing physical activity using an objective measure such as accelerometers or pedometers can provide another perspective. In one such study that used accelerometers, energy expended by older adults was positively related to satisfaction with life (Fox, Stathi, McKenna & Davis, 2007). However, findings for overall measures of life satisfaction should be interpreted with caution, because a systematic review of the research evidence failed to show that life satisfaction was any higher for the exercise groups when compared to those who did not exercise (Netz, Wu, Becker & Tenenbaum, 2005).

The effects of different types of physical activity such as light, moderate, or vigorous intensity seem to vary across the domains of quality of life. For the psychological domain, there was a positive effect for light-intensity activity over moderate and vigorous activity, whereas for the physical domain, a larger effect was seen for moderate to vigorous activity as opposed to light-intensity exercise (Gillison et al., 2009). Interestingly, the impact of physical activity on quality of life was influenced by the goal of a particular exercise intervention (e.g., disease management) or rehabilitation (e.g., cardiac rehabilitation). The greatest improvements in overall quality of life were observed for those patients undergoing rehabilitation when compared to healthy older adults or those managing a disease such as diabetes (Gillison et al., 2009). Older adults who are more physically active may be more likely to have a better quality of life when assessed using measures of physical and psychological well-being. Different intensities of physical activity have been positively associated with different aspects of quality of life in healthy older adults as well as those undergoing rehabilitation or managing a chronic disease.

Physical Activity and Psychological Well-Being

While quality of life includes many facets of one's life, psychological well-being refers to the mental aspects of quality of life. It focuses on the effect of physical activity on positive aspects of **psychological well-being** (aspects of psychological good health such as positive self-concept, happiness, and emotional well-being) rather than on mental illness. Psychological well-being is viewed as a broad term that captures diverse aspects of quality of life, including emotional well-being and positive self-perceptions (e.g., self-esteem and self-efficacy).

Physical Activity and Emotional Well-Being

Emotional well-being is a term that captures one aspect of psychological well-being, that which pertains to the emotions (e.g., vigor) or positive mental health (e.g., absence of depression) of an individual. The emotional well-being of an older adult can be viewed from many perspectives including levels of anxiety, stress, tension, anger, confusion, energy, vigor, fatigue, depression, positive affect, negative affect, and optimism (Netz et al., 2005). In a review of those research studies, positive associations have been shown between exercise and emotional well-being with the strongest effects observed for light-intensity exercise (Gillison et al., 2009). One study followed adults aged 45-69 years old prospectively for 10 years and showed that physical activity and positive mental health were associated such that those individuals who were more active reported more positive mental health (Steinmo, Hagger-Johnson, Shahab, 2014).

Additionally, in that same study, adults who also reported more positive mental health reported more physical activity (Steinmo et al., 2014). In a review of studies, a significant difference was found between those who participated in an exercise intervention and those who did not for anxiety (including stress and tension) but not for energy, positive affect, anger, or depression (Netz et al., 2005). While depression did not appear to differ in response to exercise when the results of multiple studies were combined, individual studies provide some support for the effect of exercise on depressive symptoms and the prevention of depression. In community-dwelling older adults, depressive symptoms decreased following either a walking or a low-intensity resistance/flexibility program and remained low for 60 months following the intervention (Motl, et al., 2005). In an intervention with older adults experiencing depression, a high-intensity resistance-training program (80% of 1RM) was more effective at reducing depressive symptoms than a low-intensity resistance-training program (20% of 1RM) or a standard care group (Singh et al., 2005). Research has suggested that the effect of physical activity on depression is an indirect effect whereby physical activity influences other variables such as social support, physical health, feelings of control, and self-esteem that in turn are associated with decreased depression (Cairney, Faught, Hay, Wade, & Corna, 2005). There is some evidence that exercise and physical activity may be as effective as social or education strategies for reducing symptoms of depression; however, given the limitations with the current research studies it is difficult to make more definitive conclusions at this time (Barbour & Blumenthal, 2005). The link between physical activity and emotional well-being is also seen in a sample of community-dwelling adults over 60-64 years of age (Black, Cooper, Martin, Brage, Kuh, & Stafford, 2015). In that study, individuals who walked more than one hour a week and those who reported participating in leisure time physical activity at least five times a week reported higher levels of emotional well-being than those who did not (Black et al., 2015). Engaging in physical activity has been associated generally with more positive emotional well-being overall.

Physical Activity and Positive Self-Perceptions

Self-esteem is one's positive and negative attitudes toward oneself as a whole and has been suggested to be a central aspect of psychological well-being (Rosenberg, Schooler, Schoenbach, & Rosenberg, 1995). Self-esteem is thought to be a global construct representing a component of the self or self-acceptance (Rosenberg et al., 1995). In addition to global self-esteem, subdomains that relate to specific behaviors such as academic or physical self-perceptions are also important. It is specific self-perceptions such as physical self-worth that are thought to be linked more closely to the performance of specific behaviors than perceptions of global self-esteem. However, when examining the relationship to psychological well-being, it is global self-esteem that plays the larger part (Rosenberg et al., 1995). It is thought that by influencing specific subdomains of self-esteem such as perceptions of physical self-worth, changes would occur in global self-esteem and subsequently in psychological well-being.

A review of the relationship between physical activity and self-esteem showed there was a small but reliable positive relationship, suggesting that those adults who increase their physical activity also see improvements in their global self-esteem (Spence, McGannon, & Poon, 2005). Although the relationship of physical activity to global self-esteem has been identified as being small, the link between physical activity and global self-esteem is greater when there is an accompanying improvement in physical fitness (Spence et al., 2005). Further, participants in aerobic exercise programs and lifestyle activity programs showed improvements in self-esteem, while participants in skill-training programs did not show an increase in self-esteem (Spence et al., 2005). However, given the relatively small effect between physical activity and global self-esteem, one must be cautious not to overstate this relationship (Spence et al., 2005).

In 1989, Sonstroem and Morgan developed a multidimensional model of exercise and self-esteem, which illustrated the associations between physical activity, self-perceptions, and self-esteem. This model was then revised to include physical self-worth (Sonstroem, Harlow, & Josephs, 1994; see figure 3.1 for an illustration of the variables in this model). Using this model, physical activity has been shown to be related to domain-specific self-perceptions of physical self-worth (Fox et al., 2007; McAuley et al., 2005). The effect of physical activity on global self-esteem is thought to be mediated by how one perceives her or his physical self (McAuley et al., 2005). For instance, participation in physical activity leads to changes in perceptions of physical capabilities such as strength, physical functioning, fitness levels, and even perceptions of one's body and attractiveness. These different perceptions then influence the individual's perceptions of self-worth, which in turn impacts global self-esteem. These relationships have been demonstrated in several research studies. For example, this pattern emerged where physical activity was first associated with perceptions of physical condition, attractiveness, and strength. Those perceptions were then related to physical self-worth and then, in turn, physical self-worth was related to global self-esteem (McAuley et al., 2005). Similar associations were found in another study where physical activity was related to physical self-worth through components such as perceptions of attractiveness and physical health that, in turn, may impact physical self-worth and general

perceptions of self-esteem (Moore, Mitchell, Beets & Bartholomew, 2012). In another study that assessed physical activity levels of older adults using accelerometers, overall energy expended in physical activity was related to physical self-perceptions, including perceptions of physical self-worth, physical functioning, and sport competence (Fox et al., 2007).

Not only do these links between physical activity and perceptions of physical self-worth and self-esteem appear in cross-sectional and longitudinal research, evidence from intervention studies where people start an exercise program has also emerged (Elavsky et al., 2005; Fox et al., 2007; Opdenacker, Delecluse, & Boen, 2009). For example, in response to a physical activity intervention that involved tai chi three times a week, older adults maintained their levels of physical self-perceptions while those not involved in the intervention experienced a decline (Fox et al., 2007). More positive perceptions of physical self worth and self-esteem have been shown to increase in response to a wide range of interventions including a walking intervention (Elavsky et al., 2005), home-based physical activity program (Opdenacker et al., 2009), structured group-based exercise program (Opdenacker et al., 2009), and tai chi (Fox et al., 2007). Collectively, these findings highlight the influence that physical activity has on how one perceives his or her own abilities. When older adults start an exercise program, one way they may improve their psychological well-being is by improving their perceptions of their physical self-worth and subsequently self-esteem.

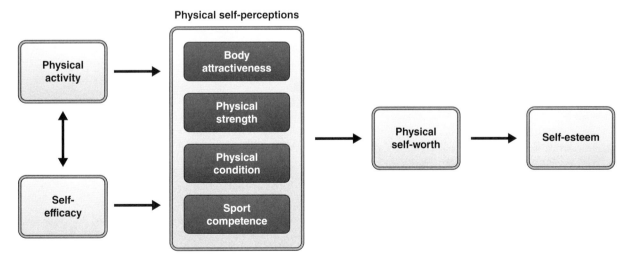

FIGURE 3.1   Summary of the relationship between physical activity, self-efficacy, and self-esteem.

Based on Sonstroem & Morgan (1989); Sonstroem, Harlow, and Josephs (1994).

Physical Activity and Self-Efficacy

A similar self-perception that has the potential to impact psychological well-being is self-efficacy. **Self-efficacy** describes one's confidence in her or his ability to perform a specific task (Bandura, 1997). These perceptions of confidence influence the choice of activities engaged in, the goals that are set, and the persistence in the chosen activities (Bandura, 1997). For example, individuals who do not think they will be able to perform a specific activity successfully (low self-efficacy) may not attempt the activity at all. Conversely, other people who are confident in their abilities may be more open to trying new activities. Self-efficacy can take many forms. Individuals can be confident in their ability to perform specific tasks such as walking for six minutes or playing a musical instrument. Another form of efficacy involves one's confidence to manage specific behaviors such as scheduling physical activity sessions. This type of self-efficacy is called self-regulatory efficacy and is thought to play a key role in whether individuals engage in healthy behaviors such as physical activity (Bandura, 2005).

Physical activity may affect the quality of life of older adults through this mechanism of perceived control or self-efficacy (White et al., 2009). Researchers have shown that older adults who are more confident in their ability to manage physical activity behaviors (higher self-regulatory efficacy) are more satisfied with their lives (Strachan, Brawley, Spink, & Glazebrook, 2010). Other researchers have shown that physical activity has a direct impact on self-efficacy, which in turn is related to more positive perceptions of self-worth (psychological well-being) and lower levels of perceived disability (White et al., 2009). Subsequently, these more positive perceptions of self-worth and lower levels of perceived disability were associated with an improved global quality of life (White et al., 2009). Several studies have shown that self-efficacy affects perceptions of physical self-worth directly regardless of any changes in physical activity itself (McAuley et al., 2005; Opdenacker et al., 2009). In one study, changes in physical activity were related to changes in self-efficacy such that those who increased their physical activity level also became more confident (McAuley et al., 2008). In turn, the improved levels of confidence were related to the

psychological well-being of the older adults. These findings highlight another way that physical activity may contribute to psychological well-being, through improving self-efficacy.

Higgins, Middleton, Winner, and Janelle (2014) reviewed 20 physical activity interventions targeting healthy adults. Physical activity interventions that included structured exercise sessions were associated with improved task self-efficacy (confidence to exercise) and longer interventions improved barriers to self-efficacy (confidence to deal with obstacles that may make it hard to exercise). McAuley and Katula (1998) reviewed the literature that examined the relationship between physical activity and self-efficacy in older adults. They concluded that most well-controlled exercise-training studies resulted in significant improvements in both the physical fitness and self-efficacy of older adults. For example, in a cross-sectional survey, older adults who had more positive perceptions of their own physical ability (self-efficacy) engaged in higher levels of leisure time physical activity (Orsega-Smith, Payne, Mowen, Ching-Hua, & Godbey, 2007).

There is growing recognition that self-efficacy not only is an important outcome of physical activity, but also may be an important predictor of sustained behavioral change in sedentary populations (Aparicio-Ting, Farris, Courneya, Schiller, & Friedenreich, 2015). For example, Aparicio-Ting and colleagues (2015) reported that self-efficacy and beliefs about the advantages and disadvantages were related to remaining physically active twelve months following a physical activity intervention in a sample of postmenopausal women. In another study, changes in self-efficacy were related not only to positive changes in physical activity but also to goals for physical activity and positive expected outcomes (White, Wojcicki, & McAuley, 2012). These findings suggest that self-efficacy also is important for the promotion of physical activity in older adults.

Fostering self-efficacy is vital when working with older adults given that their confidence to perform physical activity is often lower than that observed in young and middle-aged adults (Netz & Raviv, 2004). Bandura (1997) identifies four sources of self-efficacy perceptions including successful experiences, modeling behaviors of others, verbal persuasion, and physiological states. Understanding each of these sources is important for physical activity professionals who want to improve their clients' perceptions of self-efficacy.

Physical activity instructors can focus on providing successful experiences for their clients by planning activities that the clients will succeed at but that still challenge them. It is important not to make these activities too difficult because clients need to feel a sense of accomplishment or mastery.

Seeing other people performing the targeted activity is another way to improve self-efficacy. There are several considerations when having older adults observe models. First, models who are perceived to be similar to them, including other older adults, are often the most effective models. Second, it is acceptable if the model struggles with the activity before succeeding. Watching someone who struggles but eventually succeeds lets the clients know that it is okay if they struggle because they might achieve success as well. Using models to perform a specific task such as balancing on one leg would promote a task efficacy or confidence to perform that specific task (e.g., balancing on one leg). However, it is important to also note that you could use models who are successfully adhering to your exercise program and seeing results. This type of model would be promoting self-regulatory efficacy. To incorporate this model, you could discuss success stories of clients who have adhered to the physical activity and who describe how they have overcome some challenges. For example, part of the Go4Life campaign from the National Institute of Aging at NIH presents success stories. Once success story is from Sam, who is 84 years old:

> I started exercising regularly way back in 1960. A friend put me in touch with a personal trainer at a nearby gym, and he showed me how to lift weights. Today, at age 83, I'm still exercising to stay fit. I get up every day and exercise for 10 to 15 minutes. I lift weights followed by stretching. In the evening, I do the same routine for about 15 minutes. I'm a drummer by profession, and I do about four gigs a month. Exercise keeps my muscles strong and lets me continue to do my drumming.
>
> From Success Stories: Busy Lifestyle at http://go4life.nia.nih.gov/

Incorporating the third source of self-efficacy into your practice with older adults could be as simple as providing encouragement and telling the clients that you are confident they can perform the specific task. The final source of self-efficacy pertains to how the client is feeling and is based on the physiological states. If someone is nervous or feels their legs wobbling, they probably will feel like they will not be able to perform a specific activity. The challenge for the instructor is helping the client determine whether feeling weak or fatigued is due to being unable to the perform the activity or simply because he or she is working hard, where fatigue and feeling wobbly is a natural outcome. As a physical activity instructor, helping the client to navigate through these various physiological states is important for maintaining efficacy levels. A study of older German adults examined how these sources related to self-efficacy for physical activity, and reported that mastery experience, self-persuasion, and decreasing negative affect were key factors related to self-efficacy (Warner et al., 2014). Self-efficacy is increased by physical activity while at the same time plays an important role in increasing participation in physical activity programs. There are numerous ways to promote self-efficacy among older adults, including providing successful experiences, using models similar to them perform the behavior, giving verbal encouragement, and being aware of physiological states.

Physical Activity and Social Environment

We do not live in isolation but rather are immersed in a social environment. This social environment shapes us just as our behaviors influence our social environment. In fact, a fundamental need of humans is the need to belong (Baumeister & Leary, 1995). This need highlights the importance of social interactions and our social network to our well-being. For example, older adults who reported more social interactions along with having given and received more social support had more positive perceptions of well-being (Thomas, 2010). Not only does physical activity participation affect the physical and mental functioning of older adults, it also can contribute to such social interactions and **social functioning**. The promotion of social interactions among older adults is essential, given that social inactivity and loneliness are predictors of mortality (Tilvis et al., 2012). In a large survey of Finnish adults over 75 years of age, 46.1 percent were identified as socially isolated, 39.4 percent as having high levels of social inactivity, and 37 percent as suffering from loneliness (Tilvis et al., 2012). Only 23 percent of the sample did not report any of these negative social factors. Exercise interventions have been shown to have a positive effect on social functioning, especially individual-based interventions (Gillison et al., 2009).

Social environments are often conceptualized in two forms: the structure of the environment or the social networks of individuals (i.e., number of friends or contacts) and the processes that go on within the social environment such as the receipt of social support or social influences (House, Umberson, & Landis, 1988). Physical activity has been associated with both of these aspects of the social environment. For example, older adults who were more physically active also reported larger social networks (Vance, Wadley, Ball, Roenker & Rizzo, 2005). Those older adults who are more physically active show more positive social functioning overall (Acree et al., 2006). Further, older women who increased their exercise over the course of three years also rated their social functioning more positively than those older women who remained sedentary (Lee & Russell, 2003). In contrast, those women who stopped exercising showed decreases in their social functioning (Lee & Russell, 2003). Other researchers have shown that physical activity participation by older adults has been linked to both emotional support from others as well as involvement in social activities (Rennemark et al., 2009). To further highlight the importance of physical activity for social interactions, researchers from Brazil surveyed older adults and found that those who were more physically active were more satisfied with their relationships with family, friends, and neighbors (Benedetti, Schwingel, & Torres, 2011). Furthermore, these older adults were also more likely to engage in social groups in the community (Benedetti et al., 2011).

The social environment also has been shown to encourage participation in physical activity behaviors. The importance of others in promoting physical activity is demonstrated in a brief intervention that showed an increase in physical activity for those older adults who participated with their partner when compared to those who participated without a partner or who were single (Gellert, Ziegelmann, Warner, & Schwarzer, 2011). In focus groups conducted with older adults, the influence of family, friends, and health care professionals such as nurses, doctors, and physical therapists was identified as important for being physically active (Wilson & Spink, 2006). Others have highlighted that the support older adults receive from friends is associated with being more physically active during their leisure time (Orsega-Smith et al., 2007). Interestingly, the combination of both social support and self-efficacy may be key; older adults who had high levels of social support from friends and also had high self-efficacy were the most physically active (Warner, Ziegelman, Schuz, Wrum, & Schwarzer, 2011).

One important consideration when working with older adults is to consider their preferences for the type of social environment in which they want to be active. One study by Wilcox, King, Brassington, and Ahn (1999) reported that 67 percent of older adults preferred exercising on their own with some instruction compared to 33 percent who preferred group-based exercise classes. However, other researchers have suggested that older adults may in fact prefer some group-based classes where other class members are of similar ages (Beauchamp, Carron, McCutcheon, & Harper, 2007). Another study echoed the importance of the presence of others similar to them because older adults aged 60-67 years old preferred to exercise with others of a similar age (Burton, Kahn & Brown, 2012). This does not negate the importance of others in more informal physical activity settings. For example, Cohen-Mansfield and colleagues found that a higher percentage of older adults surveyed preferred to walk with a companion (33%) than to walk alone (18%) (Cohen-Mansfield, Marx, Biddison, & Guralnik, 2004). Further, when asked how they prefer to be active, 47 percent of older adults preferred to exercise with others, 20 percent preferred exercising alone, and 33 percent had no preference (Wilson & Spink, 2009). Several implications can be drawn from an awareness of these preferences. First, individuals with different preferences report different influences for physical activity, especially from friends (Wilson & Spink, 2009). This suggests that there is a need to tailor programs for people who have different preferences; for example, providing group programs for those who prefer to exercise with others and individual programs for those who prefer to exercise alone. Given the importance of tailoring interventions (King et al., 2006), it may also be beneficial to consider the preferred social environment when tailoring programs for older adults. A final consideration is the need for programs for older adults of similar ages, given the preference of some to participate with similarly aged others (Beauchamp et al., 2007; Burton et al., 2012). The social environment plays an important role in older adults' psychological well-being, and physical activity has the capacity to enhance the social environment. Additionally, social influences from others can help older adults initiate and maintain physical activity programs.

Physical Activity and Cognitive Function

The prevalence rate for some level of cognitive impairment has been estimated to be 22 percent of adults over 70 years of age (Brookmeyer et al., 2011). Given that this translates to one in five older adults having some level of impairment, maintaining cognitive function is vital to quality of life in later years. In a 2009 position stand, the American College of Sports Medicine highlighted that higher levels of physical activity and fitness are associated with lower risk of cognitive impairment and dementia (Chodzko Zajko et al., 2009). **Cognitive function** involves a combination of skills, including memory, attention, learning, goal setting, decision making, and problem solving. In a meta-analysis, Colcombe and Kramer (2003) organized the cognitive tasks employed in reviewed studies into four categories:

1. *Speed tasks:* Simple tasks requiring rapid responses that do not involve high-level cognition (e.g., reaction times and finger tapping)

2. *Visuospatial tasks:* Tasks that require rotating real or imaginary objects in three-dimensional space (e.g., remembering three line drawings and recreating them)

3. *Controlled processing tasks:* Tasks that require the use of effortful processing strategies and that gradually become automatic with extended practice (e.g., a choice reaction time where one key is pressed when presented with one letter and a different key for a different letter)

4. *Executive control tasks:* Tasks that require coordination, inhibition, and working memory

and that also depend on effortful processing but do not become automatic over time (e.g., a choice reaction time that also requires inhibiting conflicting cues)

The results of this meta-analysis indicated that physical activity had the greatest impact on the performance of executive control tasks, followed by controlled processing tasks, visuospatial tasks, and then speed tasks (Colombe & Kramer, 2003). A review of 29 studies on aerobic exercise in adults reported improvement in attention and processing speed, executive function, and memory (Smith et al., 2010). In another review of the literature, Kramer and Erickson (2007) showed that fitness training consistently had a positive effect on cognitive function over a series of studies. However, another review reported that there was a lack of evidence for exercise being associated with cognitive function in community-dwelling older adults (Snowden et al., 2011). One type of intervention that did show promise for improving cognitive function was cardiovascular training. Significant improvements in executive function, general cognition, memory, and language were observed (Snowden et al., 2011).

The effect of physical activity on cognitive function is not limited to just aerobic activity. Other studies have investigated the benefits of strength training and multicomponent exercise training (Snowden et al., 2011). Strength training appears to be associated with executive function and memory. Visuospatial tasks appear to show the greatest response to multicomponent interventions. One study showed that older adults who participated twice a week in resistance training exercise improved in their ability to perform a cognitive task requiring selective attention when compared with a balance-training group (Liu-Ambrose, Nagamatsu, Voss, Khan, & Handy, 2012). Improvements in the functional plasticity of the brain in response to the resistance training were also observed based on increased brain activity in the frontal cortex captured using a functional magnetic resonance imaging (fMRI) machine.

Several characteristics of the exercise itself influenced or moderated the effect of exercise on cognitive function. Characteristics included the type of training (i.e., cardiovascular only versus a combined training program), duration of the program (i.e., short or long), and session duration (short, moderate, or long) (Colcombe & Kramer, 2003). For example, findings suggested that while aerobic exercise had a moderate effect on cognitive functioning, the combination of aerobic, strength, and flexibility exercises was optimal for achieving improvements in cognitive function (Colcombe & Kramer, 2003). Programs that lasted longer than six months showed the strongest relationship with cognitive functioning. In terms of session duration, Kramer and Erickson (2007) reported that sessions lasting at least 30 minutes were necessary to see changes in cognitive function. In addition, it is also important to recognize that not all physical activity interventions have been able to demonstrate changes in cognitive function even when they show changes in physical fitness (Komulainen et al., 2010). Physical activity shows some promising links with aspects of cognitive functioning, especially executive control (i.e., planning and response inhibition). Stronger effects are seen for multicomponent fitness programs, programs with durations longer than six months, and session durations of at least 30 minutes.

One area that is receiving increasing research interest, across all age groups, is exergaming (Kamal, 2011). Exergaming can range from playing video games that require physical movement to enhancing exercise through virtual reality cycling tours. One study examined the effect of exergaming compared to traditional exercise on cognitive function in a sample of 79 older adults (Anderson-Hanley et al., 2012). In that study, older adults who participated in the cyber-cycling group showed greater improvements in executive function when compared to a traditional exercise group. Furthermore, those in the cyber-cycling group had a lower risk of developing mild cognitive impairment over the three-month intervention. One possible mechanism identified in this study was brain-derived neurotrophic factor, which is associated with plasticity in the brain.

A variety of mechanisms have been suggested to explain how physical activity may improve cognitive function, including changes in the structure of and chemicals within the brain (Coelho et al., 2013; Erickson et al., 2011; Kirk-Sanchez & McGough, 2014). In a review of animal studies, several changes in brain structure have been identified in response to physical activity and fitness (Kirk-Sanchez & McGough, 2014). One improvement in response to increased fitness or physical activity is nerve-cell proliferation and growth in regions of the brain such as the hippocampus, which is important for memory.

Other changes include increased nerve growth factors such as brain-derived neurotrophic factor (BDNF), which improves the efficiency of the nerve cells by enhancing synapse (connection between cells) efficiency. Another change in response to physical activity is improved vascularization (an increase in the number of blood vessels), making it easier to transport oxygen to the brain. In human studies, physical activity and fitness have been associated with less loss of grey matter in the frontal, temporal, and parietal lobes (McAuley et al., 2004). Further, in response to an aerobic exercise intervention, older adults showed a larger increase in the size of the hippocampus as well as higher levels of brain-derived neurotrophic factor than did a group that received a stretching intervention (Erickson et al., 2011). The impact of physical activity and fitness on cognitive function appears to be through changes in the structure of the brain that occur in response to participation in physical activity.

Promoting Physical Activity

Given the numerous physical and psychological benefits older adults receive from participating in physical activity, it is important for physical activity and health professionals to be aware of factors that promote or hinder physical activity participation in older adults. However, a complex mix of factors is related to participation in physical activity (King & King, 2010). There is also a growing recognition that individual behaviors such as physical activity are influenced both by individual and personal characteristics as well as by broader factors such as social/cultural and environmental/policy factors (King & King, 2010). As mentioned previously, personal characteristics such as self-efficacy are important factors in the promotion of physical activity (McAuley et al., 2008; White et al., 2012). Other personal characteristics associated with being more likely to participate in physical activity include being male, being a younger age, being in good health, having an absence of chronic conditions, and having a lower body mass index (Koeneman, Verheijden, Chinapaw, & Hopman-Rock, 2011). At the social/cultural level, important factors include the immediate social environment (e.g., receipt of social support) (Koeneman et al., 2011) and a physician's advice (Schutzer & Graves, 2004), as well as the broader social environment including cultural influences and media influences. Cultural differences in factors related to participation have received little attention, although they are starting to be examined. For example, different barriers are mentioned by different ethnic groups. American Indians report barriers of the physical environment and lack of knowledge more often than do Whites, Latinos, Vietnamese, Chinese, and African Americans (Mathews et al., 2010). These variations in barriers across different cultures highlight the potential need for ethnic-specific activity programming. Beyond the social/cultural environment, the impact of the physical environment (e.g., facilities, accessibility or connectivity to destinations, safety, aesthetics, convenience) on older adults' physical activity also has received limited attention in the literature (Haselwandter et al., 2015). For example, factors such as aesthetics, personal safety, and services have been associated with walking for residents in retirement villages (Nathan, Wood, & Giles-Corti, 2014). Also at the environment level, policies have the potential to affect physical activity. Such policies include increasing funding or the number of programs as well as targeting transportation and building accessibility (King & King, 2010). These differing influences highlight the complexity of promoting physical activity in older adults and of the approaches needed to increase physical activity levels.

Given the changing demographics of society, physical activity promotion has received greater attention by organizations and policy makers. In order to address the problem of low physical activity in older adults, an approach that targets multiple levels (i.e., personal, social, and environmental) will be needed (King & King, 2010). One of the main limitations is the lack of attention paid to exploring comprehensive and sustainable approaches; current interventions mostly target personal characteristics and are usually short-term in length (King & King, 2010). There is a need to adopt a multilevel approach to promoting physical activity in older adults that addresses not just the personal characteristics but also the social/cultural and environmental/policy factors.

A policy-level initiative promoting physical activity for older adults is the *National Blueprint: Increasing Physical Activity Among Adults Age 50 and Older*. This major planning document was released in May 2001 with the goal being to develop a coordinated national strategy for promoting physical activity among older people. The *National Blueprint* was developed with input from more than 60 individuals representing 46 organizations with expertise in health, medicine, social and behavioral sciences, epidemiology, gerontology and geriatrics, clinical science, public policy, marketing, medical systems, community organization, and environmental issues. A major goal of the *National Blueprint* was to identify some of the societal barriers to physical activity among older adults and to outline specific strategies for overcoming these barriers. The blueprint identifies barriers in the areas of research application, home and community programs, workplace settings, medical systems, public policy and advocacy, and marketing and communications. Some of the barriers that have the greatest relevance for health professionals and physical activity instructors in local communities are the following:

- Many neighborhoods and communities are poorly planned, unsafe, and designed in a manner that discourages regular physical activity by older adults.
- Community resources (senior centers, senior residences, community centers, neighborhoods and apartment units, schools, and places of worship) are often disconnected.
- Health organizations do not collaborate enough with professionals in urban and community planning, transportation, recreation, and design to develop strategies that can make communities more amenable to physical activity.
- Many older adults do not know how to start a safe and appropriate home-based physical activity program.
- Many older adults are isolated and lack transportation to community physical activity facilities and programs.
- Health care professionals do not have adequate, tested, and age-appropriate patient education materials on physical activity for older patients.
- Medical professionals do not have the information to make referrals to community resources. They often lack knowledge about quality programs, materials, and resources.

In addition to identifying barriers to physical activity in society at large, the *National Blueprint* proposes a number of concrete strategies to overcome these barriers. While many of the strategies are complex and will require the combined efforts of many individuals and organizations before they can be realized, several of the strategies can be implemented at the local level and have significant implications for physical activity instructors and health professionals. These strategies follow:

- Create a national clearinghouse to disseminate effective, tested public education, social marketing materials, and public policy information on physical activity and aging.

- Identify barriers to walking by adults, determine why these barriers exist, and develop specific recommendations for overcoming them.

- Establish and disseminate standards for fitness leaders who work with midlife and older populations.

- Locate examples of activity-friendly communities and home- or community-based programs, and devise a system to share best practices.

- Encourage more health, physical education, recreation, and dance professionals to become trained and certified to work with older adults.

- Obtain funding and implement physical activity programs for older adults through appropriate existing community facilities, such as YMCAs and YWCAs, community centers, senior centers, and places of worship.

- Provide community organizations with a template for good physical activity programs.

- Establish partnerships among health, aging, urban- and community-planning, transportation, environmental, recreation, social service, and private sector agencies. Encourage these groups to work together to define, create, promote, and sustain communities that support lifelong physical activity.

- Identify high-quality community sources of information on physical activity and older adults (YMCAs and YWCAs, certified trainers, fitness clubs, etc.), and provide this information to clients in health care settings.

The *National Blueprint* is a challenging document! It challenges organizations to rethink how they are addressing issues related to physical activity. It challenges them to develop partnerships to share resources and work collaboratively to begin to restructure society in such a way as to enable older adults to be more active. To evaluate the effectiveness of the *National Blueprint,* Park and colleagues (2010) interviewed both senior administration and junior staff members from several organizations that developed the document. The interviewees talked about how the blueprint influenced their own organizational missions and strategies by including goals about physical activity. Interviewees also talked about how leader behavior changed to become more in line with the blueprint as well as changes in organization behavior, beliefs, attitudes, and performance.

The blueprint also challenges each of us as individuals. It asks us to identify how we can best contribute to the redesign and restructuring of our local communities. We are challenged to become more active in creating environments that enable and promote physical activity. We are encouraged to join coalitions, form partnerships, and share our knowledge and expertise. Most important, we are challenged to think outside of the box.

There are several initiatives that are currently promoting physical activity for older adults. Two programs initially funded by the Robert Wood Johnson Foundation that have been successfully implemented in various communities are *Active Choices* and *Active Living Everyday* (Wilcox et al., 2008). *Active Choices* is a program based on telephone counseling for six months following an initial face-to-face meeting, while *Active Living Everyday* is a small-group-based program. Both of these programs include behavioral change strategies such as goal setting and self-monitoring. While originally tested in a research setting, these programs have been translated for dissemination in the community with community sites subsequently making some adaptations to tailor the programs to their specific needs or target group (Wilcox et al., 2008). An example of one such change involved shortening the *Active Living Everyday* program from 20 weeks to 12 weeks by reducing some of the material presented and lengthening the sessions from 60 to 90 minutes. By evaluating interventions within the community setting, we can determine whether the programs can be put into practice and then evaluate the challenges associated with that implementation. For both of these programs, the physical activity level of the participants significantly increased over the course of the program, suggesting that translating these interventions into the community setting was feasible and effective (Wilcox et al., 2008).

Another initiative that addresses some of the strategies highlighted by the *National Blueprint* is the Go4Life initiative led by the National Institute on Aging at the National Institutes of Health (http://go4life.nia.nih.gov/). Go4Life focuses on increasing the physical activity of older adults in their daily lives. It includes a wealth of resources that are available to older adults, including sample workouts, strategies to help with behavioral change such as goal setting, and advice for coping with barriers. It includes stories and photos of other older adults who are physically active, which may help promote self-efficacy. The target audiences include older adults as well as health care professionals and organizations. Go4Life provides resources such as posters, handouts, and informational packets for organizations and health care professionals who work with older adults. Through the provision of these resources, *Go4Life* provides social marketing materials and information as well as examples of physical activity programs for community organizations to adopt (see figure 3.2). However, Go4Life is a relatively new initiative, so it will take time to evaluate its effectiveness.

There are many ways that physical activity and health professionals can begin to think outside the box and get more involved in local efforts to promote physical activity. For example, many senior centers and continuing-care retirement communities would greatly appreciate receiving expert advice and assistance on physical activity programming from local fitness experts such as personal trainers and kinesiology faculty and graduate students. Links can also be developed between local physicians' offices and community fitness clubs and sports centers. A number of cities have established community coalitions to promote active living, in which local industry representatives, health care organizations, service agencies for older adults, transportation specialists, health and fitness professionals, local government officials, and many others meet regularly to develop programs and projects designed to reduce barriers to active living in the community. Fitness professionals should make every effort to reach out to other professionals working in

the area of healthy aging. A phone call to a local senior center or Area Agency on Aging is often an excellent way to start getting involved.

Summary

This chapter discussed the contribution of physical activity to successful aging, including relationships with quality of life, psychological well-being, social functioning, and cognitive functioning. The dissemination of information on the physical and psychological health benefits of physical activity alone is not sufficient to motivate people to be more physically active. To achieve long-term changes in behavior, it is necessary to also address a variety of social/cultural, environmental/policy, and individual factors that affect physical activity, both for the individual and for society at large. At the level of the individual, this requires applying theories of motivation and behavioral change. Physical activity instructors need to carefully assess their clients' needs and readiness to adopt physical activity (see chapter 5) and employ behavioral management techniques to help older adults successfully maintain an exercise program (see chapter 7). It is not sufficient to develop a generic exercise program and expect all older adults to fit in and participate enthusiastically. Physical activity instructors who want to tailor physical activity programs for older adults should consider their clients' perceptions of aging stereotypes, self-efficacy, preferences for being active, and other individual characteristics.

The existence of aging stereotypes and the prevalence of ageism represent a challenge that may need to be overcome before many older adults will want to increase their physical activity. In order to get potential clients to want to participate in physical activity, physical activity instructors may have to work with older adults to promote positive views of aging and realize that older adults have the potential for many physical and psychological benefits from physical activity. It is also important for instructors working with older adults to dispel the common myths by helping their clients realize that they do not have to be healthy to exercise, it is never too late to start, they do not need expensive clothing or equipment, and gains can be achieved without pain. Instructors also have an obligation to teach older adults that physical activity offers more than

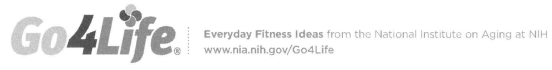

Go4Life® Everyday Fitness Ideas from the National Institute on Aging at NIH
www.nia.nih.gov/Go4Life

Making Your Fitness Center Comfortable for Members 50+

Many older adults want to be physically active. But older adults who are not used to fitness centers may feel intimidated or uncomfortable going to a facility with equipment and routines that are unfamiliar. Here are a few tips on making your facility senior-friendly.

Staff

- Everyone wants support and encouragement. Make sure staff are welcoming and positive and have a passion for working with older people.

- Ensure personal trainers are certified to work with older adults.

- Provide training on common health issues faced by older adults so that staff are better able to advise clients about beneficial exercises and helpful modifications for those living with chronic conditions.

- Some older adults may be reluctant to take a class taught by someone much younger. They may worry that they can't keep up. A teacher closer in age to the participants may encourage older adults to sign up.

Activities

- Offer classes that may have a special appeal for this age group, such as water aerobics, tai chi, balance, or low-impact strength training.

- Offer classes just for women or just for men.

- If possible, offer classes based on a variety of functional levels, or consider allowing older members to try a certain class for the first time in a more comfortable setting.

- During classes, offer appropriate modifications for those living with chronic conditions.

- You may wish to offer chair classes since many older adults have issues getting down on and up from the floor.

Scheduling

- Provide classes or activities during the middle of the day. Early morning or late afternoon classes may be too crowded or fast-paced.

- An hour-long class may be too much for some older adults. Offer some shorter classes, too.

- Consider offering a yoga class after a strength-training class to add flexibility and relaxation to the routine.

Atmosphere

- Look around your center and listen. How is your center decorated? Is music playing (if so, what kind and how loudly)?

- Does your center feel welcoming to every age group?

VISIT
www.nia.nih.gov/Go4Life

- Print useful tools.

- Order free exercise guides, DVDs, and posters for your locker rooms.

 NIH National Institute on Aging

Go4Life is a registered trademark of the U.S. Department of Health and Human Services.

FIGURE 3.2 Recommendations for organizations to address the needs of older adults.

Reprinted from National Institute on Aging. https://go4life.nia.nih.gov/sites/default/files/MakingYourFitnessCenterComfortableForMembers50%2B.pdf just physical benefits. Regular physical activity is also one of the most effective methods for improving quality of life, increasing psychological well-being, including positive self perceptions of self-efficacy and self-esteem, and maintaining cognitive function.

Given that older adult participation in physical activity is influenced at more than just the individual level, broader environmental and societal factors need to be addressed. At the societal level, much needs to be done to restructure our communities to promote physical activity. The *National Blueprint: Increasing Physical Activity Among Adults Age* *50 and Older* has identified a number of societal impediments to the adoption of physical activity among older adults. The blueprint argues that in order to bring about significant changes, partnerships and coalitions need to be developed between individuals and organizations with an interest in active aging. There is little doubt that physical activity instructors of older adults will have many opportunities to participate in such coalitions and help to integrate older adults' opportunities for physical activity into the wider social, cultural, and economic context.

Key Terms

ageism

cognitive function

psychological well-being

quality of life

self-efficacy

self-esteem

social functioning

Recommended Readings

National blueprint: Increasing physical activity among adults age 50 and older. https://www.ncoa.org/resources/national-blueprint-increasing-physical-activity-among-adults-age-50-and-older/.

King, A. & King, D. (2010). Physical activity for an aging population. *Public Health Reviews, 32,* 401-426.

Kramer, A.F., & Erickson, K.I. (2007). Effects of physical activity on cognition, well-being, and brain: Human interventions. *Alzheimer's & Dementia: The Journal of the Alzheimer's Association, 3(2),* S45-S51.

Netz, Y., Wu, M.J., Becker, B.J., & Tenenbaum, G. (2005). Physical activity and psychological well-being in advanced age: A meta-analysis of intervention studies. *Psychology and Aging, 20,* 272-284. doi: 10.1037/0882-7974.20.2.272

Study Questions

1. Why is it important to be aware of aging stereotypes?
   a. It is important that older adults learn to act their age.
   b. Perceptions of aging have been linked to mortality and health status in older adults.
   c. Choices to participate in physical activity may be associated with older adults' perceptions of age-appropriate behaviors.
   d. b and c

2. Quality of life includes the following dimension(s):
   a. physical functioning
   b. psychological well-being
   c. good quality social relationship
   d. all of the above

3. Which of the following best describes the relationship between physical activity and self-esteem?

a. Physical activity directly impacts self-esteem.

b. Physical activity influences physical self-perceptions, which then influence self-esteem.

c. Physical activity influences self-esteem, which then influences physical self-perceptions.

d. Physical activity is not related to self-esteem.

4. Which of the following best describes the social environment you might expect for someone who is physically active?

a. is socially isolated

b. has a small social network

c. is engaged with the community

d. all of the above

5. Which types of physical activity appear to be associated with cognitive function in older adults?

a. multicomponent physical activity that includes aerobic activity

b. activities lasting at least 30 minutes

c. programs lasting at least 6 months

d. all of the above

6. To promote physical activity among older adults, which of the following best describes the ideal approach?

a. Offer programs that address individual characteristics, social/cultural factors, physical environment challenges, and policy changes.

b. Offer programs that focus on providing in-depth counseling to individuals in order to tailor the programs to meet their specific needs.

c. Offer programs that consider changes to the physical environment only.

d. Offer programs that focus on organizational policy changes only.

7. In the *National Blueprint: Increasing Physical Activity Among Adults Age 50 and Over,* which of the following topics are discussed?

a. societal barriers for physical activity

b. strategies for overcoming societal barriers for physical activity

c. strategies for organizations and individuals to make changes

d. all of the above

Application Activities

1. You are a physical activity instructor in a community center and you want to increase programming for older adults. Briefly describe what strategies you would take to encourage older adults to sign up for the new programming. Consider addressing stereotypes of aging, self-efficacy, and social influences.

2. You have an 80-year-old client who is not sure about the benefits that she will gain from participating in physical activity and is also worried about being too old. Briefly describe the key points you would discuss with this client.

3. In your community, identify organizations that are important for older adults' physical activity participation. What types of strategies are they currently employing to promote physical activity? What improvements could they make to enhance the promotion of physical activity? Consider the strategies outlined in the *National Blueprint* or the resources available with Go4Life.

4

Physiological Aspects of Aging

Priscilla G. MacRae

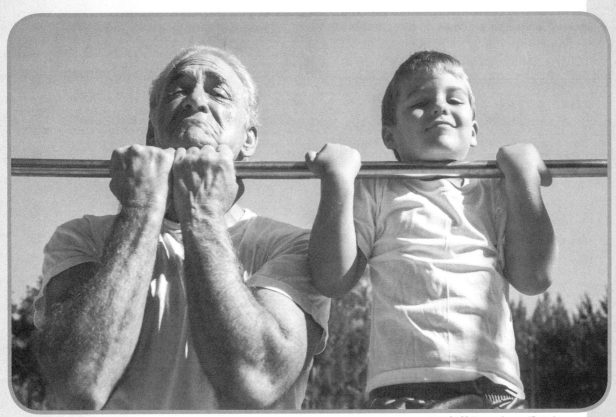

Objectives

After completing this chapter, you will be able to

1. define biological aging and distinguish between primary, secondary, and tertiary aging;
2. describe the effects of aging on the structure and function of the cardiovascular, respiratory, muscular, skeletal, and nervous systems;
3. describe how regular exercise affects physiological aging and how this knowledge informs physical activity programming for older adults; and
4. discuss the most common diseases observed in the cardiovascular, respiratory, muscular, skeletal, and nervous systems of older adults associated with changes in each body system.

Biological aging refers to the cellular, tissue, and organ decline that leads to a loss of functional capacity, a decrease in homeostasis and, consequently, an increased vulnerability to disease and death (Spirduso, Francis, & MacRae, 2005). Aging is often associated with progressive declines in physiological functions:

- A decrease in peak oxygen transport of 5 mL $\cdot$ kg^{-1} $\cdot$ min^{-1} per decade between ages 25 and 65 years

- An increase in body fat content, with decreased glucose tolerance and a deterioration of blood lipid profile

- A 25 percent decrease in peak muscle force and lean tissue from age 40 to 65, with an accelerating loss thereafter; selective atrophy of fast-twitch muscle fibers; and less coordination of muscle contractions

- A 7 percent loss of flexibility per decade of adult life

- A progressive decrease in bone calcium and deterioration of bone matrix, beginning at age 25, and accelerating for 5 postmenopausal years in women

- Decrease in balance and slowing of reaction and movement time

- Deterioration of function in special senses (vision, hearing, smell, and taste), impaired memory, poor sleep patterns, and depression

These declines can be attributed to biological aging (primary aging), negative lifestyle habits such as physical inactivity (secondary aging), and the development of disease (tertiary aging). It is important for physical activity instructors to understand the physiology of aging. This knowledge guides you in the design and implementation of the most effective exercise programs for older adults. The purposes of this chapter are to briefly summarize the effects of biological aging on the major systems of the body, discuss how exercise affects these biological changes, describe the most common diseases associated with the aging of each system, and then discuss implications for instructors of physical activity programs.

Cardiovascular Function

The cardiovascular system includes the heart, blood vessels, and blood. This system provides oxygen and nutrients to the cells of the body and removes carbon dioxide and other waste products. The cardiovascular system works closely with the respiratory system and is controlled by the nervous system. Much research has been devoted to describing differences in cardiovascular function between younger and older adults. It is clear that these aging changes are not due solely to primary aging but also to decreased physical activity or the onset of diseases.

With increasing age, one of the major changes in cardiovascular function is a decline in aerobic capacity. This decline is due to reductions in maximum cardiac output, maximum stroke volume, and maximal heart rate, as well as a reduction in oxygen delivered to, and used by, the working muscles. There are also age-associated changes in blood. These changes include a reduction in the number of both red and white blood cells and in hemoglobin, the iron-containing, oxygen-transporting part of the red blood cells. Not only does the composition of blood change, but older adults are at increased risk for blood clots and the pooling of blood in the veins of the legs. This pooling of blood in the legs is primarily caused by a breakdown of the valves in their veins. As a result of these changes, aging is always listed as a major risk factor for cardiovascular diseases such as hypertension (high blood pressure), coronary artery disease, peripheral arterial disease, and cerebral vascular disease. Though much decline occurs in the cardiovascular system with age, regular physical activity slows the decline and restores function even in the frailest older adults.

Despite age-associated changes in the cardiovascular system, regularly engaging in physical activity slows the decline and restores function even in the frailest older adults.

Aerobic Capacity

The single best measure of cardiovascular function (Nelson et al., 2007) is **aerobic capacity**, also known as work capacity. Aerobic capacity, or **maximal oxygen uptake ($\dot{V}O_2$max)**, represents the ability of the cardiopulmonary system to deliver oxygen to active muscles and the ability of those muscles to use oxygen and energy substrates to perform work during maximal physical stress. Aerobic capacity involves several physiological functions: pulmonary respiration by the lungs; central circulation by the heart and blood vessels; peripheral circulation by the arteries, veins, and capillaries; as well as aerobic respiration by the muscle mitochondria. Aerobic capacity can be expressed as an absolute value, that is, total volume of oxygen the body uses per minute of physical activity (L/min), or relative to body weight ($mL \cdot kg^{-1} \cdot min^{-1}$).

Aging is associated with a progressive decline in $\dot{V}O_2$max that stems from the functional deterioration of essentially all components of oxygen uptake, from the lungs to the mitochondria of skeletal muscle

(Hepple, 2000). Using cross-sectional data, an average linear decline of approximately 1 percent per year after age 25 in healthy, but sedentary, males and females has been reported (Fitzgerald, Tanaka, Tran, & Seals, 1997; Wilson & Tanaka, 2000). In a nine-year longitudinal study, Katzel and colleagues (Katzel, Sorkin, & Fleg, 2001) found that endurance trained 60-year-old men had a 65 percent higher $\dot{V}O_2$max than their healthy but sedentary counterparts (49.6 vs. 30.1 $mL \cdot kg^{-1} \cdot min^{-1}$, respectively). In the endurance-trained group, men who continued to train vigorously experienced no significant decline across the nine years of follow-up (<0.28% per year), while those who reduced their training declined in $\dot{V}O_2$max by approximately 2 percent per year. The healthy but sedentary men exhibited a significant decline in $\dot{V}O_2$max of 1 percent per year. These results indicate that as much as 50 percent of the so-called age-related decline in aerobic capacity may be accounted for by reduced physical activity in conjunction with the loss of muscle mass and increases in fat mass (Cunningham, Paterson, Koval, & St. Croix, 1999). While aging leads to a decline in aerobic capacity, the rate of this decline is greatly affected by the physical activity pattern of an individual.

The factors that determine $\dot{V}O_2$max include central factors, such as how much oxygen is delivered to the muscles, and peripheral factors, such as how much oxygen can be used by the muscles. Reduction in oxygen delivery, principally due to reduced maximal cardiac output and the altered distribution of cardiac output, appears to be the dominant factor in explaining the decline in $\dot{V}O_2$max up until 65 years of age. **Maximal cardiac output**, the maximal amount of blood ejected from the heart per minute (L/min) at peak exercise, and the fraction of the blood flow arriving at working muscles are reduced with aging (Lakata & Sollott, 2002). Maximal cardiac output is a function of maximal heart rate multiplied by **maximal stroke volume** (the volume of blood pumped with each heart beat at peak exercise).

Aging affects maximal heart rate and stroke volume. Although average resting heart rates of older adults are not different from young adults of similar fitness levels, the **maximal heart rate (HRmax)** (the highest heart rate a person exhibits under maximal exercise stress) decreases approximately 5 to 10 beats per decade (Wiebe, Gledhill, Jamnik, & Ferguson, 1999). No amount of training is able to halt this characteristic decline in maximal heart rate with aging. This age-related decline in maximal heart rate with age is primarily a result of reduced sympathetic drive from the nervous system (Seals, Monahan, Bell, Tanaka, & Jones, 2001). There is also a modest decline in maximal stroke volume and this, combined with the decline in maximum heart rate, contributes to the lower maximal cardiac output observed in older adults (Tanaka & Seals, 2008). In addition to the central factor of reduced maximal cardiac output (central factor), the decline in $\dot{V}O_2$max is a function of impaired distribution of cardiac output; less blood reaches the working muscles in what is termed *maldistribution* of blood (Betik & Heppel, 2008).

While reduction in oxygen delivery (central factor) contributes most to the decreases in $\dot{V}O_2$max observed in persons under the age of 65, a decline in the ability of the muscle mitochondria to use the oxygen delivered to them (peripheral factor) plays a particularly important role after age 65 (Betik & Hepple, 2008). The density, volume, respiration capacity, and oxidative enzyme activity of the mitochondria are reduced in aging muscle (Short & Nair, 2001). These mitochondrial changes greatly limit the aerobic capacity of an older adult. However, regular participation in aerobic activity attenuates these effects. Aerobic training increases mitochondrial number and improves function, thereby enabling working muscles to extract more oxygen from the blood (Holloszy, 2001; Short & Nair, 2001). This leads to improved $\dot{V}O_2$max and increased exercise capacity with less fatigue. These mitochondrial adaptations to regular physical activity are especially important for older adults with the lowest aerobic capacities (Nieman, 2010).

Aerobic capacity is so important because it determines one's ability to maintain independent function. The minimal level of aerobic capacity compatible with an independent life at age 85 appears to be about 18 milliliters per kilogram per minute (5 METs) for men and 15 milliliters per kilogram per minute (4.3 METs) for women (Paterson, Cunningham, Koval, & St. Croix, 1999). A **metabolic equivalent (MET)** is a physiological measure of the energy cost, or intensity, of a physical activity. Physical activities of light intensity, such as walking at a self-selected walking pace, would be less than 3 METs, while moderate physical activities, such as fast walking or biking, would be between 3 and 6 METS. Vigorous activity, like jogging or dancing, would be at an intensity ranging from 6 to 10 METs. The aerobic capacity of an 80-year-old who is sedentary may be reduced to such a low level that a maximal effort is required to perform simple activities of daily living, such as standing up from a chair. According to Shephard (1997), a 15 to 20 percent gain in aerobic capacity, due to regular exercise training, is equivalent to a 10-year reduction in biological age. This improvement in aerobic capacity increases the individual's ability to move freely in the environment without undue fatigue.

Heart Rate

The autonomic nervous system exerts an enormous influence over cardiovascular function, and aging is associated with a reduction in autonomic regulation of the heart, independent of physical fitness (Perini, Fisher, Veicsteinas, & Pendergast, 2002). Although resting heart rate largely remains unchanged with age, the ability of the heart to increase contraction rate in response to both submaximal and maximal exercise is reduced. Changes in the electrical conduction system of the heart or in the dynamic regulation of the heart by the autonomic nervous system contribute to decreased heart rate response to a given workload (Perini et al., 2002). Maximal heart rate (MHR) decreases by as much as 10 beats per decade following its peak at age 20. However, age alone is an inconsistent predictor of MHR (Huggett, Connelly, & Overend, 2005). MHR is often estimated using the age-predicted equation of 220 beats per minute minus the age, in years, of the individual (220 − age). Unfortunately, this equation frequently underestimates MHR for adults over 40 years of age. A more accurate equation for estimating MHR in older adults is 208 − (0.7 × age) (Tanaka, Monahan, & Seals, 2001).

MHR often is used as a measure of work intensity in order to determine training heart rates, but this may be problematic in older adults due to the effects of certain medications. Some medications, such as beta-blockers prescribed for high blood pressure and cardiac conditions, affect resting and maximal heart rate, lowering maximal heart rate by as much as 30 beats per minute (American College of Sports Medicine, 2017). Thus, a rating of perceived exertion (RPE) scale may be a more accurate way to determine exercise intensity for older clients. Refer to chapter 13 for more information on aerobic endurance training and monitoring of RPE. Another method for determining exercise intensity is the talk test (Persinger, Foster, Gibson, Fater, & Porcari, 2004). According to this protocol, if a client is exercising at a level at which they can "just respond to conversation," then the exercise intensity should be "just about right," indicating a training intensity of 60 to 80 percent of $\dot{V}O_2$max. Self-reported RPE or the ability to talk while exercising are therefore considered to be better measures of exercise intensity in older adults compared to using a percentage of predicted maximal heart rate.

Age-related changes in autonomic control of the heart rate may have other important clinical and exercise implications. Reductions in autonomic activity can lead to increased variability of heart rate and arterial blood pressure. This variability can potentially, although very rarely, lead to lethally rapid heart rates and sudden cardiac death (Seals et al., 2001). These changes in heart rate and arterial blood pressure are serious symptoms that should signal the immediate cessation of exercise.

Blood Pressure

One of the most important measures of cardiovascular function, under both rest and exercise conditions, is blood pressure. The force the blood creates against the walls of the arteries and veins as it is pumped by the heart to every part of the body is known as **blood pressure**. Blood pressure is measured in millimeters of mercury (mmHg) using a sphygmomanometer. Blood pressure is recorded as systolic (blood pressure while the heart muscle is contracting to pump blood out) over diastolic (blood pressure while the heart muscle is relaxing between beats). Blood pressure values of less than 120/80 mmHg are considered healthy. Due to age-related stiffening of large arteries, resting and exercise blood pressures rise as the life span progresses. Approximately 65 percent of Americans ages 60 or older have high blood pressure, also known as **hypertension** (blood pressure at or above 130 mmHg systolic or at or above 80 mmHg diastolic). High blood pressure is not a benign aging change because it is a potent risk factor for stroke, heart disease, and chronic kidney disease. Hypertension is more common in adults who are African American as opposed to Caucasian or Hispanic. Before 45 years of age men are more likely than women to be diagnosed with hypertension. After age 65, how-ever, hypertension affects women more often than men. In addition to age, many lifestyle factors are associated with increased risk for high blood pressure, including physical inactivity, smoking, obesity, overconsumption of alcohol, and high salt intake.

> Hypertension affects approximately 65 percent of Americans 60 years old and older.

In both young and older adults with hypertension, regular aerobic and resistance exercise training reduces blood pressure, with greater effects observed if weight loss occurs (Chodzko-Zajko et al., 2009). Beneficial changes in blood pressure are seen in aerobic exercise training intensities between 40 and 70 percent of $\dot{V}O_2$max, equivalent to 55 to 80 percent of maximal heart rate or an RPE of 12 to 15 (moderate to hard intensity). Aerobic training, performed at a frequency of three to five sessions per week, with each session lasting 30 to 60 minutes, leads to lasting blood pressure benefits (Fagard, 2001). Resistance training also reduces blood pressure in older adults with normal blood pressure, though the effect is more profound in those with hypertension (Martins, Veríssimo, Coelho eSilva, Cumming, & Teixeira, 2010). Regular aerobic and resistance training optimize blood pressure in older adults.

Exercise Training Effects on Cardiovascular Function

As recently as the 1970s, there was skepticism regarding the ability of older adults who were sedentary to substantially improve their aerobic capacity with training. Over the past three decades, however, multiple studies have documented training-induced increases of 10 to 25 percent in $\dot{V}O_2$max among adults between 60 and 80 years of age (Chodzko-Zajko et al., 2009). Such increases are similar to the percent improvements observed in younger adult populations. On average, there is a 16 percent improvement in peak $\dot{V}O_2$ for older adults who train at a sufficient intensity (>60% of pretraining $\dot{V}O_2$max), frequency (>3 days per week), and duration (>16 weeks; Huang, Gibson, Tran, & Osness, 2005). In general, training programs lasting longer than 16 weeks resulted in greater improvements than did shorter programs. It is clear that older men and women can increase their aerobic capacity with endurance training and, as a result, lead more active, independent, and fulfilling lives.

Records from World Masters competitions provide some indication of the upper limits of physiological function in older adults. While aging is primarily associated with a decline in function, older adults today are actually surpassing the performance of young adults from previous generations. For example, a 61-year-old ran a faster 100-meter sprint time and a 73-year-old marathoner ran a faster marathon time than the respective Olympic winners in 1896. These examples support the ability of the body, when not hampered by disease and disuse, to perform at high intensity. These amazing World Masters records are due to improved training methods, better health care, optimal nutrition, advances in technology (e.g., shoes, track, timing systems), and increases in leisure time and media exposure for such events. Perhaps growing old would be perceived in a more positive light if the stories of these Masters athletes were publicized more aggressively.

Age Changes in Cardiovascular Function and Implications for Instructors

Declines in cardiovascular function, measured by a decline in maximal aerobic capacity, are associated with increased risks of disability and disease, in conjunction with a reduction in cognitive function and quality of life (Chodzko-Zajko et al., 2009). Although no amount of physical activity can prevent biological aging, there is evidence that regular exercise can minimize the detrimental physiological effects of a sedentary lifestyle, increase active life expectancy, and reduce the risk for chronic disease and disability. The American College of Sports Medicine and the American Heart Association outlined physical activity recommendations for older adults to optimize health. The specific recommendations are discussed in chapter 8.

There are several considerations when monitoring exercise training in older adults. Physical activity instructors need to be aware that it takes a longer time for heart rate, blood pressure, and oxygen consumption to reach equilibrium at any given work rate in older adults, so a longer warm-up is

needed. Excessive strain on the cardiopulmonary system of older adults can become an issue at the start of an exercise session, especially if the period of warm-up activity before beginning higher-intensity exercises is inadequate (Scheuermann, Bell, Paterson, Barstow, & Kowalchuk, 2002). How to design and implement an appropriate warm-up for healthy older adults is described in more detail in chapter 10. Untrained older adults are likely to experience greater fatigue if exercise is sustained for more than a few minutes at a high intensity such as 70 to 75 percent of peak oxygen uptake, the equivalent of an intensity perceived as hard or an RPE of 7 or 8 (the Borg CR10 scale is discussed in detail in chapter 13). However, with training, older adults can safely exercise at higher intensities for longer time periods.

In many older adults, particularly those with cardiovascular disease, exercise places enormous strain on the heart and can lead to signs and symptoms (e.g., dizziness, muscle cramps, or chest pain) of dangerous conditions when exercise intensity exceeds their aerobic capabilities. Educating older adults to recognize these signs and symptoms and respond by lowering the intensity at which they are exercising or even pausing to rest is very important. In addition, the aging heart is more vulnerable to rhythm disorders, particularly **ventricular fibrillation**, a dangerously rapid and erratic heart rhythm (Billman, 2002). An older exercise participant with heart disease may experience symptoms of chest pain, shortness of breath, or other signs of exertional intolerance. These symptoms may be attributed to insufficient cardiac blood supply during the critical period at the beginning of exercise. A sufficiently long warm-up period (about 10-20 min of lower-intensity activity) allows time for the cardiopulmonary adaptations necessary for safe exercise. Equally important is an adequate cool-down period, which provides the increased recovery time necessary for older adults (American College of Sports Medicine, 2017). An inadequate cool-down period may result in venous pooling in the legs that can lead to a rapid drop in blood pressure, light-headedness, or fainting after exercise, which can result in a fall. An inadequate cool-down also increases the likelihood of postexercise cardiac rhythm disturbances brought on by high levels of circulating exercise hormones (e.g., norepinephrine) following strenuous exercise (Billman, 2002). Refer to chapter 10 for more information on designing an age-appropriate cool-down.

An adequate cool-down period is needed to prevent venous pooling in the legs that may lead to a rapid decline in blood pressure, light-headedness, or fainting postexercise.

Respiratory Function

The respiratory system, in conjunction with the cardiovascular system, provides oxygen and nutrients to the cells of the body and removes waste products. It is comprised of the nasal cavities, the lungs, and connecting structures. The structures connecting the nasal cavities to the lungs include the pharynx, larynx, trachea, bronchi, and the alveoli of the lungs (see figure 4.1). The alveoli are the structures where oxygen and carbon dioxide are exchanged between the lungs and the blood. There is modest deteriora-

tion in the structure of the respiratory system with aging, including

- loss of elasticity in the airways,
- stiffening of the chest wall due to arthritis of the ribs,
- decreased flexibility in the cartilage connecting the ribs to the sternum, and
- reduction in the alveolar-capillary surface area (Taylor & Johnson, 2010).

These changes lead to altered pulmonary function including a decrease in forced expiratory volume, forced vital capacity, and expiratory flow, as well as an increase in residual volume. These changes do not limit exercise in the majority of healthy older adults because oxygen levels in arteries supplying the lungs remain within normal ranges during low-, moderate-, and even high-intensity exercise (Taylor & Johnson, 2010).

Aging is associated with multiple changes in respiratory physiology. Pulmonary function tests

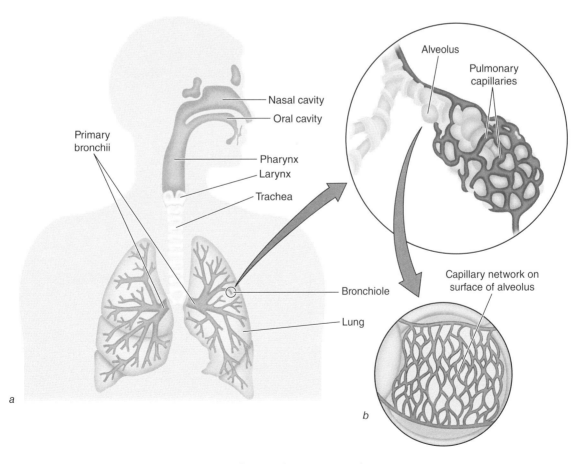

FIGURE 4.1 *(a)* The pulmonary system and *(b)* pulmonary ventilation.

utilize spirometry to determine how well the respiratory system is working. These tests measure how much air the lungs can hold, how quickly air can be moved in and out of the lungs, and how efficiently the gas exchange between the lungs and blood occurs. Important dynamic measures of lung function include forced expiratory volume and forced vital capacity. **Forced expiratory volume (FEV)** is a measure of the amount of air you can exhale with force in one breath. If measured across the first second, it is referred to as FEV1. **Forced vital capacity (FVC)** refers to the maximal volume of air that you can exhale after maximal inspiration. The best single measure of dynamic lung function is a ratio of FEV1/FVC. This ratio peaks when people are in their early 20s and declines approximately 0.5 percent per year from 30 to 65 years of age with a steeper decline thereafter (Sprung, Gajic, & Warner, 2006). A static measure of lung function is **residual lung volume**, which is the amount of air remaining in the lungs after a maximal exhalation. Residual lung volume accounts for approximately 20 percent of total lung volume at 20 years of age and 35 percent of total lung volume at 65 years of age (Sprung et al., 2006). These changes in pulmonary function of healthy older adults do not limit their ability to exercise. However, regular exercise improves some of the age-related decline in pulmonary function (Taylor & Johnson, 2010).

Pulmonary function does not usually limit exercise performance in older adults unless they have some form of chronic pulmonary disease such as asthma, chronic obstructive pulmonary disease (COPD), or emphysema (see chapter 17 for complete descriptions of these diseases). Shortness of breath, however, often causes older adults to voluntarily end exercise sessions. This exercise-induced breathlessness is tolerated less well by older individuals who are sedentary than by those who participate in moderate to strenuous physical activity. As physical activity becomes a regular habit, older clients should be less fearful of this breathlessness and be able to increase the duration and intensity of their exercise. Deep breathing exercises do not improve pulmonary function in healthy older adults. However, there is some evidence that deep, diaphragmatic breathing may be helpful in older adults with compromised respiratory function, such as those with asthma and COPD.

Muscle Function

There are approximately 700 skeletal muscles in the human body. Their main function is movement; either moving the body from one place to another or moving the body parts relative to each other. However, muscles also support and protect internal organs, serve as sphincters regulating material entering and exiting openings of the digestive and urinary tracts, and maintain body temperature. Muscles are composed of individual muscle fibers, also called muscle cells, surrounded by connective tissue. This connective tissue comes together at the end of muscles to form tendons, attaching the muscles to bones. Muscles can only function when activated by nerves.

Measuring strength, the ability to generate maximal muscle force in a single contraction, and power, the ability of muscles to generate force rapidly, assesses muscle function. **Strength** is measured by quantifying the amount of work done while **power** is measured by dividing work by time. Though muscle strength and power are positively related, they measure different aspects of muscle function. Strength is most commonly assessed by a one-repetition maximum (1RM) test. A 1RM test is performed after a sufficient warm-up, and involves lifting a maximum amount of weight one time, without regard to the speed of the lift. Power, on the other hand, refers to the ability to perform work quickly. Lower-body muscle power in older adults has been assessed using isokinetic dynamometry, vertical jumping on a force platform, and lower extremity pneumatic resistance equipment (Reid & Fielding, 2012). Muscle strength and muscle power is essential for many activities of daily living and is necessary for job-related tasks. Moderate levels of strength and power are necessary for activities such as carrying groceries, climbing stairs, getting up from a chair, and lifting grandchildren. In older adults, higher levels of muscle strength and power are associated with the reduction of many risks such as falls, osteoporosis, back pain, depression, arthritis, diabetes, and dementia (Peterson, Rhea, Sen, & Gordon, 2010).

Optimal muscle function is important for individuals of all ages and may be even more important for older adults who tend to lose muscle mass, muscle strength, and muscle power with age. A substantial loss of lower-body strength and power not only impairs walking and increases the risk for falls, but it also increases the older adults' risk for disability and death (National Center for Injury Prevention and Control, 2015). Adequate lower-body muscle power may prevent a catastrophic fall by enabling an individual to correct unexpected losses of balance by quickly stepping to regain balance or grabbing a handrail. Next we will discuss age-related changes in muscle mass, muscle strength, and muscle power. In addition, a summary of the relationships between muscle strength, muscle power, physical function, and resistance training will be examined.

Sarcopenia

There is a robust relationship between chronological age and muscle mass decline, with muscle mass peaking between 25 and 35 years of age, followed by a decline (see figure 4.2). The age of onset and rate of this decline in muscle mass is much steeper if an adult develops a chronic disease or leads a physically inactive lifestyle, as indicated by the lower line in figure 4.2 (Sayer et al., 2008). This progressive decline in skeletal muscle mass leads to a decrease in power, strength, and physical function, which increases risk for disability and loss of independence.

The term **sarcopenia** (from the Greek words *sarx,* "flesh," and *penia,* "loss"), also known as muscle atrophy, describes the age-related decrease in muscle mass (Rosenberg, 2011). Epidemiological research

has determined that 5 to 13 percent of adults between 60 and 70 years of age have sarcopenia, with as many as 50 percent of those over 80 years of age classified as sarcopenic (Cruz-Jentoft, Landi, Topinková, & Michel, 2010). Loss of muscle mass in men is gradual across the life span, while women show a more dramatic decrease following menopause. Sarcopenia is not a disease but may be classified as a geriatric syndrome, as are falls and frailty (Cruz-Jentoft et al., 2010). Moderate sarcopenia has been associated with difficulty in squatting, stooping, and kneeling, whereas severe sarcopenia may prevent older adults from getting up from a chair independently (Peterson et al., 2010). Sarcopenia represents an impaired state of health with a high personal toll. Sarcopenia not only leads to decreased mobility and increased risk of falls and fractures as well as impaired ability to perform activities of daily living, but also contributes to a marked loss of independence. This loss of independence, coupled with increased disability, reduces quality of life and increases risk of death (Cruz-Jentoft et al., 2010). However, there is hope; strong evidence supports the claim that the rate of muscle mass loss can be slowed by engaging regularly in physical activity, particularly high-intensity resistance training. There is evidence that older adults with early sarcopenia are the most likely to benefit from high-intensity resistance training combined with improved nutrition.

Sarcopenia and muscle weakness are multidimensional processes affected by and reflective of the structural, hormonal, metabolic, and neurological changes associated with aging and general disuse. This is better understood by examining elementary skeletal muscle composition. Skeletal muscle is composed of two principal types of contractile fibers. **Type I** (or slow-twitch) **muscle fibers** contract slowly but are also slow to fatigue. They are responsible for maintaining upright sitting or standing postures and are recruited for physical activities that require repetitive motions, such as walking, cycling, or swimming. In contrast, fast-twitch muscle fibers, designated as **type II muscle fibers**, are fast-contracting and quick to fatigue. Physical activities that require power, like getting up from a chair or performing the cha-cha, activate fast-twitch muscle fibers.

The cross-sectional area (size) of the contractile fibers indicates their ability to produce force, with smaller size being associated with less force. Age-related changes in muscle structure include a 1 to

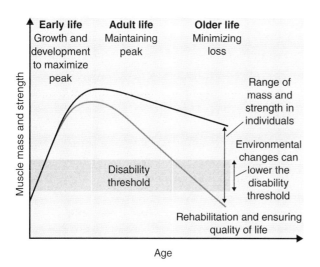

FIGURE 4.2 Life course model of sarcopenia.

Reprinted by permission from Avan Aihie Sayer, Holly Syddall, Helen Martin, Harnish Patel, Daniel Baylis, and Cyrus Cooper, "The Developmental Origins of Sarcopenia," *The Journal of Nutrition, Health and Aging* 12, no. 7 (2008): 427-432.

25 percent decrease in cross-sectional area of type I fibers, with a much larger decline of 25 to 50 percent in cross-sectional area of type II fibers (Brunner et al., 2007). This decrease in muscle fiber size, particularly in type II fibers, is due to the selective loss of large motor neurons that connect to these fast-twitch fibers and the decreased rate of muscle protein synthesis with age. Since older adults move less in general, and perform fewer quick or powerful movements requiring fast-twitch muscle fibers, this selective loss in type II fibers with age is primarily due to disuse.

Other mechanisms associated with sarcopenia include a decline in sex hormones, mitochondrial dysfunction, endocrine changes, and increased insulin resistance, a cause of type II diabetes (Cruz-Jentoft et al., 2010). Many older adults consume an inadequate amount of nutrients, which, along with increased age-related malabsorption of nutrients, also contributes to sarcopenia. Finally, an increase in chronic diseases such as osteoporosis, arthritis, cardiovascular disease, and obesity affect the onset and proliferation of sarcopenia and often lead to increased fear of injury when physical activities are performed. The causes of sarcopenia are multi-factorial and still poorly understood, but the loss of independence and metabolic complications related to sarcopenia make it a major public health issue.

Muscle Strength

Although the term *sarcopenia* specifically refers to a loss of skeletal muscle mass, it is inevitably associated with decreases in muscle function, measured by a decline in muscle strength and power. Muscle contractions may be classified as isometric or isotonic. An **isometric contraction** is produced when the muscle contracts against a fixed, immovable resistance. For example, isometric contractions are involved in holding a sleeping grandchild. **Isotonic contractions** are produced when the muscle contracts and moves an object. Isotonic contractions may be further subdivided into **concentric** (muscle contraction with muscle shortening) or **eccentric** (muscle contraction with muscle lengthening). For example, concentric contractions of the extensor muscles of the lower body occur when standing from a seated position; eccentric contractions of these same muscles occur when lowering the body back into a seated position.

In the general U.S. population, muscle strength peaks between ages 25 and 35, is maintained or declines slightly between ages 40 and 49, and thereafter declines, on average, by 0.5 to 1 percent per year after age 50 (Nelson et al., 2007). Although the rate of decline in strength is similar across all three types of contractions until about 60 years of age, a faster decline in concentric and isometric strength is observed after this age when compared to eccentric strength. As Vandervoort (2009) notes, the predicted loss of concentric strength is so great that, by 85 years of age, rising from a chair exceeds the maximal lower body strength and power of an individual.

Muscle strength is highly associated with functional activities. Loss of muscle strength is associated with slow walking speed, poor endurance, inability to rise from a chair, increased risk for falls, and higher incidence of disability and frailty in older adults (Volkers, de Kieviet, Wittingen, & Scherder, 2012). As might be expected, muscle strength is highly related to both the type and frequency of physical activity. Older adults who participate in more intense physical activity have higher levels of muscle strength. Additionally, this relationship between physical activity intensity and muscle strength may be described as a continuous, dose-response pattern. That is, those who participate in vigorous physical activities and exercise (e.g., weight lifting) demonstrate higher strength and power than those participating in moderate-intensity physical activities such as walking or gardening. Furthermore, lower-body strength quickly declines when people decrease their habitual physical activity, falling to strength levels comparable to those who are chronically inactive. Habitual inactivity and its consequent lower muscle strength significantly increase risk of disability in older adults.

Muscle Power

Although a large number of studies have established muscle strength as a determinant of functional limitations in older adults, evidence suggests that muscle power is more critical to function than muscle strength (Reid & Fielding, 2012; Reid et al., 2012). In addition, muscle power declines sooner and more rapidly than muscle strength with advancing age (Aagaard, Suetta, Caserotti, Magnusson, & Kjaer, 2010). Therefore, interventions targeting restoration of muscle power in older individuals should be a primary focus for practitioners and researchers. A comparison of the age-related muscle power changes in the leg extensors in three distinct populations showed changes in both lower-body power and muscle mass (Reid & Fielding, 2012; Reid et al., 2012):

- Older adults with mobility limitations (aged 70-85 years) had 65 percent less lower-body power and 13 percent less muscle mass compared with healthy older adults (aged 70-85 years).

- Older adults with mobility limitations (aged 70-85 years) had 95 percent less lower- body power and 25 percent less muscle mass compared with healthy middle-aged adults (aged 40-55 years).

The magnitude of the differences between the muscle power deficits compared to the muscle mass deficits indicates that factors aside from muscle atrophy are major contributors to the reductions in muscle power. For example, impairments in neuromuscular function (connections between the nervous system and the muscles), which may include a loss of motor neurons, are common in older adults (Aagaard et al., 2010). These neuromuscular changes with aging, along with changes in growth factors, circulating cytokines, and increased oxidative stress, all contribute to the loss of muscle power with aging.

Over 20 years ago, it was first reported that for older adults who were frail and institutionalized, peak leg power was more predictive of physical function (e.g., ability to get out of a chair, to climb stairs, and to walk quickly) than was muscle strength (Bassey et al., 1992). In fact, older adults with limited lower-body muscle power have a two- to threefold greater risk of mobility impairment and disability than individuals with limited lower-body strength (Reid & Fielding, 2012). Therefore, the use of resistance-training protocols that promote power, through training at a high velocity, appear to have the greatest ability to improve muscle power, thereby improving physical function and decreasing disability (see chapter 12 for a more in-depth discussion of different types of resistance training).

Resistance Training Effects on Muscle Function

Evidence suggests that adults, no matter how old or frail, can improve strength, power, and physical function with resistance training. The first studies to examine the effects of resistance training shocked many people by reporting large improvements in lower-body muscle strength (107%-227%), peak power (10%-17%) and significant **hypertrophy** (increases in muscle size) in healthy older men (65 years of age) after only three months of high-intensity resistance training (Frontera, Meredith, O'Reilly, Knuttgen, & Evans, 1988). Fiatarone and her colleagues (1994) reported similar benefits following 10 weeks of high-intensity resistance training in older adults (mean 87 years) who were frail and living in a nursing home. The following benefits were observed:

- increases in lower-body muscle strength of 113 percent

- a 3 percent improvement in muscle mass compared to a 2 percent decline in the non-exercise group

- increases in gait speed of 13 percent

- improved stair climbing power of 28 percent

These studies support the use of resistance training with the older adult population as a way to increase strength, power, and muscle mass and to improve physical function.

In a meta-analysis of 47 randomized controlled trials, the average increase in strength was 24 to 33 percent for adults 50 to 80 years of age, with similar increases for upper- and lower-body strength (Peterson et al., 2010). On average, these resistance-training programs were 18 weeks in duration; resistance training was performed an average of 2 to 3 times per week at an intensity of 40 to 85 percent of 1RM. The participants usually completed an average of 2.4 sets of 10 repetitions. This means that a total of 24 repetitions, involving eight different major muscle groups of the body, were performed. Therefore, it is clear that older adults, from healthy to frail, should be performing resistance-training exercise 2 to 3 times per week to maintain or develop strength and power and to optimize physical function.

Studies designed to maximize muscle power generally have demonstrated that high-velocity power training (i.e., doing work faster) is feasible, well-tolerated, and effective in older adults, including healthy older men and women, those with disability and mobility limitations, and even those over 80 years of age (Reid & Fielding, 2012). Not only is power training effective for increasing power (resulting in twofold increases when compared with traditional strength-training protocols), but power training also improves strength, balance, and measures of physical function to a greater extent than slow-velocity strength training (Tschopp, Sattelmayer, & Hilfiker, 2011). In addition to the improvements in strength, balance, and physical function, power training is advantageous because it requires less time and is perceived as less exhausting by older adults than is traditional strength training (slow-velocity resistance training; Sayer, 2007; Sayer & Gibson, 2010). Though concerns have been expressed that power training may lead to greater injury, a meta-analysis of strength and power training in older adults found no major adverse effects with strength or power training. Some adverse effects such as minor musculoskeletal discomfort and joint pain were reported, but no more than have been reported in other regular exercise programs such as walking (Tschopp et al., 2011).

Age Changes in Muscle Function and Implications for Instructors

Although no amount of physical activity can stop the biological aging process, there is increasing evidence that regular exercise can minimize the physiological effects of an otherwise sedentary lifestyle. Resistance training improves function and limits the development and progression of diseases and syndromes like sarcopenia. Current guidelines for physical activity in older adults developed by the American College of Sports Medicine (ACSM, 2017) state that exercise prescription for older adults should include muscle strengthening along with aerobic training and balance exercises. The minimum recommendation for older adults participating in muscle-strengthening exercises (resistance training) suggests two or more sessions on nonconsecutive days each week, performing 8 to 10 resistance exercises involving major muscle groups of the body at a moderate to high level of effort for a single set of 10 to 15 repetitions. Although these guidelines provide a basis for a beginning program of resistance training, there is now ample evidence that the old, as well as the young, can safely progress with resistance exercise toward goals of increased muscle power, strength, and muscle mass.

Skeletal Function

The skeletal system includes 206 bones along with the cartilages, ligaments, and other connective tissues that stabilize or connect them. Bones work together with muscles and nerves to produce movement. In addition to the structural support bones provide, they serve as a reservoir for minerals like calcium (98 percent of all calcium in the body is in the bones) and a site for red blood cell, white blood cell, and platelet production, as well as protection for delicate tissues and organs. Decisions early in life, such as the amount of calcium and vitamin D consumed, as well as the type and frequency of physical activity participation, affect bone health in later life.

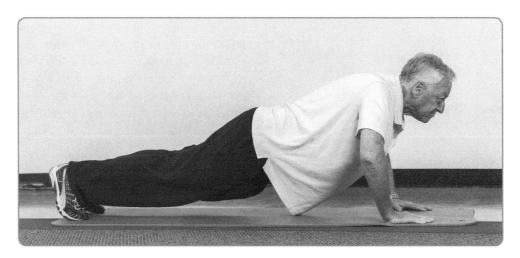

Muscle strength or power exercises are necessary for performing daily activities such as carrying groceries, climbing stairs, and lifting grandchildren or pets.

Bone Mineral Density

Both women and men lose bone mass as the skeletal system ages. At any given age, **bone mineral density (BMD)**, the proportion of deposited mineral salts to organic bone matrix, is lower in women than in men (U.S. Department of Health and Human Services, 2015). Bone mass at maturity (i.e., peak bone mass) and subsequent bone loss determine BMD. Peak BMD is usually reached by 25 years of age and in women remains fairly stable until menopause (around 50 years of age; Marcus, 2001). Women lose up to 5 percent of BMD annually in the first five years after menopause, followed by 2 to 3 percent annual loss thereafter (Gomez-Cabello, Ara, González-Agüero, Casajus, & Vicente-Rodriguez, 2012). Men start from a higher baseline than women, and lose BMD at a slower rate after age 50 (i.e., approximately 1%-2% per year).

Osteoporosis

Osteoporosis, a skeletal disease characterized by low bone density and microarchitectural deterioration of bone (see figure 4.3), is the most common cause of fractures in older adults (Gomez-Cabello et al., 2012). Bone is very active tissue that is continually being remodeled throughout life. Generally speaking, osteoporosis involves degradation of the bone that results from an imbalance between the activity of osteoblasts (bone-building cells) and osteoclasts (bone-reabsorbing cells). Hormone levels, particularly estrogen, levels of calcium and vitamin D in the blood, and stress forces produced by exercise affect the balance between bone building and bone reabsorption. The clinical diagnosis of osteoporosis is made when BMD values are 2.5 standard deviations below peak BMD for the person's age and sex. When BMD is 1.0 to 2.5 standard deviations below the peak BMD, a person is diagnosed with **osteopenia**, a precursor to osteoporosis. Thirty years ago little was known about bone disease and many doctors believed that bone fragility was just a part of old age and could not be avoided. Today we know that osteoporosis is preventable and early and consistent lifestyle choices, such as consuming sufficient dietary calcium and vitamin D, as well as participating in daily weight-bearing exercise, have the greatest effects on optimizing bone health. No matter how old or frail, it is never too late to improve one's bone health.

Approximately 10 million Americans (8 million women, 2 million men) have osteoporosis, leading to approximately 1.5 million fractures annually. Older adults who fracture a hip are at an increased risk of nursing home placement and are over four times more likely to die within three months. Osteoporosis is a major health concern in the United States because one out of every two women and one out of every four men over 50 years of age will have an osteoporosis-related fracture in their lifetime (U.S. Department of Health and Human Services, 2015). Medical expenses for osteoporosis-related fractures were $18 billion in 2005, with billions more spent in caring for these individuals or lost due to time off from work because of the fracture (U.S. Department of Health and Human Services, 2015).

Vertebral fractures, commonly experienced by older adults, often go undetected. Vertebral fractures are often associated with loss of height and postural changes including thoracic kyphosis (humpback) and persistent pain (Eagan & Sedlock, 2001). Unfortunately, many patients diagnosed with osteoporosis are told by their physicians to reduce physical activity to prevent fractures. Although exercises that involve spinal flexion (bending forward), twisting, and sudden movements should be avoided by those with osteoporosis, physical activity is essential for preserving remaining bone mass and functional mobility. Special exercise considerations for clients with osteoporosis are discussed in chapter 17.

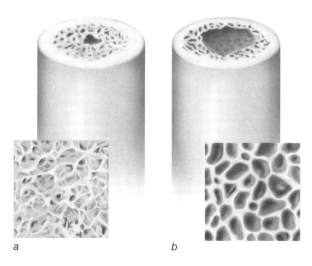

a   *b*

FIGURE 4.3 Microarchitectural changes in bone leading to osteoporosis: *(a)* normal and *(b)* osteoporotic bone.

Exercise Training Effects on Skeletal Function

Studies in older adults indicate that exercise training increases bone-related variables, or at least attenuates the decline in bone mass during aging. The focus of research over the last 30 years has been to determine the types as well as the frequency, intensity, and duration of exercise needed to optimize training effects on bone health.

The effects of aerobic training on BMD remain controversial. Walking, one of the simplest and most accessible forms of aerobic exercise, is the preferred choice of aerobic exercise among older adults. Unfortunately, most of the studies that have examined the relationship between BMD and walking in older adults reported no increases in bone parameters after training (Gomez-Cabello et al., 2012). However, the fact that regular walking may maintain or slow the loss of bone mass in older adults, along with the many other benefits associated with a regular walking program, support the continued inclusion of walking in exercise programming for older adults. Furthermore, studies show that combining aerobic training with other high-impact activities such as jogging or stepping may have more benefits for bone health. Exercise interventions that are specifically designed to maximize loading forces to optimize mechanical stress on bone are of greater benefit in improving bone mass among older adults.

Resistance training is one of the most common types of exercise used to improve bone mass in older adults. Multiple studies in older women and men have shown that resistance training increases BMD by as much as 3.8 percent, while control groups experienced declines as great as 3.6 percent (Gomez-Gabella et al., 2012). In addition, resistance training that involved greater loads and fewer repetitions resulted in greater gains in BMD than lower loads repeated more times (Metcalfe et al., 2001). The higher loads, which increase mechanical stress on the bone, increase **osteogenesis** (bone formation) to a greater extent than do lower loads. Zehnacker and Bemis-Dougherty (2007) reviewed the findings of 20 studies and concluded that weighted or resistive exercises can be beneficial in maintaining BMD in postmenopausal women and in increasing BMD of the spine and hip in women with osteopenia and osteoporosis. The greatest improvements in bone mass were achieved through resistance training that involved high-intensity lifting for two to three sets per session and at least three sessions per week (Zehnacker & Bemis-Dougherty, 2007). Although significant effects were observed after 4 to 6 months in some parts of the body, the efficacy of the training program was greater when it was extended for at least one year. Resistance training appears to be a powerful stimulus to improve and maintain bone mass during the aging process.

Multicomponent exercise training, a combination of strength, aerobic, high-impact, and weight-bearing exercise, has also been shown to be effective in improving BMD in older women and men (Gomez-Cabello et al., 2012). The greatest improvements, seen after 12 months of multicomponent exercise training in older men, resulted in increases of 1.6 percent to 2.1 percent of BMD at the lumbar spine, femoral neck, trochanter, and total hip (Kukuljian et al., 2009). In a later study, involving a multicomponent training program that included moderate-intensity weight-bearing exercise, significant bone adaptation was observed over an eight-month period in community-dwelling older women through an increment of BMD at the femoral neck (Marques et al., 2011). This research shows that combinations of different exercises can improve BMD in older men and women. In particular, a combination of aerobic, strength, and balance training optimizes bone health in older adults (U.S. Department of Health and Human Services, 2004).

Nervous System Function

The nervous system includes all the neural tissue in the body and is one of the most complex organ systems. The nervous system is subdivided into the central nervous system (CNS) and the peripheral nervous system (PNS). The CNS, composed of the brain and spinal cord, is responsible for integrating, processing, and coordinating sensory input and motor output. It also is responsible for cognitive functions, such as memory, learning, and decision-making, as well as the formulation, expression, and control of emotions. The PNS, which comprises all the neural tissue outside of the brain and spinal cord, is responsible for transmitting sensory information from inside and outside of the body to the brain and for carrying motor commands from the brain to muscles and other tissue. Along with the endocrine system, the nervous system controls and adjusts the activities of all systems of the body. You would not be able to compose a thought, form an emotion, or initiate an action without a properly functioning nervous system.

Changes in Nervous System Structure and Function

Changes in nervous system structure and function occur with increasing age. Brain volume changes throughout the full life span, with brain volume increasing during childhood and adolescence until approximately age 13 (Hedman et al., 2012). This increase appears to be mainly due to an increase in gray matter (i.e., neurons). During young adulthood, between 18 and 35 years of age, another wave of growth in brain volume occurs. This brain growth appears to be due to an increase in white matter (i.e., connections between neurons), with little change in gray matter. Between 35 and 60 years of age, there is a steady loss in brain volume of approximately 0.2 percent per year, which accelerates gradually to an annual brain volume loss of 0.5 percent after age 60 (Hedman et al., 2012). Understanding the mechanisms underlying these changes in brain volume may contribute to distinguishing progressive brain changes in psychiatric and neurological diseases from healthy aging processes.

Other major structural changes that affect brain function with age include a change in the cerebrovascular system (i.e., blood supply to the brain). Blood flow to the brain decreases with age due to a gradual narrowing of the cerebral arteries (Peters, 2006). These arteries, like many others in the body, accumulate fatty deposits in the walls of blood vessels (atherosclerosis), thereby reducing blood flow to the brain. Reduced blood flow itself does not cause a cerebral crisis, but it does increase the probability that the individual will suffer a stroke. The cumulative effect of the decrease in brain volume and blood supply to the aging brain over time increases susceptibility to disease and dysfunction.

Other changes in the aging nervous system include changes in brain chemistry as well as in sensation and speed of response. Aging is associated with changes in neurotransmitters, the chemicals released by neurons as they communicate with other neurons and target tissues, such as muscle. Growth factors, such as brain derived neurotropic factor (BDNF), important for keeping neural tissue

healthy, decrease with age. Aging also is associated with a decline in function of the special senses including vision, hearing, vestibular (balance), touch, smell, and taste. Additionally, there is decline in the general sensation known as **proprioception** or "position sense." These structural changes in the nervous system are associated with changes in function such as slower nerve conduction speed as well as reaction and movement times. In addition, reflexes (involuntary automatic responses to a stimulus) become slower and consequently less effective. All these changes contribute to an aging nervous system that is less responsive and adaptive to environmental demands, making it more subject to functional decline.

Changes in the aging nervous system can be observed structurally and are manifested in altered intellectual (cognitive), emotional, and physical function. However, the relationship between changes in structure and changes in function with increasing age is not clearly understood. Aside from structural factors, changes in nervous system function are affected by nutritional status and physical inactivity as well as intellectual and social isolation. In addition, interindividual differences in nervous system structure and function increase with age, making it difficult to describe the changes in structure and function of a "typical healthy" 65-year-old or 85-year-old.

Although there is great heterogeneity among older adults, some generalizations can be made in terms of cognitive function when compared to young adults. A slight slowing of thinking and memory seems to be a normal part of aging. Although this decline is normal, many people have misconceptions about the type and extent of this slowing. A common myth is that all older adults become senile or demented. Another myth is that the increased confusion experienced by some older adults is due to getting old, when such decline may actually be evidence of disease.

> Structural changes in the aging nervous system are manifested in changes in intellectual (cognitive), emotional, and physical function.

Changes in the structure and function of the nervous system vary greatly between individuals. Some people have many structural changes in their brain;

others have few. Structural changes characteristic of an aging brain include atrophy (loss of brain volume), presence of amyloid plaques between neurons, neurofibrillary tangles (twisted fibers within neurons), and white matter hyper-intensity, an abnormality in tissue resembling a lesion (Hedman et al., 2012). These structural changes are used as markers of neurodegeneration and are associated with an increased risk of dementia, stroke, and death. It is unclear, however, whether these structural changes are the cause of changes in cognitive, emotional, or physical function. For example, plaques and tangles are associated with Alzheimer's disease, but some people with the most severe symptoms have fewer plaques and tangles than those with mild or moderate symptoms. For the majority of older adults (approximately 85%), changes in nervous system structure do not interfere with their ability to live independently (Martini, Tallitsch, & Nath, 2017).

Changes in Cognitive Function

Cognitive ability is one of the most valued human characteristics. Cognition refers to a group of mental processes that include attention, memory, learning, problem solving, and decision-making. Two major categories of cognition are crystallized and fluid intelligence. **Crystallized intelligence**, assessed using tests of general information or vocabulary, refers to acquired knowledge such as vocabulary or facts. **Fluid intelligence**, assessed by measuring reasoning and problem solving, is considered the highest level of cognitive processing (Salthouse, 2012). Fluid intelligence (i.e., executive function), describes higher-order cognitive functions that are linked to frontal lobe activity of the brain. The frontal lobe, an area of the brain not fully developed until the late 20s, is most affected by the normal aging process and many dementias.

With aging there is a nearly linear decline in measures of fluid intelligence and executive function beginning in the 30s. On the other hand, increases in measures of crystallized intelligence continue to improve through the first five decades of life. Specifically, analytical reasoning, a measure of fluid intelligence, peaks in the 20s, and is then followed by a linear decline. Conversely, performance on the New York Times crossword puzzle, a measure of crystallized intelligence, improves until the mid-50s, after which performance remains relatively constant through the mid-70s. Therefore, it is not accurate to describe all cognitive functions as declining after 30 years of age.

An intriguing discrepancy exists between when the peak in analytic reasoning occurs, between ages 20 and 30, and the average age of chief operating officers (CEOs) in Fortune 500 companies, which is close to 60 years of age. This discrepancy suggests that declines in some cognitive ability may be offset by an improvement in other abilities (Salthouse, 2012). It is possible that the relatively narrow laboratory measurements of cognition fail to consider other types of intelligence (i.e. practical, social, or emotional). In addition, there are few reliable measures of cognitive functions like creativity and empathy, which may be important for optimizing function in real-world situations. Though younger people may have better short-term and "get-to-the-point-quickly" memory, older adults have had a greater variety of experiences and may be better able to build a wider image out of many different aspects of their memory. Essentially, older adults can make more connections because they have experienced more things over the course of their lives. Therefore, evidence of the negative consequences associated with a decline in fluid intelligence is not observed until the level of cognitive ability reaches pathological limits, such as occurs with dementia (Salthouse, 2012).

Exercise Training Effects on Nervous System Function

The cognitive benefits of physical fitness through cardiovascular and resistance training are demonstrated in cross-sectional and longitudinal studies as well as in intervention studies, thereby constituting one of the most reliable messages about successful aging (Flegal & Reuter-Lorenz, 2010). The notion that exercise training is associated with improved cognitive performance in older adults has been investigated for over 40 years. The pioneer studies by Spirduso (Spirduso, 1975; Spirduso & Clifford, 1978) reported that active older men, who ran or played a racquet sport three times a week, had significantly better cognitive performance (i.e., faster reaction times and movement times) than inactive older men. The active older men exhibited performances comparable to that of inactive men 40 years younger. Similar results were documented in older women (MacRae, Feltner, & Reinsch, 1994), and other studies have reported that regular exercise can be beneficial for many aspects of cognition, with the greatest benefit observed for the high-level processing involved in executive function (Colcombe & Kramer, 2003).

Regular moderate exercise, not medication, improves cognitive function, decreases dementia risk, and slows dementia progression. For example, as little as three months of regular aerobic exercise improved cognitive scores in healthy older adults and those with mild cognitive impairment or dementia, with greater improvements observed after 12 months of training (Ahlskog, Geda, Graff-Radford, & Petersen, 2011; Erickson & Kramer, 2009; Voss, Nagamatsu, Lui-Ambrose, & Kramer, 2011). In addition, adults who routinely engaged in exercise, sports, or general physical activity in midlife were shown to reduce their risk for dementia by 28 percent (Ahlskog et al., 2011). Individuals with mild cognitive impairment or dementia who participated in high-intensity aerobic exercise improved on the Alzheimer's Disease Assessment Scale—Cognitive subscale, while the control group, who performed stretching exercises, declined in performance on this subscale (Ahlskog et al., 2011). These studies, along with many others, indicate that regular aerobic exercise improves cognitive function in healthy and cognitively impaired older adults, thereby decreasing the risk or progression of dementia.

Older adults derive cognitive benefits from engaging in not only aerobic training but also resistance training. In a study of community-dwelling older women, those who engaged in resistance training for two sessions per week for 12 months improved their cognitive performance. Not only was cognition improved in these women, but positive blood flow changes occurred in the frontal cortex, an area of the brain associated with executive function (Liu-Ambrose, Nagamatsu, Voss, Khan, & Handy, 2012). No improvement in cognition or blood flow was observed in older women who engaged in resistance training only once a week. Since resistance training has an established role in optimization of bone health, prevention of falls, reduction of injurious falls, and moderation of the development of sarcopenia, it should be promoted as an essential component in any exercise program designed for older adults. Resistance training, combined with aerobic training, appears to offer the greatest benefit for optimizing cognitive function in older adults.

In addition to aerobic and resistance training, there is some evidence that motor skill training improves motor fitness, which positively affects cognitive performance and brain activation patterns in older adults. In one study, motor fitness, which is measured by indices of movement speed, balance, motor coordination, and flexibility, as well as physical fitness, measured by cardiovascular fitness and muscle strength, was positively associated with cognitive functioning in older adults (Voelcker-Rehage & Niemann, 2013). Additionally, functional brain imaging revealed that physical and motor skill fitness affected different areas of the brain, each in a unique way. Therefore, at least three components of exercise training—aerobic, resistance, and motor skill training—contribute to brain health and the optimization of cognitive function with increased age. The challenge is to improve dissemination of this information and develop strategies to empower adults of all ages to incorporate these types of physical activities into their daily routines.

Changes in Vision, Hearing, and Touch

There are many changes in the special senses of vision and hearing with aging. One of the earliest signs of vision decline with increased age is an impaired ability to read a book or newspaper clearly. This near-sightedness (presbyopia) results from a stiffening of the lens of the eye, such that it no longer is able to accommodate focusing on objects that are near. Most people first notice this impairment in the early to middle 40s. There is a 10-fold decline in near focus from age 20 to 70; what is adequately clear at 4 inches (10 cm) for the young person must be placed at almost 40 inches (100 cm) for the older individual (Farage, Miller, Ajayi, & Hutchins, 2012). After age 80, less than 1 percent of the population has 20/20 vision.

Other changes in vision with age include a reduced sharpness of focus, increased sensitivity to glare, inability to distinguish certain colors, and a narrowing of the visual field. As the pupil becomes smaller and less light is able to enter the eye, more illumination is needed in order to see sharply. This need increases progressively with age, so that a 60-year-old with normal vision needs twice the illumination to see as well as a 20-year-old (Farage et al., 2012). Older adults are more sensitive to glare and have greater difficulty adjusting to changing lighting conditions, such as when moving from indoors to outdoors and vice versa. Older adults need greater contrasts in order to distinguish surfaces or discriminate between objects, such as the edge of a step and the step below it. With age, the ability to perceive color diminishes, particularly in the violet-blue-green portion of the visible light spectrum. Older adults discern and discriminate bright, warm colors (red and yellow) more easily than cool colors (blue and green). Beginning around age 40, peripheral vision begins to narrow, causing older adults to compensate by increasing their vigilance and using more frequent head turning. These compensation techniques can increase the overall instability of an older person due to the greater rotations of the head and neck required for scanning the environment. As an instructor of older adults, keep these vision changes in mind. For example, when giving visual presentations to older adults, maximize the contrast between font and background, minimize glare, and use bright, warm colors in order to optimize the clarity of what you are trying to communicate.

Hearing loss can affect an older adult's life in many ways. Gradual hearing loss (presbycusis) is characterized by a loss in the ability to hear low-intensity sounds or tones and poses significant challenges for older adults when moving about in crowded, noisy environments. Some form of hearing impairment is found in 60 percent of people age 55 or older, and 20 percent of those over age 80 require a hearing aid (Farage et al., 2012). The ability to perceive high-pitched sounds also declines, making male voices a better option than female voices for general announcements. Older adults struggle with discerning high-pitched consonants, such as "ch," "sh," and "z." Additionally, older adults are more likely to suffer from tinnitus, a hissing or ringing in the ear. To aid auditory perception and recognition by older adults, sound signals of at least 60 decibels are needed (conversational speech is 50 decibels), high frequencies should be avoided, and background noise should be limited. In conversation with an older adult, one should speak clearly, use shorter sentences, and pause more often to facilitate comprehension. Pausing when speaking to older adults with hearing impairments allows them to rely more on body language or other context cues to overcome their hearing difficulties and provides them with more time to process information. Loss of hearing with age can be a most isolating experience, greatly affecting an individual's engagement in society and quality of life.

The perception of touch, pressure, and vibration declines with age, especially in an older individual's hands and feet. Lower sensitivity to pressure makes it harder to sense when the body has made full contact with a surface (such as being fully seated) or when a small surface has been depressed (such as an elevator button or keyboard key). The decline in sensitivity to touch, pressure, and vibration becomes apparent by the fifth decade and progresses exponentially after age 65 or 70 (Farage et al., 2012). However, the rate of decline differs by body site, with touch on the face remaining relatively unchanged while sensitivity to touch on the hands and feet declines rapidly. This decline is more severe for the lower extremities and may contribute to the increase in falls observed in older adults.

Age Changes in Nervous System Function and Implications for Instructors

Regular physical activity, whether aerobic, resistance, or more complex motor skills, has been shown to positively affect the aging nervous system. The ability to see, hear, remain aware of body position, and respond to external feedback is essential for safe mobility. Areas where older adults are participating in physical activity should be well lit to compensate for age-associated visual deficits. Using a large font for written instructions and speaking slowly and clearly, perhaps using a microphone, for verbal instructions are more effective techniques with older adults. It also is helpful to limit written instructions to one page and make these available to clients as a handout. Asking an older adult to be a model and demonstrate a skill allows the instructor to assist other clients who may be experiencing difficulty learning the new skill. During organized group fitness classes, instructors should offer plenty of opportunities for questions, and should divide their time among each client in order to check each client's comprehension. If a client has a history of frequent falls or postural instability, he or she can perform physical activity with external support (e.g., chair, wall bars). If a client's balance is severely impaired, exercises may be modified and performed in a seated position. Impaired sight and hearing, poor balance, slower reaction times, slower movement times, impaired righting reflexes, and less-powerful muscles make older adults increasingly susceptible to falls during exercise. Given all the challenges older adults face, instructors should look for ways they can highlight the achievements of their participants and provide motivation. Older adults, like most clients in an exercise program, find it rewarding and motivating to keep a written record of their accomplishments, such as the exercises they performed during the session. In addition, periodic progress assessments add additional incentive for continuing with exercise training.

Older adults with motor and sensory impairments, but whose judgment and cognitive abilities remain intact, are aware of the difficulties imposed by their functional limitations. Consequently, they are able to interact with their environment in an efficient and effective manner, even under novel circumstances. They are also less likely to engage in behavior that jeopardizes their safety. In contrast, older adults with cognitive impairments may engage in dangerous behaviors that place them at high risk of a fall or injury. Those with cognitive impairments can be more impulsive, experience difficulty following directions, and show an inability to accurately perceive or respond to changes in their environment. Therefore, it is very important to obtain thorough information about each client's medical conditions before she or he begins any exercise class (see chapter 5 for a more in-depth discussion of the recommended preexercise screening process).

Summary

The functions of most body systems decline with age. These changes progressively limit the functional capacity of older adults and increase their risk for various diseases and injuries. The normal effects of aging are worsened by age-related decreases in habitual physical activity and the onset of chronic disease to the extent that functional declines are due mostly to the cumulative burden imposed by sedentary lifestyles and chronic diseases, not aging alone. Cardiovascular capacity, respiratory function, muscle integrity, joint mobility, bone mass, and neurological function all decline with age but much more so in physically inactive older adults and those afflicted with chronic conditions involving these systems. Furthermore, because threshold levels of aerobic capacity, lung function, and muscle strength determine one's ability to live independently, declines in the body systems contribute to and perpetuate functional mobility deficits and disability.

However, a well-designed physical activity program for older adults can increase function by a similar percentage as in young adults. The optimal program should provide aerobic activities to enhance cardiorespiratory function, resistance exercises to strengthen the major muscle groups, weight-bearing exercises to strengthen the bones, range-of-motion exercises to increase flexibility in the major joints, and activities designed to enhance balance. Although the aging process is not reversed by physical activity, it is slowed, and at any given age, gains in functional capacity can counteract the adverse effects of 10 to 20 years of aging. Enhanced function also extends independence and improves quality-adjusted life expectancy.

Key Terms

aerobic capacity

biological aging

blood pressure

bone mineral density (BMD)

concentric

crystallized intelligence

eccentric

fluid intelligence

forced expiratory volume (FEV)

forced vital capacity (FVC)

hypertension

hypertrophy

isometric contraction

isotonic contraction

maximal cardiac output

maximal heart rate (HRmax)

maximal oxygen uptake ($\dot{V}O_2max$)

maximal stroke volume

metabolic equivalent (MET)

osteogenesis

osteopenia

osteoporosis

power

proprioception

residual lung volume

sarcopenia

strength

type I muscle fibers

type II muscle fibers

ventricular fibrillation

Recommended Readings

Chodzko-Zajko, W.J., Proctor, D.N., Fiatarone Singh, M.A., Minson, C.T., Nigg, C.R., Salem, G.J., & Skinner, J.S. (2009). American College of Sports Medicine Position Stand. Exercise and physical activity for older adults. *Medicine & Science in Sports & Exercise, 41*, 1510-1530. doi: 10.1249/MSS.0b013e3181a0c95c

Taylor, A.W., & Johnson, M.J. (2008). *Physiology of exercise and healthy aging*. Champaign, IL: Human Kinetics.

Study Questions

1. The maximal oxygen uptake of a 50-year-old man has decreased by 20 percent over the past 10 years. How should this be interpreted?

   a. This is a fairly typical rate for the aging of oxygen transport.

   b. The rate is slower than normal; the client should be congratulated on a healthy lifestyle.

   c. This individual will be unable to participate in regular physical activity.

   d. The normal effects of aging have probably been exacerbated by a decrease in daily activity and an accumulation of body fat.

2. Which of the following does NOT contribute to the decrease in cardiac output in an older person?

   a. loss of elasticity in the airways

   b. a decrease in filling of the ventricles

   c. a decrease in maximal heart rate

   d. a decrease in stroke volume

3. Why would a sedentary 60-year-old woman complain of severe breathlessness when exercising on a cycle ergometer, even at a light to moderate level of exercise intensity?

   a. She has reached maximal effort.

   b. Because of her sedentary lifestyle, she has no recent experience with sensations associated with vigorous effort.

   c. She has some form of acute respiratory disease.

   d. There is some technical error in the pulse counter.

4. A 60-year-old woman claims to have maintained a constant body weight over the past 10 years, although she engages in little physical activity. What would you think is the most likely explanation of this?

   a. She has managed to avoid an accumulation of fat by careful dieting.

   b. Her activities of daily living are sufficient to control her weight.

   c. There is little tendency for most people to accumulate fat over the second half of adult life.

   d. Fat accumulation has been masked by the loss of an equal mass of lean tissue.

5. Which of the following would be unlikely to contribute to maintenance of bone density in an older adult?

   a. weight-supported activities such as pool exercises

   b. a resistance-training program

   c. a high-calcium diet

   d. ingestion of vitamin D supplements

6. An 80-year-old man has a maximal oxygen uptake of 15 milliliters per kilogram per minute. What comment would you make to him?

    a. This is an above-average value for your age. Keep up the good work!

    b. You have allowed your level of aerobic fitness to drop to a level where you will soon have difficulty living independently.

    c. Given the level of fitness that you have reached, you should have no difficulty completing a Masters marathon this summer.

    d. Your aerobic fitness is good, but you should engage in more resistance exercises.

7. A 90-year-old woman has engaged in resistance exercises for 10 weeks. What changes would you expect to see?

    a. No changes in muscle strength can be achieved at this age.

    b. Strength can be enhanced, but no gains are likely to be seen in less than a year of steady activity.

    c. Strength will increase, but there will be little if any increase in lean tissue mass in such a period of time.

    d. Her muscle bulk will be restored to that of someone 10 to 20 years younger.

Application Activities

1. Now that you better understand the effects of age-related changes in various body systems, make a list of all the important things that you, as an instructor, must do to ensure that the exercise environment is safe for older adults. Which types of exercises are appropriate for older adults, and which might prove unsafe for them because of age-related physiological changes?

2. What elements of program design would you emphasize to improve the overall health and fitness of a recently retired, relatively sedentary 67-year-old man referred by his physician? In general, his health is good, although he is slightly overweight. His former career was very stressful and time-consuming, and he has not participated in any regular physical activity for many years.

3. What elements of program design would you emphasize to improve the overall health and fitness of a frail 85-year-old woman who entered an assisted-living residence this year? She has been diagnosed with osteoporosis and has a history of wrist fracture. What special considerations or accommodations should you make because of her condition? Which types of exercises would be both safe and beneficial for her? Which types would be inappropriate?

PART

II

Screening, Assessment, and Goal Setting

Training Module 1:
Overview of Aging and Physical Activity

Training Module 9:
Ethics and Professional Conduct

Training Module 2:
Psychological, Sociocultural, and Physiological Aspects of Physical Activity and Older Adults

Training Module 8:
Client Safety and First Aid

Training Module 3:
Screening, Assessment, and Goal Setting

International Curriculum Guidelines for Preparing Physical Activity Instructors of Older Adults

Training Module 7:
Leadership, Communication, and Marketing Skills

Training Module 4:
Program Design and Management

Training Module 6:
Teaching Skills

Training Module 5:
Program Design for Older Adults With Stable Medical Conditions

Now that you have a basic understanding of the aging process and the psychological, sociocultural, and physiological aspects of physical activity, and know more about the expanding field of gerokinesiology, the next step is learning how to collect information that is specific to the goals and preferences of your prospective clients. The second part of the book addresses training modules 3 and 4 of the *International Curriculum Guidelines for Preparing Physical Activity Instructors of Older Adults*. Module 3 recommends areas of study that include information on selection, administration, and interpretation of preexercise health and activity screening along with fitness and mobility assessments appropriate for older adults. Module 3 also recommends areas of study that include information on establishing, with client input, realistic and measurable short-, medium-, and long-term goals. This information will provide the basis for exercise program design and appropriate referrals to other health professionals. Module 4 recommends areas of study that include information about how to use the results obtained from screening, assessment, and client goal-setting activities to make appropriate decisions regarding individual and group physical activity and exercise program design and management. These topics are addressed in chapters 5 through 7.

- Chapter 5 presents guidelines for the choice and use of screening tools to determine the overall health, physical activity, and disability status of older adult participants. A screening tool to identify risk factors of coronary heart disease is also introduced in this chapter. How to share screening results with clients and how to maintain confidentiality is also discussed in this chapter.

- Chapter 6 introduces you to the Functional Fitness Framework that can be used to guide the selection of sound field-based assessment tools. These tools are used to assess physical impairments and functional limitations among older adults. This chapter describes several assessment tools that are appropriate for use in field settings as well as guidelines for the administration of the various assessments in group-based settings.

- Chapter 7 describes the major personal, environmental, and program-related factors that influence older adults' motivation to be physically active. Important theories of behavioral change that guide the planning, delivery, and evaluation of physical activity programs are also discussed. The cognitive and behavioral strategies presented for both group and individual settings will help you motivate older adults to make physical activity an integral part of their lives. Finally, you will learn how to develop an individualized behavioral modification plan, which includes short- and long-term goal development, progress monitoring, problem-solving skills to help clients overcome obstacles to physical activity, and rewards and incentives to support behavioral change.

Preexercise and Health Screening

Debra J. Rose

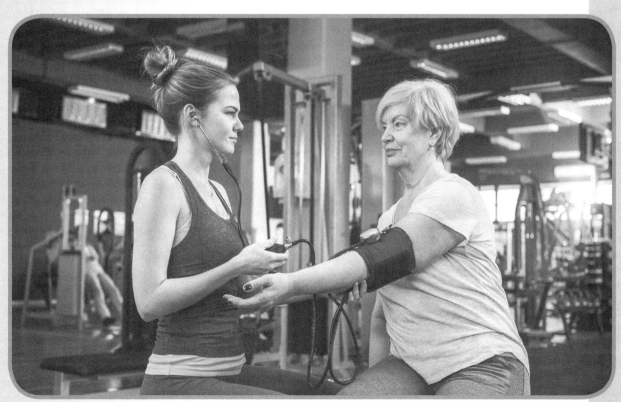

Objectives

After completing this chapter, you will be able to

1. select, administer, and interpret the results of screening tools to determine the health, physical activity, and disability status of older adult participants;
2. evaluate the risk factors for coronary artery disease, which restricts blood flow to the heart;
3. identify medical conditions that require referral to a physician;
4. recognize the signs and symptoms of diseases that place an individual at risk during functional performance testing and exercise;
5. design and administer a health history and activity questionnaire;
6. design and administer informed consent and physician consent documents; and
7. identify when screening should be repeated to determine changes in health status.

An important responsibility of physical activity instructors of older adults is to conduct a thorough preexercise screening of potential clients to evaluate their current health, physical activity, and disability status. The risk of injury during physical activity is present for all people but is particularly high for older adults who have one or more chronic medical conditions, have been physically inactive for a prolonged period of time, or have enrolled in an exercise program that exceeds their physical capabilities. Given this risk, it is important to conduct an initial screening of all older adults who are interested in joining your physical activity program. The screening will help you identify your clients' (1) health and disability status, (2) signs and symptoms associated with certain diseases, and (3) risk factors that predispose them to certain diseases. A systematic approach to screening is essential in order to optimize the older adult's safety during performance testing and exercise and to develop effective exercise prescriptions.

Preexercise screening is a process whereby you obtain information from a potential client before he or she completes performance testing or begins an exercise program. The primary goal of this process is to become familiar with the physical condition of each older adult who wishes to join your program. The screening process also helps you determine whether a client is ready to participate in physical

activity. The screening tools needed include an informed consent form (which explains the purpose, procedures, risks, and benefits of performance testing and your program in simple language and which must be signed by the client to indicate his or her written consent to participate in testing or exercise), a physician consent form, the **Physical Activity Readiness Questionnaire for Everyone** (**PAR-Q+**), a screening tool to determine a client's readiness to participate in a low- to moderate-intensity exercise program, a health history and physical activity questionnaire, and other tools to evaluate a client's coronary artery disease risk factors, body composition, and blood pressure. Also known as ischemic heart disease, **coronary artery disease** is caused by the narrowing of the coronary arteries (atherosclerosis), which decreases the supply of blood to the heart (myocardial ischemia). In certain moderate- to high-risk cases, a physical exam and additional laboratory tests may also be necessary. The electronic version of the PAR-Q+ questionnaire can be completed by the potential client and reviewed by a qualified exercise or health care professional.

This chapter focuses on the procedures for conducting preexercise health screenings. It will assist you, as the physical activity instructor, to recognize conditions that place an individual at risk during performance testing or exercise and conditions that require medical referral before the individual can participate in an exercise program. You will learn when it is appropriate to repeat the screening process to determine any changes in health status. Examples of each of the screening forms are also presented in this chapter.

Preexercise Screening

The screening process identifies clients who (1) have diseases, symptoms, or risk factors that require medical examination and clearance before starting an exercise program, (2) are at risk of a cardiac event while exercising, (3) should be excluded from participation in your exercise program, or (4) should participate in a medically supervised exercise program because their relative risk is too great or because they have clinically significant disease. In addition to identifying individuals at risk of a cardiac event during exercise, the screening process provides valuable information to address a variety of other important programming issues. Screening also helps you to identify clients who may need additional attention or accommodation in your program. For example, you may need to prescribe aquatic exercise rather than a walking program for someone with severe osteoarthritis.

A review of the client's medical history reveals the number, types, and dosages of medications (both prescription and nonprescription) the client takes. This can help you identify any medical conditions that are being supervised by a physician and any potential adverse effects from medication that may occur during exercise participation. For example, taking sedatives or narcotics can reduce alertness, and blood-pressure-lowering medication may lead to hypotension during exercise. (Refer to chapter 17 for additional information on this topic.)

Previous or current injuries that place the client at greater risk of an accident or re-injury during exercise can also be identified during screening. For example, you may find that a client has sustained a previous ankle fracture or a neck injury during a car accident. Screening helps you determine contraindicated exercises that place the client at risk of re-injury. In addition to the health and disability status of your client, determining his or her current physical activity level (frequency, duration, and intensity) and the types of activities your client enjoys helps you to choose appropri-

ate fitness and functional testing and to develop an individualized exercise prescription that will increase compliance.

Why Screen?

- Learn as much as you can about the person in order to provide a safe and effective exercise program.
- Identify relevant health problems, the amounts and types of medications used, and current level of physical activity.
- Identify risk level and determine the need for additional screening or medical referral.
- Choose the correct type of follow-up fitness and mobility tests.
- Identify the client's goals, interests, barriers, motivators, quality of life, family support, and psychological state.

Recommendations for Exercise Preparticipation Health Screening

In 2015, the American College of Sports Medicine (ACSM) published updated exercise preparticipation health screening recommendations based on studies showing that existing exercise preparticipation health screening guidelines (ACSM, 2013) were resulting in excessive physician referrals, thus creating a barrier to participation in exercise. Following the convening of a scientific roundtable by ACSM in 2014, a new evidence-informed model to guide the conduct of exercise preparticipation health screenings was adopted. Unlike previous recommendations, risk-factor profiling is no longer included in the preexercise screening process. Instead, the updated recommendations are based on three important factors: presence of signs or symptoms of or known cardiovascular, metabolic, or renal disease; current physical activity level; and desired exercise intensity. According to the authors of the consensus statement, "these variables have been identified as risk modulators of exercise-related cardiovascular events" (p. 2473). See the

Recommended Readings list for further information about the current exercise preparticipation health screening process algorithm developed by ACSM.

Risk Factors for Coronary Artery Disease

The most serious risk associated with vigorous exercise is sudden cardiac death (Thompson et al., 2007). Although the risk of sudden cardiac death is elevated during vigorous activity, the long-term benefits of physical activity on cardiac risk far outweigh the temporary elevation in risk during exercise. In fact, the incidence of death from coronary artery disease is much less among adults who are physically active than among those who are sedentary (Soares-Miranda, Siscovick, Psaty, Longstreth, & Mozaffarian, 2016). The cardiac risks are primarily associated with vigorous exercise when the individual has an existing medical condition that can precipitate a medical emergency during exercise. It is further believed that individuals who have risk factors are more likely to develop coronary artery disease that may go undetected for some time. Individuals with undetected heart disease are at greater risk of sudden death while participating in performance testing or exercise. However, once these risk factors are identified, several of them can be reduced through behavioral and lifestyle modification. The risk factors to consider include the following:

- *Age.* Men over the age of 45 and women age 55 or older are at higher risk.
- *Family history.* Having a father or male sibling with cardiovascular disease who experienced myocardial infarction (heart attack), coronary revascularization, or sudden death before age 55 or a mother or other first-degree female relative with the same condition before age 65 indicates higher risk.
- *Cigarette smoking.* A participant who currently smokes cigarettes on a daily basis or who quit within the previous six months or is or was exposed to environmental tobacco smoke is at higher risk.
- *Hypertension.* A participant with high blood pressure, or hypertension (defined as someone with a reading at or above 130 mmHg systolic or at or above 80 mmHg diastolic) or is taking antihypertensive medication is at greater risk. **Systolic blood pressure** is the pressure in the arteries during the contraction phase of the heart cycle, and **diastolic blood pressure** is the pressure in the arteries during the resting phase.

- *Dyslipidemia.* Cholesterol is a fatty substance found in nerves and other tissues, and high levels are associated with elevated risk for heart disease. Risk factors include having a **low-density lipoprotein** cholesterol (LDL-C) reading greater than or equal to 130 milligrams per deciliter *or* having a **high-density lipoprotein** cholesterol (HDL-C) reading less than 40 milligrams per deciliter *or* taking a lipid-lowering medication. A total serum cholesterol (if that is the only value available) of 200 milligrams per deciliter or higher is a risk factor.

- *Prediabetes.* Prediabetes is a risk factor if an individual has impaired fasting glucose (IFG) *or* impaired glucose tolerance (IGT).

- *Obesity.* **Body mass index (BMI)** is a measure of body weight relative to body height (weight in kilograms divided by height in meters squared) that is used to evaluate body composition. A BMI of greater than or equal to 30 *or* waist girth greater than 40 inches (102 cm) for men and greater than 35 inches (88 cm) for women is a risk factor.

- *Sedentary lifestyle.* Not participating in a minimum of 30 minutes of moderate-intensity physical activity at least three days per week for at least three months increases risk.

Several tools are available to identify these risk factors. For example, a health history and activity questionnaire can be used to determine age, family history of heart disease, medication use, history of smoking, and sedentary lifestyle. Blood pressure can be measured to detect hypertension. A blood profile can identify individuals with high cholesterol or with high glucose (or blood sugar) levels associated with **diabetes**. Body mass index (BMI) and measures such as waist-to-hip ratio or waist circumference that indicate an individual's abdominal fat can be used to identify obesity. Each of these measurement tools is described later in this chapter.

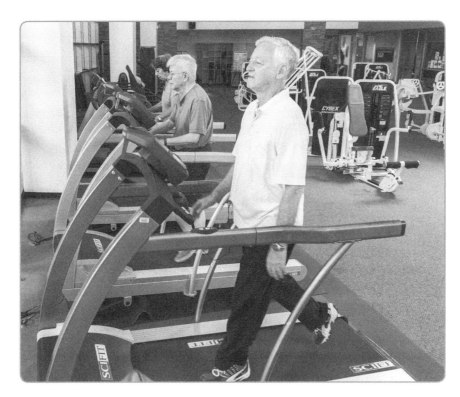

Staying physically active later in life reduces the incidence of coronary artery disease.

Screening Steps

Many different approaches have been taken to pre-exercise screening procedures. As a physical activity instructor of older adults, you should become familiar with at least one approach to screening potential program participants. To keep the process simple, this discussion is limited to five essential steps. Some additional screening tools are discussed in the next section; you may want to consider incorporating them into your screening process if you have the resources available and the time to administer these additional tests.

Step 1: Informed Consent

Before you allow potential clients to participate in any performance testing or a moderate-intensity physical activity program, it is important that they read and complete an informed consent form. The purpose of **informed consent** is to ensure the participant's autonomy in deciding whether or not to take part in the performance testing or program

activities. True informed consent involves an ongoing process of communication between the physical activity instructor and participants to ensure that all elements of a program or testing procedure are clearly understood. The informed consent document is not only part of that communication process but constitutes a *legal obligation* to your exercise participants. Federal law mandates the administration of an informed consent document anytime an individual may be exposed to possible physical, psychological, or social injury as a result of participating in a physical activity program. Although an informed consent document won't protect you from legal action, it will improve your defense and increase the odds of a favorable outcome of any legal action if your program is supervised by qualified individuals and operated according to an established set of guidelines.

Typically, informed consent documents are reviewed by an institutional review board (IRB) or a risk management unit that is responsible for reviewing an organization's protocols to ensure that appropriate laws and ethical standards are met. If your organization does not have a mechanism for reviewing these types of documents, you should consult with a lawyer to ensure that your informed consent document conforms to legal and ethical requirements. Many sample consent forms are available that can be tailored for use in exercise settings and that address performance testing as well as exercise program issues. Figure 5.1 provides an example of an informed consent form that addresses both performance testing and exercise program issues.

Informed consent is typically obtained by having the participant read and sign a document that describes the performance tests and exercise program. The informed consent document, therefore, has two basic components: information and consent. The information provided is not meant simply to disclose information but also to educate participants. The informed consent document normally includes a description of the objectives of the screening procedures and performance tests, a description of the physical activity program, a summary of the risks and benefits, a statement that the participant is voluntarily choosing to participate and is free to withdraw from the program without prejudice at any time, a statement concerning confidentiality, a description of medical coverage (even if there is none) in case of injury, an offer to answer any questions, and the contact information of someone who can answer questions or address concerns (ACSM, 2017). It is important that you provide participants with sufficient time to read and complete this form and to ask any questions they might have about any aspect of the form, the program, or the performance tests to be conducted. You should also allow them time to consider their involvement in the context of their other daily commitments and to discuss their involvement

---

Healthy Aging Center, Longevity State University
Older Adult Fitness Program

Participant Consent Form

In response to the growth in the programs addressing the needs of older adults, Longevity State University has developed a new Healthy Aging Center. The director of the center is Betty Wellness, PhD. Through its educational, research, and service activities, the center has as its mission the promotion of health, vitality, and well-being in later years. The Older Adult Fitness Program is one of several programs under the direction of the center. The center provides a safe environment where people 50 years of age and over can engage in health promoting activities and programs.

Purpose: I understand that the purpose of this exercise program is to improve my functional fitness and health. During this program I may perform exercises to improve the capacity of my heart and lungs, my muscle strength and endurance, my joint flexibility, my body composition (amount of fat and lean tissue), and my balance, agility, and mobility.

Procedures: The fitness classes will meet for 12 weeks, three times per week for 90 minutes. Each class will be instructed by trained students and supervised by faculty with extensive education and experience in Kinesiology/Exercise Science and aging. The class consists of a 15-minute warm-up followed by four 15-minute exercise stations, including aerobic, strength, flexibility, and neuromotor fitness. The class ends with a 15-minute cool-down. Before participating in the older adult fitness program, I will be asked to complete a medical and activity history questionnaire and obtain medical clearance to participate based on responses provided on the PAR-Q+ questionnaire. I will also be asked to participate in a series of functional fitness tests to identify weaknesses in my physical ability to do activities of daily living and to allow the class supervisors to more effectively prescribe appropriate exercises. These tests will include a six-minute walk (walking as far as I can in six minutes) or a two-minute step-in-place

(continued)

FIGURE 5.1   Sample informed consent form.

(stepping in place for two minutes); an eight-foot (2.4-meter) up-and-go (standing up from sitting in a chair, walking eight feet [2.4 meters], turning around a cone, and returning to the chair as quickly as possible); walking speed (walking 50 feet, or 15.2 meters); a chair sit-and-reach (reaching toward my foot while seated in a chair with my leg straight); a back-scratch test (reaching over my shoulder and behind my back); a 30-second chair stand (standing from sitting in a chair as many times as I can in 30 seconds); and a 30-second arm curl (lifting a five-pound [2.3-kilogram] weight for women or an eight-pound [3.6-kilogram] weight for men as many times as I can in 30 seconds).

Risks: The risks associated with the classes are minimal, but the exercises performed during the testing and exercise sessions may cause me some immediate and delayed muscle soreness and physical fatigue. If I experience any physical discomfort (chest pain, leg pain, muscle discomfort, etc.) during the class or testing, I should immediately inform the class supervisor.

I understand that I am being asked to exercise within my own comfort level. During exercise my body may show signs that I should stop exercising. I understand that it is my responsibility to report any of these signs or symptoms to my instructor and doctor. These signs include

- light-headedness or dizziness;
- chest heaviness, pain, tightness, or angina;
- palpitations or irregular heartbeat;
- sudden shortness of breath not due to increased physical activity; or
- discomfort or stiffness in muscles and joints persisting for several days after exercise.

Benefits: I understand that the results of these tests will help determine my fitness levels, which will be useful in developing my individualized exercise prescription.

All questions that I have about these procedures have been answered to my satisfaction. If I have additional questions, I can contact Dr. Betty Wellness at 715-555-9595. I understand that participation in the program is completely voluntary, and I am free to stop participation at any time. I understand that the center does not provide compensation for injuries that I may sustain. If I am accidentally injured during the classes, the program personnel will be unable to offer treatment, and I will be required to seek treatment with my own physician. I understand that any information obtained in this program will remain confidential and will not be disclosed to anyone other than my physician or those responsible for my exercise prescription without my written permission. I agree that results from these tests can be used for research purposes. My name will not be directly associated with any of the results in a published report.

My signature indicates that I have carefully read the information provided in this document and have voluntarily decided to participate. Furthermore, I, for myself and my heirs, fully release from liability and waive all legal claims against Longevity State University and all testing and training personnel for injury or damage that I might incur during participation in the Senior Fitness Program.

Signature of participant _____ Date _____

Signature of witness _____ Date _____

FIGURE 5.1 *(continued)*

with family and friends. Therefore, you may want to provide this document to your clients before the day when performance testing or the exercise program is to commence, thus allowing them time to consider their participation.

Comprehension is a key element of the informed consent document. The participant must be able to read and comprehend the document. First, the document should be as short as possible while still containing all the necessary elements. Second, although these documents have some legal merit, they are not to be written in legalese. Rather, they are to be written at approximately an eighth-grade reading level. This helps to overcome many problems with literacy and understanding. Third, when preparing these (and other) documents for older adults, it is better to make the print size larger than normal to accommodate visual limitations. A font size of 14 or 16 points is usually sufficient.

Step 2: The Physical Activity Readiness Questionnaire for Everyone (PAR-Q+)

The Physical Activity Readiness Questionnaire for Everyone (PAR-Q+; see figure 5.2) replaces the PAR-Q that was first developed by the Canadian Society for Exercise Physiology in 1994 and subsequently revised in 2002. Over time, a number of limitations associated with the PAR-Q were identified (Jamnik et al., 2011; Warburton et al., 2011), and the PAR-Q+ was developed to address those. The PAR-Q+ is intended to enhance the risk stratification process by including additional questions about chronic medical conditions that can be further probed by a qualified exercise professional. It replaces the one-page form, considered to be a minimal evaluation of individuals prior to beginning a *low- to moderate-intensity* exercise program, with a four-page form. While the PAR-Q is still widely used in the United States, its overly conservative format has been shown to result in a number of false-positive responses that promote barriers to participation in physical activity among older adults. The PAR-Q is also limited to use with individuals between the ages of 15 and 69 years. These two significant limitations, among others, prompted the development of the PAR-Q+ (Jamnik et al., 2011; Warburton et al.,

2011). Both the PAR-Q and PAR-Q+ are self-report questionnaires.

The PAR-Q+ contains a range of questions aimed at identifying any possible restrictions or limitations to participating in physical activity. The entire process requires approximately five minutes to complete. If an individual answers *no* to each of the seven questions provided on page 1, then he or she is cleared for unrestricted physical activity participation. If, however, the individual answers *yes* to one or more of the questions, he or she must then complete pages two and three of the PAR-Q+. As shown in figure 5.2, the follow-up questions on these pages are related to specific chronic conditions (e.g., cardiovascular disease, cancer, type 1 diabetes) and, based on the participant's responses, will (1) lead to being cleared to exercise or (2) trigger a referral to a qualified exercise professional or (3) require the participant to complete an electronic version of a more comprehensive medical screening tool called the electronic Physical Activity Readiness Medical Examination (ePARmed-X+).

It is recommended that you include the new PAR-Q+ questionnaire as part of the screening to help identify individuals who are at risk. Adoption of this more comprehensive preexercise screening process may reduce the number of potential clients needing to obtain medical clearance prior to participating in your physical activity program.

Step 3: Physician Consent

In addition to obtaining the consent of the participant, the international curriculum guidelines for preparing physical activity instructors recommend obtaining a physician's consent for the client to participate. The consent document for the physician should describe the exact nature of the performance testing to be conducted and the major components of the program. It should also include contact information so that the physician can contact you, or another responsible person such as the facility director, if he or she has any questions about the program. The document should have a place for the physician's endorsement of his or her patient's participation, with or without any conditions for participation, and a place for denial of endorsement with an option to state the reason or reasons. Figure 5.3 provides a sample physician's consent letter.

2018 PAR-Q+

The Physical Activity Readiness Questionnaire for Everyone

The health benefits of regular physical activity are clear; more people should engage in physical activity every day of the week. Participating in physical activity is very safe for MOST people. This questionnaire will tell you whether it is necessary for you to seek further advice from your doctor OR a qualified exercise professional before becoming more physically active.

GENERAL HEALTH QUESTIONS

Please read the 7 questions below carefully and answer each one honestly: check YES or NO.	YES	NO
1) Has your doctor ever said that you have a heart condition ☐ OR high blood pressure ☐?	☐	☐
2) Do you feel pain in your chest at rest, during your daily activities of living, **OR** when you do physical activity?	☐	☐
3) Do you lose balance because of dizziness **OR** have you lost consciousness in the last 12 months? Please answer **NO** if your dizziness was associated with over-breathing (including during vigorous exercise).	☐	☐
4) Have you ever been diagnosed with another chronic medical condition (other than heart disease or high blood pressure)? **PLEASE LIST CONDITION(S) HERE:** _____	☐	☐
5) Are you currently taking prescribed medications for a chronic medical condition? **PLEASE LIST CONDITION(S) AND MEDICATIONS HERE:** _____	☐	☐
6) Do you currently have (or have had within the past 12 months) a bone, joint, or soft tissue (muscle, ligament, or tendon) problem that could be made worse by becoming more physically active? Please answer **NO** if you had a problem in the past, but it *does not limit your current ability* to be physically active. **PLEASE LIST CONDITION(S) HERE:** _____	☐	☐
7) Has your doctor ever said that you should only do medically supervised physical activity?	☐	☐

☑ **If you answered NO to all of the questions above, you are cleared for physical activity.**
Please sign the PARTICIPANT DECLARATION. You do not need to complete Pages 2 and 3.

- ▶ Start becoming much more physically active – start slowly and build up gradually.
- ▶ Follow International Physical Activity Guidelines for your age (www.who.int/dietphysicalactivity/en/).
- ▶ You may take part in a health and fitness appraisal.
- ▶ If you are over the age of 45 yr and NOT accustomed to regular vigorous to maximal effort exercise, consult a qualified exercise professional before engaging in this intensity of exercise.
- ▶ If you have any further questions, contact a qualified exercise professional.

PARTICIPANT DECLARATION
If you are less than the legal age required for consent or require the assent of a care provider, your parent, guardian or care provider must also sign this form.

I, the undersigned, have read, understood to my full satisfaction and completed this questionnaire. I acknowledge that this physical activity clearance is valid for a maximum of 12 months from the date it is completed and becomes invalid if my condition changes. I also acknowledge that the community/fitness centre may retain a copy of this form for records. In these instances, it will maintain the confidentiality of the same, complying with applicable law.

NAME _____ DATE _____

SIGNATURE _____ WITNESS _____

SIGNATURE OF PARENT/GUARDIAN/CARE PROVIDER _____

◉ **If you answered YES to one or more of the questions above, COMPLETE PAGES 2 AND 3.**

⚠ **Delay becoming more active if:**

- ✓ You have a temporary illness such as a cold or fever; it is best to wait until you feel better.
- ✓ You are pregnant - talk to your health care practitioner, your physician, a qualified exercise professional, and/or complete the ePARmed-X+ at **www.eparmedx.com** before becoming more physically active.
- ✓ Your health changes - answer the questions on Pages 2 and 3 of this document and/or talk to your doctor or a qualified exercise professional before continuing with any physical activity program.

(continued)

FIGURE 5.2 The Physical Activity Readiness Questionnaire for Everyone (PAR-Q+).

Reprinted with permission from the PAR-Q+ Collaboration and the authors of the PAR-Q+ (Dr. Darren Warburton, Dr. Norman Gledhill, Dr. Veronica Jamnik, and Dr. Shannon Bredin).

2018 PAR-Q+

FOLLOW-UP QUESTIONS ABOUT YOUR MEDICAL CONDITION(S)

1. Do you have Arthritis, Osteoporosis, or Back Problems?

If the above condition(s) is/are present, answer questions 1a-1c   If **NO** ☐ go to question 2

1a.	Do you have difficulty controlling your condition with medications or other physician-prescribed therapies? (Answer **NO** if you are not currently taking medications or other treatments)	YES ☐ NO ☐
1b.	Do you have joint problems causing pain, a recent fracture or fracture caused by osteoporosis or cancer, displaced vertebra (e.g., spondylolisthesis), and/or spondylolysis/pars defect (a crack in the bony ring on the back of the spinal column)?	YES ☐ NO ☐
1c.	Have you had steroid injections or taken steroid tablets regularly for more than 3 months?	YES ☐ NO ☐

2. Do you currently have Cancer of any kind?

If the above condition(s) is/are present, answer questions 2a-2b   If **NO** ☐ go to question 3

2a.	Does your cancer diagnosis include any of the following types: lung/bronchogenic, multiple myeloma (cancer of plasma cells), head, and/or neck?	YES ☐ NO ☐
2b.	Are you currently receiving cancer therapy (such as chemotherapy or radiotherapy)?	YES ☐ NO ☐

3. Do you have a Heart or Cardiovascular Condition? *This includes Coronary Artery Disease, Heart Failure, Diagnosed Abnormality of Heart Rhythm*

If the above condition(s) is/are present, answer questions 3a-3d   If **NO** ☐ go to question 4

3a.	Do you have difficulty controlling your condition with medications or other physician-prescribed therapies? (Answer **NO** if you are not currently taking medications or other treatments)	YES ☐ NO ☐
3b.	Do you have an irregular heart beat that requires medical management? (e.g., atrial fibrillation, premature ventricular contraction)	YES ☐ NO ☐
3c.	Do you have chronic heart failure?	YES ☐ NO ☐
3d.	Do you have diagnosed coronary artery (cardiovascular) disease and have not participated in regular physical activity in the last 2 months?	YES ☐ NO ☐

4. Do you have High Blood Pressure?

If the above condition(s) is/are present, answer questions 4a-4b   If **NO** ☐ go to question 5

4a.	Do you have difficulty controlling your condition with medications or other physician-prescribed therapies? (Answer **NO** if you are not currently taking medications or other treatments)	YES ☐ NO ☐
4b.	Do you have a resting blood pressure equal to or greater than 160/90 mmHg with or without medication? (Answer **YES** if you do not know your resting blood pressure)	YES ☐ NO ☐

5. Do you have any Metabolic Conditions? *This includes Type 1 Diabetes, Type 2 Diabetes, Pre-Diabetes*

If the above condition(s) is/are present, answer questions 5a-5e   If **NO** ☐ go to question 6

5a.	Do you often have difficulty controlling your blood sugar levels with foods, medications, or other physician-prescribed therapies?	YES ☐ NO ☐
5b.	Do you often suffer from signs and symptoms of low blood sugar (hypoglycemia) following exercise and/or during activities of daily living? Signs of hypoglycemia may include shakiness, nervousness, unusual irritability, abnormal sweating, dizziness or light-headedness, mental confusion, difficulty speaking, weakness, or sleepiness.	YES ☐ NO ☐
5c.	Do you have any signs or symptoms of diabetes complications such as heart or vascular disease and/or complications affecting your eyes, kidneys, **OR** the sensation in your toes and feet?	YES ☐ NO ☐
5d.	Do you have other metabolic conditions (such as current pregnancy-related diabetes, chronic kidney disease, or liver problems)?	YES ☐ NO ☐
5e.	Are you planning to engage in what for you is unusually high (or vigorous) intensity exercise in the near future?	YES ☐ NO ☐

FIGURE 5.2   *(continued)*

2018 PAR-Q+

6.   **Do you have any Mental Health Problems or Learning Difficulties?** *This includes Alzheimer's, Dementia, Depression, Anxiety Disorder, Eating Disorder, Psychotic Disorder, Intellectual Disability, Down Syndrome*

If the above condition(s) is/are present, answer questions 6a-6b   If **NO** ☐ go to question 7

6a.	Do you have difficulty controlling your condition with medications or other physician-prescribed therapies? (Answer **NO** if you are not currently taking medications or other treatments)	YES ☐ NO ☐
6b.	Do you have Down Syndrome **AND** back problems affecting nerves or muscles?	YES ☐ NO ☐

7.   **Do you have a Respiratory Disease?** *This includes Chronic Obstructive Pulmonary Disease, Asthma, Pulmonary High Blood Pressure*

If the above condition(s) is/are present, answer questions 7a-7d   If **NO** ☐ go to question 8

7a.	Do you have difficulty controlling your condition with medications or other physician-prescribed therapies? (Answer **NO** if you are not currently taking medications or other treatments)	YES ☐ NO ☐
7b.	Has your doctor ever said your blood oxygen level is low at rest or during exercise and/or that you require supplemental oxygen therapy?	YES ☐ NO ☐
7c.	If asthmatic, do you currently have symptoms of chest tightness, wheezing, laboured breathing, consistent cough (more than 2 days/week), or have you used your rescue medication more than twice in the last week?	YES ☐ NO ☐
7d.	Has your doctor ever said you have high blood pressure in the blood vessels of your lungs?	YES ☐ NO ☐

8.   **Do you have a Spinal Cord Injury?** *This includes Tetraplegia and Paraplegia*

If the above condition(s) is/are present, answer questions 8a-8c   If **NO** ☐ go to question 9

8a.	Do you have difficulty controlling your condition with medications or other physician-prescribed therapies? (Answer **NO** if you are not currently taking medications or other treatments)	YES ☐ NO ☐
8b.	Do you commonly exhibit low resting blood pressure significant enough to cause dizziness, light-headedness, and/or fainting?	YES ☐ NO ☐
8c.	Has your physician indicated that you exhibit sudden bouts of high blood pressure (known as Autonomic Dysreflexia)?	YES ☐ NO ☐

9.   **Have you had a Stroke?** *This includes Transient Ischemic Attack (TIA) or Cerebrovascular Event*

If the above condition(s) is/are present, answer questions 9a-9c   If **NO** ☐ go to question 10

9a.	Do you have difficulty controlling your condition with medications or other physician-prescribed therapies? (Answer **NO** if you are not currently taking medications or other treatments)	YES ☐ NO ☐
9b.	Do you have any impairment in walking or mobility?	YES ☐ NO ☐
9c.	Have you experienced a stroke or impairment in nerves or muscles in the past 6 months?	YES ☐ NO ☐

10.   **Do you have any other medical condition not listed above or do you have two or more medical conditions?**

If you have other medical conditions, answer questions 10a-10c   If **NO** ☐ read the Page 4 recommendations

10a.	Have you experienced a blackout, fainted, or lost consciousness as a result of a head injury within the last 12 months **OR** have you had a diagnosed concussion within the last 12 months?	YES ☐ NO ☐
10b.	Do you have a medical condition that is not listed (such as epilepsy, neurological conditions, kidney problems)?	YES ☐ NO ☐
10c.	Do you currently live with two or more medical conditions?	YES ☐ NO ☐

PLEASE LIST YOUR MEDICAL CONDITION(S) AND ANY RELATED MEDICATIONS HERE: _____

_____

GO to Page 4 for recommendations about your current medical condition(s) and sign the PARTICIPANT DECLARATION.

Copyright © 2018 PAR-Q+ Collaboration   3 / 4
01-11-2017

(continued)

FIGURE 5.2   *(continued)*

2018 PAR-Q+

☑ **If you answered NO to all of the FOLLOW-UP questions (pgs. 2-3) about your medical condition, you are ready to become more physically active - sign the PARTICIPANT DECLARATION below:**

▶ It is advised that you consult a qualified exercise professional to help you develop a safe and effective physical activity plan to meet your health needs.

▶ You are encouraged to start slowly and build up gradually - 20 to 60 minutes of low to moderate intensity exercise, 3-5 days per week including aerobic and muscle strengthening exercises.

▶ As you progress, you should aim to accumulate 150 minutes or more of moderate intensity physical activity per week.

▶ If you are over the age of 45 yr and **NOT** accustomed to regular vigorous to maximal effort exercise, consult a qualified exercise professional before engaging in this intensity of exercise.

⬡ **If you answered YES to one or more of the follow-up questions about your medical condition:**

You should seek further information before becoming more physically active or engaging in a fitness appraisal. You should complete the specially designed online screening and exercise recommendations program - the **ePARmed-X+ at www.eparmedx.com** and/or visit a qualified exercise professional to work through the ePARmed-X+ and for further information.

⚠ **Delay becoming more active if:**

✓ You have a temporary illness such as a cold or fever; it is best to wait until you feel better.

✓ You are pregnant - talk to your health care practitioner, your physician, a qualified exercise professional, and/or complete the ePARmed-X+ **at www.eparmedx.com** before becoming more physically active.

✓ Your health changes - talk to your doctor or qualified exercise professional before continuing with any physical activity program.

● You are encouraged to photocopy the PAR-Q+. You must use the entire questionnaire and NO changes are permitted.
● The authors, the PAR-Q+ Collaboration, partner organizations, and their agents assume no liability for persons who undertake physical activity and/or make use of the PAR-Q+ or ePARmed-X+. If in doubt after completing the questionnaire, consult your doctor prior to physical activity.

PARTICIPANT DECLARATION

● All persons who have completed the PAR-Q+ please read and sign the declaration below.

● If you are less than the legal age required for consent or require the assent of a care provider, your parent, guardian or care provider must also sign this form.

I, the undersigned, have read, understood to my full satisfaction and completed this questionnaire. I acknowledge that this physical activity clearance is valid for a maximum of 12 months from the date it is completed and becomes invalid if my condition changes. I also acknowledge that the community/fitness center may retain a copy of this form for records. In these instances, it will maintain the confidentiality of the same, complying with applicable law.

NAME _____   DATE _____

SIGNATURE _____   WITNESS _____

SIGNATURE OF PARENT/GUARDIAN/CARE PROVIDER _____

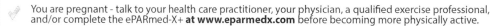

─────── **For more information, please contact** ───────
www.eparmedx.com
Email: eparmedx@gmail.com

Citation for PAR-Q+
Warburton DER, Jamnik VK, Bredin SSD, and Gledhill N on behalf of the PAR-Q+ Collaboration. The Physical Activity Readiness Questionnaire for Everyone (PAR-Q+) and Electronic Physical Activity Readiness Medical Examination (ePARmed-X+). Health & Fitness Journal of Canada 4(2):3-23, 2011.

Key References
1. Jamnik VK, Warburton DER, Makarski J, McKenzie DC, Shephard RJ, Stone J, and Gledhill N. Enhancing the effectiveness of clearance for physical activity participation; background and overall process. APNM 36(S1):S3-S13, 2011.
2. Warburton DER, Gledhill N, Jamnik VK, Bredin SSD, McKenzie DC, Stone J, Charlesworth S, and Shephard RJ. Evidence-based risk assessment and recommendations for physical activity clearance; Consensus Document. APNM 36(S1):S266-s298, 2011.
3. Chisholm DM, Collis ML, Kulak LL, Davenport W, and Gruber N. Physical activity readiness. British Columbia Medical Journal. 1975;17:375-378.
4. Thomas S, Reading J, and Shephard RJ. Revision of the Physical Activity Readiness Questionnaire (PAR-Q). Canadian Journal of Sport Science 1992;17:4 338-345.

The PAR-Q+ was created using the evidence-based AGREE process (1) by the PAR-Q+ Collaboration chaired by Dr. Darren E. R. Warburton with Dr. Norman Gledhill, Dr. Veronica Jamnik, and Dr. Donald C. McKenzie (2). Production of this document has been made possible through financial contributions from the Public Health Agency of Canada and the BC Ministry of Health Services. The views expressed herein do not necessarily represent the views of the Public Health Agency of Canada or the BC Ministry of Health Services.

Copyright © 2018 PAR-Q+ Collaboration   4 / 4
01-11-2017

FIGURE 5.2   *(continued)*

Healthy Aging Center
Longevity State University
Older Adult Fitness Program

Medical Clearance by Personal Physician

Your patient, _____, has expressed an interest in participating in the Older Adult Fitness Program, one of the programs offered by the Healthy Aging Center at Longevity State University. The center, under the direction of Betty Wellness, PhD, has offered health promotion programs for older adults for the past 20 years.

We would appreciate your medical opinion and recommendations concerning this individual's suitability for participation in moderate-intensity physical activity. If you feel that this individual might benefit from participation in the program, we would greatly appreciate your endorsement of his or her participation.

Assessments: The program participants are required to complete a health history and activity questionnaire, followed by a series of functional fitness assessments. This is done to identify weaknesses in physical parameters associated with activities of daily living and to more effectively prescribe appropriate exercise.

Physical Parameters	Assessments	Approval
Cardiovascular	Six-minute walk	yes___ no___
	Two-minute step-in-place	yes___ no___
Muscle strength and endurance	30-second chair stand	yes___ no___
	30-second arm curl	yes___ no___
Flexibility	Chair sit-and-reach	yes___ no___
	Back scratch	yes___ no___
Balance and gait	8-foot (2.4-m) up-and-go	yes___ no___
	50-foot (15.2-m) walking speed	yes___ no___

Exercise program: The intensity of the program is based on the individual capabilities of each participant. The class meets two times per week for 90 minutes. Each class will be instructed by trained graduate students and supervised by faculty with extensive education and experience in Kinesiology/Exercise Science and aging. The class will consist of a 15-minute warm-up; four 15-minute stations including aerobic, strength, flexibility, and neuromotor fitness (i.e., balance, agility, and coordination); and a 15-minute cool-down.

Exercise class approval: yes _____ no _____

Please list any modifications or comments for testing and exercise class. (If approval was denied, you may, at your option, give the reason[s].)_____
_____

Patient's last blood pressure reading: _____ / _____

Please indicate by your signature below that your patient is medically cleared to participate in the specific testing and training described. Please call Dr. Betty Wellness at 715-555-9595 if you have any questions concerning the program.

_____	_____	_____
Signature of physician	*Print name of physician*	*Date*

Physician's phone #: (_____) _____ - _____

FIGURE 5.3 Sample physician's consent letter.

Step 4: Health History and Activity Questionnaire

One of the most important steps in the preexercise screening process is to identify any **contraindications** to performance testing and exercise and to determine any risks or limitations that may be relevant to the exercise program. This step is typically accomplished by administering a questionnaire. The participant usually completes the questionnaire on her or his own. After reviewing the information, you can then follow up with specific questions to gain further clarification where needed. This information, combined with the results of the PAR-Q+ questionnaire, will help you determine whether the individual is ready to participate in the exercise program you are offering.

Figure 5.4 provides an excellent example of a health history and activity questionnaire developed at the Center for Successful Aging at California State University, Fullerton. The questionnaire asks for information about demographics; existing chronic or acute diseases, including risk factors for cardiovascular disease (questions 1-4); assistive devices such as eyeglasses, hearing aids, canes (questions 5-8); medications (question 9); previous emergency care and/or injuries (questions 10-11); fall history (questions 12-14); perceived health status (question 15); functional limitations and disability (questions 16, 18-20); and current levels of activity (questions 21-23). Question 17 asks participants about their perceived mental well being and is the 14-item version of the Warwick-Edinburgh Well-Being Scale (Tennant et al., 2007) while question 18, an expanded version of the Composite Physical Function (CPF) scale, is used to evaluate a participant's ability to perform a wide range of activities, from basic activities of daily living such as dressing and bathing to advanced activities such as aerobic dance and other strenuous exercise (Rikli & Jones, 1998, 2013). The higher the score (i.e., maximum score = 60), the higher the level of perceived physical function.

While some health history and activity questionnaires can be very extensive, they do not need to inquire about every disease and disorder that could possibly exist. They need only help you categorize an individual's level of risk in more general terms. The participant's health and activity history enables you to identify conditions that may place him or her at risk and to detect any contraindications to performance testing and exercise.

From your participants' questionnaire responses you can also identify whether they are taking any medications, such as beta-blockers, bronchodilators, or insulin, that could affect their ability to exercise or their response to exercise in general (e.g., heart rate or blood pressure). If an individual has a medical condition or is taking a medication that is unfamiliar to you, be sure to obtain more information from an appropriate medical or pharmaceutical resource before allowing that individual to participate in performance testing or exercise. (Refer to chapter 17 regarding exercise considerations for common medical conditions.)

The questionnaire provides you with the following additional information about your clients: (1) previous and current exercise activities, (2) ability to participate in an exercise program, (3) exercise preferences, (4) risk of suffering a medical emergency during exercise, and (5) risk of falls and disability. Depending on the purpose of your program and the staff available for health behavior counseling, you might ask for additional information, such as alcohol and caffeine consumption, drug use, driving record, occupational history, recreational pursuits, nutritional patterns, sleep habits, and stress levels. This information can identify participants who are at risk for heart attack, stroke, cancer, and other diseases and accidents such as falls.

Information gathered from the preactivity screening (PAR-Q+), health and physical activity questionnaire, and physical and mobility assessments (see chapter 6) also facilitates the development of realistic and achievable goals and a safer and more individualized physical activity program for your participants. Many chronic, degenerative diseases are related to lifestyle. Although it is impossible to change certain risk factors such as age, sex, and family history, many other factors can be positively affected by behavioral and lifestyle modifications. For example, many of the risk factors associated with coronary artery disease, including smoking, high blood pressure, elevated cholesterol, and a sedentary lifestyle, can be addressed through behavioral modification techniques such as smoking cessation, reduction of fat intake, and regular exercise. Although helping your clients with behavioral modification may not be feasible because of time constraints or lack of expertise, you can suggest that they ask their physicians for a referral.

Date: _____

Health/Activity Information

Center for Successful Aging, California State University, Fullerton

Name:_____

Address: _____

City _____ State:_____ Zip:_____

Home phone #: (____) _____ - _____ Gender: Male _____ Female _____

Cell phone #: (____) _____ - _____ Email: _____

Date of birth: ___ / ___ / _____ Height:_____ Weight:_____

Ethnicity: _____ Highest level of education:_____

Whom to contact in case of emergency: Phone #: (____) _____ - _____

Relationship of emergency contact: _____

Name of your physician: _____

Physician phone #: (____) _____ - _____

1. **(A) Have you ever been diagnosed as having any of the following conditions?**

   If YES, indicate year of diagnosis.

Heart attack	_____ Yes	_____ No	_____
Transient ischemic attack	_____ Yes	_____ No	_____
Angina (chest pain)	_____ Yes	_____ No	_____
Stroke	_____ Yes	_____ No	_____
Peripheral vascular disease	_____ Yes	_____ No	_____
Sensory neuropathies (problems with sensation)	_____ Yes	_____ No	_____
Respiratory disease	_____ Yes	_____ No	_____
Parkinson's disease	_____ Yes	_____ No	_____
Multiple sclerosis	_____ Yes	_____ No	_____
Polio or postpolio syndrome	_____ Yes	_____ No	_____
Other neurological conditions	_____ Yes	_____ No	_____
Osteoporosis	_____ Yes	_____ No	_____
Rheumatoid arthritis	_____ Yes	_____ No	_____
Other arthritic conditions	_____ Yes	_____ No	_____
Visual or depth perception problems	_____ Yes	_____ No	
Inner ear problems or recurrent ear infections	_____ Yes	_____ No	_____
Cerebellar problems (ataxia)	_____ Yes	_____ No	_____
Other movement disorders	_____ Yes	_____ No	_____
Chemical dependency (alcohol or drugs)	_____ Yes	_____ No	_____
Depression	_____ Yes	_____ No	_____

(continued)

FIGURE 5.4 Health history and activity questionnaire.

© Debra J. Rose, Center for Successful Aging at California State University-Fullerton.

1. **(B) The following questions relate to your risk for cardiovascular disease.**
   Do you have a personal history of any of the following?
   Cigarette smoking _____ Yes _____ No
      Packs per day _____   *Number of years smoked* _____
   Obesity or highly overweight _____ Yes _____ No
   Physical inactivity _____ Yes _____ No
   High blood pressure (at or above 130/80 mmHg) _____ Yes _____ No
      Current blood pressure _____
   High cholesterol (over 200 mg/dL) _____ Yes _____ No
      Cholesterol level _____
   Diabetes or high blood sugar (over 110 mg/dL) _____ Yes _____ No
      Blood glucose level _____   *Year diagnosed with diabetes* _____
   Family history of heart attack or stroke, at young age _____ Yes _____ No
      Indicate family member and age: _____

2. **Have you ever been diagnosed as having any of the following conditions?**
   Cancer _____ Yes _____ No
      If YES, describe what kind: _____
   Joint replacement _____ Yes _____ No
      Year(s): _____
      If YES, how many times?   Right hip   _____
                                 Left hip   _____
                                 Right knee   _____
                                 Left knee   _____
   Cognitive disorder _____ Yes _____ No
      If YES describe condition: _____
   Uncorrected visual problems _____ Yes _____ No
      If YES describe type: _____
   Any other type of health problem? _____ Yes _____ No
      If YES describe condition: _____

3. **Do you currently suffer any of the following symptoms in your legs or feet?**
   Numbness _____ Yes _____ No
   Tingling _____ Yes _____ No
   Arthritis _____ Yes _____ No
   Swelling _____ Yes _____ No

4. **Do you currently have any medical conditions for which you see a physician regularly?** _____ Yes _____ No
   If YES, describe condition: _____

FIGURE 5.4   *(continued)*

5. **Do you require eyeglasses?** _____ Yes _____ No

   If YES, what type of glasses do you wear?

   _____ Bifocals   _____ Magnification only

   _____ Graded lenses   _____ Trifocals

6. **Do you have your eyesight checked at least once a year?** _____ Yes _____ No

7. **Do you require hearing aids?** _____ Yes _____ No

   If YES, which ear? _____ Left _____ Right _____ Both

8. **Do you use an assistive device for walking?**

   _____ Yes _____ No _____ Sometimes

   If YES or SOMETIMES, what type of assistive device do you use?

   _____ Single-point cane   _____ Rolling stand walker

   _____ Three-point cane   _____ Three-wheel walker with seat

   _____ Quad cane

9. **List all medications that you currently take (including all "over-the-counter" and "alternative medicines"). Please attach an additional page to the questionnaire if insufficient space to list all medications in the table below.)**

Type of medication	For what condition

10. **Have you required emergency medical care or hospitalization in the past year?**

    _____ Yes _____ No

    If YES, please list when this occurred and briefly explain why: _____

    _____

11. **Have you ever had any condition or suffered any injury that has affected your balance or ability to walk without assistance?** _____ Yes _____ No

    If YES, please list when this occurred and briefly explain condition or injury:

    _____

12. **How many times have you fallen within the past year?**

    If you have fallen in the **past year**, please provide a detailed description of each incident as you remember it.

    Fall #1 within the last year:

    (a) Date:_____

    (b) Location (e.g., bathroom, garden, grocery store):_____

    (c) Reason for fall (e.g., uneven surface, going downstairs): _____

    (d) Did you require medical treatment? _____ Yes _____ No

(continued)

FIGURE 5.4 *(continued)*

Fall #2 within the last year:

(a) Date:_____

(b) Location (e.g., bathroom, garden, grocery store):_____

(c) Reason for fall (e.g., uneven surface, going downstairs): _____

(d) Did you require medical treatment? _____ Yes _____ No

13. **How concerned are you about falling?**

1	2	3	4	5
Not at all	A little	Moderately	Very	Extremely

14. **As a result of this concern, have you stopped doing some of the things you used to do or liked to do?** _____ Yes _____ No

15. **How would you describe your health?**

_____ Poor _____ Fair _____ Good _____ Very good _____ Excellent

16. **In the past 4 weeks, to what extent did health problems limit your everyday physical activities (such as walking and household chores)?**

_____ Not at all _____ Slightly _____ Moderately

_____ Quite a bit _____ Extremely

17. **Following are some statements about feelings and thoughts. Please place an "X" in the box that best describes your experience of each statement over the last 2 weeks.**

Statement	None of the time	Rarely	Some of the time	Often	All of the time
I've been feeling optimistic about the future.					
I've been feeling useful.					
I've been feeling relaxed.					
I've been feeling interested in other people.					
I've had energy to spare.					
I've been dealing with problems well.					
I've been thinking clearly.					
I've been feeling good about myself.					
I've been feeling close to other people.					
I've been feeling confident.					
I've been able to make up my own mind about things.					
I've been feeling loved.					
I've been interested in new things.					
I've been feeling cheerful.					

FIGURE 5.4 *(continued)*

18. Please indicate your ability to do each of the following by placing an "X" in the most appropriate box.

Statement	Can do (5 points)	Can do with some difficulty (4 points)	Can do with a lot of difficulty (3 points)	Cannot do without help (2 points)	Cannot do at all (1 point)
Take care of own personal needs (e.g., dressing yourself)					
Bathe yourself, using tub or shower					
Climb up and down a flight of stairs (e.g., second story)					
Do light household activities (e.g., cooking, dusting, washing dishes, sweeping a walkway)					
Do heavy household activities (e.g., scrubbing floors, vacuuming, raking leaves)					
Do own shopping for groceries or clothes					
Walk outside one or two blocks					
Walk 1/2 mile (6-7 blocks)					
Walk 1 mile (12-14 blocks)					
Lift and carry 10 pounds (4.5 kg; e.g., a full bag of groceries)					
Lift and carry 25 pounds (11 kg; e.g., medium-to-large suitcase)					
Do strenuous activities (e.g., hiking, calisthenics, moving heavy objects, bicycling, aerobic dance activities, strenuous digging in garden)					

19. In general, do you currently require household or nursing assistance to carry out daily activities? _____ Yes _____ No

If YES, please check the reasons(s):

_____ Health problems   _____ Lack of strength or endurance

_____ Chronic pain   _____ Lack of flexibility or balance

_____ Other reasons: _____

(continued)

FIGURE 5.4 *(continued)*

20. **In a typical week, how often do you leave your house (to run errands, go to work, meetings, classes, church, social functions, etc.)?**

_____ less than once per week   _____ 3-4 times per week

_____ 1-2 times per week   _____ almost every day

21. **Do you *currently* participate in regular physical exercise (such as walking, sports, exercise classes, house work, or yard work) that is strenuous enough to cause a noticeable increase in breathing, heart rate, or perspiration?**

_____ Yes _____ No

If YES, how many days per week?

_____ One _____ Two _____ Three _____ Four _____ Five _____ Six _____ Seven

22. **When you go for walks (if you do), which of the following best describes your walking pace?**

_____ Strolling (easy pace, takes 30 min or more to walk a mile)

_____ Average or normal (can walk a mile in 20-30 min)

_____ Fairly brisk (fast pace, can walk a mile in 15-20 min)

_____ Do not go for walks on a regular basis

23. **Did you require assistance in completing this form?**

_____ None (or very little)

_____ Needed quite a bit of help   Reason: ________________________________

FIGURE 5.4 *(continued)*

Step 5: Feedback to Clients and Confidentiality

Once you have gathered and interpreted the information from the preactivity screening, you should share the results with the client. This feedback is very valuable. It allows you to educate the client about his or her health and disability status. It also enables you and the client to establish goals and discuss how participation in specific activities can help meet those goals (see chapter 7 for more information on how to establish meaningful goals with clients).

Screening information should be discussed privately with each client. The results and interpretation of the screening assessment should be explained in language that is easily understood by the client. Be sure to avoid unfamiliar, technical terms. Telling a client that she or he is at increased risk of disease is never good news. To motivate the client to participate in an activity program, explain the results in a positive manner that does not scare or intimidate him or her. Share the good news: Many things can be done to improve the client's current health. Identifying appropriate, low-risk activities and periodically reevaluating his or her health status encourage participation and help to convince the client that better health can be achieved.

The five prescreening exercise steps are the following:

1. Informed consent
2. Physical Activity Readiness for Everyone questionnaire
3. Physician's consent
4. Health history and activity questionnaire
5. Feedback to clients and confidentiality

A separate folder (in print or electronic format) containing each client's health and medical informa-

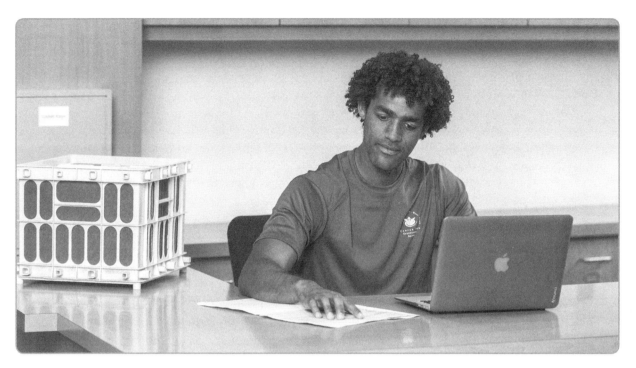

Clients' health and medical records need to be safely stored in a password-protected database.

tion should be permanently maintained. This allows you to refer to previous screening results and compare assessments over time. A good filing system allows you to easily update information when necessary, such as a change in medications. Remember, the information that you collect during screening is confidential. It is to be shared only with the client and the appropriate staff members as needed for risk identification and program management. You may choose to give a copy of the results to the client so that he or she can share them with his or her physician. However, the information is not to be shared with other clients, even if requested by another client. The information must be kept secure and not left in an area with unrestricted access. Folders containing this confidential information should be kept in a locked cabinet that is accessible only to you and other designated staff members. If the information is stored electronically, it must be in a password-protected database.

Additional Screening Tools

It is not feasible, or necessary, to conduct a thorough battery of laboratory tests on every individual who wishes to join an exercise program. However, relatively easy-to-use screening tools can provide valuable information about clients' blood pressure and body composition.

Blood Pressure

When possible, measuring a client's blood pressure should be part of the screening. Because high blood pressure is an important risk factor to recognize before performance testing or exercise participation begins, measuring a client's blood pressure can help you assess a participant's health and risk of an exercise-related medical event. If a client's blood pressure reading is high, he or she should be immediately referred to a physician for further consultation before any performance testing or exercise participation.

Blood pressure is measured in millimeters of mercury (mmHg). The reading typically is recorded as two numbers or a ratio: Systolic pressure (the pressure while the heart contracts) is expressed first, or on top, and the diastolic pressure (the pressure while the heart relaxes between beats) is given second, or on the bottom. Resting systolic blood pressure that is below 120 mmHg and diastolic blood pressure below 80 mmHg is considered normal. According to the revised blood pressure classification, individuals with systolic blood pressure values between 120 and 139 mmHg or diastolic blood pressures between 80 and

89 mmHg are categorized as being prehypertensive. While the report states that this classification does not constitute a disease category, it can be used to identify adults at high risk of developing hypertension and alert both the individual and the physician to the need for immediate intervention in order to prevent or delay disease onset. Lifestyle modifications (e.g., diet, physical activity) are recommended for individuals classified as prehypertensive. A person is considered to have Stage 1 hypertension when their systolic blood pressure is 130-139 mmHg or their diastolic pressure is 80-89 mmHg. They shift into Stage 2 hypertension when their systolic blood pressure is 140 mmHg or higher and their diastolic reading is at 90 mmHg or higher. The classification system for the severity of hypertension is shown in table 5.1. Older adults with hypertension should have their blood pressure monitored using either an automatic or a manual blood pressure cuff, both during and after exercise to ensure that it is under control.

Body Mass Index

A commonly used measurement that provides a rough indication of obesity is the body mass index (BMI). The BMI is a quick and easy method of determining the appropriateness of a client's body weight in relation to his or her height. The BMI can be calculated by dividing body weight in kilograms (kg) by height in meters squared (m^2):

$$BMI = kg/m^2$$

To convert body weight to kilograms, divide the body weight in pounds by 2.2. To determine height in meters, divide the height in inches by 39.4. For example, if an individual weighs 160 pounds (160 pounds/2.2 = 72.7 kilograms) and is 5 feet 6 inches tall (66 inches/39.4 = 1.7 meters), you would divide 72.7 by 2.89, resulting in a BMI of 25.2.

A BMI between 18.5 and 24.9 for men or women is desirable (Expert Panel on the Identification, Evaluation, and Treatment of Overweight and Obesity in Adults, 1998). When the BMI is between 25 and 29.9, an individual is considered to be overweight and is at a slightly elevated risk of developing obesity-related medical conditions, including heart disease, hypertension, and diabetes. It is recommended that individuals in this category who have no other cardiovascular disease risk factors not gain additional weight. Those with two or more obesity-related risk factors, such as hypertension and diabetes, should be advised to lose weight. A BMI of 30 or higher indicates obesity and is associated with an elevated risk of mortality from all causes. Individuals with a BMI ≥30 should also lower their weight. Moreover, when BMI values are combined with above-normal waist circumference values, the risk of disease is further elevated (Flint et al., 2010).

The BMI is a good starting point for determining body composition because it is easy to calculate and can be used to evaluate change. However, it should be used in conjunction with the waist-to-hip ratio or waist circumference (discussed in the following section), or even visual inspection, since the BMI does not discriminate between fat and nonfat tissue. As a result, the BMI for individuals with high muscle mass must be interpreted with caution since their BMI may incorrectly indicate that they are overweight, or even obese. Although this is rarely an issue in older adult populations, it may apply to some master-level athletes, especially those involved in heavy resistance exercise.

Table 5.1   Blood Pressure Categories

Blood pressure category	SBP (mmHg)		DBP (mmHg)
Normal	Less than 120	and	Less than 80
Elevated	120-129	and	Less than 80
High blood pressure (hypertension) stage 1	130-139	or	80-89
High blood pressure (hypertension) stage 2	140 or higher	or	90 or higher
Hypertensive crisis (consult your doctor immediately)	Higher than 180	and/or	Higher than 120

SBP = systolic blood pressure; DBP = diastolic blood pressure.

Reprinted with permission www.heart.org ©American Heart Association, Inc.

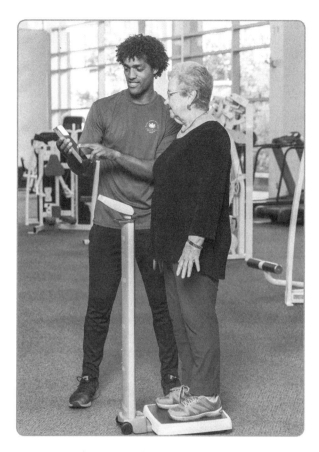

A quick way to determine if clients are overweight or obese is to measure their body mass index (BMI).

- The BMI is based on a client's body weight in relation to his or her height.
- The BMI can be calculated by dividing body weight in kilograms by the square of height in meters.
- A BMI between 18.5 and 24.9 is desirable for men and women.
- A BMI above 30 indicates obesity and is associated with an elevated risk for mortality from all causes.

Waist-to-Hip Ratio and Waist Circumference

Two other methods to evaluate obesity are waist-to-hip ratio and waist circumference. These measures indicate an individual's amount of abdominal fat (android obesity), high levels of which are associated with greater risk of heart disease, type 2 diabetes, and hypertension. To determine the **waist-to-hip ratio**, simply divide the client's waist circumference by hip circumference. The **waist circumference** is measured at the narrowest part of the trunk between the bottom of the sternum and the belly button. The hip measurement is taken at the largest circumference around the buttocks. According to the World Health Organization (2008), waist-to-hip ratios of 0.90 or less in men and 0.85 or less for women are considered to be healthy.

Implications for Program Design and Management

Preactivity screening provides information about individuals *before* they participate in performance testing or exercise classes. Clearly, many factors that can affect, for better or worse, an individual's health status, require a change in the exercise program. How often should the information gained from screening be updated? A basic rule of thumb is that whenever a client has a recognized decline in health or function that suggests an elevation in risk, he or she should be reevaluated. For example, if a client experiences acute symptoms such as dizziness or fatigue, the exercise intensity should be lowered to a level that does not produce the symptoms. If a client begins to experience chronic symptoms (e.g., chest pain indicative of heart disease) that are aggravated by exercise, he or she should be referred to a physician and reevaluated before resuming the exercise program. In addition, each client's health information should also be updated whenever there is a recognized change in care or status. For example, if the physician prescribes a new medication, the individual's confidential, permanent health information should be updated to reflect that change. Clients are advised to have an annual medical examination, regardless of health status, and all preactivity screening tests and forms should be repeated or renewed annually, including the physician's consent form, the health history and activity questionnaire, BMI measurement, blood pressure measurement, and so on.

One challenge that physical activity instructors of community-based programs face is accommodating walk-ins, people who would like to participate immediately but have not been screened. Although it is recommended that you screen all participants following the steps in this chapter, it is not always possible to do this in some exercise class settings. In such cases, have the participants complete the PAR-Q+ to quickly identify those at the greatest risk of injury. As for any client, if a walk-in answers yes to any of the questions, his or her participation should be delayed until further screening can be performed.

Screening is an essential component of all exercise programs for older adults. Not only is screening a legal responsibility, but the client's safety and the program's effectiveness depend on it. Some people are reluctant to provide health or personal information. An open line of communication between you and each participant is extremely important. You should do your best to educate all prospective clients about the importance of providing accurate information during screening and the need for further medical screening if it is indicated. Without this information, it is impossible to determine whether a person is at a high risk of injury or death while participating in performance testing or exercise. If you feel you need more information as you conduct the screening process, do not hesitate to refer clients to their physicians. Because safety is paramount, you should exclude from participation those individuals with cardiovascular disease who do not complete recommended medical evaluations and those who fail to complete the screening questionnaires.

Summary

An initial screening of participants to identify those with symptoms of disease and those at increased risk of disease is essential to optimize safety during performance testing and exercise and to develop an effective exercise prescription. In addition, screening establishes a baseline of health and fitness parameters that can be used to monitor future progress. Thus it is also an invaluable motivational tool for older adults. By following the five steps of the screening process described in this chapter, you can identify those individuals who need a medical check-up before participating in performance testing or exercise.

The basic tools required for preactivity screening include consent forms for the participant and his or her physician and questionnaires for the participant to complete. Several items must be covered by the participant's consent form, including a description of the risks, benefits, and procedures of the exercise program. The PAR-Q+ can serve as an evaluation tool for minimal screening of individuals before a low- to moderate-intensity exercise program or for initial screening of walk-ins. In addition, the health history and activity questionnaire provides you with information about an individual's health history, lifestyle, and physical activity.

Other screening tools, such as blood pressure and BMI, can improve your understanding of a client's health status. Guided by the information that you obtain during the preactivity screening, you can recognize conditions that put an individual at risk during performance testing or exercise and conditions that require medical referral before participation. Furthermore, documenting the information that you gather during screening reduces your risk of liability and improves your ability to individualize each participant's exercise prescription. Updating this information at least yearly allows you to gauge progress and determine whether an individual's exercise program should be modified.

Key Terms

body mass index (BMI)

contraindications

coronary artery disease

diabetes

diastolic blood pressure

high-density lipoprotein (HDL)

informed consent

low-density lipoprotein (LDL)

Physical Activity Readiness Questionnaire for Everyone (PAR-Q+)

systolic blood pressure

waist circumference

waist-to-hip ratio

Recommended Readings

Riebe, D., Franklin, B.A., Thompson, P.D., Garber, C.E., Whitfield, G.P., Magal, M., & Pescatello, L.S. (2015). Updating ACSM's recommendations for exercise preparticipation health screening. *Medicine & Science in Sports & Exercise, 47,* 2473-2479.

Warburton, D.E.R., Gledhill, N., Jamnik, V.K., Bredin, S.S.D., McKenzie, D.C., Stone, J., . . .Shephard, R.J. (2011). Evidence-based risk assessment and recommendations for physical activity clearance: Consensus Document. *Applied Physiology, Nutrition, & Metabolism, 36,* S266-S298.

Study Questions

1. Which of the following individuals should have a medical exam prior to starting a moderate walking program?

   a. 22-year-old male student with a father who died at age 50 from a heart attack

   b. 35-year-old sedentary woman with high blood pressure

   c. 52-year-old man who smokes, has high serum cholesterol, and has chest pain and difficulty breathing when climbing stairs

   d. all of the above

2. Which of the following factors should be considered when classifying an individual's risk status prior to exercise?

   a. diagnosed high blood pressure

   b. serum cholesterol over 240 milligrams per deciliter

   c. family history of heart disease in parents or siblings before age 55 for male relatives and age 65 for female relatives

   d. all of the above

3. The Physical Activity Readiness Questionnaire for Everyone (PAR-Q+)

   a. can be used as a minimal screening for entry into a low- to moderate-intensity exercise program

   b. can be used as a minimal screening for entry into a high-intensity exercise program

   c. is recommended for screening people of any age

   d. should never be used for walk-ins

4. Which is *not* a positive risk factor for heart disease in men?

   a. blood pressure of 146/95 mmHg

   b. waist circumference of 90 centimeters

   c. father died of heart attack at age 54

   d. HDL cholesterol of 25 milligrams per deciliter

5. Which of the following does *not* need to be included as part of an informed consent document?

   a. explanation of risks and benefits

   b. name of a physician to contact in case an injury occurs

   c. statement that participation is voluntary

   d. contact information of someone who can answer questions

6. The BMI indicates a client's
   a. body weight in relation to height
   b. percentage body fat
   c. blood cholesterol
   d. waist circumference

7. An individual with a resting blood pressure of 165/85 mmHg has
   a. prehypertension
   b. stage 1 (mild) hypertension
   c. stage 2 (moderate) hypertension
   d. normal blood pressure

Application Activities

1. George is a 72-year-old man who is 5 feet 9 inches tall and weighs 210 pounds. Determine his BMI. In which category does this place him: desirable body composition, overweight, or obese?

2. While reviewing a female client's health history and activity questionnaire, you note that she has reported on the Composite Physical Function scale that she can dress and bathe independently, walk up and down stairs, cook and dust, go shopping, and walk six blocks outside. However, she finds it difficult to walk a mile, lift and carry a bag of groceries or a large suitcase, and rake leaves. In addition, she cannot perform strenuous activities such as hiking or bicycling. Based on this information, how would you classify her functional ability?

3. The following individuals are interested in joining your exercise program. Based on the following results of their preexercise screenings, evaluate their eligibility to participate in your physical activity program and any further actions that should be taken.
   a. Phil is a 50-year-old postal letter carrier. He estimates that he walks approximately 90 minutes while delivering the mail on five days each week. He is 5 feet 8 inches (173 cm) tall and weighs 142 pounds (64 kg). He smokes one pack of cigarettes a day. His blood pressure is 124/85 mmHg, his cholesterol level is 190 milligrams per deciliter, and his HDL is 60 milligrams per deciliter. He has no family history of heart disease or any other metabolic disorders.
   b. Nancy is a 67-year-old retired secretary who is 5 feet 6 inches (168 cm) tall, weighs 132 pounds (59 kg), and has never smoked. She recently retired from her job and wants to begin an exercise program to improve her health. Her blood pressure is 120/70 mmHg, her cholesterol level is 180 milligrams per deciliter, and her HDL is 44 milligrams per deciliter. She has no family history of heart disease or any other metabolic disorders.
   c. Maria is a 71-year-old retired retail store manager who is 5 feet 9 inches tall (175 cm) and weighs 206 pounds (93 kg). She has been a heavy smoker all of her life, smoking a pack a day. She has type 2 diabetes, a resting blood pressure of 160/90 mmHg, a cholesterol level of 250 milligrams per deciliter, and an HDL level of 28 milligrams per deciliter. Maria's mother had a heart attack when she was 63.

Physical and Functional Assessments

C. Jessie Jones
Roberta E. Rikli

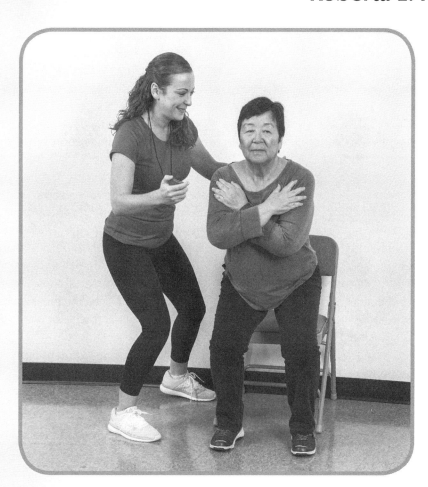

Objectives

After completing this chapter, you will be able to

1. describe the purpose and benefits of conducting physical performance assessments,
2. explain the Functional Fitness Framework,
3. summarize the major criteria for the selection and evaluation of sound assessment tools,
4. distinguish the strengths and limitations of common field tests used to measure physical performance,
5. recognize the difference between norm-referenced and criterion-referenced standards and how to interpret them, and
6. understand processes for effective group testing.

Physical activity instructors can play a critical role in not only helping to reduce the disability span but also increasing active life expectancy so that the aging process can be a positive experience. It is important to understand that *active* means more than just being physically active or having a life free from disability. According to the World Health Organization (WHO, 2002) **active aging** "is the process of optimizing opportunities for health, participation, and security in order to enhance quality of life as people age" (p.12). The definition implies that the word *active* "refers to continuing participation in social, economic, cultural, spiritual, and civic affairs, not just with the ability to be physically active or to participate in the labor force" (WHO, 2002, p. 12). Although active life expectancy has a multitude of contributing factors (e.g., personal, social, economic, health and social services, and behavioral), continuing to be physically active and physically fit are major determinants of an active life expectancy. Thus, being physically active and physically fit can help reduce functional decline and onset of chronic diseases, while at the same time promote independence, social contacts, mental health, economic benefits, and overall quality of life.

As discussed in previous chapters, much of the physical decline that leads to disability is preventable and even reversible through the early detection of **physical impairments** and **functional limitations** and the initiation of targeted physical activity programs. Physical performance assessments can help you to (1) identify and predict who is or will be at risk for mobility problems, falls, and disability; (2) determine if your program is appropriate for a particular older adult; (3) motivate your clients to set personal behavioral goals; (4) select exercises that address an older adult's specific needs; (5) provide meaningful feedback to participants; (6) determine if a referral to the client's physician is indicated; and (7) evaluate the effectiveness of your physical activity or fitness program.

Unfortunately, very few physical activity instructors actually conduct the types of assessments needed to appropriately individualize programs for their clients. Common reasons reported for this omission include (1) lack of time, space, and budget; (2) absence of a requirement by facility management; (3) insufficient personnel; (4) lack of appropriate assessment tools to address the wide range of functional levels; and (5) lack of training in administering tests and interpreting their results. The purpose of this chapter is to provide knowledge necessary to select and use appropriate assessment tools to measure important physical and functional performance variables, including fall risk in older adults.

Functional Fitness Framework

The **Functional Fitness Framework** (Rikli & Jones, 1999a, 2013b) identifies the physical fitness parameters associated with the functional abilities that are required for the performance of various activities of daily life. Some common activity goals are listed in the last column of figure 6.1 (e.g., personal care, shopping, housework). These activity goals cannot be achieved unless certain motor functions, such as those listed in the middle column (e.g., walking, stair climbing, lifting), can be performed. These functions in turn require an adequate level of one or more of the physical fitness parameters identified in the first column (e.g., strength, endurance, flexibility).

Disability is defined as difficulty in the performance of socially defined roles and tasks, such as personal care, household chores, socializing with friends, working, and recreation. The information in figure 6.1 on the Functional Fitness Framework can be used as a guide in selecting appropriate assessment tools to identify physical impairments that may affect your clients' ability to perform activities of daily living or engage in recreational pursuits.

Considerations for Test Selection and Evaluation

Although numerous scales and tests have been developed to measure physical disabilities in frail older adults, far fewer assessment tools have been developed that can be used to measure physical performance and functional ability levels in the healthier, community-dwelling older adult population (VanSwearingen & Brach, 2001). Before we describe recommended assessment methods, it is important that you become familiar with the criteria used to select sound measurement tools. Unfortunately, not all published assessment tools have the scientific rigor necessary to ensure their reliability and validity for the intended population. The following sections present two major categories of criteria for the selection and evaluation of test instruments: (1) practicality of use and (2) psychometric properties (the degree to which tests meet established test construction guidelines).

Practicality

Practicality, also referred to as the usability or feasibility of the test, should be considered when

Physical Fitness Parameters	Functional Abilities	Activity Goals
Muscle strength/endurance	Walking	Personal care
Aerobic endurance	Stair climbing	Shopping or errands
Flexibility	Standing up from chair	Housework
Motor ability	Lifting or reaching	Gardening
• Balance	Bending or kneeling	Sports
• Coordination	Jogging or running	Traveling
• Speed and agility		
• Power		
Body composition		
Physical impairment →	Functional limitation →	Physical disability

FIGURE 6.1 Functional Fitness Framework. A physical performance framework demonstrating the progressive relationship between physiological parameters, functional performance, and activity goals.

Reprinted by permission from R.E. Rikli and C.J. Jones, "Development and Validation of a Functional Fitness Test for Community-Residing Older Adults," *Journal of Aging and Physical Activity* 7, (1999a): 129-161.

selecting assessment tools. A practical test is one that is usable within the conditions at hand. Many factors influence the usability of a test item, including (1) the type of equipment and space needed, (2) the time needed to administer and score the test, (3) the personnel and expertise needed to conduct the test, (4) the level of fatigue caused by a particular test or test item, (5) whether the test is socially acceptable and meaningful to your clients, and (6) whether the test is safe to use without medical clearance. For example, although one of the preferred means of measuring upper-body strength might be administering the chest press (using a plate weight machine), this may not be practical for use in most field settings because of the cost of this specialized equipment or because of the time it would require to measure a large number of clients on the same day. Similarly, a strenuous test (e.g., an exercise stress test that measures $\dot{V}O_2$max) that requires physician approval would not be practical in settings when participants do not have easy access to physicians.

Psychometric Properties

The selection and evaluation of test items should also be based on its **psychometric properties** (i.e., the degree to which the test meets test construction guidelines with respect to reliability, validity, discrimination power, and performance standards). For example, in assessing older adults, it usually is important that test items be able to provide accurate (reliable and valid) measures of current ability and be able to assess future risk for mobility problems, falls, or disability.

Reliability

Reliability indicates the degree to which two test scores would be similar if the test were repeated under identical conditions, meaning that the test is relatively free of measurement error and provides dependable and consistent scores. This type of consistency in a score is also referred to as *test–retest reliability*. Reliability (i.e., the correlation between two sets of scores) should be greater than .80. In collecting baseline measures, it is especially important that a test provide a reliable baseline score; otherwise you can never be sure that a change in score reflects an actual change in performance over time or whether the change was due to unstable (unreliable) measures. The reliability of a test item is

always determined using trained test administrators. Therefore, it is extremely important that all testers are trained to administer each test item according to its published protocol. If more than one tester will administer the same test item, then each tester should practice administering and scoring the test item with the same small set of clients. The scores obtained by each tester for the same clients should be compared for accuracy. When scores obtained by multiple testers are very similar (are highly correlated), the test is considered to have good **inter-rater reliability**.

Validity

The most important characteristic of any test is its **validity**. A valid test is one that has been shown to measure what it is intended to measure. One way to evaluate a test's validity is by comparing its scores with scores on another criterion measure that is already known to be valid (sometimes referred to as a *gold standard*). For example, a test to measure lower-body strength such as the 30-second chair stand (see figure 6.2), discussed later in this chapter, was validated by comparing older adult performances on this measure with their performances on a proven laboratory-based measure of lower-body strength, a one-repetition maximum (1RM) leg press. The scores of the two tests were statistically compared using correlation analysis. Tests are generally considered to have acceptable **criterion-related validity** when the correlation values are greater than .70.

A test's validity can also be assessed through content analysis. **Content validity**, often referred to as *face* or *logical validity,* is the degree to which a test measures the domain of interest. No statistical procedures are needed to determine whether a test has content validity; experts in the field only need to agree that the test measures a particular domain of interest. For example, the domain of interest of the Berg Balance Scale (BBS) is balance (Berg, Wood-Dauphinee, Williams, & Gayton, 1989; Berg, Wood-Dauphinee, & Williams, 1992). Experts in the field have agreed that the items on the BBS do indeed measure different dimensions of balance.

When a test can predict future conditions or behaviors, such as falling or disability, the test is said to have **predictive validity**. For a test to have predictive validity, research findings must demonstrate statistically that its score is highly related to

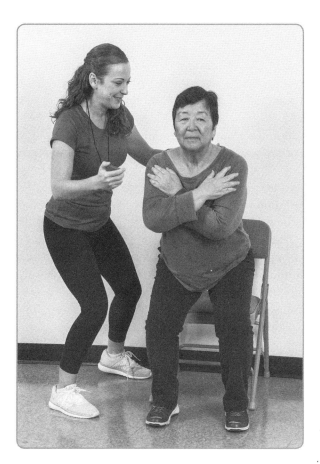

FIGURE 6.2   The 30-second chair stand, an item in the Senior Fitness Test battery, is a reliable and valid field-based measure of lower-body strength.

Reliability: The degree to which two test scores are similar when the test is repeated under similar conditions.

Interrater reliability: The degree to which two or more test administrators are able to produce the same scores for the same clients.

Validity: The ability of a test to measure what it is intended to measure.

Criterion-related validity: The degree to which a test correlates with a proven criterion measure (a recognized gold standard).

Content validity: The degree to which a test measures the intended domain of interest.

Predictive validity: The ability of a test to predict future outcomes.

a future outcome, such as falls, loss of functional mobility, or disability. For example, people who score 25 points or lower out of 40 on the Fullerton Advanced Balance Scale have been shown statistically to have a high risk of falls (Hernandez & Rose, 2008). Other popular field test measures, such as the single item gait speed test and the Short Physical Performance Battery (SPPB) provide meaningful standards that can be used to predict disability rates, nursing home admittance, and survival rates in older adults (Cesari et al., 2011; Guralnik et al., 2000; Studenski et al., 2011).

Discrimination Power

When a test is able to discriminate among different levels of an attribute or ability, or can detect small but meaningful changes in performance, it is said to have good **discrimination power**. To assess a change in performance over time or in relation to a particular intervention, a test needs to measure performance levels on a continuum, with minimal floor or ceiling effects. A **floor effect** occurs when a test is too difficult for many of the clients performing it (e.g., using the 1-mile [1.6-km] walk or run for frail older adults). A **ceiling effect** occurs when a test is too easy for most clients. For example, the Berg Balance Scale (Berg, et al., 1989) tends to exhibit ceiling effects when administered to high-functioning older adults (Rose, Lucchese, & Wiersma, 2006). Many community-residing older adults achieve the maximum score of 56 points on the Berg test, despite reporting balance problems. Receiving a maximum score at baseline on a test would make it impossible to demonstrate improvement over time.

In other words, a subcomponent of discrimination power is the **responsiveness** of a measure, which is its ability to detect small but important changes over time. The smaller the change in performance detected by the measure, the higher the responsiveness and the more confident the instructor can be about detecting changes at the end of the exercise program. Tests that use continuous scoring systems (e.g., the timed eight-foot [2.4 m] up-and-go, which is reported in seconds; Rikli & Jones, 1999a, 2013b) are inherently more sensitive to changes in performance than tests that use only categorical scores (e.g., pass/fail or good, average, and poor). For example, the SPPB (previously mentioned), which is a popular field test with excellent predictive properties for such things as mortality or admission to nursing homes, is limited in its ability to detect gradual change in individual performance over time because it uses a categorical 1-4 ranking system rather than a continuous-scale method of scoring. In addition, the SPPB contains items that have been found to be too easy (side-by-side balance task) or too difficult (5-times chair stand) to be effective performance discriminators for up to 20 to 50 percent of community-residing older adults (Guralnik et al., 1994; Seeman et al., 1994) and for as much as 75 percent of assisted living or residential care patients (Giuliani et al., 2008).

Performance Standards

After clients are tested, it is important to interpret the scores and then explain them to your clients. **Performance standards** provide a useful way of interpreting test results. There are two types of performance standards: norm referenced and criterion referenced. Tests with **norm-referenced standards** (typically presented as percentile norms) make it possible to evaluate performance by comparing a person's score with others of the same age and sex. **Criterion-referenced standards**, on the other hand, provide a means of evaluating performance in relation to a particular reference point or goal

---

Discrimination power: The ability of a test to distinguish different levels of an attribute or ability, including changes that occur over time.

Floor effect: Occurs when a test is too difficult for much of the population of intent, thus making it impossible for these people to receive a score.

Ceiling effect: Occurs when a test is too easy for a large part of the population, causing many people to "top out" in the scoring scale, which limits the discrimination power of the test.

Performance standards: Can be either norm-referenced (where an individual's scores are compared to others within a particular group) or criterion-referenced (where scores are compared to some point of interest, such as physical independence).

---

of interest, such as having the fitness level needed to remain physically independent. Although both types of standards provide important comparison information, criterion-referenced fitness standards are especially helpful in identifying people at risk for mobility problems or loss of physical independence. For example, research has shown that if a 70- to 74-year-old female is unable to complete at least 14 chair stands in 30 seconds, this indicates she likely has insufficient lower-body strength for her age, thus putting her at risk for loss of mobility and independence in later years (Rikli & Jones, 2013a, 2013b). Physical independence generally requires having the physical capacity needed to perform common everyday activities on one's own (without additional assistance) such as simple housework, lifting and carrying objects, negotiating steps, and walking far enough to do one's own shopping and errands.

Recommended Assessment Tools

This section briefly describes two assessment tools designed to measure physical capacity and functional abilities in older adults. Both tests meet the basic criteria for sound tests discussed in the previous section. The tests described in this section are capable of measuring various aspects of the physical fitness parameters or motor functions needed to achieve the activity goals described in the Functional Fitness Framework presented in figure 6.1. Based on feedback from hundreds of practitioners in the field, these tests are practical and easy to use in terms of training, equipment, space, and time requirements. Plus, they have met the scientific requirements for good reliability and validity.

The Senior Fitness Test

The Senior Fitness Test (SFT) (Rikli & Jones, 2013b) measures the underlying physical parameters needed to perform functional tasks of daily living (e.g., ambulation, reaching, rising from a chair, climbing stairs). The test battery, originally referred to as the Fullerton functional fitness test (Rikli & Jones, 1999a, 1999b) utilizes common functional tasks such as standing up from a chair to assess important physical fitness parameters such as lower body strength. Because each of the SFT items is practical and relevant, participants who complete the test find the experience meaningful and motivating. In addition, the test items have been well-documented for their reliability and validity and have published performance standards, both percentile norms and criterion-referenced fitness standards (Rikli & Jones, 1999b, 2013a, 2013b). A brief description of each test item is presented in table 6.1, along with age-group fitness standards.

The *Senior Fitness Test Manual* (Rikli & Jones, 2013b) provides detailed information on administering and scoring the test in individual and group settings and explains how to provide feedback to participants about their results using both percentile

Table 6.1 Summary of the Senior Fitness Test Items With Age-Group Fitness Standards

Test item	Purpose	Brief protocol	Age-group fitness standards for men (M) and women (W)
30-Second Chair Stand	To assess lower-body strength needed for numerous tasks such as climbing stairs; walking; and getting out of a chair, tub, or car	Number of full stands that can be completed in 30 seconds with arms folded across chest	# stands in 30 seconds: 60-64 (M=17; W=15) 65-69 (M & W = 15) 70-74 (M=15; W=14) 75-79 (M=14; W=13) 80-84 (M=13; W=12) 85-89 (M & W =11) 90+ (M & W = 9)
Arm Curl	To assess upper-body strength needed for performing household tasks and other activities involving lifting and carrying things such as groceries, suitcases, and grandchildren	Number of biceps curls that can be completed in 30 seconds holding a hand weight of 5 pounds (2.27 kg) for women; 8 pounds (3.63 kg) for men	# curls in 30 seconds: 60-64 (M=19; W=17) 65-69 (M=18; W =17) 70-74 (M=17; W=16) 75-79 (M=16; W=15) 80-84 (M=15; W=14) 85-89 (M & W=13) 90+ (M & W= 11)
6-Minute Walk	To assess aerobic endurance, which is important for such tasks as walking distances, climbing stairs, shopping, and sightseeing	Number of yards (or meters) that can be walked in 6 minutes around a 50-yard (45.7 m) course	# of yards walked: 60-64 (M=680; W=625) 65-69 (M=650; W=605) 70-74 (M=620; W=580) 75-79 (M=580; W=550) 80-84 (M=530; W=510) 85-89 (M=470; W =460) 90+ (M & W = 400)
2-Minute Step Test	Alternate aerobic endurance test for use when space limitations or weather prohibits taking the 6-Minute Walk Test	Number of full steps completed in 2 minutes, raising each knee to a point midway between the patella (kneecap) and iliac crest (top hip bone); score is number of times right knee reaches the required height	# of steps: 60-64 (M=106; W=97) 65-69 (M=101; W= 93) 70-74 (M=95; W=89) 75-79 (M=88; W=84) 80-84 (M=80; W=78) 85-89 (M=71; W=70) 90+ (M & W = 60)

(continued)

Table 6.1 *(continued)*

Test item	Purpose	Brief protocol	Age-group fitness standards for men (M) and women (W)
Chair Sit-and-Reach	To assess lower-body flexibility, which is important for good posture, normal gait patterns, and various mobility tasks such as getting into and out of a bathtub or car	From a sitting position at the front of a chair, with leg extended and hands reaching toward toes, the number of inches (cm) (+ or -) between extended middle fingers and tip of toe	Standards have not been determined for this test item.
Back Scratch	To assess upper-body (shoulder) flexibility, which is important in tasks such as combing hair, putting on overhead garments, and reaching for a seat belt	With one hand reaching over the shoulder and one up the middle of the back, the number of inches (cm) between extended middle fingers (+ or –)	Standards have not been determined for this test item.
8-Foot Up-and-Go	To assess agility and dynamic balance, which are important in tasks that require quick maneuvering such as getting off a bus in time, getting up to attend to something in the kitchen, or getting up to go to the bathroom or to answer the phone	Number of seconds required to get up from a seated position, walk 8 feet (2.44 m), turn, and return to seated position	Seconds to complete task: 60-64 (M=4.8; W=5.0) 65-69 (M=5.1; W=5.3) 70-74 (M=5.5; W=5.6) 75-79 (M=5.9; W=6.0) 80-84 (M=6.4; W=6.5) 85-89 (M & W =7.1) 90+ (M & W = 8.0)

Fitness standards reflect the criterion score (level of fitness) on each test item that is associated with being able to perform the common everyday activities that will be needed for mobility and physical independence until late in life. Progressively higher standards are required for younger older adults (those in their 60s, 70s, and even 80s) so that normal age-related declines will not cause them to fall below the fitness level needed to remain independent at age 90+. More complete descriptions, tables, and charts illustrating these fitness standards can be found in Rikli and Jones (2013a, 2013b).

Reprinted by permission from R.E. Rikli and C.J. Jones, *Senior Fitness Test Manual,* 2nd ed. (Champaign, IL: Human Kinetics, 2013).

norms and criterion-referenced fitness standards. The manual's appendixes include reproducible sample forms, charts, tables, and posters for instructors to use with their programs. Also available for use with the SFT is an instructional video on how to administer the SFT items and computer software for recording and analyzing the results. A summary of the SFT's benefits is as follows:

- The SFT battery was designed to meet the practical and psychometric properties (reliability, validity, and discrimination) and conditions previously discussed.

- It is convenient and practical to use in terms of equipment, training, space, and time requirements.

- It assesses a wide range of physical abilities.

- It uses continuous-scale scoring so that significant differences can be detected in functional levels immediately and over time.

- Older adults can perform test items safely without the need for a medical release in most cases.

- Its norm-referenced standards provide a way of interpreting scores relative to age and gender-matched peers.

- Its criterion-referenced standards provide fitness goals associated with physical independence.

Fullerton Advanced Balance Scale

The Fullerton Advanced Balance (FAB) Scale was developed to measure multiple dimensions of balance in different sensory environments (Rose, 2010; Rose, Lucchese, & Wiersma, 2006). The test was developed for use with higher-functioning older adults. The FAB Scale is comprised of 10 test items that are scored using a 0-to-4 ordinal scale (see table 6.2). The highest score possible on the test is 40 points. items include standing on foam with eyes closed, walking with head turns, stepping up and over an obstacle (figure 6.3), and a two-footed jump for distance. The FAB Scale is easy to use in a community setting, has demonstrated high test–retest reliability, intra- and interrater reliability (when administered by trained professionals), and construct validity. In addition, the FAB Scale is predictive of risks for falls (Hernandez & Rose, 2008). The procedures for administering and scoring the test are described in *FallProof! A Comprehensive Balance and Mobility Training Program* (Rose, 2010).

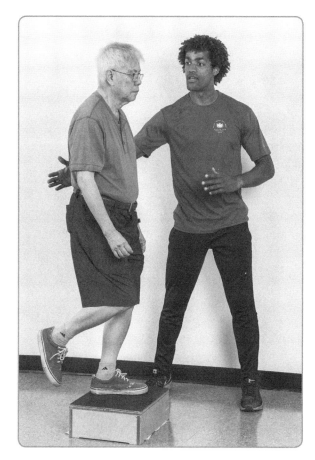

FIGURE 6.3 Participant steps up and over a 6-inch-high bench, an item on the FAB Scale that measures anticipatory postural control and dynamic balance.

Table 6.2 Fullerton Advanced Balance (FAB) Scale

Test item	Dimension(s) of balance measured
1. Stand with feet together, eyes closed	Sensory organization (somatosensory inputs)
2. Reaching forward to retrieve object	Anticipatory postural control, forward limits of stability
3. Turning in a full circle to right and left	Sensory organization, dynamic balance
4. Stepping up and over bench	Anticipatory postural control, dynamic balance
5. Tandem walk	Dynamic balance in reduced base of support
6. Standing on one leg, eyes open	Static balance in reduced base of support
7. Standing on foam, eyes closed	Sensory organization (vestibular inputs)
8. Two-footed jump for distance	Dynamic balance, whole-body motor coordination
9. Walk with head turns	Sensory organization (visual-vestibular inputs)
10. Unexpected backward release	Reactive postural control

Adapted by permission from D.J. Rose, *Fallproof. A Comprehensive Balance and Mobility Program,* 2nd ed. (Champaign, IL: Human Kinetics, 2010), 65-66.

Guidelines for Group Physical Performance Testing

This section provides some basic guidelines to help ensure safe, reliable, and efficient physical performance assessments in a group setting. A number of tasks must be completed both prior to and on the actual assessment day. Two important tasks to be completed prior to assessment day are training test administrators and scheduling clients for testing.

Administrator Training

Once you have selected the test items that are appropriate for your setting, you need to assemble the necessary equipment and tools and then become very familiar with how to administer the test. It is best to practice administering and scoring the tests with a group of clients you know well. After you are comfortable with your skills in administering the test items, you have to decide how many assistants you need to administer the test items efficiently and effectively in a group setting. The next step is to train each test administrator until he or she can conduct the test and record the score reliably. It is best for you and your assistants to practice measuring the same group of clients and then comparing scores to check their accuracy. It is extremely important to follow the test protocol exactly as written and to treat all clients the same. If clients are unable to perform a test item using the exact protocol, allow them to complete the test as best they can (if safe) and mark down the score and any adaptations used in the "note" section of the scorecard. Scores of clients using modified protocols should not be compared to the performance norms, since they technically would score a zero (0) if using the proper protocol. However, their adapted scores can be used in evaluating their own personal changes in performance over time.

Scheduling Assessments

Before scheduling the assessments, you need to establish how many clients you can accommodate in a single testing period. Whether you conduct individual or group assessments, each participant needs to complete a health history and activity questionnaire and an informed consent form and receive medical clearance if necessary before the assessment (see chapter 5).

Prior to performing any relatively strenuous test item (such as the SFT chair stand, 6-minute walk, or 2-minute step test), a client with any of the following conditions should get medical clearance:

- A physician has previously advised the client not to exercise because of a medical condition.
- The client currently experiences chest pain or dizziness or has angina (chest tightness, pressure, pain, heaviness) following exertion or during exercise.
- The client has experienced congestive heart failure.
- The client has high and uncontrolled blood pressure (160/100 mmHg or above).

Participants should also be reminded on the informed consent form to monitor their physical exertion level, to perform all test items within their comfort zone (i.e., never to a point of overexertion or beyond what feels safe), and to notify the instructor if they feel any discomfort or experience any unusual symptoms. In addition, before assessment day, participants should be given written instructions to avoid heavy exertion and alcohol use for 24 hours before testing, to eat a light meal one hour before testing, to wear clothing and shoes appropriate for physical activity, and to bring a hat and sunglasses for walking outside. As a reminder, the assessment date and time can also be written on the top of the instruction sheet.

Assessment Day

Arrive early on assessment day to make sure that each test station is set up correctly, scorecards are ready, and all equipment is in working order. Double-check that your assistants understand their responsibilities. Clients should not be allowed to participate in any assessments if their health history and activity questionnaires or informed consent forms have not been completed. Before conducting the assessments, you or another physical activity instructor should lead the participants through 8 to

10 minutes of general warm-up and flexibility exercises. The measures of functional status described in this chapter do not require a warm-up period longer than this. Before starting, participants should be instructed to do the best they can but never to push themselves to overexertion or beyond what they feel is safe for them. The participants can then be evenly divided and sent to one of the stations to begin testing (see figure 6.4). Testing stations should be planned so that one test item does not overly fatigue the participant prior to the next test item. It works best if the testing coordinator is not assigned to a specific test station so that person can be free to move around the room to monitor the pace of the testing and to spot-check for assistants' accuracy in test administration and scoring.

After all testing is completed, check each recorded score for readability and completeness. It is extremely important that you treat all data (client information and scores) as confidential, preferably keeping the data in a cabinet that locks. Detailed information for group testing, data management, and interpreting SFT scores can be found in the *Senior Fitness Test Manual* (Rikli & Jones, 2013b). For information about administering the FAB Scale and interpreting scores refer to *FallProof!* (Rose, 2010).

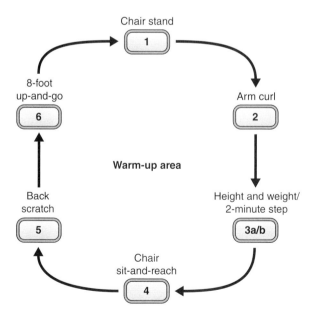

FIGURE 6.4   Testing stations allow you to measure more people at one time.

Reprinted by permission from R.E. Rikli and C.J. Jones, *Senior Fitness Test Manual,* 2nd ed. (Champaign, IL: Human Kinetics, 2013), 79.

Interpreting Test Results

After testing your clients, they are almost certainly going to ask "How did I do?" There is no single best way to share test results with your clients, but you need to consider the individual and inspire hope no matter how poorly she or he performed on the test. You need to communicate that everyone can improve with exercise and that it is never too late to improve. Refer to the test manuals to see whether performance norm-referenced and criterion-referenced standards are available for interpreting scores. Depending on the test item, there are three basic ways to interpret scores:

1. *Pre- and posttesting.* If performance norm-referenced or criterion-referenced standards for a test item are not available, you must use your professional judgment to interpret the initial scores. After your clients have participated in your program for a certain period of time (at least eight weeks), you can administer the same test again and compare the raw data scores from the pretest to the posttest. You also could express the difference in scores as a percentage of improvement and share that information with each participant. Pre- and posttesting also let you know how effective your program intervention is at improving the physical and functional status of your clients.

2. *Norm-referenced standards.* If the test you use has performance norms it will allow you to compare clients' scores with others of the same age and sex. However, it is important to remember when interpreting scores that norms are based on average scores for a particular group of people. For example, the norms for the SFT battery are based on the scores of over 7,000 community-dwelling older adults in the United States between 60 and 94 years of age who volunteered to be tested at a local facility. The volunteers were 89 percent white and 11 percent nonwhite, fairly well-educated, and generally active individuals (about 60 percent reporting that they participated at least three times per week for at least 30 minutes per day in moderate physical activity). Although

you should be able to generalize the normative values to scores of similar older adults, you must take care in interpreting scores for individuals who are different from those represented in the normative study. Unlike table 6.1, which shows criterion-referenced performance scores (see next list entry), table

6.3 provides normal range scores for men and women, with *normal* defined as the middle 50 percent of the population. Participants scoring above the normal range would be considered *above average* for their age and gender, while those scoring below the range would be *below average*.

Table 6.3   Senior Fitness Test Normal Range of Scores for Men and Women

Test item	Men (age in years)						
	60-64	**65-69**	**70-74**	**75-79**	**80-84**	**85-89**	**90+**
	Normal range of scores						
30-sec chair stand (no. of stands)	14-19	12-18	12-17	11-17	10-15	8-14	7-12
30-sec arm curl (no. of reps)	16-22	15-21	14-21	13-19	13-19	11-17	10-14
6-min walk (no. of yards)	610-735	560-700	545-680	470-640	445-605	380-570	305-500
2-min step test (no. of steps)	87-115	86-116	80-110	73-109	71-103	59-91	52-86
Chair sit-and-reach (inches + or –)	–2.5-+4.0	–3.0-+3.0	–3.5-+2.5	–4.0-+2.0	–5.5-+1.5	–5.5-+0.5	–6.5-+0.5
Back scratch (inches + or –)	–6.5-+0.0	–7.5--1.0	–8.0--1.0	–9.0--2.0	–9.5--2.0	–10.0--3.0	–10.5--4.0
8-ft up-and-go (seconds)	3.8-5.6	4.3-5.7	4.2-6.0	4.6-7.2	5.2-7.6	5.3-8.9	6.2-10.0
Test item	Women (age in years)						
	60-64	**65-69**	**70-74**	**75-79**	**80-84**	**85-89**	**90+**
	Normal range of scores						
30-sec chair stand (no. of stands)	12-17	11-16	10-15	10-15	9-14	8-13	4-11
30-sec arm curl (no. of reps)	13-19	12-18	12-17	11-17	10-16	10-15	8-13
6-min walk (no. of yards)	545-660	500-635	480-615	430-585	385-540	340-510	275-440
2-min step test (no. of steps)	75-107	73-107	68-101	68-100	60-91	55-85	44-72
Chair sit-and-reach (inches + or –)	–0.5-+5.0	–0.5-+4.5	–1.0-+4.0	–1.5-+3.5	–2.0-+3.0	–2.5-+2.5	–4.5-+1.0
Back scratch (inches + or –)	–3.0-+1.5	–3.5-+1.5	–4.0-+1.0	–5.0-+0.5	–5.5-+0.0	–7.0--1.0	–8.0--1.0
8-ft up-and-go (seconds)	4.4-6.0	4.8-6.4	4.9-7.9	5.2-7.4	5.7-8.7	6.2-9.6	7.3-11.5

Normal is defined as the middle 50 percent of the population. Those scoring above this range would be considered above average for their age and those below the range as below average.

3. *Criterion-referenced standards.* If a test item has criterion-referenced performance standards, scores can be compared to a threshold score (cut-point) that helps to identify people at risk for such things as mobility problems, falls, and loss of physical independence. As indicated in table 6.1, the Senior Fitness Test has criterion-referenced fitness standards (fitness goals) needed for maintaining mobility and physical independence on five of its seven test items: 30-second chair stand, 30-second arm curl, 6-minute walk, 2-minute step test, and 8-foot up and go. Refer to Rikli and Jones (2013a) for technical details about the development and validation of the standards and to Rikli and Jones (2013b) for more user-friendly descriptions of the standards and for related performance tables and charts (see figure 6.5 for an example) and instructions on how to interpret individual scores and provide client feedback.

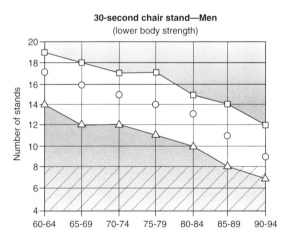

30-second chair stand—Men
(lower body strength)

FIGURE 6.5 Sample performance chart showing normal range of scores and functional fitness standards for men on the 30-second chair stand. Similar charts for other test items can be found in Rikli and Jones (2013).

Reprinted by permission from R.E. Rikli and C.J. Jones, *Senior Fitness Test Manual,* 2nd ed. (Champaign, IL: Human Kinetics, 2013), 93.

Summary

Being able to select, administer, and interpret physical performance tests is a critical skill for all physical activity instructors of older adults. The benefits of assessments include the ability to (1) identify and predict which clients are at risk for mobility problems, (2) determine if your physical activity program is appropriate for particular clients, (3) motivate clients, (4) individualize the physical activity program, (5) provide meaningful feedback to clients, (6) determine if a medical referral is necessary, and (7) evaluate program outcomes.

The selection and evaluation of test items or test batteries should be based on their practicality of use and their psychometric properties (reliability, validity, and discrimination power). The availability of performance standards further aids in the interpretation of the scores. When a test has norm-referenced standards, an individual's score can be compared to scores of others of the same age and sex. A criterion-referenced standard is a threshold score that has been associated with (referenced to) a particular goal of interest, such as maintaining mobility and physical independence.

Although other measurement instruments are available for assessing physical performance in older adults, the Senior Fitness Test (SFT) battery and the Fullerton Advanced Balance (FAB) Scale have been featured because of their strong psychometric properties and ease of use in assessing independent, community-dwelling older adults. Procedures in efficient group testing include obtaining necessary equipment, practicing administering and scoring test items, training assistants, scheduling assessments, having clients complete the necessary paperwork, preparing scorecards, and setting up test stations. Methods for evaluating and interpreting client scores include use of pre- and posttest comparisons, norm-referenced performance standards, and criterion-referenced performance standards.

Key Terms

active aging

ceiling effect

content validity

criterion-referenced standards

criterion-related validity

disability

discrimination power

floor effect

Functional Fitness Framework

functional limitations

interrater reliability

norm-referenced standards

performance standards

physical impairments

practicality

predictive validity

psychometric properties

reliability

responsiveness

validity

Recommended Readings

Rikli, R.E, & Jones, C.J. (2013). *Senior fitness test manual* (2nd ed.). Champaign, IL: Human Kinetics.

Rose, D. (2010). *FallProof! A comprehensive balance and mobility training program* (2nd ed.). Champaign, IL: Human Kinetics.

Study Questions

1. Active aging is defined by the World Health Organization as

   a. the process of optimizing opportunities for health, participation, and security in order to enhance quality of life as people age

   b. the process of optimizing participation in physical activity in order to enhance quality of life as people age

   c. the process of optimizing health and physical well-being in order to enhance quality of life as people age

   d. the process of optimizing health and physical well-being to help prevent disability in later life

   e. the process of optimizing opportunities for health and well-being in order to enhance quality of life as people age

2. When two or more test administrators obtain very similar scores for the same clients, the test is said to have acceptable

   a. predictability

   b. validity

   c. discrimination power

   d. interrater reliability

   e. sensitivity

3. _____ provide(s) a means of evaluating performance against a particular standard or goal of interest, such as physical independence.

   a. Criterion-referenced performance standards

   b. Physical fitness–referenced performance standards

   c. Norm-referenced performance standards

   d. Pre- and posttesting

   e. Practicality

4. If you wanted to compare your client's performance with what is expected for someone of the same age and sex, you would use

   a. criterion-referenced performance standards

   b. norm-referenced performance standards

   c. pre- and posttesting

   d. practicality

   e. discrimination

Application Activities

1. Develop a short presentation to deliver to the administration of a senior center or assistive care facility to explain the importance of conducting physical performance measures on its clients.

2. Make and execute a plan to administer one of the test batteries discussed in this chapter to a small group of older adults at different physical fitness levels. Provide them with feedback about their results, and explain how they might use these results to improve their physical fitness and ability to perform activities associated with daily living.

Goal Setting and Behavioral Management

Sara Wilcox
Abby C. King

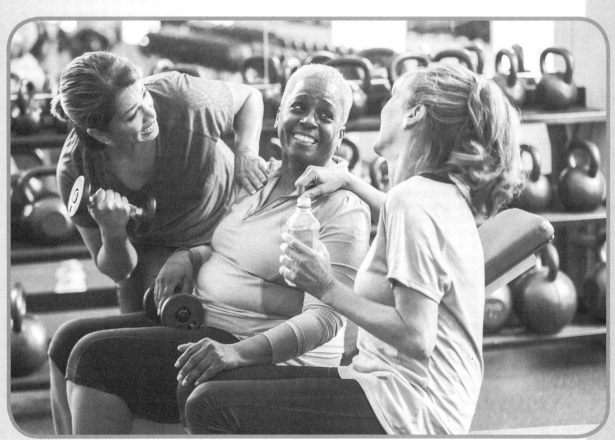

Objectives

After completing this chapter, you will be able to

1. summarize the major personal, environmental, and program-related factors that affect older adults' exercise participation;
2. describe several key theories and models of behavioral change and how they apply to exercise by older adults;
3. develop an individualized behavioral modification plan that includes key cognitive and behavioral change strategies;
4. assist older clients in developing short- and long-term goals, monitoring progress, and modifying goals as needed; and
5. incorporate cognitive and behavioral change strategies into your exercise programs for older adults.

It is as important to understand the psychosocial factors that increase or decrease older adults' likelihood of adopting and maintaining an exercise program as it is to understand their health, fitness, and mobility status. According to self-report surveillance data, almost one quarter (23.7%) of adults in the United States age 65 years and older report no physical activity, and only 39.3 percent meet recommendations (Centers for Disease Control and Prevention, 2007). Objective data indicate that the percentage meeting recommendations is likely to be much smaller (Troiano et al., 2008). In addition, dropout rates from exercise programs are high. In 2004, the American College of Sports Medicine issued a best practices statement regarding physical activity programs and behavioral counseling in older adult populations (Cress et al., 2005). The statement concluded that including a comprehensive behavioral management strategy can enhance recruitment, increase motivation, and minimize attrition. The strategies that were highlighted in this statement were social support, self-efficacy, active choices (tailoring to the needs and interests of the client), health contracts, perceived safety, regular performance feedback, and positive reinforcement. The purpose of this chapter, therefore, is to provide the physical activity instructor with strategies to maximize exercise **adoption** (i.e., beginning a program) and **adherence** (i.e., maintaining a program) by older adults. Specifically, we discuss the factors that influence the adoption and maintenance of

exercise in older adults, strategies for promoting behavioral change and adherence, and implications of these issues for program design and management.

Factors Influencing Older Adults' Exercise Participation

No single factor can predict whether or not an older adult will initiate and maintain an exercise program. Rather, exercise behaviors are determined by multiple interacting factors. These factors can be grouped into three general categories: personal characteristics, program-related factors, and environmental factors (see reviews by Picorelli, Pereira, Pereira, Felicio, & Sherrington, 2014; Van Cauwenberg et al., 2011; Wilcox, Tudor-Locke, & Ainsworth, 2002).

Personal Characteristics

The most consistent demographic factors that are negatively associated with exercise participation by older adults include being female, being in an ethnic minority group, older age (especially those 85 years old or older), rural residence, and low socioeconomic status. While exercise programs obviously cannot modify any of these factors, awareness of them can help you guide and tailor programs to address the unique barriers faced by these subgroups of older adults.

Health-related factors also affect exercise participation. Older adults in poor physical condition and poor health are less active than their healthy counterparts, and illness has been shown to be a strong predictor of poor adherence to exercise programs. Arthritic pain is a significant barrier to exercise by older adults, despite the benefits of exercise for people with arthritis. Older adults who smoke and those who are overweight also tend to be less active than their nonsmoking, average-weight peers.

Attitudes, knowledge, and beliefs, as well as psychological factors, also influence exercise behaviors of older adults. An individual's willingness to make changes in his or her physical activity level is typically a necessary but not sufficient factor for exercise adoption. Older adults who perceive greater benefits of exercise, as opposed to fewer barriers to exercise, are more likely to be active. Older adults have reported a number of motivations for physical activity (perceived benefits). The desires to improve health, prevent disease and disability, manage chronic illness, and improve mobility are commonly reported health-related motivations for exercise by older adults. Another motivation is the desire to improve mental health or mood, for example, by decreasing stress, depression, and anxiety and by improving energy and engagement in life. Older adults, like younger adults, cite appearance-related benefits as another motivation for exercise. Exercise enjoyment has also been associated with higher levels of physical activity and may be especially important for older adults. Exercise self-efficacy, or confidence in one's ability to undertake regular exercise successfully even when faced with obstacles, is a strong predictor of exercise adoption in older age. Finally, previous experience with exercise is associated with current exercise participation.

It is important to remember that older adults, especially older women, may hold more negative attitudes and beliefs about physical activity than younger adults because of inexperience, misconceptions, and stereotypes. Commonly cited barriers to physical activity by older adults, especially older women, include the fear of falling or suffering an exercise-related injury such as a heart attack, lack of self-motivation or willpower, psychological distress (e.g., depression and anxiety), low exercise self-efficacy, and lack of knowledge or experience with the activity. Lack of time is a frequently cited barrier to physical activity by adults in general (Sallis & Owen, 1999; Trost, Owen, Bauman, Sallis, & Brown, 2002). Justine, Azizan, Hassan, Salleh, and Manaf (2013) explored barriers to participation in physical activity and exercise among Asian middle-aged (45-59 years) and older (≥60 years) adults. Employing the Health Belief Model (HBM) to guide their inquiry, the researchers found the most common external barriers (i.e., barriers beyond an individual's control) reported across both age groups to be factors such as "not enough time," "no one to exercise with," and "lack of facilities," while the internal barrier (i.e., factors determined by an individual's personal decision) reported most often by both groups was being "too tired." Consistent with previous research findings, the older adult group also cited "lack of motivation" as a common barrier to participating in physical activity.

Program Factors

Program-related factors include the structure, format, complexity, intensity, convenience, and financial and psychological costs associated with the activity. The majority of older adults prefer moderate-intensity activities instead of more vigorous ones. Physical activities that are convenient, inexpensive, and noncompetitive also tend to be preferred. For example, older adults most often cite walking and gardening as preferred physical activities. Contrary to expectations and stereotypes, many older adults prefer physical activities that can be undertaken outside of a formal class or group setting (Brown, Finkelstein, Brown, Buchner, & Johnson, 2009). Structured group exercise programs have been found to be less appealing to older adults if their fellow exercisers are dissimilar in age to themselves (i.e., much younger in age) (Beauchamp, Carron, McCutcheon, & Harper, 2007) or the group program is not tailored to their individual needs or preferences (Dunlop & Beauchamp, 2013). Although the immediate health and functional outcomes are similar between well-designed community-based group exercise and supervised home exercise programs (Lewis, Peiris, & Shields, 2017), adherence to supervised home-based programs is typically higher than adherence to class or group programs (Ashworth, Chad, Harrison, Reeder, & Marshall 2005; King, Pruitt, et al., 2000).

Environmental Factors

Social and physical environmental factors also influence exercise participation. **Social support** (defined as assistance received through social relationships) from friends, family, and health professionals is positively associated with exercise adoption and maintenance. Social support appears to be, in general, more important to older women than to men, yet many older women do not perceive that they receive support from their physicians and families to be physically active. Physical environmental factors such as the travel distance required for exercise, climate and weather, neighborhood safety, neighborhood walkability, availability of facilities for physical activity (e.g., parks, walking and jogging paths), and aesthetics can also affect physical activity by older adults (King et al., 2011). However, these factors have received relatively little systematic investigation. A review of 31 studies found few consistent associations between physical activity and environmental variables in older adults and called for more diverse and higher-quality research in this area (Van Cauwenberg et al., 2011).

Potential personal, program-related, and environmental barriers to exercise and motivations for exercise by older adults are summarized in the sidebar. By better understanding how these factors affect older adults in general and your clients in particular, you can more effectively select strategies to help your clients overcome or minimize their barriers and enhance their motivations for exercise. We now turn to a description of strategies to promote exercise in older adults.

Theoretical Frameworks for Behavioral Change

Behavioral theories offer systematic ways of viewing relations among variables that are often used to explain and predict behavior as well as guide interventions or program. For senior fitness instructors, theory can be used to systematically guide the choice of elements to include in exercise programs as well as guide what to measure in order to assess the program's impact. In this chapter, we describe four theories or models that have been widely applied to health behavioral change, including physical activity behavior; have been used with older adult samples; lend themselves to intervention strategies by senior fitness instructors; or include a combination of these criteria. These theories and models include the Transtheoretical Model, social cognitive and learning theories, the theory of planned behavior, and relapse prevention models. At the end of this section, we suggest a six-step process based on these four model for helping older adults initiate and maintain behavioral change.

Transtheoretical Model

Changing a behavior such as physical activity can be difficult for adults of any age. The Transtheoretical Model is useful for understanding people's readiness and motivation for change (Prochaska, DiClemente, & Norcross, 1992; Prochaska & Marcus, 1994). The model states that behavioral change is a process that comprises five stages (see figure 7.1). In the precontemplation stage, people have no **intention** to adopt or change a behavior because they may not be aware of the problem, they may be in denial about the problem, or they may be unwilling or uninterested in changing. In the contemplation stage, people are thinking about adopting or changing a behavior in the near future. They are aware of the benefits of the behavior but are also acutely aware of the difficulties of changing. In the preparation stage, people intend to take action to change their behavior in the immediate future and have generally taken initial steps toward change. For example, they may have purchased walking shoes, joined a gym, or begun to take short walks in the neighborhood. In the action stage, people have made consistent changes in their behavior but have not yet maintained the behavior for a long period of time. Finally, people in the maintenance stage have been participating in the desired behavior for at least six months. Self-efficacy (or confidence to perform a behavior), which is described in more detail in the next section, generally is assumed to increase across the different stages of change. Decisional balance, or the weighing of pros and cons in considering an active lifestyle, may also change across stages from a greater proportion of cons (e.g., "I don't have time for physical activity") in the early stages of change, to an increasing proportion of pros ("Physical activity helps me reduce stress") in the later stages of change. Most clients seen by physical activity instructors are in the preparation,

Exercise Barriers and Motivations for Older Adults

Barriers to Exercise

Health and Medical
- Illness or injury
- Pain or discomfort
- Lack of strength or stamina

Knowledge
- Lack of knowledge
- Lack of ability

Motivational or Psychological
- Lack of time
- Lack of self-motivation (feeling lazy or unmotivated)
- Not a priority
- No enjoyment
- Fear of injury
- Low self-efficacy or confidence
- Exercise perceived as inappropriate or unnecessary for older adults
- Poor body image
- Depression or anxiety

Program Related
- Lack of age-appropriate classes
- Intensity too high
- Inconvenient class times or hours of operation
- Program cost

Environmental
- Lack of access to services, public transportation, and recreation facilities
- Low walkability of neighborhood
- Unsafe environment (crime, traffic, etc.)
- Poor weather
- Lack of support from family, friends, health care providers

Data from Brittain et al. (2002).

Motivations for Exercise

Health and Medical
- To feel good physically
- To improve overall health
- To reduce risk of disease
- For rehabilitation
- To maintain or improve mobility
- To maintain or improve ability to do activities of daily living
- To reduce risk of falls
- To improve fitness
- To improve strength
- To reduce or manage body weight

Mental Health
- To have more energy
- To reduce stress and anxiety
- To reduce depression
- To enjoy life more fully
- To feel good mentally

Appearance Related
- To maintain or improve appearance
- To reduce or manage body weight

Social
- For social contact and interaction
- Encouragement by family or friends
- Recommendation of health care provider

Other
- For enjoyment of activity
- For competition or personal challenge

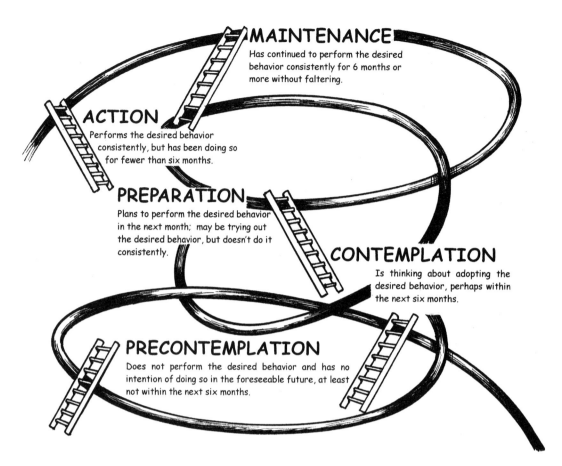

FIGURE 7.1   Stages of change from the Transtheoretical Model.

From the Centers for Disease Control, *Promoting Physical Activity: A Guide for Community Action* (Champaign, IL: Human Kinetics, 1999), 59.

action, or maintenance stage because they have begun to take action toward change. Keep in mind that your clients may not always move forward from one stage to the next. For example, a person who is in the action or maintenance stage of change may relapse to an earlier stage of change when faced with a health or personal crisis.

Perhaps one of the most important lessons from the Transtheoretical Model is that interventions are most successful when they are tailored to the client's general stage of readiness for change. For example, setting specific exercise goals would likely not be useful for a client who is in the precontemplation stage, because the client is not ready to change his or her behavior. It would be more helpful to provide this client with information about exercise that addresses common myths concerning exercise and highlights the utility of regular physical activity for different types of people. Marcus and Forsyth (2003) have described practical ways to apply the Transtheoretical Model to physical activity promotion.

Social Cognitive and Learning Theories

Social cognitive and learning theories (Bandura, 1986a; Bandura, 1977; Baranowski, Perry, & Parcel, 2002) view human behavior as the result of reciprocal interactions between behavior, personal factors, and environmental influences (social and physical). These theories emphasize that people have the ability to change their behavior by setting short-term, intermediate, and long-term goals; monitoring their progress toward reaching these goals; reinforcing their progress toward goals through rewards and incentives; using problem-solving skills to overcome obstacles; and altering their social and physical environments to support their behaviors. These theories emphasize the importance of observational learning of behaviors through role models. They also indicate that people are more likely to attempt a behavior if they believe the behavior will lead to a desired outcome (referred to as outcome expectations or expectancies) and if they are confident that they will be able to successfully perform the behavior, even in the face of barriers or obstacles (referred to as self-efficacy). Many of the behavioral strategies that are described later in this chapter are derived from social cognitive and learning theories.

Self-efficacy, a key construct in social cognitive theory (Bandura, 1982, 1986b, 1997), is strongly related to exercise and other health behaviors in older adults. For clients who have low self-efficacy, there are four ways in which self-efficacy can be learned and enhanced. The most potent way is through performance accomplishments (see list below), because self-efficacy increases when a person successfully executes the specific behavior being targeted. By encouraging clients to set realistic goals that they can meet, physical activity instructors can increase their clients' self-efficacy.

These are four strategies to increase your clients' self-efficacy:

1. *Performance accomplishments.* Encourage realistic goals, and start with activities that your client is likely to have success with. For example, it is often worthwhile to ask what the client has enjoyed doing in the past.

2. *Persuasion.* Encourage clients, and express your confidence in their abilities.

3. *Observational learning.* Demonstrate desired behavior using older adults whom clients can relate to as role models.

4. *Reduced emotional arousal.* Provide appropriate ongoing instruction, demonstration, supervision, and reassurance.

Another way in which self-efficacy can be positively influenced is through persuasion. We have all probably accomplished something we initially thought was very difficult because someone encouraged us to try it and to persist in our attempts. Physical activity instructors can encourage clients over time and express confidence in their abilities.

Of course, it is important that this expressed confidence be genuine. Self-efficacy is also enhanced through observational learning. That is, we often learn by observing another person's behavior and its outcomes and then modeling that behavior. People tend to be most persuaded when the individual they are watching is perceived as similar to themselves (called coping models), when the individual being observed initially struggles with the behavior but ultimately succeeds, and when the individual being observed is rewarded for his or her behavior. Using other older adults as models can be very motivating. A woman who has never exercised could be introduced to a woman who had a similar history but is now regularly active. Finally, emotional arousal that is too high tends to decrease self-efficacy. Our confidence is lowered when we feel nervous or negative about a task or situation. Older adults may have concerns about injuring themselves through exercise, and basic education and reassurance about the risks and benefits of exercise might be useful. For example, some older adults find even small increases in heart rate, respiration, or perspiration concerning, fearing that it is unsafe. Reassurance concerning these types of experiences can help to assuage fears and empower older adults to stick with such activities. Similarly, instruction and supervision in the use of exercise equipment can reduce feelings of anxiety and self-consciousness that an older adult may feel. Enhancing self-efficacy appears to be particularly useful in the initial adoption stage of exercise.

Theory of Planned Behavior and Reasoned Action

The theory of reasoned action (Ajzen & Fishbein, 1980; Fishbein & Ajzen, 1975), which was later expanded into the theory of planned behavior (Ajzen, 1991, 2011), focuses on how beliefs, attitudes, intention, and behaviors are related. The theory states that the most important determinant of behavior is a person's behavioral intention. In other words, a client who intends or plans to start a walking program in the next month is much more likely to do so than another client with low intentions. According to the theory, a client's attitude toward the behavior, **subjective norms** (belief about whether people approve or disapprove of the behavior), and **perceived behavioral control** (perceived control over the behavior, similar to self-efficacy) all influence intentions. When a person has a positive attitude about physical activity, thinks that important people in his or her life approve of the behavior, and thinks that he or she can overcome obstacles to becoming more active, the individual should have increased intention to be active. Furthermore, this theory says that perceived behavioral control can have a direct effect on intention. That is, even when attitude and subjective norms are positive, events outside of one's direct control (e.g., injury, poor weather) can prevent the target behavior from occurring.

Figure 7.2 shows the relations between these theoretical constructs. It also reflects the expectancy-value nature of this theory. That is, attitudes are formed by behavioral beliefs (a belief that performing the behavior is associated with certain attributes or outcomes) combined with evaluation of those behavioral beliefs (value attached to the attribute or outcome). Therefore, attitudes toward physical activity should be most positive when a person believes that physical activity will lead to certain outcomes and these outcomes are rated favorably. For example, an older adult may believe that physical activity will improve his mobility, and improvements in mobility are valued. Similar expectancy-value constructs operate for subjective norms and perceived behavioral control. In research settings, initial elicitation studies are conducted to learn the behavioral beliefs, normative beliefs, and control beliefs most salient to the population of interest. These beliefs then serve as targets for interventions. In practice settings, you can better understand these constructs and guide your approach by asking older adults the following questions: What are the good and bad things that would come from being more physically active (behavioral beliefs)? How important are these outcomes to you (evalu-

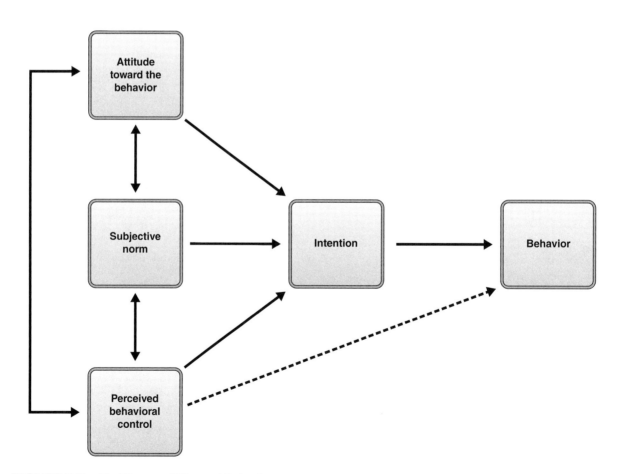

FIGURE 7.2   The Theory of Planned Behavior.

Reprinted from I. Ajzen, "The theory of planned behavior," *Organizational Behavior and Human Decision Processes* 50, (1991): 182.

ation)? Do people important to you, such as your family, friends, or physician, think you should or should not be physically active (normative beliefs)? How motivated are you to do what these people think you should do (motivation to comply)? What are some things that help you or get in the way of you taking part in physical activity (control beliefs)? How strong or how powerful are each of these factors (perceived power)?

Note that while the theory of planned behavior has been studied frequently in observational investigations, it has been applied less systematically than social cognitive and learning theories in developing actual interventions or programs in the physical activity area. In addition, evidence suggests that intentions to be active do not always translate into actual increases in physical activity. An example of this is the so-called New Year's Resolution Effect. In fact, if intentions were sufficient to lead to sustained physical activity increases, most of the U.S. population, including older adults, would be sufficiently active. Unfortunately, this is not the case.

Relapse Prevention Models

Models of relapse prevention (Marlatt & Gorden, 1985) originate from the study of addictive disorders. According to these models, when a person encounters a high-risk situation and has adequate coping responses, self-efficacy will be increased, and a relapse back to unwanted behaviors will be unlikely. However, without a coping response, the person's self-efficacy will decline and he or she will focus on the positive aspects of the undesirable behavior. For example, after a stressful day (the high-risk situation) the person might focus on how eating a large meal and watching television would be more pleasant than going for a walk. As a result, the person will likely engage in the undesirable behavior, forgo the desirable behavior, or both, and then may experience a loss of control and feelings of guilt. This lapse in behavior combined with the negative emotions associated with the lapse will lead to an increased probability of a full-blown relapse (i.e., complete cessation of physical activity). Later in this chapter, we discuss strategies that can reduce the likelihood of relapse.

Based on the models and theories described earlier, a six-step process is suggested for helping older adults initiate and maintain behavioral change.

Step 1: Explore Initial Expectations and Exercise Objectives

Clients enter an exercise program with vastly different expectations about exercise and what it will do for them (i.e., outcome expectations or perceived benefits). It is important for these initial expectations to be explicitly discussed for at least two reasons. First, these expectations should dictate the type of exercise program that is recommended. Clearly, different programs should be recommended to an overweight older adult who wants to lose weight, to a frail older adult who wants to improve balance and reduce the risk of falls, and to a healthy but less active older adult who wants to run a 10K race. Second, a discussion of expectations can indicate how realistic these goals are. A client who expects to lose 20 pounds (9 kg) in two months through a walking program is likely to be very disappointed after two months of hard work and little weight loss. You can correct clients' misconceptions that are revealed during your initial screening and discussion and thus prevent later disappointments that could cause them to drop out of the program.

Step 2: Help Each Client Set Personalized and Realistic Goals

The next step is to assist each client in setting goals for achieving her or his overall objectives. In goal setting, your role is to help direct the client toward appropriate goals. It is critical, however, that the client take primary responsibility for setting his or her own goals. The role of the physical activity instructor is to ask questions ("How likely is it that you can meet that goal next week?"), request clarification ("What days will you exercise next week?" "What time of day works best for you?"), and make suggestions ("I've found that focusing only on weight loss can be frustrating for many people. I suggest that we work together to set goals around your actual walking—goals that you have more control over. We'll keep your longer-term objective in mind when setting these goals."). Ideally, exercise goals should not be prescribed or dictated by the instructor, given that the client's buy-in and commitment to the goals is essential for successful behavioral change.

Characteristics of Effective Goals

An important role of the physical activity instructor is to ensure that goals meet four requirements: They should be measurable, specific, realistic, and behavioral. First, ask yourself, "Will my client know when he or she has met his or her goal?" That is, can the goal be measured? An example of a measurable goal is, "I will attend an exercise class three days per week for the next month." An example of a goal that cannot be easily measured is, "I will exercise more." It is not clear how *more* is defined here. Goals must also be specific. A specific goal, such as, "I will attend the 10:00 a.m. exercise class on Mondays, Wednesdays, and Fridays," helps the client plan his or her behavior and increases the likelihood of meeting the goal.

Next, a goal must be realistic. People are likely to be very motivated when they first begin an exercise program and may set unrealistically high goals. Although you do not want to dampen your clients' enthusiasm, you also want to be sure that their goals are realistic. In general, it is best for clients initially to set small goals that they are quite certain can be achieved. If goals are not met, clients are likely to feel that they have failed and to be at increased risk of dropping out of the exercise program. Overly ambitious goals can also lead to soreness or injury.

Finally, although clients often focus on physiological or performance-related outcomes, such as weight loss or improved strength and fitness, physical activity instructors should encourage clients to set behavioral outcome goals, such as attending three aerobic exercise classes and two strength-

> Your client's goals should have these characteristics:
>
> *Measurable*. Your client should be able to determine whether or not the goal was met.
>
> *Specific*. Your client should specify when he or she will perform the exercise.
>
> *Realistic*. Goals that your client is sure to achieve will enhance self-efficacy.
>
> *Behavioral*. Your client has more direct control over goals that are behavioral (e.g., walking three times per week) than goals that are outcome-oriented (e.g., losing 10 pounds).

training sessions per week. Physiological and performance-related outcome goals, such as weight loss, often take a long time to achieve, and the client may feel frustrated if progress is slow. In contrast, clients have much more control over their behavior than over these types of outcomes of their behavior. Encourage clients to view exercise as important in and of itself, with an array of benefits that go well beyond weight loss and similar outcomes.

Short-Term and Long-Term Goals

Both short-term and long-term exercise goals are important. Clients often focus on long-term goals. For example, they may want to increase strength by a certain percentage, lose 50 pounds (23 kg),

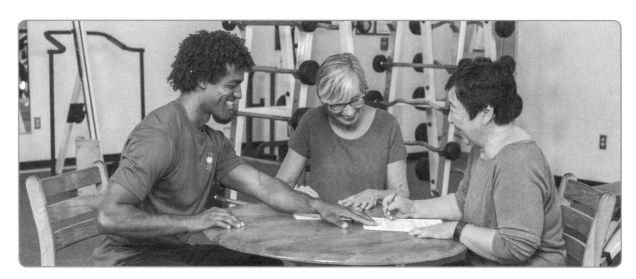

Assist your clients in setting short- and long-term goals.

be able to touch their toes, or run a 5K road race. However, when initiating a new behavior, the client must set short-term goals that are almost certain to be achieved. It is hard to stay motivated when your only goal is to lose 50 pounds, because this goal takes time to achieve. Encourage clients to set daily and weekly exercise goals. Your clients will experience a sense of accomplishment and mastery when they achieve what they set out to do. Achieving these short-term goals is also the most potent way for your clients to increase their self-efficacy, an important determinant of future behavior. Monitor your clients' progress on longer-term goals and adjust short-term goals. Like short-term goals, long-term goals should have a behavioral focus. For example, one woman's short-term goal might be to attend two aerobic exercise classes per week for the next two weeks. Her long-term goal might be to increase her frequency to three aerobic exercise classes per week and to engage in upper- and lower-body resistance training two days per week by the sixth month of her program. Goals should be discussed, monitored, and adjusted regularly based on the client's progress, health status, and long-term objectives.

Step 3: Provide Feedback and Monitor Goals

Physical activity instructors often help their clients to set goals but then never review their progress toward these goals. Regularly review your clients' goals, their successes, and their struggles. Focusing on successes as well as struggles shows you what factors help clients meet their goals. You can then point out these helpful factors to your clients during periods when they struggle. Goals should be frequently reviewed (every week or two) with your clients at the start of a program and less frequently (monthly or bimonthly) after they have succeeded in meeting some of their goals.

Encourage clients to use a log for self-monitoring (such as the exercise log shown in figure 7.3) where they can record the activity, its duration, its intensity, and any other information that may be relevant to the program (e.g., their mood or energy level). Many online and mobile self-monitoring tools are now available and may be of interest to more technology-savvy older adults. Pedometers, or step counters, are a low-cost and potentially effective way to

Day	Description of physical activity	Duration of activity (minutes)	Heart rate or RPE*	Other comments
Sunday				
Monday				
Tuesday				
Wednesday				
Thursday				
Friday				
Saturday				
My exercise goals for next week:				

* Rating of perceived exertion using the Borg CR10 scale.

FIGURE 7.3 Sample exercise log.

self-monitor a walking program. Research has shown that clients who engage in more self-monitoring are more likely to change their health behaviors (Burke, Wang, & Sevick, 2011; Conroy et al., 2011).

In addition to providing feedback and monitoring progress toward goals, conducting a behavioral analysis with your older adult clients can be useful. A **behavioral analysis** is a systematic way of examining the factors that increase or decrease the likelihood of exercising. An easy way to remember how to conduct a behavioral analysis is to focus on the ABCs of behavioral change. "A" represents the antecedents to behavior. **Antecedents** are cues or prompts that set the stage for target (exercise) or nontarget (sedentary) behavior. They include thoughts, emotions, perceived barriers and motivators, and factors in the physical and social environment that affect behavior. Some antecedents increase the likelihood of the target behavior. For example, leaving walking shoes by the bed serves as a reminder to walk the next morning and increases the likelihood of walking. Conversely, emotional antecedents such as feeling stressed or tired decrease the likelihood of exercising. Encourage clients to use cues and prompts in their environment that increase the likelihood of exercise (for example, having a coworker or spouse ask about their exercise program). "B" represents the behavior itself. The type, intensity, location, and purpose of the activity (e.g., for the purpose of recreation as opposed to transportation) have differing antecedents and consequences that can, in turn, influence future behaviors. "C" represents the **consequences** of the behavior; that is, those circumstances that immediately occur surrounding a behavior. These consequences can be reinforcing or punishing. Receiving praise for exercising or enjoying the social aspects of an exercise group are examples of reinforcing consequences that increase the likelihood of future exercise. It's important to understand that most people are influenced much more by the *immediate* consequences of their actions (e.g., how they feel after exercising) rather than by more distant consequences (e.g., losing weight or reducing the risk of chronic disease). Examples of punishing consequences are feeling uncomfortably fatigued after exercise or having a spouse complain that you are never around because of your new exercise program. Punishing consequences decrease the likelihood of future exercise. The choice of the behavior itself can impact the

types of consequences experienced. For example, vigorous exercise may cause muscle soreness or injury, which reduces the likelihood of adhering to the program. Walking in a park, on the other hand, may be very pleasant, increasing the likelihood that older adults will continue this type of activity. Finally, walking that is done for transportation rather than exercise has different antecedents and consequences. Of particular note, whether consequences are perceived as rewarding and motivating as opposed to unpleasant and punishing depends on each specific individual. It's therefore important to listen to each client's perspectives related to finding rewarding, immediate consequences for him or her. For example, while one client may find participating in exercise groups to be motivating and fun, another client may find such groups to be overwhelming, intimidating, or inconvenient.

When conducting an individualized behavioral analysis, focus on the ABCs:

- Identify *antecedents* to your client's behavior. Antecedents are thoughts, emotions, perceived barriers and motivators, and aspects of the environment that set the stage for or "cue" target (exercise) versus nontarget (sedentary) behavior.

- Assess the *behavior* linked with the antecedents. For example, does your client skip his or her exercise session on days he or she finds stressful? What type of behavior does your client choose? Is the activity enjoyable to and realistic for your client?

- Examine whether the immediate *consequences* of your client's behavior are reinforcing or punishing.

Your behavior as the instructor is also important in the ABC model. Providing appropriate warm-up and cool-down exercises; matching the exercise intensity to the abilities of the clients; providing regular praise, encouragement, and a nonjudgmental attitude; and displaying warmth to clients are examples of instructor-related antecedents, behaviors, and consequences that can affect your clients' exercise behaviors. Chapter 16 offers more in-depth discussion of the qualities associated with good leadership and instruction.

An individualized behavioral analysis involves exploring with the client the events, feelings, and situations that tend to trigger exercise or sedentary behavior, aspects of the exercise itself that increase or decrease exercise (e.g., the type, intensity, and setting of the exercise), and the reinforcing or punishing consequences of exercise (see table 7.1). This can be done through a discussion with the client, a short questionnaire that asks about these issues, or the client's keeping a log or diary for a week that records the factors that facilitate or impede physical activity. Once these relationships are outlined, you can work with the client to modify the antecedents of the behavior, aspects of the behavior itself, and the consequences of the behavior in order to increase the likelihood of continuing to exercise. The reinforcing antecedents and consequences change over time, so it is important to reexamine this framework throughout the program.

Another way to help clients attain their exercise goals is to encourage them to seek out social support for exercise. It has consistently been found that social support is related to exercise participation; those who receive more social support for exercise have higher rates of adherence than those who receive less social support. Social support can come from the client's family, friends, coworkers, exercise classmates, or physical activity instructor. Social support provided by an exercise partner can be very useful to some individuals, but social support can take many other forms. As a physical activity instructor, you have valuable *informational support* to share with clients: advice, suggestions, and information regarding exercise. *Instrumental* or *tangible support* is another type of social support that is often practical in nature, for example, a spouse's help in preparing dinner to free up more time for walking or a friend's offering a ride to attend an exercise program. *Emotional support* generally refers to expressions of love and empathy and can include encouragement for being active. Many people are reluctant to ask for help. It can be useful to discuss with clients the type of support they need and then brainstorm ways to get this support. You can also convey encouragement and genuine concern for your clients through your actions and by fostering a supportive program environment.

Once the client has identified his or her objectives, set short- and long-term goals, and developed a plan for modifying behavioral antecedents and consequences, it can be useful for the client to sign

Table 7.1 Behavioral Analysis

Antecedent	Behavior	Consequence
The likelihood of exercising decreases		
Spouse complains that client never spends time with him because she is always exercising.	Client misses exercise session.	Client receives attention and affection from spouse.
Client is in a hurry and does not do any warm-up exercises.	Client completes exercise session.	Client experiences muscle soreness the following day.
Client is busy during the holidays.	Client skips exercise sessions.	Client feels guilt and a sense of failure.
The likelihood of exercising increases		
Client lays out exercise clothes for the next day at bedtime.	Client attends morning exercise class.	Client enjoys the social interaction of the class.
Client reminds himself or herself of the health benefits of exercise when not in the mood to exercise.	Client completes exercise session.	Client's children praise him or her for adhering to the exercise program.
Client's spouse offers to walk with him or her.	Client and spouse walk together.	Client enjoys the interaction and feels supported.

a written **behavioral contract** (Gerber, Bloom, & Ross, 2010; Haber & Rhodes, 2004; Heneman et al., 2005). This contract should explicitly outline the client's specific goals, how they will be measured, and the consequences of the client's behavior. How will the client be rewarded when the goals are met? What will happen if goals are not met? Both the instructor and the client should receive a copy of the contract, and this contract should be referred to and updated regularly. Behavioral contracts increase a client's commitment to behavioral change and serve as a concrete reminder of the behavioral plan. Figure 7.4 is a sample behavioral contract.

Step 4: Use Rewards and Incentives

Reinforcement has a greater impact on behavior than does **punishment**. Clients should be encouraged to reward themselves for meeting their behavioral goals. You can ask clients, "What will you do to reward yourself when you reach this goal?" It is important that the client choose his or her own rewards, since what is reinforcing for one person may not be reinforcing for another. Physical activity instructors can also build reinforcements into their programs, such as praising clients, offering incen-

---

Exercise is important to me because (list the benefits you hope to receive from exercising):

My specific exercise goals for the next two weeks are to (list your goals; be sure that they are measurable):

To reach these goals, I will exercise (list specific days and times):

To record my behavior, I will:

When I reach my goals, I will reward myself by:

If I don't reach my goals, I will:

My longer-term exercise goals (for the next three to six months) are to:

I agree to work hard toward reaching my exercise goals. I will contact my exercise instructor for assistance if I am having trouble reaching my goals.

Signed: _____ Date: _____

Witness: _____ Date: _____

FIGURE 7.4 Sample behavioral contract.

tives for class attendance, and providing formal recognition. When a person initiates a new behavior, reinforcements should be frequent and consistent. Over time, however, reinforcements should become less frequent, tapering to just occasional. As exercise becomes habitual, the client will ideally find exercise reinforcing in and of itself (intrinsic motivation) and will rely less on external reinforcements (extrinsic motivation).

Step 5: Use Problem Solving to Overcome Obstacles

Even when all these steps are followed, clients will inevitably encounter barriers to adhering to their exercise program. Many of the same techniques described for behavioral analysis can be used to engage the client in problem solving. For example, a client who is always too tired and unmotivated to

---

Client-Generated Problem Solving

Problem

A 68-year-old retired client comes to your office frustrated that he has not been able to exercise all week because he has been baby-sitting for his grandchildren every night (he usually exercises at night). How should you approach this client?

Possible Solutions

- You think of an easy solution to this barrier. Share your solution with the client.
- Ask your client if he has any ideas for overcoming the barrier.

Recommended Approach

Your client can probably come up with a solution on his own, and he is more likely to act on a solution he generates. Try to elicit a solution from your client, and reflect back any emotions you perceive.

Sample Script

Instructor: "It seems that before you started baby-sitting, you were exercising regularly. I can see why you are frustrated. Do you have ideas about how you can get back into your exercise program even though you have this new responsibility?"

Client: "Not really . . ."

Instructor: "So it seems that there is really no way around this barrier?"

Client: "Well, I'm not sure I'd go that far. My exercise program is important to me; it's just that I really like exercising at night, and now I can't."

Instructor: "So it's not an ideal situation, but it sounds as if you might have an idea for getting around it."

Client: "I guess I might be able to exercise in the morning."

Instructor: "OK, that's one option. How confident are you that you could exercise in the morning?"

Client: "I'd say probably 80 percent."

Instructor: "That's not bad. Are you willing to try to adjust your schedule this week and let me know how it goes next week?"

Client: "Yes, I can do that."

exercise at the end of the day might consider exercising first thing in the morning. Again, if barriers are the problem, solutions that are generated by the clients themselves are most likely to be successful. It is often difficult for physical activity instructors to refrain from giving advice. However, clients are more likely to act on their own solutions. Furthermore, this approach reduces the likelihood of the "yes but" struggle between the instructor and client, when the instructor provides a suggestion and the client responds with why it will not work. An example of how to facilitate problem solving with clients is provided in the sidebar "Client-Generated Problem Solving."

Step 6: Promote Long-Term Adherence

The choice of whether or not to exercise is a daily decision. Although a person's risk of dropping out of an exercise program is often lower when he or she has maintained participation for six months or longer, **lapses** (i.e., missing several exercise sessions) and **relapses** (i.e., returning to a sedentary state) are the rule rather than the exception for many. Once your client has incorporated an exercise program into his or her lifestyle, it is a good time to introduce relapse prevention strategies.

Helping clients to view lapses and relapses as a normal part of behavioral change can be useful. Encourage clients to identify situations when they are likely to experience lapses or relapses in their exercise program. The most common situations include travel, holidays, illness, stress, fatigue, poor weather, and competing family obligations. When clients anticipate these high-risk situations and develop strategies (both cognitive and behavioral) to deal with them, they are better prepared in the actual situations and tend to have higher self-efficacy in coping with them. Illness and family obligations, particularly caregiving, are especially relevant for older adults. It can be difficult for anyone to restart an exercise program after recovering from a cold or flu, but it is particularly challenging for older adults, who tend to remain ill longer and may experience a greater loss of function during this period.

Many thoughts go through a person's mind when deciding whether or not to exercise. Thoughts such as "I'm too tired" and "I'm not in the mood" often precede (i.e., are antecedents to) the decision to not exercise. An important part of relapse prevention is helping people question their "all-or-nothing" thinking. After missing an exercise session or two, a person often feels as though he or she has completely failed. This person might decide to wait until the following week or the following month or even the following year to resume their program. In addition, it is common to feel discouraged when goals are not met and outcomes are not reached. These thoughts can lead to a brief lapse in an exercise program or to quitting the program altogether.

Clients can be taught to replace their negative thoughts with more realistic or positive ones. The first step is for the client to be aware of his or her thoughts and how thoughts lead to behaviors. Encourage clients to challenge their thoughts. A useful technique is to ask what the client would say to a friend with the same thought, and encourage the client to focus on similar advice. You can also model healthy thoughts by emphasizing that adherence is not an all-or-nothing phenomenon. For example, when a client says, "I had a stressful week and only exercised twice—I really blew it," you can respond, "I think it's great that you were still able to get in two sessions, despite your stressful week!" It is important that neither you nor the client forgets that engaging in *some* level of physical activity is better than engaging in *no* physical activity.

Although it is important to brainstorm ways to overcome barriers and high-risk situations, there will inevitably be times when it is nearly impossible for a person to exercise. One strategy that may initially seem counter to your natural instincts is to schedule a brief, planned lapse with your client. It is important that the time frame of the lapse be defined very specifically. Also, the client should have a very specific plan for resuming the exercise program after the lapse. Otherwise, it can be difficult to start up again after the scheduled time has passed. A planned lapse gives the client permission to stop exercising, and thus the client is less likely to feel guilty or to view herself or himself as a failure, which is a common trigger for a relapse.

Finally, an important aspect of relapse prevention is helping clients to differentiate between a lapse and a relapse. The all-or-nothing trap is powerful, and clients should be reminded to view exercise and adherence as a continuum. This more realistic view reduces negative thoughts and emotions associated with lapses, thus reducing the likelihood of a complete relapse. A summary of cognitive and behavioral strategies to increase exercise adherence is shown in table 7.2.

Physically Active Lifestyles

As a supplement to increasing participation in regularly scheduled, leisure-time physical activity, all participants should be encouraged to look for additional, more routine forms of physical activity to add to their day. Given that overall volume of physical activity is positively related to a range of positive health outcomes (PAGAC, 2018), clients should be encouraged to find ways of increasing their energy expenditure and reducing the time spent in sedentary behaviors (e.g. sitting, watching TV) outside their formal exercise group or personal training program. Given that older adults are at the highest risk for sedentary lifestyles and are the most sedentary segment of the American population (i.e., 60% of their waking hours is spent in sedentary behaviors), it is particularly important that you help your older adult clients identify physical activities they can do outside of your structured physical activity program (Matthews et al., 2008). For instance, taking stairs rather than elevators, parking farther from stores to allow more walking, and other ways to increase walking during daily chores and routine activities should all be encouraged as part of a well-rounded physical activity program. The Active for Life program tested, in community settings, two evidence-based programs that aim to increase lifestyle physical activity: Active Living Every Day and Active Choices. Both programs, when implemented in community settings across the United States by nonacademic groups, were shown to increase physical activity and improve other parameters of quality of life in midlife and older adults (Wilcox et al., 2008).

You should also encourage your clients to reduce the amount of time they spend in daily sedentary activities such as sitting, watching television, and using computers. A growing body of literature shows that sedentary behaviors are predictive of negative health outcomes, particularly diabetes and cardiovascular disease, independent of how physically active people

Table 7.2 Cognitive and Behavioral Strategies to Increase Exercise Adherence

Strategy	Explanation
Behavioral analysis	Conduct a behavioral analysis, and work with clients to determine ways to modify antecedents and consequences of their exercise behavior.
Behavioral contract	Use a behavioral contract that specifies exercise goals and the consequences of both reaching and not reaching those goals.
Social support	Encourage clients to enlist social support for their exercise program from family, friends, exercise classmates, and fitness instructors. Provide support and encouragement to clients in your exercise program, and identify ways to promote support in exercise classes.
Self-efficacy	Aim to increase clients' self-efficacy by ensuring that their goals are realistic and can be met, providing peer role models, offering encouragement, and providing instruction to decrease anxiety and self-consciousness.
Cognitive	Encourage clients to replace unhelpful thoughts (e.g., all-or-nothing views of adherence) with more productive thoughts.
Preparation for lapses and relapses	Prepare clients for lapses and relapses, develop strategies to reduce their occurrence, and consider scheduling planned lapses.
Reassessing and adjusting goals	Periodically reassess clients' exercise goals and help them adjust goals as needed.
Reassessing physical performance	Periodically reassess clients' physical performance and help them adjust exercise goals as needed.

are (Proper, Singh, van Mechelen, & Chinapaw, 2011). A small pre–post study conducted with older adults showed that using strategies similar to those described in this chapter (e.g., goal setting, self-monitoring) were effective in reducing sedentary time and increasing physical activity in a sample of older Australian adults (Gardiner, Eakin, Healy, & Owen, 2011).

Implications for Program Design and Management

The cognitive and behavioral strategies described in this chapter can be applied in many different settings, to a variety of physical activities, and across a range of older adults' functional levels. For example, the strategies described in this chapter have been successfully applied in supervised home-based programs as well as in group programs; in resistance training, fall prevention, aerobic conditioning, and active lifestyle programs; using face-to-face communication as well as communication through print, telephone, and different communication technologies; and among populations ranging from frail older adults to high-functioning, healthy older adults (Ettinger et al., 1997; Hughes et al., 2006; Jette et al., 1999; King et al., 2007; King, Haskell, Taylor, Kraemer, & DeBusk, 1991; King, Pruitt, et al., 2000; Kolt et al., 2012; Kolt, Schofield, Kerse, Garrett, & Oliver, 2007; Martinson et al., 2010; Opdenacker, Boen, Coorevits, & Delecluse, 2008; Opdenacker, Delecluse, & Boen, 2011; Pahor et al., 2006; Rejeski et al., 2003; Stewart et al., 1997; Stewart et al., 2001; van Stralen, de Vries, Mudde, Bolman, & Lechner, 2011). There have also been a growing number of studies showing that peer volunteers can be trained to effectively implement these types of behavioral programs (Buman et al., 2011; Castro, Pruitt, Buman, & King, 2011; Layne et al., 2008; West et al., 2011).

As noted in the preceding section, the strategies across these studies can be delivered through different formats. For example, behavioral change strategies and action plan progress can be reviewed in person at the individual or group level, via telephone, mail, or other electronic methods (e.g., email, texts). Alternatives to in-person contact can be particularly useful for older adults, who may have more difficulty attending group programs due to transportation problems, scheduling conflicts, or family caregiving responsibilities.

A critical requirement in all these various situations is that you tailor the program and strategies to each client's needs, physical and cognitive abilities, interests, and preferences. These strategies cannot be applied in a one-size-fits-all manner. Therefore, you must possess the flexibility and creativity required to meet clients at their level. Most physical activity instructors enjoy working with older adults and are interested in helping people. These are two of the most important characteristics that you can possess, but they are not enough. Researchers have found a number of characteristics of helping professionals that predict positive behavioral outcomes, regardless of the type of intervention or treatment (Goldstein & Higginbotham, 1991; Marzano, 2007). These characteristics include being a good listener and having empathy, flexibility, openness, genuineness, and competence. Important instructor characteristics are described in greater depth in chapter 16.

The specific ways in which strategies described in this chapter can be integrated into exercise programs depend on the nature and format of the program. In some, though not all, exercise programs, the instructor has an opportunity to meet with clients individually and focus on goal setting and behavioral analysis. Prepared worksheets, such as the behavioral contract and self-monitoring log shown in this chapter, help facilitate this process and make it more time efficient. These worksheets also provide the client with something to take home as a reminder of the goals and behavioral plan. In group exercise programs, self-monitoring logs and behavioral contracts can be distributed before or after class.

Exercise instructors can also focus on a different behavioral strategy at each session. For example, during the cool-down portion of an exercise class, the instructor might discuss social support and strategies to increase it. Topics can be presented in rotation. Praising clients, facilitating group cohesion by using clients' names, and arriving early to class to talk with clients are also good ways to incorporate reinforcement and social support into your program. For group or facility-based programs, the physical environment should reinforce cognitive and behavioral strategies. Bulletin boards can be used to highlight a "client of the month" and to present behavioral strategies. For telephone-based interventions, semi-structured telephone scripts can be used to review progress toward goals. When clients are not meeting goals, you can encourage them to use problem-solving strategies, review antecedents to their behavior, and use positive reinforcement. Phone calls can also emphasize the importance of social support and relapse-prevention strategies. For mail-based monitoring, tear-off reply forms or postcards can be used for the client to indicate progress toward established goals, any new goals, and how they are dealing with barriers. Prepared mailings (e.g., tip sheets on common barriers) can then be sent to address the specific issues indicated by the client.

The effectiveness of your behavioral interventions should be monitored and evaluated. Relevant questions that your evaluation could address include, "Are clients' needs being met?" "Are clients improving their health and well-being?" and "What strategies do clients find most and least useful?" Evaluations do not need to be expensive or time-consuming to conduct. For example, client surveys, suggestion boxes, and monitoring attendance before and after implementing a behavioral modification strategy are relatively simple ways to evaluate your program.

Summary

Despite the many benefits that can be achieved through regular physical activity, dropout rates from exercise programs remain high. Factors that influence the adoption and maintenance of physical activity are multidimensional and include personal characteristics, program factors, and environmental characteristics (social and physical).

Cognitive and behavioral strategies, many of which are derived from theoretical models of behavioral change, can enhance exercise adoption and maintenance. These strategies can be used in individual and group settings. A client's readiness for change and self-efficacy are characteristics that should be assessed very early in a program. The next step is to explore clients' initial expectations about exercise and their overall objectives and to use this information to guide the choice of activities and goals. Goals should be generated by clients rather than by instructors, although instructors can facilitate goal setting. Regularly reviewing progress and revising goals, encouraging the use of self-monitoring logs, helping clients assess the antecedents and consequences of their behavior (behavioral analysis), using behavioral contracts, and encouraging clients to enlist social support for change are techniques to enhance goal attainment. Finally, long-term maintenance of physical activity is critical. Relapse prevention strategies include helping clients to identify high-risk situations, to view lapses as a normal part of behavioral change, to reduce all-or-nothing thinking regarding adherence, and to schedule planned lapses in some circumstances.

The cognitive and behavioral strategies discussed in this chapter can be applied to different types of clients, settings, and physical activities. However, they must be tailored to the client's individual needs, abilities, and interests. Physical activity instructors can incorporate behavioral strategies into group exercise programs as well as individual programs by presenting behavioral strategies during the class (e.g., during warm-up or cool-down), distributing self-monitoring logs and behavioral contracts, creating a physical environment that emphasizes behavioral strategies, and creating a social environment that supports and encourages clients. Physical activity instructors are encouraged to use cognitive and behavioral strategies in their programs for older adults in a flexible and individualized manner.

Key Terms

adherence

adoption

antecedents

attitudes

behavioral analysis

behavioral contract

consequences

intention

lapses

perceived behavioral control

punishment

reinforcement

relapses

social support

subjective norms

Recommended Reading

Marcus, B.H., & Forsyth, L.H. (2009). *Motivating people to be physically active.* (2nd ed.). Champaign, IL: Human Kinetics.

Study Questions

1. Which factor or factors influence the initiation and maintenance of physical activity?
   a. personal characteristics
   b. program factors
   c. environmental characteristics
   d. all of the above

2. Which demographic factor or factors are associated with sedentary behaviors?
   a. female sex
   b. male sex
   c. low socioeconomic status
   d. both a and c

3. Your client sets a short-term behavioral goal to "exercise more." Which of the following characteristics does this goal lack?
   a. specific
   b. realistic
   c. measurable
   d. a and c

4. Which of the following is true about exercise goals?
   a. Short-term goals should focus on behavioral outcomes (e.g., exercise), whereas long-term goals should focus on physiological outcomes (e.g., weight loss).
   b. Short-term goals should focus on physiological outcomes, whereas long-term goals should focus on behavioral outcomes.
   c. Both short- and long-term goals should focus on behavioral outcomes.
   d. Both short- and long-term goals should focus on physiological outcomes.

5. Which of the following is the best description of behavioral analysis?
   a. examining the antecedents and consequences of a behavior
   b. examining ways to decrease undesirable behavior
   c. examining ways to increase desirable behavior
   d. developing a system of rewards and punishments for behaviors

6. Your client has never done strength-training exercises before and is convinced that she cannot do them. Although all of the following strategies would increase her self-efficacy, which one is expected to be *most* effective, according to social cognitive theory?
   a. encouraging and persuading her to try
   b. having her start by lifting very light weights so that she can experience success in strength training
   c. demonstrating how to do each of the exercises
   d. having her watch a peer do each of the exercises

7. According to the theory of planned behavior, what is the best predictor of physical activity?

    a. intentions to be physically active

    b. a positive attitude about physical activity

    c. the belief that others approve of physical activity

    d. situations that support physical activity

8. You are working with a client whom you believe is at risk for having a relapse in her physical activity. Which of the following strategies is unique to relapse prevention models?

    a. tell the client that it is very important that she stick with her program

    b. help the client identify situations that make physical activity difficult and develop a plan to deal with them

    c. tell the client that relapses are very rare

    d. be encouraging and supportive to the client

Application Activities

1. Keep a self-monitoring log for two weeks to get a better sense of what this experience is like for your clients. What did you like and dislike about keeping the log? After you have completed the log, ask one of your clients to keep a log for two weeks. Review the completed log with your client and discuss his or her experiences with keeping the log.

2. Ask one of your new clients to complete a behavioral contract. Practice how you would assist your client in setting measurable, specific, realistic, and behavioral goals and choosing appropriate reinforcements.

3. How would you approach a client who tells you that she is going to drop out of your exercise group because she is not making the progress that she expected? Focus on your listening rather than advice-giving skills.

4. Choose four behavioral change strategies and develop brief descriptions that you can present during the cool-down portion of your exercise classes. Discuss one strategy per class.

PART

III

Core Program Principles and Training Methods

Training Module 1:
Overview of Aging and Physical Activity

Training Module 9:
Ethics and Professional Conduct

Training Module 2:
Psychological, Sociocultural, and Physiological Aspects of Physical Activity and Older Adults

Training Module 8:
Client Safety and First Aid

International Curriculum Guidelines for Preparing Physical Activity Instructors of Older Adults

Training Module 3:
Screening, Assessment, and Goal Setting

Training Module 7:
Leadership, Communication, and Marketing Skills

Training Module 4:
Program Design and Management

Training Module 6:
Teaching Skills

Training Module 5:
Program Design for Older Adults With Stable Medical Conditions

Now that you possess the knowledge and skills to screen and assess your clients and to incorporate cognitive and behavioral change strategies into your exercise programs, the next step in the successful design and implementation of effective physical activity programs for a heterogeneous older adult population is understanding the core exercise principles and training methods. These are presented in part III. Chapters 8 through 14 address content presented in training modules 4 and 5 of the *International Curriculum Guidelines for Preparing Physical Activity Instructors of Older Adults*. Module 4 recommends areas of study that include information about how to use results from screening, assessment, and client goals to make appropriate decisions regarding individual and group physical activity and exercise program design and management. Module 5 recommends areas of study that include information on common medical conditions of older adults, signs and symptoms associated with medication-related negative interactions during physical activity, and how to adapt exercise for clients with different fitness levels and stable medical conditions to help prevent injury and other emergency situations.

- Chapter 8 discusses the relevance of the disability model to physical activity programming for older adults and the potential functional benefits of different types of physical activities that should be included in a well-rounded exercise program for older adults. You will learn how to apply basic exercise principles (e.g., specificity and overload) for effective program design. Some important exercise principles that are unique to the older adult population are also considered.

- Chapter 9 is new to this edition and introduces readers to the concept of whole-person wellness and each of the six dimensions (physical, emotional, intellectual, vocational, spiritual, and social) that contribute to whole-person wellness. The chapter first describes research investigating the role of each of the dimensions in promoting wellness and then presents practical strategies for purposefully and seamlessly integrating each of the six dimensions into a physical activity program.

- Chapter 10 describes acute physiological changes in the neuromuscular, cardiopulmonary, and metabolic systems that occur during the warm-up and cool-down components of an exercise program. Examples of appropriate warm-up and cool-down activities for older adults that engage participants emotionally, socially, cognitively, and spiritually are also presented.

- Chapter 11 provides a discussion of age-associated changes in joint and muscle flexibility and how these changes affect older adults' ability to perform various activities of daily living. Critical ranges of joint flexibility required for these basic activities are also identified. The remainder of the chapter provides examples of dynamic and static flexibility exercises for all the major muscle groups and joints in the body. The dynamic flexibility exercises described are recommended for inclusion in the warm-up, while the static flexibility exercises can be easily incorporated into the cool-down component of the class or performed as a stand-alone component.

- Chapter 12 introduces you to important resistance-training principles (e.g., progressive overload and specificity) and the exercise variables that govern the development of muscle strength, power, and endurance (e.g., resistance, exercise order, sets, number of repetitions, and rest and recovery periods). You will also learn how to design a safe and effective resistance-training component that meets the personal goals and preferences of older adult clients.

- Chapter 13 provides an overview of the exercise principles and variables that must be considered when designing and implementing the aerobic endurance component of a physical activity program. Guidelines for accommodating older adults with different fitness levels and functional abilities are also presented in this chapter.

- Chapter 14 describes how age-associated changes in multiple body systems are likely to affect various dimensions of balance and mobility. This chapter identifies the four essential skills needed for good balance and mobility and then provides a set of progressive balance and mobility exercises that address each of these essential skills. You will learn how to adjust the challenge level of balance exercises to accommodate clients with different balance and mobility skills.

Important Considerations When Designing Exercise Programs for Older Adults

Debra J. Rose

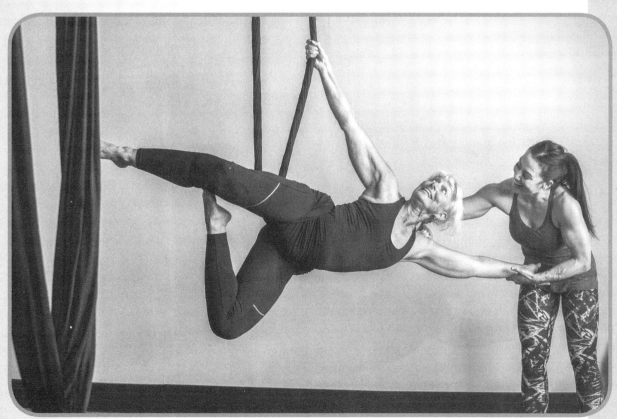

Objectives

After completing this chapter, you will be able to

1. describe an age-appropriate approach to designing and implementing physical activity programs for older adults,
2. discuss current recommendations relative to physical activity for older adults,
3. explain how various types of exercise relate to specific physical functions and activities, and
4. apply exercise principles when developing physical activity programs for older adults.

Designing and implementing exercise programs for older adults requires a thoughtful approach, one that addresses each individual's needs, preferences, and abilities. Traditional approaches to exercise programming for younger adults have generally focused on improving specific physiological parameters, such as cardiorespiratory endurance or muscle strength. These programs are often designed for people with specific goals in mind, such as athletic performance, fitness, body sculpting, or weight reduction. Although these goals may be appropriate for some older adults, alternative goals may be helpful to accommodate the needs of an older adult population that is considerably more diverse. Although many people remain relatively healthy and fit throughout their lives, others experience declines in health, fitness, and overall function. Thus, the older adult segment can range from those who compete as master athletes to those who have difficulty getting up from a chair. The approach presented in this book considers this variability by focusing on functional training and utilization of several senior-specific principles when designing safe and effective exercise programs for older adults across the continuum of function.

This chapter begins by briefly describing the heterogeneity of the older adult population and reasons why some older adults do not age well. I then discuss how this information, combined with screenings and assessments, can guide the planning of physical activity programs for older adults. How different types of activities can affect various dimensions of physical functioning will also be discussed. Currently published national physical activity guidelines and recommendations that address the specific needs of older adults are then summarized. Finally, important exercise principles specific to older adults and how to apply them in the development and implementation of group-based physical activity programs are described.

Heterogeneity of Older Adults

A major shift in the leading causes of death in all groups, including older adults, occurred over the course of the past century. Instead of acute and infectious diseases being the major contributors to death, chronic diseases and degenerative illnesses are now the more common causes of death in the 21st century. Many adults are also aging with multiple chronic conditions, which places a considerable burden on health care resources in the United States and other developed countries. In the United States, it is estimated that two out of three older adults live with multiple chronic conditions (Centers for Disease Control and Prevention, 2013); the leading causes of death due to chronic disease include heart disease, cancer, respiratory diseases, stroke, and Alzheimer's disease. Although many older adults experience multiple chronic conditions, it is important to remember that a good percentage of older adults have no chronic diseases and live very long and healthy lives. It is therefore important that we do not make erroneous assumptions about an older adult's capabilities and design one-size-fits all physical activity programs as a result.

> Chronic diseases and degenerative illnesses as opposed to acute and infectious diseases are now the more common causes of death in the 21st century.

In addition to having variation in the number and types of medical conditions, older adults exhibit a wide range of physical functioning (Seeman, Merkin, Crimmins, & Karlamangla, 2010). **Physical functioning** refers to an individual's ability to perform basic physical actions such as walking, climbing stairs, bending, and reaching. Even among those 75 years of age and older, 32 percent of men and 25 percent of women report no difficulty in functional limitations (Jindai, Nielson, Vorderstrasse, & Quinones, 2016). Similar variation among older adults is found in performance tests of physical functions such as walking or lifting heavy objects (Dumurgier, et al., 2009; Rikli & Jones, 2013). The major practical implication for physical activity instructors is that exercise programs need to be tailored and adapted to accommodate diverse health conditions and physical abilities of older adult clients.

> Most older adults have at least one chronic health condition and some limitation in physical functioning. However, some older adults have no chronic conditions and good functioning. This variation is found even among people 80 years of age and older.

Optimizing Physical Function Through Exercise

The disablement process model described by Verbrugge and Jette (1994; see figure 8.1) is an adaptation of a model originated by Saad Nagi (1976, 1991). According to this model, pathology such as chronic health conditions or injury can lead to impairments in body systems—cardiovascular, musculoskeletal, cognitive, sensory, and motor. Eventually, the accumulated impairments can lead to functional limitations (e.g., problems with walking or stair climbing), and ultimately to disability. **Disability** is an umbrella term that includes impairments, activity limitations, and participation restrictions. The term describes the negative aspects of the interaction occurring between a person (with a health condition) and that person's contextual factors (personal and environmental) (World Health Organization, 2011). As a specific example of this process, loss of muscle strength (a body system impairment) can lead to slower walking times (a limitation in physical functioning), and limitations in walking ability without intervention can lead to disability. However, early identification of emerging impairments and functional limitations, together with appropriately tailored physical activity, can delay or prevent subsequent decline (Daniels, vanRossum, de Witte, Kempen, & van den Heuvel, 2008). In addition, research has shown that exercise can reverse functional decline (Pahor et al., 2006).

A second theoretical perspective suggests that there is a threshold of physical or physiological fitness below which a person becomes dependent on others for help with daily tasks, that is, disabled (Shephard, 1993; Vita, Terry, Hubert, & Fries, 1998). According to this view, people gradually decline but accommodate or compensate for losses; however, below some critical point, they can no longer perform certain daily activities without assistance. According to Shephard (1993), sedentary people generally reach this threshold at about age 80 years, while active people often do not reach this threshold for 10 to 20 more years. Additional markers for physical fitness thresholds are described in chapter 6.

These two theoretical perspectives highlight the critical importance of optimizing physical functioning through exercise. Physical activity instructors can help clients maintain or improve their physical functioning, regardless of where the clients are on the functional continuum. Comprehensive screenings and assessments, as described in chapters 5 and 6, provide physical activity instructors with knowledge about each participant's physical impairments (e.g., reduced aerobic endurance or muscle

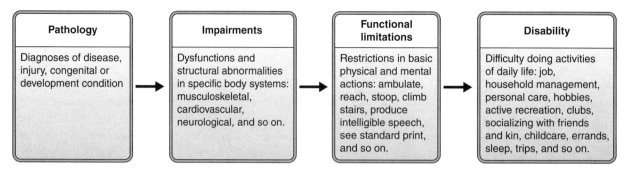

FIGURE 8.1   Disablement process model: The main pathway of a larger model.
Adapted from Verbrugge and Jette (1994).

strength), limitations in physical functioning (e.g., difficulty walking, climbing stairs, bending, or lifting), and disabilities (e.g., difficulty performing tasks such as personal care or shopping errands). Based on results obtained from the initial screening and assessment, physical activity instructors can begin to individualize and prioritize the most appropriate types of exercise for their clients.

Functional Benefits of Exercise

As mentioned earlier, the goals of exercise programs for older adults may differ from the goals for younger adults. One key difference is that many older adults can use exercise to improve or maintain their physical functioning and thus help them stay independent, or avoid disability. For instance,

a certain level of lower-body strength is needed to get out of a bathtub or to climb stairs, and adequate levels of agility, power, and dynamic balance are needed to move out of the way of an approaching car (Rikli & Jones, 2013). Some functional tasks that may be made easier by performing different types of exercise are shown in table 8.1.

Exercise benefits can be made more salient to older adults if the benefits can be directly linked to the ability to remain independent. The physiological (fitness) benefits derived from exercise may be too abstract or uninteresting for some older adults. Many clients may be motivated more by self-identifying important tasks and activities of daily life and recreation and then having a physical activity instructor explain how various types of exercises can help them maintain or improve their ability to do these activities.

Table 8.1   Functional Tasks That May Improve With Exercise Training

Type of exercise training	Functional tasks
Aerobic endurance	Walk in order to complete errands or attend events, perform activities requiring stamina such as vacuuming and raking, climb stairs
Resistance exercise for upper body and trunk	Lift and hold a grandchild, place luggage in overhead storage during travel, carry groceries, open heavy doors, perform garden work such as pulling weeds, perform housework such as washing windows
Resistance exercise for lower body	Stand up from the floor, get into and out of a chair or bathtub, climb stairs, pick up a package from the floor, step onto a curb
Flexibility exercise for upper body	Turn head to look at traffic while driving or walking, fasten a zipper on the back of a dress, scratch an itch on the back, reach overhead to a cupboard, comb hair
Flexibility exercise for lower body and trunk	Put on socks and shoes, inspect feet, cut toenails
Neuromotor fitness activities, including balance, agility, coordination, and gait training	Walk the dog, avoid obstacles, negotiate curbs, climb stairs, pull weeds in the garden, respond appropriately to unexpected losses of balance

Exercise and Physical Activity Guidelines for Older Adults

In 1998, the American College of Sports Medicine (ACSM) published its first position stand on the importance of exercise and physical activity for older adults. The key message from the position stand was that regular exercise and physical activity can improve functional capacity and health and lead to greater independence and quality of life for older adults. Citing strong supportive evidence, the ACSM noted that older adults who participate in regular endurance exercise (such as walking, running, swimming, and cycling) and resistance training can gain many benefits related to healthy aging. Although the position stand reviewed experimental evidence of the benefits of exercise for older adults, it provided very little guidance for physical activity instructors on how best to set exercise variables such as frequency and duration for older adults other than frail and very old individuals. A second position stand was subsequently published by ACSM in 2009 that provided more concrete programming guidelines for physical activity instructors based on evidence related to the benefits of regular physical activity for older adults (Chodzko-Zajko et al., 2009). More specific and global recommendations relative to exercise frequency, intensity, and type were provided for aerobic, resistance, and flexibility exercise. No recommendations were given for balance exercise other than stating that it be included in any program serving "frequent fallers or individuals with mobility problems" (p. 1511).

In 2011, Garber and colleagues published an updated position stand that included specific recommendations for incorporating **neuromotor fitness** training into any exercise prescription designed for older adults. The authors recommended that older adults engage in comprehensive exercise programs that include components aimed at improving cardiorespiratory function, muscle strength, flexibility, and neuromotor fitness. As explained by the authors, neuromotor fitness training "incorporates motor skills such as balance, coordination, gait, agility, and proprioceptive training" (p. 1345). The updated recommendations were intended for all adults, regardless of age and functional ability. Based on the available evidence, it was recommended that apparently healthy adults, irrespective of age, engage in neuromotor fitness training at least two to three days per week for at least 20 to 30 minutes each day. The types of activities recommended include exercises that involve motor skills (e.g., balance, agility, coordination, and gait) as well as proprioceptive exercises and multifaceted activities such as tai chi and yoga. Unfortunately, insufficient evidence was available for any recommendations to be made with respect to exercise intensity, volume, or progression.

> ACSM (2011) recommends that older adults participate in neuromotor fitness activities two to three days per week for at least 20 to 30 minutes each day.

Since their publication in 2008, the national **Physical Activity Guidelines for Americans** (PAGA) have been widely disseminated and used to guide the design of a number of physical activity interventions (U.S. Department of Health and Human Services, 2008; PAGAC, 2018). According to the guidelines, individuals should engage in 150 minutes of moderate-intensity exercise, 75 minutes of vigorous-intensity exercise, or an equivalent combination of moderate- and vigorous-intensity aerobic exercise per week. In addition to aerobic activity, at least two days of resistance training should also be undertaken. In a subsequent update, the American College of Sports Medicine (ACSM) and American Heart Association (AHA) further stated that these guidelines are to be considered minimum requirements for preventing disease, with higher levels of physical activity recommended to gain advanced protection against inactivity-related chronic disease.

Despite the nationwide campaigns to promote the guidelines and the health benefits derived from physical activity in general, the percentage of older adults currently meeting both recommended guidelines remains very low. Using 2011 Behavioral Risk Factor Surveillance System (BRFSS) survey data, Harris et al. (2013) reported that the prevalence of meeting both the aerobic and resistance training guidelines ranged from 30.7 percent in adults between 18 and 24 years of age to 15.9 percent in adults aged 65 years and older (CDC, 2013). Using a more objective physical activity measurement (i.e., body-worn accelerometers), Tucker, Welk, and Beyler (2011) reported even lower levels of physical activity among adults in the United States, estimating that fewer than 10 percent met the 2008 PAGA criterion for aerobic endurance. Their data was drawn from the National Health and Nutrition Examination Surveys (NHANES) 2005-2006.

In his editorial that appeared in the World Health Organization Bulletin, de Souto Barreto (2013) called for a shift in the approach used to promote physical activity participation. He argued that the current physical activity guidelines should still provide a goal to be achieved but not a mandatory one, given that a large number of older adults, particularly those living with multiple chronic diseases or disability, lack the functional capacity to achieve such an insurmountable goal. Similarly, many older adults may simply lack the motivation or be reluctant to engage in moderate- to vigorous-intensity physical activity for fear of injury. Providing data in support for this shift in approach, Loprinzi, Lee, and Cardinal (2015) demonstrated that older adults who engaged in more than 300 minutes per week of what they defined as lifestyle light-intensity physical activity (LLPA) derived significant health benefits (e.g., reduced body mass index, waist circumference, C-reactive protein levels, insulin resistance) when compared to older adults engaging in less than 300 minutes per week. The higher LLPA group also had fewer chronic diseases. A particular strength of this study was that physical activity levels were determined based on accelerometer data obtained from a nationally representative sample of older adults participating in the 2003-2006 National Health and Nutrition Examination Surveys (NHANES). On the basis of their findings the authors called for the refining of the current physical activity guidelines to include light-intensity recommendations in addition to current moderate- to vigorous-intensity physical activity (MVPA) recommendations.

Becoming familiar with the recommendations advanced in the most recent position stand published by the American College of Sports Medicine (ACSM, 2017) as well as the guidelines presented in the 2008 Physical Activity Guidelines for Americans (PAGA; U.S. Department of Health and Human Services, 2008) can help you in at least three ways. The recommendations and guidelines provide (1) evidence-based recommendations for exercise testing and prescription that you can use to design safe and effective exercise programs for older adults, (2) exercise options that can help you

address the individual needs and interests of your clients, and (3) documentation of what constitutes safe practice according to experts in the field, which can help protect you from litigation when followed. Legal issues related to exercise programming are discussed in chapter 18.

Exercise Principles for Program Design

Two major principles of exercise, overload and specificity, need to be addressed when designing exercise programs. The principle of **overload** states that "in order for a training adaptation to take place (an increase in muscular strength or muscle size) a greater-than-normal stress (force or load) must be applied to produce this adaptation" (ACSM, 2018, p. 112). The load can be progressively increased by manipulating the type or mode of exercise selected, the position in which the exercise is performed, or other exercise variables such as the frequency, duration, or intensity of a particular exercise. For example, to improve the cardiovascular system, an older adult could gradually increase the number of days walks are taken, the walking distance, the walking speed, or the incline of the walking surface.

The principle of **specificity** states that the training effects derived from physical activity are specific to the type of exercise and muscles involved (ACSM, 2017). For example, a low-resistance and high-repetition exercise increases the oxidative capacity of the muscle but does little to strengthen the muscle. In contrast, a high-resistance, low-repetition exercise increases strength and muscle size but does little to increase muscle endurance.

Specific Exercise Principles for Older Adults

In addition to the traditional principles of exercise, overload and specificity, experts in gerokinesiology recommend applying three additional principles when designing and implementing physical activity programs for older adults: (1) functional relevance, (2) challenge, and (3) adaptation/tailoring (Gillis

& Stewart, 2005). Your ability to understand and implement these principles exemplifies the specialized knowledge and practical training needed to become an effective physical activity instructor of older adults.

Functional Relevance

The principle of **functional relevance** encourages selecting exercises that simulate the movements of everyday activities to be performed in environments that are similar to those regularly encountered by program participants (Rose, 2010). For instance, during the neuromotor fitness component, participants can practice walking on a variety of surfaces that mimic everything from a thickly carpeted floor to a slick surface similar to an icy sidewalk. To make strengthening activities more functionally relevant, participants could practice picking up a weight such as a bag of groceries, carrying it across the room, and placing it on a shelf. Functional relevance is similar to the exercise principle of specificity, but its focus is on functional activities that simulate movements performed in daily life. The functional relevance principle makes your older adult clients more aware of the connection between their exercise sessions and activities they perform in their daily lives.

> The functional relevance principle encourages the selection of exercises that simulate the movements of everyday activities to be performed in environments that are similar to those regularly encountered by program participants.

Challenge

A second exercise principle related to the functional training of older adults is the **challenge** principle. Selected activities or exercises need to challenge, but not exceed, an individual's intrinsic capabilities (e.g., strength, cognition, sensorimotor ability). For example, the level of challenge can be altered by changing the task demands (seated, standing, or moving; single or multiple task) or the environmental demands (surface type, lighting, visual flow; Rose, 2010) associated with a set of

activities. Additional information about assessing an individual's intrinsic capabilities and then matching them to the task and environmental demands presented in an exercise program is presented in chapters 6 and 15. For a client who has serious balance problems, for example, you should challenge each of the systems that contribute to balance and mobility (i.e., sensory, motor, cognitive) but at the same time provide a safe environment (i.e., a stable surface) so that he or she does not fall. This client could begin walking on a stable surface initially and then gradually progress to more challenging surfaces or to negotiating obstacles in reduced lighting conditions. The challenge could also be manipulated by adding a second cognitive task, such as counting while walking (Rose, 2010). In the resistance-training example of lifting, carrying, and putting away groceries, a participant might start with a light weight and place it on a low shelf and then progress to lifting a heavier weight onto a higher level shelf.

> The principle of challenge emphasizes the need to select activities or exercises that challenge but do not exceed an individual's intrinsic capabilities. The level of challenge of an exercise can be adjusted by changing the task or environmental demands or both simultaneously.

There is a fine line between exercises that challenge a person enough to produce positive effects and those that place a client at risk of injury. The more information you have about your clients' medical conditions, physical status, and psychological state (e.g., exercise self-efficacy, anxiety, mood) the more effective you can be in providing the right amount of challenge safely. Your clients' healthcare providers should be involved as needed. While some of your clients may want to take unnecessary risks, others may prefer to remain within their comfort zones and be reluctant to increase the workload or participate in more challenging exercise progressions. It is important to remind the risk takers to progress more slowly, but it is equally important to gently prompt other clients to challenge themselves a little more (within a safe range). The challenge principle is discussed in more detail in chapter 15.

Adaptation/Tailoring

A third exercise principle that is important to consider when designing exercise programs for older adults is **adaptation/tailoring**. This principle states that highly individualized exercise prescriptions and solutions coupled with appropriate modifications to session goals, structure, or exercise content are necessary to accommodate age- and disease-specific changes that place older adults at higher risk for adverse events in exercise settings. The overload principle informs us that to cause a training effect, an exercise needs to challenge the system beyond what is usual; however, with older adults it is also important to apply the adaptation/tailoring principle. This will ensure that the type of exercise selected and the overall structure of the exercise session acknowledges the fluctuations in health that often occur with the aging process and the wider range of fitness levels that will be observed in group-based exercise settings.

Designing one-size-fits-all physical activity programs are completely inappropriate when the target audience is older adults. Instead, highly individualized exercise prescriptions and solutions that are tailored to the individual needs and preferences of older adults should be a prerequisite for any physical activity program designed for older adults. At all times, physical activity instructors of older adults should also have a graded set of exercise progressions in their instructional toolkit that can be readily matched to each individual client's functional capabilities in any given exercise session. For example, a person experiencing significant changes in the cardiovascular, musculoskeletal, or nervous system may need to be prescribed a longer and more gradual warm-up and a greater rest-to-work ratio when performing the interval conditioning component of the aerobic endurance segment (see chapters 10 and 13 for specific examples on how to tailor/adapt one or both components). A client who may feel comfortably challenged by performing a particular resistance exercise protocol one day may experience very painful knee joints on another day. This fluctuating pain is common among people who have arthritis and other musculoskeletal disorders. To ensure that participants do not attempt to perform at the same level each time regardless of how they

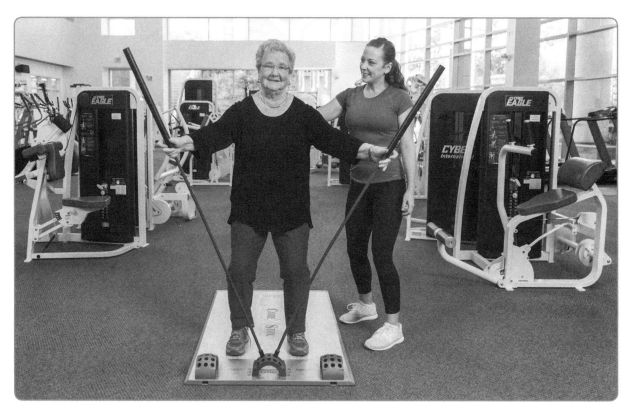

Exercise prescriptions need to be tailored to the individual needs and preferences of your older adult clients.

feel, they should be encouraged to become skilled at listening to their bodies and understanding the signs and symptoms of overexertion.

> According to the adaptation/tailoring principle, modifications to exercise session content and structure, coupled with the provision of individualized exercise prescriptions and solutions, are necessary to accommodate for the fluctuations in health associated with the aging process and wider range of fitness levels observed among older adults.

There are numerous practical implications of these exercise principles for physical activity instructors and personal trainers who wish to tailor programs for their clients. Teaching a group of older adults is generally more challenging because it requires accommodating a wide range of abilities and medical concerns. As such, the chapters that follow in this part of the book primarily focus on group instruction. However, much of the material can also be applied to personal training environments.

Summary

Working with older adults provides unique rewards and challenges for physical activity instructors, stemming from the broad range of states of health and physical functioning of older adults and the focus on maintaining or improving all components of fitness and specific physical functions that affect day-to-day activities. Appropriate aerobic endurance, resistance exercise, flexibility, and neuromotor fitness activities that include balance and mobility may help older adults maintain their independence well into their later years. By understanding the process of disablement and the role of physical activity in preventing or delaying disability, physical activity instructors can select particular types of exercises that meet their clients' goals and needs. By knowing each client's level of functioning, instructors can further tailor or adapt specific types of exercise to target the most essential functions (e.g., lower-body strength training to improve a person's ability to get up from chairs and to walk). The evidence-rich position stands commissioned by the American College of Sports Medicine (Chodzko-Zajko et al., 2009; Garber et al., 2011), coupled with the 2008 Physical Activity Guidelines for Americans (PAGA; U.S. Department of Health and Human Services, 2008) can help instructors become more confident in designing and implementing well-rounded exercise programs with the input of their older adult clients.

Through the judicious application of the exercise principles of specificity, overload, functional relevance, challenge, and adaptation/tailoring, instructors can better help their clients achieve optimal outcomes safely. The following chapters encourage you to adopt this age-appropriate approach when designing group exercise programs that focus on the functional benefits of exercise training. Functional training involves various physical activities that ultimately make the tasks and activities of daily living easier, safer, and more efficient.

Key Terms

adaptation/tailoring

challenge

disability

functional relevance

neuromotor fitness

overload

Physical Activity Guidelines for Americans

physical functioning

specificity

tailoring (*see* adaptation/tailoring)

Recommended Readings

Garber, C.E., Blissmer, B., Deschenes, M.R., Franklin, B.A., Lamonte, M.J., Lee, I.M., . . . Swain, D.P. (2011). *Quantity and quality of exercise for developing and maintaining cardiorespiratory, musculoskeletal, and neuromotor fitness in apparently healthy adults: Guidance for prescribing exercise.* Available at www.acsm.org/public-information/position-stands.

U.S. Department of Health and Human Services. (2008). *Physical activity guidelines for Americans.* Available at www.health.gov/paguidelines/.

Study Questions

1. The disablement process model defines disability as

    a. difficulty or inability to perform complex activities in various domains of life

    b. physical impairments of body systems

    c. functional limitations, such as limitations in walking or bending

    d. a common consequence of aging

2. According to Shephard (1993), sedentary adults generally reach a threshold of physical or physiological fitness at

    a. 90 years of age or older

    b. about 80 years

    c. about 65 years of age

    d. approximately 70 years of age

3. The selection of exercises that simulate movements from everyday activities performed in practice environments that are similar to those regularly encountered by program participants embodies which exercise principle?

    a. challenge

    b. adaptation/tailoring

    c. functional relevance

    d. specificity

4. According to the challenge principle, the level of challenge can be manipulated by presenting which of the following task and/or environmental demands?

    a. perform a task from a seated position versus a standing position

    b. dim the lighting in the room

    c. recite a poem while performing a walking task

    d. all of the above

5. According to the 2008 PAGA guidelines, the minimum level of aerobic physical activity that should be performed each week is

    a. 150 minutes of moderate-intensity physical activity

    b. at least 300 minutes of light-intensity aerobic activity

    c. 75 minutes of vigorous-intensity physical activity

    d. both a and c are correct

6. Potential functional benefits of upper-body strengthening exercises include

    a. improved ability to lift and carry groceries

    b. improved upper-body strength

    c. improved ability to walk

    d. all of the above

Application Activities

1. You are working with an older woman who has just completed the 30-second chair stand test. She was able to complete three chair stands in the 30 seconds, and she commented that it is difficult for her to get up from chairs and couches. Her physician told her that she could perform moderate-intensity exercise, and she has no medical conditions that would cause her difficulty getting up from the chair. Develop a list of discussion topics or questions that can determine (1) her interest in improving her ability to sit down on and get up from chairs, (2) whether she has difficulty in other activities that she does or would like to do, and (3) what types of activities or exercise training could lead to functional benefits that address these areas of concern. Also prepare an explanation that can help her link those types of training to the specific functional benefits, and include in your explanation at least one concept from either of the theoretical perspectives on how older adults become disabled.

2. Applying the principle of functional relevance, plan the activities for an exercise session for an independently living female client age 76. When asked how she spends her time each week, she said that she lives alone and spends a fair amount of time doing household tasks such as laundry and light housekeeping. She typically eats her meals at a nearby senior center, where she volunteers in the art studio. She would like to try a dance or tai chi class at the senior center but knows that some days her balance just isn't as good as it used to be. Her physician has encouraged her to stay active without any restrictions. How might you apply the challenge and adaptation/tailoring principles when designing the balance and mobility component of her program?

3. An older man is interested in starting an exercise program and has asked you what types of exercise are recommended for older adults. He is going to talk to his doctor at an upcoming physical exam and wants some background information about appropriate exercises. Summarize the recommendations from the ACSM position stands (Chodzko-Zajko et al, 2009; Garber et al., 2011) and 2008 Physical Activity Guidelines for Americans (PAGA) resources (U.S. Department of Health and Human Services, 2008; PAGAC, 2018) for him to give to his doctor.

Whole-Person Wellness for Successful Aging

Janis M. Montague
Debra J. Rose
Judy Aprile

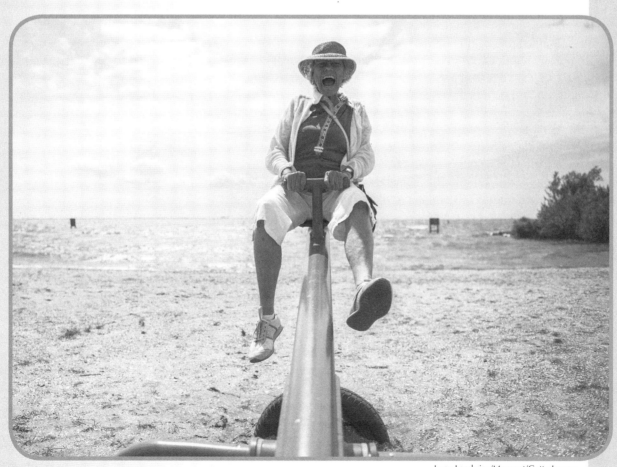

Objectives

After completing this chapter, you will be able to

1. define whole-person wellness and successful aging,
2. describe the multiple dimensions and attributes of whole-person wellness, and
3. integrate a whole-person wellness approach for successful aging into physical activity classes and programs.

The Internet, news sources, social media, and even greeting cards—all are constantly reminding us that the population is aging. Never before in recorded history have we had so many older people living so long. In the United States, life expectancy at birth has increased by as much as 30 years, from 47 years of age in 1900 to 78 years of age in 2010 (Centers for Disease Control and Prevention, 2013). In 1980 there were 25.7 million individuals 65 and older in the United States and by 2050 this group is projected to reach 83.7 million people, or 39.1 percent of the population (United States Census, 2014). Since everyone is aging from birth, this demographic shift has numerous implications for all individuals who want and expect to age well across their life course. So what is required to equate a long life with a successful aging experience? Dr. George Vaillant (2014) states in *Aging Well: Thoughts From a 75-Year-Old Study* that "aging well includes the following characteristics: caring about others; being open to new ideas; and, within the limits of physical health, maintaining social utility, never complaining when you can no longer help others. Aging well means retaining a sense of humor and capacity for play." In this chapter, we will examine how the concept of whole-person wellness for successful aging is becoming a leading model for health management.

Wellness: A Change in Perspective and Perception

To be well, individuals are encouraged to intentionally shift behaviors and perceptions toward a wellness rather than an illness perspective. Older adults benefit in many ways from adopting a positive, wellness-based perception and focusing on what is going right in their lives. For example, Levy and colleagues (Levy, Slade, Kunkel, & Kasl, 2002) found that life expectancies of older adults who held positive views about getting older were as much as 7.5 years longer when compared to their negative-thinking peers. Sarkisian, Prohaska, Wong, Hirsch, and Mangione (2005) found that older adults who had low expectations for aging well were much less likely to adopt preventive lifestyle behaviors (e.g., eating a balanced diet, minimizing alcohol and tobacco use, getting regular physical exams), including physical activity. This change in perspective and perception toward health management requires individuals to take more responsibility for their personal well-being. Wellness depends upon the combination of factual health information, realistic optimism, and appropriate action steps.

> Individuals are encouraged to intentionally shift their behaviors and perceptions toward a wellness rather than an illness perspective in order to be well.

Unfortunately, many people have found the idea of *wellness* difficult to understand because the fundamental concept of wellness for the whole person has been misrepresented. To add to the confusion, the term *wellness* has even been used to describe a wide variety of health enhancing treatments, oils, herbal remedies, beverages, devices, programs, centers, and classes (Miller, 2005). However, wellness is more than a product, service, or intervention. It is a reflection of one's perceived state of positive health and well-being (McMahon & Fleury, 2012). The Merriam-Webster dictionary defines **wellness** as "the quality or state of being in good health especially as an actively sought goal" (Merriam-Webster website, 2016). Basically, a wellness perspective asks individuals to perceive their lives as a glass half full instead of half empty.

> Health is a state of complete physical, mental, and social well-being and not merely the absence of disease or infirmity.
>
> World Health Organization, 1946.

Even though the concept can be confusing, the topic of *wellness* has become so widespread that it is being promoted at professional conferences, featured on blogs, and included in news stories (Global Wellness Institute, 2016). In addition, wellness-focused programming and education has now been woven into drugstore offerings, health insurance incentives, and government-sponsored programs (e.g., the federal Administration on Aging's health, prevention, and wellness programs; Medicare's Annual Wellness Visit; Rite Aid's Wellness + Card, Wellness Stores, and Wellness Ambassadors; AARP Walgreens Way to Wellness; Anthem Health and Wellness for Baby Boomers and Seniors; HumanaVitality Wellness Rewards for Eligible Humana Medicare Members). The ICAA Active-Aging Industry Development Survey 2015 reported several trends in wellness and program development (International Council on Active Aging, 2015). The survey respondents included professionals from senior-living communities and organizations that provide programs and services to older individuals. Survey respondents were asked what plans they had for wellness programs for older adults during the next two years. Results showed that 82 percent of the respondents planned to add more activities, classes, or programs; 42 percent planned to increase the budget for wellness activities; and 36 percent planned to hire new staff.

Consequently, physical activity instructors of older adults would benefit from learning about and embracing a whole-person wellness perspective. As role models, physical activity instructors have the unique opportunity to show their clients that wellness only happens when we change our perspective and view our lives from a positive, strengths-based approach and not through an illness, deficit-based lens. Physical activity instructors can intentionally encourage clients to change their perspective toward health and well-being. They can motivate clients during classes and encourage them to seek out wellness-focused medical and health professionals to partner with them in their quest for successful aging. Therefore, physical activity instructors who can embody whole-person wellness beliefs into their own lives and integrate those concepts into their professional practice will be in great demand.

> Physical activity instructors who can incorporate whole-person wellness beliefs into their own lives and integrate those concepts into their professional practice will be in great demand.

Defining Wellness: A Historical Perspective

Web MD (2016) defines wellness in the following way: "the achievement of that sweet spot in the pendulum where balance exists in its purest form. Wellness is not a one-time thing. It is a living thing. You don't just get there and say you've done it. You need to keep creating it. It may change over time. And it is different for everyone. We can be happier and healthier for however long we have to live." A comprehensive view of wellness reflects the integration of mind, body, and spirit throughout life's journey. Simply stated, what you do, think, feel, and believe has an impact on your health and well-being. The concept of wellness was not actively promoted until Dr. Halbert Dunn advanced the concept as a teacher, physician, statistician, and public administrator from the 1930s through the 1970s. In his book *High Level Wellness,* Dr. Dunn defined wellness as, "an integrated method of functioning which is oriented toward maximizing the potential of which the individual is capable within the functioning environment" (Dunn, 1961, pp. 4-5). Through his research, writings, and lectures, Dunn promoted a model for comprehensive well-being. He showed the interrelatedness of the mind, body, and spirit with altruism, social connectedness, self-perception, life balance, and environmental influences. Those of us interested in advancing wellness strategies to enhance successful aging owe a great deal to the teachings of Halbert Dunn. In the following excerpt from *High Level Wellness*, it is clear that over sixty years ago, Dr. Dunn was a strong advocate for promoting high-level wellness and utilizing appropriate wellness testing for older members of society.

> medical assessments . . . tell us how a patient is at a particular moment in time . . . blood analysis, urine analysis, blood pressure . . . and we have a number of functional tests. But we do not have in medicine anything that's analogous to the performance test. We do not wear a person out to see how durable he is! The only performance test that we can apply to human beings is that of living over a period of years, and finding out how the person stands up to the wear and tear of life. Longevity might be considered such a performance test, particularly if it is associated in the older years with high productivity and a state of well-being. A group of oldsters between 80 and 90, for instance, who are alert, well, active, and participating in many ways in their social structure, undoubtedly should be classified as enjoying high-level wellness. (p. 203)

In 1976, Dr. Bill Hettler, cofounder of the National Wellness Institute (NWI), the principal organization for wellness education, training, and research in the United States, defined wellness as "an active process through which people become aware of, and make choices towards, a more successful existence" (National Wellness Institute, 2016). The NWI has chosen to define six dimensions that embody personal wellness. They include the emotional, intellectual, physical, social, spiritual, and vocational dimensions. The overarching philosophy of the NWI is that wellness is the "pathway to optimal living." To guide instructors and program developers, NWI created the following three questions to assess the level to which programs and offerings are reflective of wellness principles:

1. Does this (program or activity) help people achieve their full potential?
2. Does this (program or activity) recognize and address the whole-person multidimensional approach?
3. Does this (program or activity) affirm and mobilize people's positive qualities and strengths?

It should be noted that individuals, organizations, countries, and cultures are always free to define and describe the multiple dimensions and concepts of wellness for successful aging to best meet their particular needs (Fry, 2012). For some people it is easier to use a mind, body, and spirit approach. Others might choose to add dimensions, such as environmental or financial. The choice is yours. However, the focus should always be on wellness for the whole person and not merely the pieces and parts of the individual.

Whole-Person Wellness: A Comprehensive Perspective

Simply defined, **whole-person wellness** is multidimensional, positive health leading to a satisfying quality of life and a sense of well-being (Montague & Frank, 2007). The whole-person wellness model invites individuals to enhance their quality of life by focusing positive perceptions and actions into their emotional, intellectual, physical, social, spiritual, and vocational dimensions (Edelman & Montague, 2006, 2008). It involves a proactive lifestyle environment based on knowledge of and self-responsibility for our multidimensional lives; realistic optimism; resiliency; a can-do attitude; positive self-talk; a focus on personal strengths; and strong social connections. Whole-person wellness provides the lens, or pathway, through which one perceives her or his level of well-being. This approach to life-balance is individualized, dynamic, and relative to each person's abilities, health status, and health behavior stage (McMahon & Fleury, 2012).

Whole-Person Wellness and Successful Aging: A Winning Combination

It is clear the concept of wellness for the whole person is not a new one, so why is this conscious change in perspective occurring now? Several factors are contributing to society's radical shift to a whole-person wellness focus for successful aging. These factors include changing demographics; the high cost of health care; relevant research on successful aging; and an increased understanding of appropriate health behavioral-change techniques. This change in perspective will help individuals remain healthier, positive, and proactive while aging (Rose, 2013). A framework for the study of aging and quality of life was described in *Successful Aging* (Rowe & Kahn, 1998), a book that summarized a series of studies funded by the MacArthur Foundation. Spearheaded by John W. Rowe and Robert L. Kahn, the studies were designed to examine the factors responsible for the positive aspects of aging. As stated in the introduction to the book, their research goals were "to move beyond the limited view of chronological age and to clarify the genetic, biomedical, behavioral, and social factors responsible for retaining—and even enhancing—people's ability to function in later life" (Rowe & Kahn, 1998, p. xii).

To fund this groundbreaking series of studies, the MacArthur Foundation provided more than 10 million dollars in support. Thousands of older adults participated in one or more of the interdisciplinary studies that were conducted over a 10-year period. The collective results of these studies provided the best evidence that a successful aging experience is not solely determined by genetic inheritance. Instead, results from the Successful Aging studies showed that maintaining a high level of mental function is directly related to the development and maintenance of a strong social support system; participation in regular physical activity; the desire to learn new things and develop new interests; having a belief in one's ability to handle what life has to offer; and to consciously reduce one's feelings of isolation, whether they are actual or perceived. Moreover, the older adults who participated in regular physical exercise and activities showed increased muscle strength and flexibility, aerobic endurance, and physical balance. Significant reductions in the risk factors associated with coronary heart disease, high blood pressure, colon and rectal cancer, diabetes, arthritis, and osteoporosis were also observed. Finally, the research data showed a direct relationship between aging successfully and study participants who demonstrated high self-esteem and resilience and who approached life with a "Yes, I can!" attitude.

For many older adults, participation in programs and activities that promote wellness for the whole person slows the aging process and promotes independence (Vaillant, 2002). Proponents of a successful aging model cite data that indicate older people have increased knowledge and awareness about the importance of health management—including both traditional and alternative medicine techniques. They are also aware that a comprehensive wellness model that addresses the multiple aspects of the whole person can lead to lower health care utilization, improved health, and a better quality of life (Poon, Gueldner, & Sprouse, 2003). Today's older adults have the desire for optimal health, to be engaged with life, and to be functionally capable for as long as possible. In their 2003 report, Strawbridge and Wallhagen identified the predictors of successful aging as a positive outlook on life; acceptance of aging and oneself; not smoking; not being obese; feeling very satisfied with personal relationships; having little or no hearing impairments; staying physically active; and volunteering often.

> Lower health care utilization, improved health, and a better quality of life can result from the adoption of a comprehensive wellness model that addresses the multiple aspects of the whole person.

Defining the Dimensions of Wellness

Now, let's review a research rationale and basic description of each dimension of wellness (see figure 9.1). For more in-depth definitions and descriptions of the six dimensions, please visit the National Wellness Institute's website.

Emotional Wellness

The **emotional dimension** emphasizes an awareness and acceptance of one's feelings. It reflects the degree to which an individual feels positive and enthusiastic about one's self and life. This dimension involves the capacity to manage feelings and

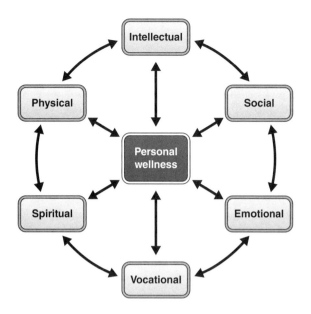

FIGURE 9.1   The Whole-Person Wellness Model.
Whole Person Wellness ©1994 Jan Montague.

behaviors, accept oneself unconditionally, assess limitations, develop autonomy, and cope with stress.

For many individuals, participation in regular physical activity can be a catalyst for personal wellness (Rose, 2013). Sometimes our mood and emotional outlook can positively or negatively influence our participation in physical activity. An effective way to address clinical depression is through participation in physical activity programs. Research clearly shows that older adults with clinical symptoms of depression can reduce the effects and severity through structured exercise programs (Bridle, Spanjers, Patel, Altherton, & Lamb, 2012).

Intellectual Wellness

In *The Six Dimensions of Wellness and Cognition in Aging Adults,* Strout and Howard (2012) concluded that cognition may be protected by pursuing wellness through multiple dimensions, such as physical activity, purpose in life, spirituality, healthy nutrition, midlife occupational complexity, motivational ability, marriage, social networks, and intellectual activities. To date, researchers have not yet identified the level at which cognition is impacted through physical activity frequency, intensity, and duration (Bherer, Erickson, & Liu-Ambrose, 2013). However, data clearly show that physical activity is protective against cognitive decline (Guure, Ibrahim, Adam, & Said, 2017; Kramer et al., 1999).

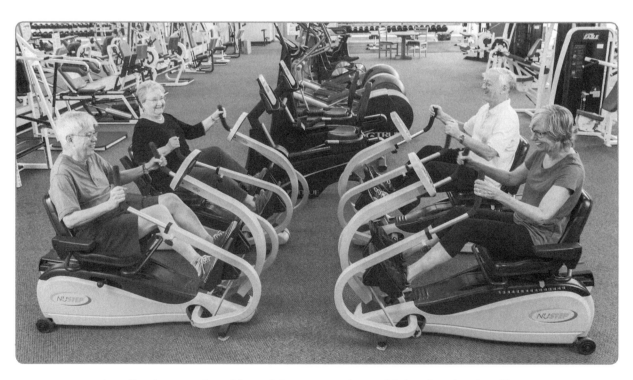

An effective way for older adults to experience higher levels of wellness across multiple dimensions is to participate in structured group exercise programs.

The **intellectual dimension** promotes the use of one's mind to create a greater understanding and appreciation of oneself and others. It involves one's ability to think creatively and rationally. This dimension encourages individuals to expand their knowledge and skill base through a variety of resources and cultural activities (Edelman & Montague, 2006).

Physical Wellness

The 2015 White House Conference on Aging Policy Brief on Healthy Aging states that older adults, regardless of ability, can experience a longer and higher quality of life by exercising regularly, eating nutritious meals, and receiving recommended health screenings (www.whitehouseconference onaging.gov/blog/policy/file). However, older adults can reap these benefits only if they actively participate in their personal wellness. More research is needed in multilevel approaches, such as behavioral change strategies and technologies that might contribute to physical activity participation in older adults (Rose, 2016).

The multifaceted **physical dimension** is relative to each person's abilities. The physical dimension encourages participation in activities that improve cardiovascular endurance, muscle strength, and flexibility. It promotes increased knowledge for achieving healthy lifestyle habits and discouraging negative, excessive behavior. The physical dimension engages individuals in activities that lead to high-level wellness, personal safety, proactive self-care, and the appropriate use of the medical system (Edelman & Montague, 2006).

Social Wellness

One's perception of being socially isolated can produce stress, which can be a powerful predictor of ill health (Kahana & Kahana, 2012). Therefore, it is imperative for physical activity instructors to incorporate positive intervention strategies to promote social engagement in activity classes.

The **social dimension** is defined as humanistic, emphasizing the creation and maintenance of healthy relationships. It enhances interdependence with others and nature, and encourages the pursuit of harmony within the family. This dimension furthers positive contributions to your human and physical environment for the common welfare of your community (Edelman & Montague, 2006).

Spiritual Wellness

Individuals who report being both spiritually and physically active have a higher perceived quality of life, health status, and well-being (Konopack & McAuley, 2012).

The **spiritual dimension** involves seeking meaning and purpose in human existence. It involves developing a strong sense of personal values and ethics. This dimension includes the development of an appreciation for the depth and expanse of life and natural forces that exist in the universe (Edelman & Montague, 2006).

Vocational Wellness

The UnitedHealth Group Health and Volunteering Study (2013) showed volunteerism plays an important role in health for older adults. Their data revealed good health requires more than measuring heart rate, cholesterol, and BMI. Perceived wellness reflects the integration of multiple dimensions such as physical health, emotional well-being, sense of purpose, and vocational contributions.

The **vocational dimension** emphasizes the importance of giving and receiving. It is the process of determining and achieving personal and occupational interests through meaningful activities. This dimension encourages goal setting for one's personal enrichment. Vocational wellness is linked to the creation of a positive attitude about personal and professional development (Edelman & Montague, 2006).

Applying the Dimensions of Wellness

Incorporating whole-person wellness dimensions and beliefs into classes and programs must be intentional and purposeful. Take the time to create lesson plans that will provide the needed structure to promote wellness during your classes and programs. Over the past three years the Center for Successful Aging (CSA) at California State University at Fullerton has begun integrating more wellness activities into each of the physical activity programs that it offers. To guide the graduate student instructors who currently deliver these classes, lesson plans were created that addressed each of the six dimensions. The goal was to purposefully and seamlessly introduce into each class simple, wellness-based activities that complemented the core physical activities being delivered. Over time, both the graduate student instructors and clients have embraced these complementary activities and now view them as being integral and desirable components of the programs. In the following sidebar, we have provided a small sample of the lesson plans we have successfully used in the CSA that address three (i.e., emotional, intellectual, spiritual) of the six dimensions of wellness described earlier. Each lesson plan is structured according to the program schedule used in the CSA. Clients attend classes on a Monday-Wednesday schedule or a Tuesday-Thursday schedule, and are presented with one new idea or activity per class each week. You will also note that the activity presented often coincides with

and is related to a national celebration or event (e.g., Thanksgiving, Active Aging Week, Older Americans Month) or health-related event (e.g., National Nutrition Month, Brain Awareness Week, National Heart Health Month). Finally, the instructor will announce the theme for the coming week prior to ending the second class of the week as a way to get the clients thinking about that particular dimension of wellness or the event that will be celebrated in the coming week.

Here are some additional ideas for content that can be integrated into your physical activity classes for the other three dimensions of aging:

- *Physical dimension:* Provide clients with a handout that explains how and why antioxidants are important to various aspects of our health and to the prevention of disease. The handout should describe what antioxidants are and how they help in promoting and maintaining health. You could then list the best food sources for antioxidants or even provide

---

Integrating Whole-Person Wellness Activities Into Physical Activity Classes

Lesson Plan: Emotional Dimension

This week's activities are very appropriate as we head into the Thanksgiving holiday. Encourage clients to continue this activity beyond this week by building it into their daily routine.

Quotation of the Week

Gratitude is the fairest blossom which springs from the soul. (Henry Ward Beecher)

Activities

Mon/Tues

Suggest to your clients that before retiring to bed tonight, think of one thing that happened on that day for which they are thankful. Each subsequent day, try to think of one new thing that happened for which they are thankful.

Wed/Thur

We call this activity "The Gratitude Tree." On the mirrored wall there will be a drawing of a tree trunk. Invite clients to add a branch to the tree, writing one thing for which they are grateful in their lives. This can be done anytime throughout the class period.

A Look Ahead to Next Week

Next week we will begin a set of activities to promote vocational wellness.

Lesson Plan: Intellectual Dimension

In celebration of National Nutrition Month and Brain Awareness Week, we will focus on activities that promote brain health, continue with our discussion of the benefits of foods high in antioxidants, and introduce other brain health foods for you to try.

Quotation of the Week

The more you use your brain, the more brain you will have to use. (George Dorsey)

Activities

Mon/Tues

Express to the clients that you hope they enjoyed last week's sampling of brain healthy nuts. Ask them if they have considered ways to incorporate more nuts into their diet for healthy fats and vitamin E. This activity can be introduced prior to the warm-up and clients can be asked to share how they plan to incorporate more nuts into their diets while holding those long stretches during the cool-down phase of the class.

Wed/Thur

Continuing with the theme of brain health, in today's class I will present a variety of brain games that will help you in the following ways:

- Find words quickly and effortlessly
- Sharpen your analytical skills
- Strengthen your visual memory for shapes and colors
- Stimulate problem-solving skills and improve focus and attention

A Look Ahead to Next Week

We will celebrate International Happiness Day, which occurs on March 20th.

Lesson Plan: Spiritual Dimension

We conclude this month of spiritual activities with one that invites serenity.

Quotation of the Week

Nowhere can a person find a retreat more full of peace than one's own soul. (Marcus Aurelius)

Activities

Mon/Tues

Conclude the class with a deep breathing and relaxation activity. You may use your own breathing exercises, a recording of guided breathing, or the attached script.

Wed/Thur

End the cool-down with rhythmic breathing. Ask the clients to open their minds and hearts to nature. Devote three minutes to focusing on the breath and quietude. Follow this activity by reading the spiritual poem about nature titled *Where Peaceful Waters Flow*, by Keith Burroughs. Conclude with three more minutes of focused breathing and quietude.

A Look Ahead to Next Week

Next week we will begin a set of activities to promote social wellness.

samples for clients to try at the end of class. You could also ask clients what foods they currently include in their diets or what they will add to increase their intake based on what they learned from the handout.

- *Social dimension:* As each client arrives for class, provide him or her with a name tag that you have prepared beforehand. Each name tag will have the client's name covered with a temporary label that shows a word or phrase (e.g., *antioxidant* will be on the label on one client's name tag and *blueberries* will be on the label on another client's name tag; *heart-healthy food* on one, *dark chocolate* on another; *Mayberry—Aunt Bee*, etc.). Before the end of class, each client will find the person who has the matching word or phrase and both will remove the temporary labels, revealing their names. This matching game is a particularly good one to introduce during the first or second class so clients can get to know each other.

- *Vocational dimension:* Invite clients to consider ways they can donate their time to a worthy cause. Develop and share a list of different ways they could provide service that requires little time (e.g., delivering the mail to a neighbor, offering to transport a neighbor to the supermarket when you are planning to go, tutoring a student who needs help in a subject area in which you have knowledge or expertise). This dimension could be introduced during the warm-up and the ideas shared while the clients are performing cool-down activities.

As you begin incorporating lesson plans, or even creating your own lesson plans, focused on each of the wellness dimensions, be sure they are flexible and easy to integrate into the type of class you are teaching. Take the time to become thoroughly familiar with the planned content, especially if you did not develop the lesson plan yourself, so that you are confident in your delivery. Finally, it is also important to remember that each client is unique and often at a different stage of health behavior. As a result, their perception of the wellness dimensions will vary and shape the type of response they exhibit to the presented activities. We have found that regularly asking our clients for feedback relative to the wellness topics and activities that have been presented, those they would like to see presented, or those they would like to see repeated has been, and continues to be, extremely helpful in shaping the lesson plans we create and deliver during the various classes we offer.

In addition to the three structured lesson plans and content ideas we have presented in this chapter, think of a few simple things you can do to promote whole-person wellness during each class and interaction with clients. First and foremost, it is important that you be the role model for each of the dimensions and purposefully create an environment that promotes each dimension of wellness. We have listed some ideas in table 9.1 to stimulate your creative juices.

Once you have mastered the concept of weaving individual wellness dimensions into classes, consider incorporating all of the whole-person wellness dimensions and principles into a single physical activity (see the following sidebar for an example).

Summary

Whole-person wellness is a life-growth process that embodies the philosophy of holistic health—the whole is greater than the sum of the parts. Effective whole-person wellness programs incorporate the wellness dimensions (emotional, social, intellectual, physical, spiritual, and vocational) with personal wellness concepts that include self-responsibility, realistic optimism, self-directed approach, self-efficacy, proactive behaviors, positive attitudes, and appropriate lifestyle choices. These concepts are intended to change the focus from what people can't do to what they can do. Therefore, age, chronic illness, terminal illness, or physical or mental ability need not limit the perceived level of wellness one can achieve; the level of wellness is always relative to one's own perspective and perception of well-being. The result of this approach is fully integrated wellness of mind, body, and spirit throughout life's journey. Simply stated, what you do, think, feel, and believe has an impact on your health and well-being.

The desire to be well and functionally able for as long as possible has older adults embracing the concepts of wellness as a leading model of successful aging. Today, people of all ages are more likely to be defined by what they can do rather than what they can't do. Older adults are becoming role models for younger cohorts because they are achieving

Table 9.1 Wellness Programming Considerations

Dimension	Actions for the instructor
Emotional	Be the role model and create an emotionally healthy class environment. This can be accomplished by being mindful of interactions with clients. For example, pause to be intentionally loving, caring, and optimistic by smiling, listening, and asking. Spend time, even for a moment, talking with, recognizing, and addressing each participant in an attentive and positive manner.
Intellectual	Offer clients appropriate information to increase their knowledge base for wellness and successful aging. First, verify that your wellness resources reflect whole-person wellness principles. Then, make available handouts that include medically sound websites; locations of libraries with free online services; links to community classes, services, and seminars; a list of evidenced-based computer programs designed to enhance cognition, and current research findings.
Physical	Deliver an appropriate physical activity class and encourage each person to recognize areas of need while reminding them to maintain their focus on strengths and abilities. Always use positive words, affirmations, facial expressions, and body language to provide a warm, positive, fun, and supportive environment.
Social	Begin each class by welcoming clients or participants in a thoughtful manner. Many of us switch into auto-pilot mode and ask everyone the simple question "How are you today?" Unfortunately, we often ask this question without expecting or wanting a true answer. A more appropriate greeting might include one of these options: "Hello, it's good to see you today," "Good morning," "Good afternoon," "I am glad to see you," or, "Isn't it a beautiful day?" Whatever greeting is used with clients or class participants, always remain positive and respectful. And remember to only ask the question "How are you today?" when you have the time to stop, listen attentively, and respond appropriately.
Spiritual	Include a few minutes during each class for participants to reflect, meditate, practice mindfulness, express gratitude, or pray.
Vocational	Invite class participants to discuss and share their interests, gifts, skills, hobbies, and talents with others in the class.

Whole-Person Wellness Walk

A whole-person wellness walk is a great way to incorporate personal wellness concepts and the multiple dimensions of wellness into one enjoyable activity. Follow the simple steps outlined below, and you can start walking the path to wellness without delay.

1. Determine your walking path, preferably in a park or other safe, outdoor, peaceful area (reflects self-responsibility, self-efficacy, and making choices).

2. Invite a friend, colleague, or family member to accompany you on the wellness walk (reflects the social dimension).

3. Do your homework! Review the types of trees, plants, flowers, birds, and so on you may see along the way (reflects the intellectual dimension).

4. Determine a personal goal that you wish to accomplish while on your wellness walk (reflects the vocational dimension).

5. Prior to starting your wellness walk, take a few minutes to warm up your muscles. At the conclusion of the wellness walk, take a few minutes to cool down. We recommend that you walk at a leisurely pace to remain mindful of your surroundings (reflects the physical and spiritual dimensions).

6. During your walk, find a quiet place to meditate on one of nature's wonders. Relax and be fully present in the moment (reflects the spiritual dimension).

desirable health outcomes by combining whole-person wellness principles with self-responsibility for health.

Current research is showing that the whole-person wellness model is not a passing fad. In the coming years, more and more senior living communities and senior service organizations will adopt whole-person wellness as their core operational philosophy. These organizations will set the new standard by promoting cultures, environments, and opportunities for successful aging. We must continue to focus on the promotion of individual well-being, whole-person involvement, and the implementation of programs and services that encourage people to be healthy in mind, body, and spirit throughout their life span. No one is ever too young, too old, too fit, or too frail to embrace a whole-person wellness perspective.

Key Terms

emotional dimension

intellectual dimension

physical dimension

social dimension

spiritual dimension

vocational dimension

wellness

whole-person wellness

Recommended Readings

Dunn, H.L. (1961). *High level wellness.* Arlington, VA: Beatty Press.

Rose, D.J. (2013). Aging successfully: Predictors and pathways. In J.M. Rippe (Ed.), *Lifestyle medicine* (2nd ed., pp. 1247-1267). Boca Raton, FL: CRC Press.

Rose, D.J., (2016). The future of aging research: Should the focus be on not growing old or growing old better? *Kinesiology Review, 5,* 65-74.

Vaillant, G. (2002). *Aging well: Surprising guideposts to a happier life from the landmark Harvard study of adult development.* Boston: Little Brown.

Study Questions

1. The term *wellness* describes

   a. a wide variety of health-enhancing treatments

   b. the quality or state of being in good health

   c. life as a glass that is half-empty

   d. a service that is provided to optimize a person's health

2. Research has shown that older adults who hold positive views about the aging process live

   a. as much as 7.5 years longer than their negative-thinking peers

   b. much happier lives

   c. no longer than older adults who hold negative views of aging

   d. more than 10 years longer than their negative-thinking peers

3. The spiritual dimension of wellness involves

   a. one's ability to think creatively and rationally

   b. having an awareness and acceptance of one's feelings

   c. seeking meaning and purpose in human existence

   d. giving and receiving

4. The whole-person wellness model developed by Montague includes the following dimensions of wellness.

   a. emotional, spiritual, physical, social, and vocational

   b. intellectual, emotional, physical, environmental, and spiritual

   c. physical, emotional, social, vocational, environmental, spiritual, and intellectual

   d. physical, social, intellectual, spiritual, emotional, and vocational

Application Activities

1. Develop an activity that focuses on one of the dimensions of whole-person wellness and present it to a group of older adults.

2. Develop a short presentation to be delivered to an older adult audience that addresses each of the dimensions of whole-person wellness and how each dimension can be incorporated into their daily lives.

Principles of the Warm-Up and Cool-Down

Mary Ann Kluge

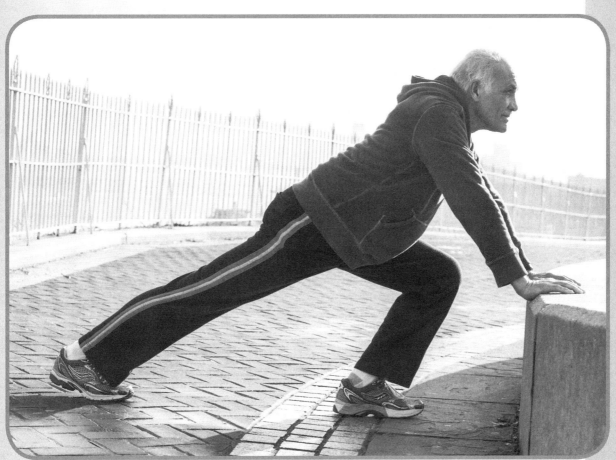

Warm-up and cool-down exercises are important for all age groups but they are essential for older adults to prevent injury and facilitate the most efficient function possible. Warm-up and cool-down exercises are designed to provide a safe transition to and adequate recovery from moderate- to vigorous-intensity exercise. This chapter provides an overview of the acute physiological changes that occur while warming up and cooling down. Practical strategies for creating safe and effective warm-ups and cool-downs for older adults are described. In addition, this chapter discusses how to use the warm-up and cool-down phases of an exercise class to engage clients in the multiple dimensions (physical, social, emotional, spiritual, intellectual, vocational) of wellness.

There is high variability in older adults with regard to functional ability, health status, joint mobility, and joint integrity. Connective tissue changes are normal throughout the lifespan. Connective tissue is known to lose extensibility as part of the aging process; a change believed to be caused by adaptation in collagen architecture (Reid & McNair, 2011). In fact, it is not uncommon for older adults to have compromised joint integrity due to accumulated disuse, misuse, abuse, or diseases of the musculo-skeletal system (Ferrini & Ferrini, 2012). Combine these changes with the tendency for most people, no matter what age, to start higher-intensity physical activity without warming up or curtail moderate- to high-intensity exercise without cooling down, and the likelihood of joint or muscle discomfort or risk for injury increases.

Warming Up

The warm-up phase is a good time for you as the physical activity instructor to assess the physical, mental, and emotional health status of your older adult clients, many of whom experience changes in blood pressure, energy levels, joint pain, mobility, and even attentional focus from one day to the next. Recommendations for warm-up include increasing the body's temperature through engagement in low-intensity, large-muscle movements and easy range-of-motion activities. During this time, the physical activity instructor should ask participants to perform a **body scan**, where they "take a look inside" for tight places, restricted movement, and even pain. At this time, participants can be asked to assess their energy levels as well. Research shows that bodily fatigue can be a precursor to injury, especially in older adults. With sleep problems being common (Inoue et al., 2013) and differing chronobiology (Kluge & Savis, 2000), it is not unusual for older adults to arrive at class in a fatigued state. Of course, fatigue in and of itself should not be a barrier to participating in exercise; there is a plethora of evidence that once older adults get moving, they feel better in numerous ways (Bean, Vora, & Frontera, 2013; Hogan, Mata, & Carstensen, 2013).

Here's how to instruct your clients to perform a body scan:

1. Look in the mirror. There are many opportunities during the day, especially when using the lavatory.

2. After noticing your outward appearance, take another "look" inside and ask yourself some of the following questions:

- How do I feel? What sensations am I aware of?

- What do my heartbeat and breathing feel like?

- What sensations am I aware of in my muscles and joints? Do I sense any stiffness or tightness? Do I feel flexible and supple?

Once clients have been introduced to the body scan during the warm-up, they should be encouraged to continue to do it themselves between classes and report their levels to the instructor before warm-up begins. This scan can also be encouraged during an exercise class to ensure that class participants are not experiencing "ouch pain" when performing the aerobic, resistance, or balance training components. Encouraging clients to pay attention to variability in energy, strength, pain or discomfort levels, and mood during workout sessions and during the day encourages mindfulness. Although we have limited knowledge about the effects of mindfulness and mind-body exercises on health and well-being, current research in this area is expanding (Ullman, 2012).

Physiological Changes Associated With the Warm-Up

Warming up increases the internal body temperature, resulting in changes that prepare the cardiopulmonary, neuromuscular, and metabolic systems for higher-intensity exercise. A warm-up increases the efficiency of numerous body systems; for example, it increases lung circulation and improves delivery of oxygen to working muscles. It also affects nervous system function, improving coordination and reaction time. Warming up results in increased blood saturation of the muscles, tendons, and joints, thereby significantly reducing their susceptibility to injury. See table 10.1 for a summary of the benefits to multiple systems.

The warm-up prepares the body for more intense physical activity by facilitating the transition from rest to exercise (Speer, 2005). This can be accomplished through **passive warm-up** (using external agents such as hot showers, saunas, ultrasound, or myofascial release) or **active warm-up** (using body movements). An active warm-up is generally preferred to a passive warm-up, regardless of the mode of exercise for which an older adult is preparing. However, passive heating in the form of a hot shower may be indicated for older adults with arthritis before they engage in fitness activities. Refer

Table 10.1 Physiological Benefits of Warming Up

System	Specific benefits
Cardiovascular	Improves cardiac blood flow, which decreases risk of myocardial ischemia. Also reduces pulmonary resistance, which increases lung circulation and leads to more efficient aerobic metabolism
Nervous	Increases blood flow to brain, which improves coordination and reaction time and increases alertness and cognitive function
Muscular	Increases blood flow and internal body temperature, which increases delivery of oxygen and nutrients to muscles, speeds up muscle contraction, improves mechanical efficiency and power by reducing muscle viscosity, increases muscle elasticity, and reduces susceptibility to injury
Skeletal	Increases range of joint motion
Connective tissue	Facilitates elongation of connective tissue; increases flexibility of muscle-tendon units
Cartilage	Facilitates diffusion of lubricating fluid into joint space

Based on DeVries and Housh (1994); Nieman (1999).

to chapter 17 for additional information on exercise adaptations for chronic medical conditions.

Components of a Safe and Effective Warm-Up

Many different forms of activity can be used to increase the internal body temperature and safely prepare older adult clients of different functional abilities for higher-intensity exercise. Examples include walking (on land or in water), performing rhythmic movements while seated or standing, and using cardiovascular equipment such as treadmills, stationary bikes, or recumbent steppers. Whenever possible, incorporate large-muscle movements into the warm-up that are similar to those you plan to introduce later in class, but at a slower tempo and lower intensity. For example, if the arms will be pushed overhead during the aerobic conditioning component of the class or during resistance-training activities, have your clients perform the same movement through a similar range of motion but more slowly during the warm-up.

It is important to remember that many older adults are taking medications intended to control heart rate and blood pressure; therefore, heart and breathing rates may not increase in older adults in a similar fashion to younger populations. It is therefore important for physical activity instructors to review each participant's medication list provided on the health history and activity questionnaire (see chapter 5) in order to determine if they are taking any medications (including nonprescription medications) that are likely to negatively influence their response to exercise. Also, older adults experience many medication changes so it is important that you encourage your participants to let you know when these changes occur so that you can revise their medication list. It is also imperative that you know and be able to monitor signs of exercise intolerance in older adults (see chapter 5).

Guidelines for Developing the Warm-Up

This section provides important guidelines for developing the warm-up component of the class and applies the senior-specific principles of challenge and adaptation/tailoring that were first discussed in chapter 8. It is important to remember that your primary goal during the warm-up is to match the activities to the physical abilities of the participants. Important guidelines to follow include matching the duration of the warm-up to the functional abilities of participants, monitoring exercise intensity and joint pain, and establishing an environment that is both physically and psychologically comfortable for participants.

Determine the Duration of the Warm-Up Component

The ideal duration of a warm-up is difficult to determine without first assessing the functional abilities of each class participant (see chapter 6). The needs of lower-functioning or frail older adults are *very different* from those of higher functioning (especially athletic) older adult needs. While some community-based programs include ongoing assessments of fitness and function at regular intervals, most do not. When clientele have been primarily sedentary and are significantly deconditioned, or new to exercise, it is important to understand that the warm-up, in and of itself, can be a workout.

For younger older adults who are active during the day or have not experienced compromises to joint integrity, it is recommended that the warm-up last between 5 and 15 minutes. For older adults who are deconditioned, however, the duration of the warm-up may need to vary (Chodzko-Zajko et al., 2009). For those not familiar with exercise or are less motor proficient, a 15-minute time period may tax them physically, cognitively, and socially. Making sure that the movement skills and physical effort are safely progressed during the early stages of the exercise program will enhance participants' efficacy.

Monitor Exercise Intensity and Joint Pain

Ultimately, your goal as an instructor is to have participants be able to self-regulate, which means be able to engage in safe, effective physical exercise without the need for constant monitoring. To achieve this, participants need to learn how to check their heart rates and use a standard **rating of perceived exertion** (**RPE**; a subjective rating of how hard they feel they are exercising) during and after the warm-up so they can be aware of how their bodies are responding to exercise that day. Use the same verbal cues each time you have clients take a pulse rate or determine an RPE, and make sure that your cues are clear and direct. Borg's (1998) RPE scale is a common scale used to evaluate the participant's perceived effort. When using the Borg scale to monitor intensity levels during the warm-up, it is important that healthy older adults not exceed an RPE of 1 to 2 on the CR10 scale, while frailer older adults should not exceed an RPE of 0.5 to 1.

Another strategy to evaluate client responses to the exercise intensity is to periodically use a circle formation during the warm-up. This allows you to watch closely for signs of overexertion. Ask your clients how they are doing or how the room temperature feels, and casually administer the **talk test** (a simple conversational assessment to guard against overexertion) to one or two clients during the warm-up. To pass the talk test, the client should be able to respond without gasping for air to a direct question that requires

more than a one-word answer (e.g., "What are your plans after class today, Anthony?"). Periodically, and whenever new clients join the class, take time during the warm-up to review the procedures for monitoring exercise intensity. It is also imperative that clients know that if they come to an exercise session late, to ensure their safety they must perform the entire warm-up routine by themselves before they will be allowed to join the group exercises. Refer to chapter 13 for more detailed information on managing aerobic training risks in general.

Choose an Appropriate Environment

If the room temperature seems warmer than normal, it is important to closely monitor your participants' responses and watch for signs of overexertion such as a flushed face or unusually rapid breathing. An ambient room temperature ranging between 68 to

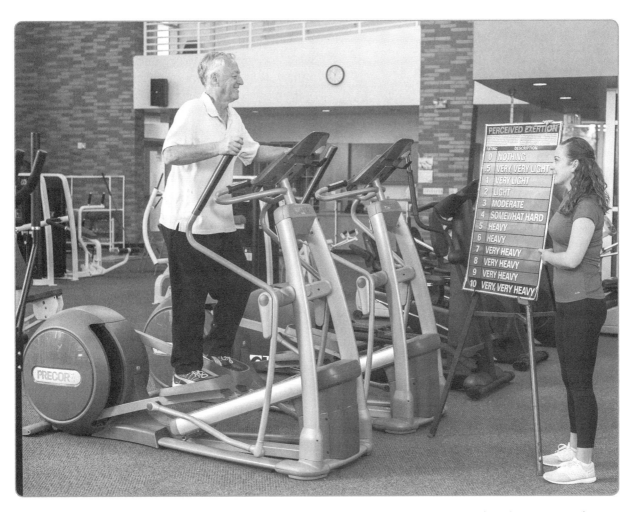

It is important to teach your clients how to rate their perceived exertion so that they can evaluate how hard they are working during the warm-up and aerobic training components of a class.

72 degrees Fahrenheit (20-22 °C) is considered to be safe (American College of Sports Medicine, 2012). An exercise environment that is too hot places your clients (especially those with high blood pressure) at a greater risk for cardiac problems. If clients become flushed, perspire easily, or mention how hot the room feels during the warm-up, it is probably too hot for the aerobic component. Modify the class to include little or no aerobic conditioning and substitute coordination, balance, flexibility, and relaxation exercises until the conditions change or a more suitable exercise space is located.

The Benefits of a Warm-Up

- Increases blood flow to the working muscles
- Lessens risk for injury
- Improves range of motion
- Improves performance

Be sure to structure the warm-up to provide numerous opportunities for feelings of accomplishment and success in movement. Try to create a noncompetitive and safe environment where participants are encouraged to work at their own level. Frequently demonstrate variations appropriate for different ability levels. Remember, even with adaptations, many people will either attempt to perform the end-goal of an activity regardless of their ability to succeed or may experience embarrassment and a lack of motivation because they can't do the activity the "right" way. Warm-up activities provide the physical activity instructor with her or his first opportunity to enhance mastery (Kluge & Savis, 2001). Provide positive reinforcement for all accomplishments and efforts, and downplay the need to be on the "right" foot at the "right" time. Once your clients are able to successfully meet small challenges, their self-esteem and confidence in their abilities will be heightened (Wise & Trunnell, 2001).

Goal Setting

Once participants are comfortable and able to perform the movements safely during the warm-up, the physical activity instructor may want to engage them in establishing mini-goals for that day's class or workout session. For example, clients may want to set a goal to perform a simple coordination sequence they already know at a faster tempo or perhaps with additional steps added to the sequence. You can also engage clients cognitively by having them identify the working muscle groups and their role in activities of daily living. Then invite them to think of an exercise goal for themselves. This approach at the beginning of class prompts participants to engage their minds as well as their bodies in the exercise.

Assessing Participant Readiness

An effective strategy for assessing participants' readiness for increased activity levels and to simultaneously help them focus and develop group cohesion is to incorporate any number of simple (and fun) warm-up activities or games. Music can facilitate this endeavor. Be aware, however, of variances among individual participants; not all people enjoy the same kind of music, have the same rhythmic abilities, or can hear verbal directions while music is playing. Moreover, adding rhythmic activities can create increased cognitive load that may not be the primary goal of the warm-up. While double dipping (i.e., having more than one objective for an activity) can lead to positive outcomes, it is important to remember that the focus of the warm-up should remain primarily on preparation for higher-intensity movements. If you do decide to add music, it is important to select songs that were popular when class participants were young adults or music with a strong beat and moderate tempo, particularly during classes early in the program. Be sure to play music at a moderate volume and turn the music down or off when explaining a new exercise or changing to a lower-intensity portion of the warm-up. Straining to hear verbal instructions over the music can be very frustrating for participants.

Increasing the Challenge

As your class participants become more comfortable with the activities presented in the warm-up, begin gradually incorporating small challenges into your warm-up by adding more complex arm movements to simple, well-learned footwork. Recall that this senior-specific principle was also discussed in chapter 8. Practice coordination sequences that require the limbs to move in unison and in opposition. If you are preparing for aerobic routines, create short routines that can fit in various places in a song and alternate them with a "home step" such as marching in place. Periodically add one or two new sets of steps lasting eight to sixteen counts to an established routine. These instructional strategies help to keep participants engaged cognitively by challenging their memory recall skills while still allowing success in movement. Research shows that successfully meeting challenges in one area of life often translates into increased confidence in one's ability to meet challenges in other areas of life (Bandura, 1997).

Engaging Participants Socially and Emotionally

The warm-up period during an exercise class is the perfect time to establish important social and emotional connections between the instructor and clients and among the clients themselves in a group setting. The warm-up provides an opportunity to converse with clients and encourage interaction, learn names, and get to know the clients better. Warm-up time can also be used to introduce new participants to the group when appropriate (Van Norman, 2005).

An example of a group warm-up activity that will provide the physical activity instructor with an opportunity to build relationships with the clients and learn more about the kinds of activities they are engaged in outside of class is "Have You Ever?" This is a simple and fun activity with origins in adventure education. Place vinyl spots or carpet squares (with rubber backing) in a circle on the floor such that there is one less spot than the number of class participants. This game is played much like musical chairs. One person (often the instructor) starts in the middle of the circle and asks the group, "Have you ever . . . (for example, gone on a cruise)?" Participants are directed to move to another spot if they have (gone on a cruise). Participants cannot merely move to a spot next to them. They must move at least two spots away. The individual who started in the middle must find a spot on the outer circle, thus

leaving someone without a spot to go to. This person becomes the leader in the middle and announces the next "have you ever" invitation to move. The game continues for approximately 5 minutes. You can vary the activity by asking the participants to use any number of different locomotor skills to move between the spots (e.g., on toes or on heels).

In addition to getting to know the clients better, this activity also allows the physical activity instructor to observe the quality of each participant's movements, including motor planning, as participants must dodge one another when moving to the open spots. Another strategy for newcomers is to have the instructor begin with a "have you ever" that includes different types of exercises, such as "Have you ever . . . (for example, done yoga)?" With this information, the instructor can find out what past experiences participants have engaging in different types of physical activity.

Guidelines for Conducting an Effective Warm-Up

- Perform ten to 20 minutes of progressive physical activity, gradually increasing the size or speed of movement and adding movement sequences.

- Use continuous, rhythmic activities (e.g., easy walking, light marching).

- Incorporate specific joint mobility exercises (joint readiness and dynamic stretching).

- Monitor intensity (on the CR10 scale, RPE between 1 and 2 for healthy older adults or between 0.5 and 1 for frailer older adults).

- Select age-appropriate music with a steady and easily distinguished beat and do a rehearsal (step-by-step at slower tempo). The tempo of the music will vary based on the fitness level of your participants but should generally range from 115 to 120 beats per minute during the warm-up.

- Include activities that promote multiple dimensions of wellness: physical, social, emotional, intellectual, vocational, and spiritual.

New Warm-Up Strategies

Older adults experienced in being physically active have likely been told for years to engage in static stretching before exercise. Research indicates, however, that joint readiness activities and **dynamic stretching** (or muscle activation) are preferred to static stretching, especially for older adults who experience passive stiffness (Page, 2012). Moreover, there is evidence that static stretching may produce "stretch-induced strength loss" (Page, 2012). Joint readiness activities and dynamic stretching are thought to effectively reduce passive stiffness and increase range of motion prior to exercise. Therefore, after completing approximately five minutes of general warm-up exercises to elevate body temperature and increase heart rate and breathing rate, performing joint readiness activities and dynamic stretching is highly recommended.

Joint Readiness

Muscles and connective tissue (the structures that connect muscles to bone and to each other) have nerves called *somatoreceptors*. Somatoreceptors need to be activated in order for the musculoskeletal system to function smoothly and efficiently. Performing **joint readiness** activities increases the circulation of synovial fluid (the fluid that lubricates joints) and prepares connective tissue (which has a blood supply) for movement. Joint readiness activities also help activate two additional sensory systems, the vestibular system (inner ear) and the visual system. When these sensory receptors are activated, they are better able to provide accurate information about body position in space.

Example of a Joint Readiness Routine

After you complete approximately five minutes of a general, whole-body warm-up, instruct your participants to remain standing (or rise from their chairs) and pretend that they are an ice-cream cone. The feet are the bottom, or tip, of the cone and the head is the top of the cone. Begin at the feet. Lead your participants through the following joint readiness activities for approximately 30 to 45 seconds each, completing the movements six to eight times in each direction.

Foot pressure rolls. Stand with feet firmly planted on the ground, hip-width apart. Without lifting the feet, increase the downward pressure on the floor by slightly rotating the ankles in a clockwise and counterclockwise direction, shifting weight from the toes to the outside of the foot, to the heels, to the inside of the foot, and back around to the toes. Encourage your clients to feel the changing pressure under the feet.

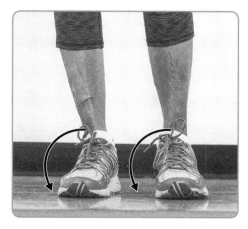

Knee circles. Bend knees and place hands on knees with the chest lifted and chin parallel to the floor. Without lifting the feet, gently lift the chest up slightly, rotate, and sink back down to the starting position. Repeat in the other direction.

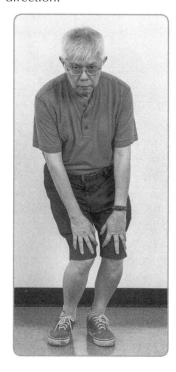

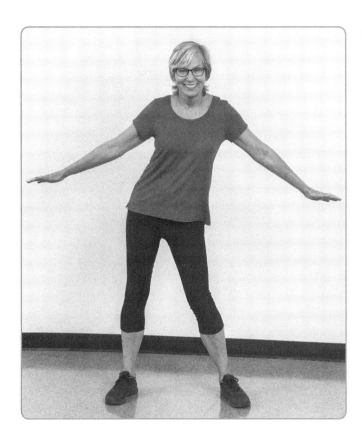

Hip circles. Just like using a hula hoop, circle the hips in a clockwise direction for a set number of rotations and then in a counterclockwise direction, starting small and increasing diameter of circles.

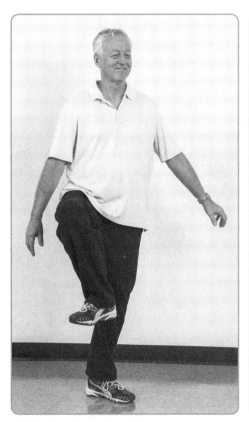
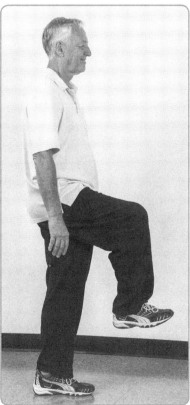

Standing leg raises or "fire hydrants." Balancing on one leg, gently bend the knee of the other leg up in front of the body, toward the stomach. Keeping that leg raised, rotate it out to the side of the body and touch it down to the floor. Reverse the process by lifting that same leg up again and rotating it back into body alignment. Lower the foot back down to the ground. Switch legs.

Trunk rotations. Stand with feet shoulder-width apart and arms by sides. *Slowly* rotate side to side, keeping arms loose against the body or swinging gently as the trunk rotates. Turn head to look over shoulder in direction of the turn.

Arm circles. Stand with feet shoulder-width apart and raise both arms out to the sides with the palms facing down. Begin slowly circling both arms toward the front for a set number of circles before circling them in the opposite direction. Slowly increase the size of the circles on each repetition. Now turn the palms up and repeat the circles in both directions.

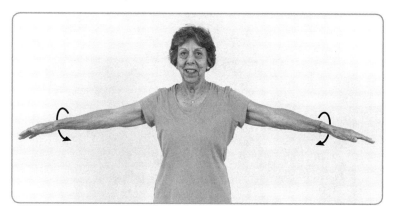

Dynamic Stretching

Dynamic warm-up, also called dynamic stretching or muscle activation, involves compound movements that increase muscle temperature while gently and simultaneously stretching muscle groups that will be used during activity (Melone, 2014). The key to a dynamic warm-up is to move in ways that mimic the types of movements that will be required during planned exercise routines. It is important when instructing older adults with arthritis and other forms of compromised joint integrity or with specific movement limitations following an injury that you encourage them to use a smaller range of motion and remain within their ability levels and pain thresholds. Examples of appropriate dynamic stretching activities are described as follows.

Wrist circles. Slowly rotate both hands at the same time, isolating the movement to the wrist joints. Repeat in the opposite direction.

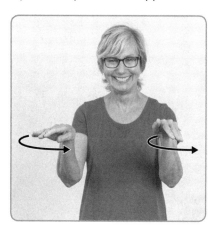

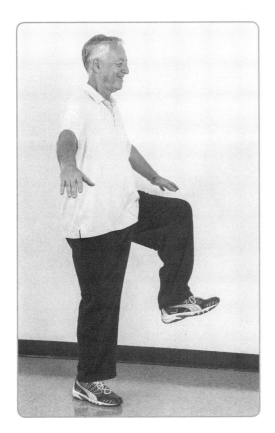

High knees. Pick up one foot, knee bent to waist level (if possible; otherwise to comfort level). Place foot down and repeat to the other side. Encourage use of arms for balance and attention to alignment. When participants put their foot down, have them make sure their knee is in alignment over their ankle (not their toe). Stride length is not as important as knee height for this exercise. High knees warms up the hip flexors while gently stretching the gluteal and hamstrings muscle groups.

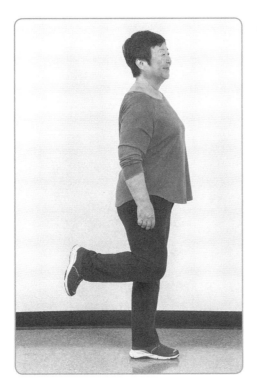

Butt kicks. Lean forward. Balancing on one foot, slide the other foot out behind, scuffing the floor while moving forward and bending the knee up and back towards the buttocks. Walk (or jog for elite levels), "kicking" up behind. Keep the chest lifted throughout the exercise. Butt kicks activate the hamstrings and gluteal muscles while gently stretching the quadriceps.

Side-step "jumping jacks." Feet are placed a little more than shoulder-width apart, arms at the side. Raise the extended arms to shoulder height, step one leg to one side and "gather" the other leg in. Tap it down and lower the arms to the sides. Now raise the extended arms again and step to the other side, again "gathering" the other leg in and tapping it on the ground. Variation: For higher functional levels, substitute a sideways shuffle for the step; not a low, tight shuffle, but a relaxed shuffle that is intended to loosen up the muscles of the inner and outer thighs and arms.

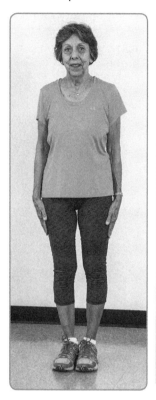
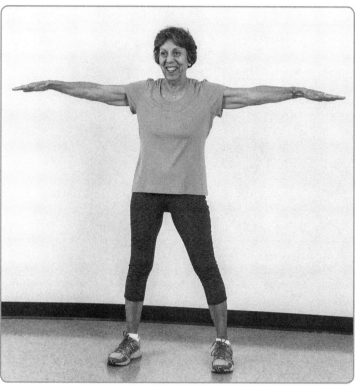

Toy soldiers. With each step walking forward, participants straighten their front leg and raise it toward the ceiling before stepping forward onto that foot. They keep a slight bend in the base leg (to protect the back). Remind participants to maintain good posture (ears above shoulders), eyes looking forward. When the front foot lands on the ground, they make sure the knee and ankle are in alignment. Not only does this activity warm-up and activate the leg muscles (front and back), it also activates the torso, which is needed in balance.

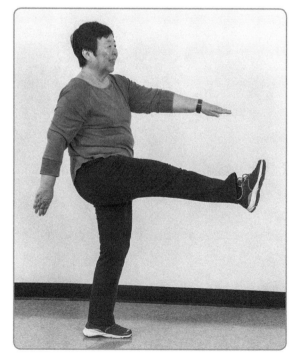

Bowing. With each step walking forward, participants place the front leg straight out in front, with the heel on the ground and the toes pointing up toward the ceiling. Then they bend forward while pushing their buttocks back. With their hands on the flexed (base) leg, they lean over the forward, straightened leg, activating the calf muscle in the back of the base leg. This activity also gently activates and stretches the gluteal, hamstrings, and calf muscles of the front leg.

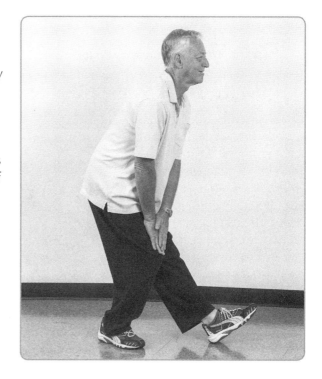

Kick-backs (sometimes called "B" walks). Participants are instructed to walk backward and with each step, "pull" their knee up and toward the stomach. After achieving an upright position with the leg raised toward the stomach, the next move is to thrust or "kick" the raised leg out and backward, gently landing on the ball of the foot. The same sequence of movements is repeated on the other side by "sitting back" in a sense, onto the now back leg, raising the other knee up in front toward the stomach, "kicking" it back, landing, and repeating. *Note:* This is a complex activity. Many people are not used to using their "back space." Reminding participants to maintain good posture and move only within a range of motion that feels comfortable cannot be emphasized enough. Beginners may need a spotter who walks alongside with one arm up in front of the participant and the other behind.

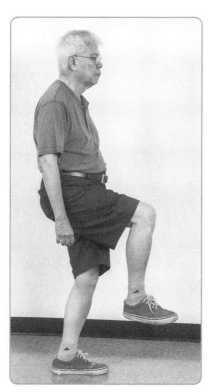
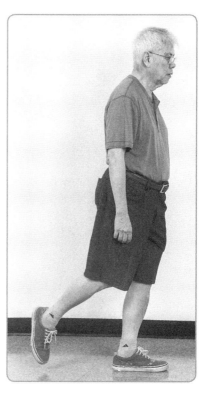

Some of the arm movements described in the next section can be added to the lower-body warm-up activities described in the preceding section once adequate strength, balance, and coordination has been achieved. For beginners, however, it is important to perform the lower- and upper-body activities separately, again, focusing time on those movements that will be introduced in the main components of the exercise class.

Goal posts. Begin with both arms out to the sides of the body, elbows bent at right angles. Keeping elbows in the same place, drop the hands down near hip level. Repeat the exercise, switching from hands up to hands down.

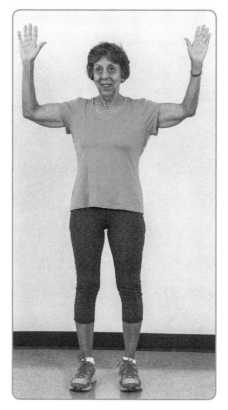
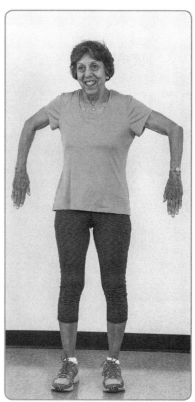

Arm kick-backs. Lean slightly forward, bending from the waist. Bend and tuck arms into the body with fists near shoulder level. Then, straighten both arms, "kicking" them back so arms are extended behind the body. Bend elbows and extend arms at the same time or alternately.

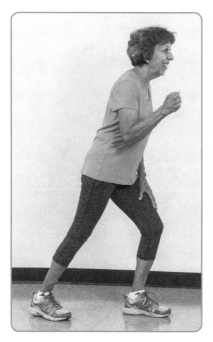
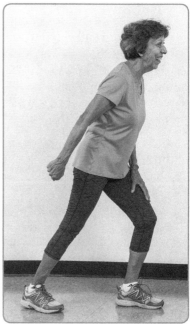

Wrists circles, hand stretches. With arms at sides or out in front, rotate wrists clockwise and then counterclockwise, then open and close hands (fingers spread out and then into a fist) repeatedly.

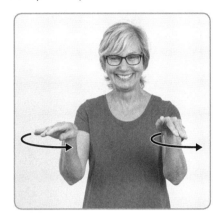

Cooling Down

The cool-down is basically the warm-up in reverse, but with the primary focus being on flexibility and relaxation. **Cooling down** involves gradually reducing the intensity of the exercise to allow for appropriate adjustments in circulation and the return of heart rate and blood pressure to near resting levels (Speer, 2005). Cooling down can also decrease muscle soreness and help prevent potential exercise-related problems such as dizziness and cardiac irregularities that can occur in high-risk populations. Reinforcing social connections and helping class participants make a conscious transition to the rest of the day are also important aspects of a cool-down. It is important to allow enough time for a proper cool-down (at least 10 minutes) and to discourage participants from leaving class before it ends.

Physiological Changes Associated With the Cool Down

Mild, continuous activity following exercise keeps the leg muscles contracting, promoting venous return and reducing the fainting and dizziness that can occur when activity is abruptly halted. Less blood pooling also reduces delayed muscular stiffness after exercise and helps reduce the level of lactic acid in the muscles, thereby promoting faster recovery (Speer, 2005).

Cooling down after aerobic activity helps to slowly decrease the level of **catecholamines** (epinephrine and norepinephrine) in the blood. High levels of catecholamines can cause cardiac irregularities among high-risk individuals, most often after as opposed to during exercise (Speer, 2005). Although such exercise-related irregularities of the heart are relatively rare, a carefully constructed cool-down is an important safety precaution.

Physiological Benefits of a Cool-Down

Decreases body temperature

Enhances venous return

Facilitates dissipation of body heat

Increases the removal of lactate

Decreases the level of catecholamines (epinephrine and norepinephrine) in the blood

From DeVries and Housh (1994); D.C. Nieman, *Exercise Testing and Prescription: A Health-Related Approach* (Mountain View, CA: Mayfield, 1999).

Developing a Cool-Down Routine

Use low-intensity, continuous movements for five to seven minutes to allow the body to adjust from exertion to rest. Use small steps from side to side and forward and backward, low marches in place, and heel presses and toe touches to the front and sides at progressively lower intensity to return the heart rate and respiration back to normal. Keep arm movements small and relaxed and predominantly below shoulder level. Mix gentle, dynamic stretches and coordination activities with low-intensity, continuous movement. See the sidebar for a sample routine.

Before your clients leave class, instruct participants to either monitor their pulse for at least 15 seconds or rate their level of perceived exertion to ensure that they have fully recovered. If partici-

Sample Low-Impact Cool-Down for Healthy Older Adults

Music: Harry Belafonte "Banana Boat Song" (109 beats per minute)

A   In a circle holding hands, low-intensity march in place (two counts of 8)

Alternating step touches, moving forward and backward (two counts of 8)

Drop hands and walk backward for more space; stay in circle formation

B   Alternating toe touches front (two counts of 8)

Alternating heel presses front (two counts of 8)

Alternating toe touches side to side (two counts of 8)

Swing arms (very little) in opposition

C   March in place (two counts of 8)

Large circle of the arms up, over the head, and down (once)

Shoulder rolls (one count of 8 forward and one count of 8 backward)

D   Alternating toe touches side to side, arms in opposition (two counts of 8)

March in place (one count of 8)

Toe touches side to side, swinging arms in unison (two counts of 8)

Repeat, swinging arms in opposition and in unison

Move together to hold hands in circle; tap the right toe in front 8 to 16 times until everyone has the right foot free to move to the right

E   Step sideways to the right, still in the circle (one count of 8)

Step to the left (one count of 8)

Repeat right and left (two counts of 8)

Step right (counts 1-4)

Step left (counts 5-8)

Repeat right and left (one count of 8)

Step right (counts 1-2)

Step left (counts 3-4)

Repeat right and left (counts 5-8 and again 1-8)

Repeat full sequence

Note: Be sure to cue in advance for the changes in direction. If participants get confused, just march in place, then tap the right toe until everyone has the right foot free to move to the right, and begin again. Music should have a slow, distinct beat (110 beats per minute).

Repeat A-D

F   Holding hands in a circle, alternate marching in place with standing upper- and lower-body stretches like reaching arms overhead, Achilles tendon stretch (lunge), shoulder stretch (arm crossing in front and then in back), hamstrings stretch (extending heel to front and flexing forward at hip). This is a great time to make personal contact with participants, asking them about their day, their families, or what they are going to do after class, sharing interesting news, and so on.

G   After 8 to 10 minutes of active cool-down, check pulse and RPE, and then progress to static flexibility exercises. Sitting on a mat or in a chair, perform flexibility exercises (see chapter 11 for exercise ideas).

H   End with relaxation breathing. Lie on your back, eyes closed, and take deep breaths. Quiet instrumental music and visualization of pleasant scenes can enhance relaxation.

pants have to leave class early, make it a standard policy that they complete the main activities 5 to 10 minutes early and then cool down until their heart and respiration rates are lower. If someone leaves class unexpectedly, be sure to have an assistant or another class participant follow that person to determine if he or she is experiencing a health problem.

It is important to set the right mood for the cool-down. Use a mat or pad to enhance comfort when performing floor exercises. Healthy older adults benefit from flexibility routines performed, in part at least, on the floor so that one muscle group can be isolated for stretching while the rest of the body is relaxed. In classes designed for older adults who are physically frail, have them perform continuous movements in a seated position and mix in gentle static stretches. While your clients are still seated, introduce activities that systematically stretch all areas of the body from the head down to the feet (i.e., neck, shoulders, arms, hands, back, hips, legs, and feet). Use relaxation strategies between stretches and at the end of class. If music is playing, it should be soothing and at a low volume. In addition, the lights can be dimmed to foster the right mood for visualization and active breathing, a simple technique to increase body awareness and lung capacity and promote relaxation. See the sidebar for a sample active breathing routine. Refer to chapter 11 for specific flexibility exercises that you can include in the cool-down component of the class.

Active Breathing Relaxation Routine

A   Place the hands on the abdomen and become aware of how the area moves while breathing.

Take a medium breath, allowing the abdomen to expand while inhaling and relax inward while exhaling.

B   Picture the lungs filling with air, pushing the diaphragm down and the abdomen out.

C   Practice slowly with medium breaths for one to two minutes; then take several very deep breaths, inhaling and exhaling slowly.

D   Slowly raise the arms above the head while inhaling *through the nose,* and lower the arms to the sides while exhaling completely *through the mouth.*

E   When comfortable with active breathing, visualize something positive or pleasant and set an intention for the day.

Using the Cool-Down to Reinforce the Wellness Connection in Group Classes

The cool-down is also the perfect time for participants to reconnect with others in the class and for you to reinforce one or more of the dimensions of wellness. For example, holding hands in a circle while performing low-intensity cool-down activities is an excellent strategy for connecting clients socially. Activities that reinforce social connection emphasize the positive nature of being part of a group, help end the class on a positive note, and help your clients begin to prepare for the rest of the day. Ending the class with the reading of an inspirational quote also reinforces the spiritual dimension of wellness. Review chapter 9 for more simple ideas on how to incorporate wellness activities into your physical activity classes.

Using the Cool-Down to Transition to the Day

Before the relaxation phase of the cool-down, make any necessary announcements. Then, after relaxation, have participants spend the final minutes of the cool-down making a thoughtful transition to the rest of the day. You may guide this reflection by suggesting a review of individual and group goals accomplished during class. You may want to invite participants to identify a personal goal for the day that connects with the functional features of the exercises they did during their exercise session. Inviting participants to share ideas and thoughts for the day supports social and emotional connections and fosters group identity. A group shoulder massage may also bring participants together and is a fun way to bring the class to a close!

Guidelines for an Effective Cool-Down

- Continuous rhythmic exercises progressively decreasing in intensity for 5 to 10 minutes, depending on participants' fitness levels
- A stretching phase that includes a focus on flexibility
- A variety of simple mind–body activities, such as yoga and tai chi
- Activities that reinforce social, emotional, and cognitive connections
- A relaxation phase to facilitate the transition from the exercise class to the rest of the day

---

Summary

The warm-up and cool-down are essential components of an exercise class for older adults. The warm-up should be carefully designed to increase body temperature for optimal performance and reduced risk of injury. In contrast, the cool-down is designed to return the body systems to their pre-activity states. The warm-up and cool-down also provide the instructor with an opportunity to engage participants socially, emotionally, cognitively, and spiritually in the exercise experience. Facilitating the psychosocial elements of physical activity can improve clients' self-efficacy, both inside and outside class, and enhance their motivation to continue attending class.

Key Terms

active warm-up	joint readiness
body scan	passive warm-up
catecholamines	rating of perceived exertion (RPE)
cooling down	talk test
dynamic stretching	warming up

Recommended Readings

Page, P. (2012). Current concepts in muscle stretching for exercise and rehabilitation. *The International Journal of Sports Physical Therapy, 7,* 109-119.

Speer, K.P. (Ed). *Injury prevention and rehabilitation for active older adults.* Champaign, IL: Human Kinetics.

Study Questions

1. How does the body usually signal that it is physiologically warmed up?
   a. heavy perspiration
   b. slight increase in heart rate
   c. light perspiration
   d. dramatic increase in heart rate

2. The warm-up positively affects the neuromuscular system by
   a. increasing blood saturation
   b. increasing muscle elasticity
   c. making the muscle contraction–relaxation cycle more efficient
   d. all of the above

3. Warming up influences pulmonary blood flow by
   a. increasing the resistance to blood flow
   b. decreasing the resistance to blood flow
   c. creating a more constant resistance
   d. allowing wider variation in resistance

4. Passive warm-up refers to
   a. applying external heating agents to the body, such as hot showers or heating pads
   b. another person's moving the client's arms or legs through an easy range of motion to prepare the client for exercise
   c. engaging in whole-body movement to increase body temperature
   d. slowly moving the arms and legs through a limited range of motion

5. The purpose of the cool-down is to slowly decrease _____ to preactivity levels.
   a. respiration
   b. body temperature
   c. heart rate
   d. all of the above

6. Mild, continuous activity following exercise
   a. prevents blood from pooling in the extremities
   b. reduces levels of lactic acid in muscles
   c. increases levels of epinephrine
   d. a and b

7. Which of the following are relevant and valuable to discuss during warm-up or cool-down?

   a. goal-setting

   b. socialization

   c. reminders about safety (e.g., proper alignment, how to rate exertion)

   d. all of the above

Application Activities

1. Design the first 10-minutes of a warm-up for a group of independent-living older adults to prepare them for 20 minutes of resistance training. Write down the specific activities you plan to include, the overall intensity and duration of the warm-up, and an appropriate rationale for the selected activities.

2. Design a 10-minute warm-up suitable for a group of frail older adults who are beginning their first week of a chair exercise class. Develop a list of general body warm-up and joint readiness activities you plan to include in your warm-up. How you will decide which activities to include? Approximately how long will the warm-up last? Will you use music? Why or why not? What information would you plan to share that is relevant to the success of the warm-up?

3. Design a five-minute cool-down for a low-impact aerobics class for independent older adults. Write down the sequence of activities and the music you plan to use.

Flexibility Training

Debra J. Rose

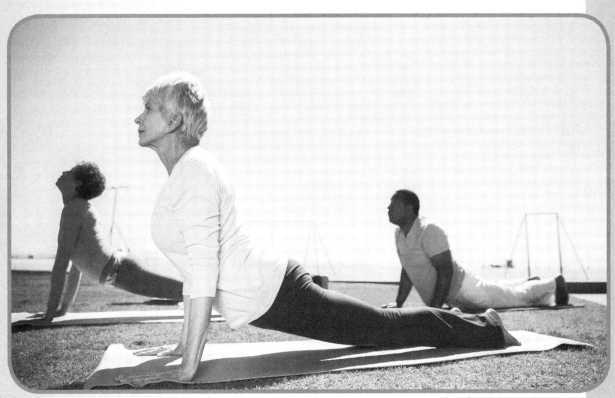

Objectives

After completing this chapter, you will be able to

1. describe the age-associated changes in joint and muscle flexibility,
2. identify the critical ranges of joint flexibility required for the performance of basic activities of daily living,
3. describe the benefits of flexibility training for daily function,
4. identify the two types of stretching techniques and when to use them in an exercise session, and
5. incorporate flexibility training into a physical activity program for older adults.

Flexibility, a term that describes the range of movement or motion possible at one or multiple joints, is important at all ages. When we were young, most of us enjoyed freedom of movement in all of our joints. Children have no difficulty breaking into a run spontaneously or picking up a stick and throwing it because their joints move freely. As we age, however, many factors contribute to a decline in flexibility (e.g., increased joint stiffness, changes in connective tissue, osteoarthritis). Indeed, for some older adults, the loss in joint flexibility can be so severe that the performance of daily activities becomes compromised. The good news is that exercises specifically designed to improve flexibility have been shown to be very effective for older adults. Although exercise alone is not likely to restore the movement potential that was present at a younger age, improvements in flexibility can result in enhanced physical function. Improved flexibility also helps older adults feel better by reducing pain and stiffness, an additional benefit above and beyond the physiological benefits achieved.

The aim of this chapter is to describe age-associated changes in flexibility, the functional consequences of a loss in flexibility, and the minimal ranges of motion that should be maintained or restored at certain joints to improve older adults' performance of daily activities. In addition, a number of dynamic and static flexibility exercises designed to improve joint range of motion are presented.

Age-Associated Changes in Flexibility

Declines in joint **range of motion (ROM)**, defined as the total excursion that is possible at a joint from the beginning of movement to the end of movement, are inevitable as a result of aging, but the rate of decline appears to be joint specific (Bell & Hoshizaki, 1981; Einkauf, Gohdes, Jensen, & Jewell, 1987; Stathokostas, McDonald, Little, & Paterson, 2013). For example, spinal extension declines, on average, by approximately 50 percent between the second and seventh decades (Einkauf et al., 1987), while hip extension and knee flexion ROM decline on average by only 20 percent and 2 percent, respectively, over the same time period. The decline in joint ROM is also generally more evident in lower-body than in upper-body joints, consistent with the decline in muscle strength. Reduced flexibility in the lower-body joints has important implications for general mobility. Lower hamstrings flexibility declines in both genders by approximately 14.5 percent, or one inch (2.5 cm) per decade (Golding & Lindsay, 1989), while losses of 15 percent (external rotation) and 11 percent (abduction) in ROM have been reported for the hip joints. Small but significant age-related changes have been reported in ankle dorsiflexion ROM. Small ROM changes independent of larger muscle strength losses have been observed (Nigg, Fisher,

Allinger, Ronsky, & Engsberg, 1992), and ankle dorsiflexion strength has been shown to decrease by approximately 30 percent between the middle-age and the older adult years (Vandervoort et al., 1992). Changes in ankle dorsiflexion ROM has been shown to be a significant factor in predicting the incidence of disability among community-dwelling older women (Tainaka, Takizawa, Katamoto, & Aoki, 2009). Any reduction in ankle ROM and strength also increases the likelihood of trips and falls during the swing phase of gait.

With age, **stiffness** in all joints and muscle tissues also increases. Stiffness is defined as the force required to move a joint through a specified ROM (Holland, Tanaka, Shigematsu, & Nakagaichi, 2002). None of the tissues associated with mobility are impervious to aging, whether it is the tendons, ligaments, fascia, joint capsules, or the fast- and slow-twitch muscles. Even muscles that are used routinely (e.g., calf muscles) show an increase in stiffness (James & Parker, 1989; Lung, Hartsell, & Vandervoort, 1996; Buckwalter et al., 1993). This increased stiffness is probably the most common complaint of older adults and results in a decline in ROM at most of the major joint complexes (Svenningsen, Terjesen, Auflem, & Berg, 1989; Vandervoort et al., 1992; Walker, Sue, Miles-Elkousy, Ford, & Trevelyan, 1984).

A number of biological factors appear to contribute to the increased muscle stiffness and reduced range of motion observed with age. These factors include an increase in the amount of inter- and intramuscular connective tissue, a change in the chemical composition of the connective tissue matrix and collagen, and breakdown of articular cartilage that increases arthritis in major joint complexes (Hall, 1976). In fact, it has been demonstrated using radiography that by the age of 75 years, 85 percent of older adults have osteoarthritic changes in the weight-bearing joints of the body (Moskowitz, 1989). As muscles age, they also lose mass as a result of the decline in the actual number of muscle fibers (Rosenberg, 2011). The age-associated loss of muscle mass is a syndrome referred to as **sarcopenia**. Subsequently, the connective tissue surrounding and within muscles increases (Eddinger, Cassens, & Moss, 1986).

Because connective tissue is composed primarily of collagen, it has much less elasticity than skeletal muscle. Thus, more collagen within and around muscles results in reduced ROM. With age, collagen fibers also change such that there are more cross-links between fibers, making the collagen less extensible or more resistant to deformation (Cetta, Tenni, Zanaboni, & Maroudas, 1982). Connective tissue also contains a gelatinous material called matrix, which holds water and gives connective tissue its resilience. The collagen-associated matrix within all connective tissue also undergoes a change in chemical composition such that the material responsible for holding water (chondroitin sulfate) is lost with age. The loss of water also contributes to making connective tissue less extensible and more resistant to being deformed (Buckwalter et al., 1993). These changes in connective tissue undoubtedly make it more difficult to move freely in old age.

A loss of muscle strength occurs concomitantly with the increase in stiffness. As a result, older adults have to use more muscle power to overcome their own inertia. For example, functional activities such as getting out of bed in the morning, getting dressed, bathing, and rising from low chairs become increasingly difficult with age. Because it is more challenging and, in some cases, painful to move, many older adults begin to move within a smaller range of motion, thereby using less and less joint flexibility. As a result of this disuse, the joint becomes less capable of reaching what is considered to be a normal **active range of motion** (the range of movement through which a person can actively [without assistance] move a joint using the adjacent muscles). In fact, because their range of motion is inadequate, it is not uncommon to find a number of community-dwelling men and women who cannot perform essential daily activities, such as putting on clothes requiring an overhead motion, rising from a low chair, or turning their head far enough when reversing a car or looking to see whether a car is in the next lane before switching lanes.

Although an age-related change in flexibility is inevitable, the magnitude of the decline is highly modifiable. Physical inactivity plays a particularly important role in the loss of flexibility with age and probably contributes more to the reduction in movement potential than normal age-related changes and pathological processes. Consequently, an important component of any well-rounded physical activity program for older adults should include flexibility training.

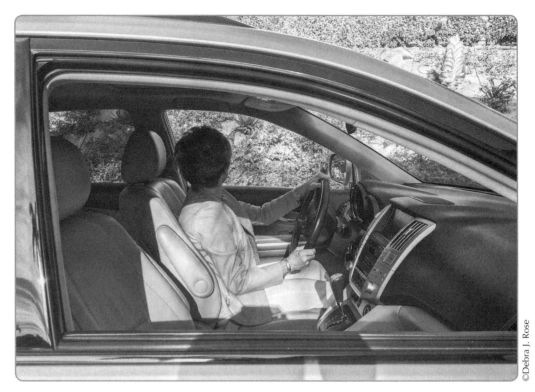

©Debra J. Rose

The loss of active range of motion in the cervical region can hinder the performance of essential daily activities such as driving a vehicle.

Flexibility and Function

The consequences of reduced flexibility are numerous. Activities of daily living most affected include those that require reaching overhead, getting into and out of a car (especially one with bucket seats), reaching into low cabinets, bending down to pick up an object from the floor, and stepping onto or down from a high step or curb. Other functional consequences of a limited range of motion include the inability to put on an article of clothing with zippers or fasteners in the back (e.g., a dress or bra) due to limited shoulder internal rotation. A reduction in shoulder elevation can restrict the ability to put on sweatshirts, T-shirts, or any other item of clothing that requires a significant amount of shoulder elevation. Inadequate knee flexion coupled with limited trunk flexibility can make it more difficult, if not impossible, for older adults to put on shoes and socks.

As the number of functional limitations due to reduced flexibility increases, an older adult's functional independence becomes more and more compromised. Not as readily apparent are the consequences of limited flexibility for balance

and strength. Both of these important domains are influenced by joint excursion. In addition, men and women with limited flexibility are more likely to sustain a muscle injury.

The association between muscle strength and flexibility in older adults has not been well defined. It is apparent, however, that when older adults gain flexibility, they typically experience an increase in strength also (Brown, Sinacore, Ehsani, Binder, & Holloszy, 2000). Perhaps the effort expended to gain range of motion is sufficient to challenge the surrounding musculature, thereby increasing muscle strength. Alternatively, increasing a joint's range of motion may release the muscles to such an extent that they can be used more readily. Regardless of the mechanism of change, improving your clients' flexibility will enable them to use skeletal muscle more efficiently.

An increase in muscle strength typically occurs when older adults improve their joint flexibility.

For a variety of reasons, older adults are more susceptible to muscle injury than younger adults. Although direct evidence is lacking, one likely major factor is limited joint and muscle excursion (Lindsay, Horton, & Vandervoort, 2000; Ploutz-Snyder, Giamis, Formikell, & Rosenbaum, 2001). A good amount of research evidence indicates that the muscles of young men and women with limited ranges of motion are more prone to injury than muscles of individuals who have normal ranges (McHugh et al., 1999; Noonan & Garrett, 1999). It should also be noted that older muscles may not recover from injury as quickly as young muscles (Brooks & Faulkner, 1996). It is therefore important for older adults to maintain as full a range of motion as possible, not just to prevent injury but also to minimize the accompanying loss in strength or aerobic capacity should an injury occur. The 2008 Physical Activity Guidelines for Americans provide an excellent set of recommendations for older adults who want to engage in regular physical activity while avoiding the risk of injury (U.S. Department of Health and Human Services, 2008).

In addition to the functional benefits associated with improved flexibility, your clients will also feel better as a result of increasing their joint ROM. Improved flexibility can have a beneficial effect on posture that, in turn, can reduce pain, improve balance, heighten the sense of well-being, and enhance self-efficacy. Improved spinal flexibility and the abil-ity to stand more erectly also reduce breathlessness, as there is more room for chest expansion.

Critical Ranges of Flexibility

To date, few **critical ranges** (absolute minimum range of joint motion required to perform a certain activity) for flexibility have been published for daily activities. Ranges that have been reported for tasks such as walking, climbing stairs, getting onto and off a toilet, and getting dressed are presented in table 11.1. Critical ranges are important to keep in mind when designing exercise programs to improve function. It is important as well to remember that some conditions do not permit reestablishing critical ranges. For example, older adults with total hip replacements are typically unable to bend the hip farther than 90 degrees. Knee joint replacements or prostheses rarely bend beyond 110 degrees.

The Benefits of Exercise and Flexibility Training

Although this component of fitness has not been well studied over the years, there is some research evidence that older adults with range-of-motion deficits can improve their flexibility. Significant improvements in joint range of motion have been noted following a variety of different exercise types

Table 11.1 Critical Ranges of Flexibility

Activity	Shoulder joint	Hip joint	Knee joint	Ankle joint
Putting on clothing overhead	90° elevation (including flexion, abduction) 45° external rotation			
Fastening or unfastening clothing in back	45° abduction, 70° internal rotation, 10° extension			
Walking at 3 mph (4.8 km/h)		30° flexion 10° extension	70° flexion	10° dorsiflexion
Ascending stairs		70° flexion	90° flexion	10° dorsiflexion
Getting onto and off toilet		110° flexion	115° flexion	10° dorsiflexion
Getting down onto and up from floor, into and out of tub		120° flexion	135° flexion	10° dorsiflexion

including passive proprioceptive neuromuscular facilitation (PNF) (Klein, Stone, Phillips, Gangi, & Hartman, 2002), traditional flexibility exercises (Christiansen, 2008; Gajdosik, Vander Linder, McNair, Williams, & Riggin, 2005; King et al., 2000; Stanziano, Roos, Perry, Lai, & Signorile, 2009), dance (Keogh, Kilding, Pidgeon, Ashley, & Gillis, 2009), and tai chi (Taylor-Piliae, Haskell, Stotts, & Froelicher, 2006). In some studies significant improvements in functional outcomes were also observed (Batista, Vilar, De Almeida Ferreira, Rebelatto, & Salvini, 2009; Cristopoliski, Barela, Leite, Fowler, & Rodacki, 2009; Stanziano et al., 2009). What matters most is stressing the **end range** of joint motion (i.e., the maximal distance a joint can be moved until a point of discomfort) using exercises or physical activity that is both safe and enjoyable.

Types of Stretching Techniques

Many different types of stretching techniques can be beneficial if applied correctly and at the right time during an exercise session. These different techniques can be divided into two main categories: **static stretching** and **dynamic stretching**. Static stretching generally focuses on a particular muscle group and involves moving the joint through a single movement plane until a given end point is reached. The joint is then held in that position for a period of time (anywhere from 10 to 90 seconds). Static stretching is intended to improve muscle length in muscles that are tight or restore muscle length following an injury or period of immobilization. Static stretching can also promote improved stretch pain tolerance and muscle relaxation poststretch (Ashwell, Foulcher, & Baker, 2014). Static stretches are very safe to perform and present little likelihood of injury if performed correctly. In contrast, dynamic stretching involves moving into and out of the stretch using a smooth and sustained motion rather than holding the joint in an end position for any period of time. Unlike static stretching, the goal of this stretching technique is to progressively increase joint ROM with each subsequent movement repetition and thereby prepare the muscles for subsequent physical activities.

A certain joint or muscle group might be targeted for stretching through a single plane of motion (single-joint dynamic stretching), or multiple joints

and muscles might be recruited and then moved through a single movement plane or multiple movement planes in task-specific patterns (multiple-joint dynamic stretching). This latter stretching technique constitutes a very functional approach to flexibility training and is beneficial for the performance of daily activities, which are usually dynamic and often require movement in multiple planes (e.g., reaching into the dishwasher to retrieve objects and then placing them on the counter, reaching into the back of a cupboard, cleaning windows, planting flowers). This approach to flexibility training nicely complements the functional resistance training described in chapter 12.

To date, no high-quality research studies have been conducted to determine which type of flexibility training is most beneficial for older adults and when it should be performed during an exercise class. However, there is general consensus among the experts that dynamic stretching is the more appropriate technique to use early in a class to facilitate warming up the body and muscles and increase blood flow to the working muscles. In contrast, static stretching should be reserved until the body is at its warmest, when muscles and joints are most receptive to being stretched. This might be at the end of an extended warm-up, immediately following the aerobics section of the class and before resistance training, or during the cool-down.

It is recommended that dynamic stretches be performed early in the class to warm up the body and increase blood flow to the working muscles, while static stretches should be reserved for a later time when the body is at its warmest and the muscles and joints are more receptive to being stretched.

Incorporating Flexibility Training Into the Exercise Program

Flexibility training can be incorporated into your physical activity program in many different ways. The warm-up provides a nice opportunity for dynamic stretching techniques, while a section of the cool-down can include static stretching techniques (see chapter 10 for examples of warm-up and cool-down routines). A stand-alone flexibility component within your program is also an option. In addition to the more traditional flexibility exercises described in this chapter, there are other ways for your older adult clients to improve joint range of motion, such as certain types of dance, tai chi, Pilates, and yoga.

The Warm-Up

As indicated in the previous section, the best type of flexibility exercise to use in the early stages of the warm-up is dynamic. Dynamic stretching can often be achieved just by moving the limbs through a progressively larger ROM as the warm-up progresses. When the muscles are warmer (after approximately 10 to 20 minutes), you can perform specific dynamic stretches that involve the muscle groups that will be used in the movements planned for the next section of the class. It is further recommended that the range of motion through which the joint is moved should not exceed the range through which subsequent activities will be performed. Examples of single-joint and multiple-joint dynamic stretches that involve both the upper and lower body include the following.

Seated Activities

Floor reach: Sit on the edge of a straight-backed chair with no armrests or a chair with no backrest. Keep back upright. Arms are outstretched forward to 90 degrees. Knees should be together and flexed about 90 degrees. Bend forward toward floor, reaching as far as possible toward the floor or touching the floor if ROM permits.

Seated trunk rotation: Sit on the edge of a chair with hands in front of the body holding an imaginary steering wheel. Slowly rotate trunk and head to the right until you can see an imaginary car in the right lane. Repeat rotation to the left side.

Seated abduction: Sit on the edge of a chair with hands holding onto chair. Alternate abducting and adducting a single leg, increasing the range of motion on each repetition. Perform the same movement with both legs simultaneously to increase the challenge.

Alternate knee to chest: Sit on the edge of a chair. Bring one knee up toward the chest. Grasp the knee and encircle it with both hands. Using both hands, bring the knee gently up toward the chest, touching the chest if possible. Repeat with opposite knee.

Standing Activities

Reach and curl: From a standing position, reach arms overhead with palms facing up to ceiling; then tuck chin onto chest and curl down into a crouched position, hands touching floor. Repeat in a controlled manner slowly and continuously five times.

Picking apples: Reach up with single arm to pick imaginary fruit, and return to imaginary bag at hip level. Encourage clients to rise up onto balls of the feet if balance is good. Reach in a new direction with each repetition (e.g., same side of body, across body). Repeat with opposite limb after five repetitions.

Climbing rope: Clients climb an imaginary rope. Emphasize good upward stretch with arms and trunk. Pulling an imaginary rope in a horizontal direction as would be used in tug-of-war also requires trunk rotation. Opposite leg lifts with each arm raise. Repeat five times. Encourage a larger ROM with each repetition.

Knees up, Mother Brown: Exaggerated march in place. Arms and legs move in opposition. One arm is raised to 90 degrees of flexion, while the opposite leg is brought up into as much hip, knee, and ankle flexion as possible.

Side lunges with (a) *arm reach across body,* (b) *arm reach to same side of body, and* (c) *forward arm reach:* Alternate movements on each subsequent repetition.

Walking, with six to seven alternating bouts of long and short strides: Opposite arm should be raised with exaggerated, wooden-soldier-like movement. To make this activity more challenging, have clients walk with slightly flexed knees. Incorporate activities that simulate those to be performed later in class.

The Cool-Down

In contrast to the warm-up, static flexibility exercises are preferred during the cool-down or at another point in the class when the internal body temperature is elevated and the muscles are thoroughly warmed up. This is necessary because stretches that require longer holds will be more effective and safer to perform when the muscles are warm. You can use the time while clients hold a longer stretch to review aspects of the class with them, solicit feedback from them, and encourage them to do flexibility exercises even on the days they do not attend class (but remind them to warm up first).

General Precautions

Like any other program component, the flexibility exercises you select must be appropriate for your clients and performed correctly. Special precautions should be followed when selecting flexibility exercises for clients with certain medical conditions (e.g., osteoporosis, rheumatoid arthritis, and osteoarthritis; refer to chapter 17 for exercise contraindications). Because static and dynamic stretching techniques can improve flexibility, both can be included in an exercise prescription. For example, a single static stretch is more comfortable than multiple repetitions of a dynamic stretch for a person who has significant joint disease and pain, at least in the early stages of an exercise program. On the other hand, for someone with poor body awareness, repeating limb movements multiple times may be helpful.

It is important that you encourage your older adult clients to move at their own pace to avoid injury. If any of the flexibility exercises presented in this chapter cause the client pain, an alternative exercise should be selected that stretches the target muscle or joint without discomfort. A client who has poor balance should perform exercises in a seated position or with the additional support of a ballet barre, chair, or wall.

Flexibility Exercise Guidelines

Here is an appropriate set of guidelines to follow when designing and delivering flexibility exercises during a physical activity class:

- Select flexibility exercises on the basis of which joints have obvious range limitations and which muscles are stiff.
- Emphasize good body alignment.

- Perform dynamic stretches during the warm-up to facilitate warming up the body and muscles.
- Do not perform static stretches until the body is at its warmest and muscles and joints are receptive to stretch.
- Move slowly into a static stretch position.
- Stretch to a point of gentle tension, but not pain.
- Do not jerk, bounce, or force a stretch, because this could result in injury.
- Hold a static stretch for 10 to 90 seconds.
- Inhale before the start of the stretch, exhale during the stretch, and breathe evenly while holding the stretch at its end position.

Examples of Flexibility Exercises

Many of the flexibility exercises described in this section can be performed in a variety of different positions (e.g., sitting in a chair or on the floor, lying prone or supine, standing, kneeling with hands on the floor). You should choose flexibility exercises on the basis of information you glean from each client's preactivity screening and performance assessment. Each exercise has a simple name to facilitate recollection of the exercise. Over time, most of your older adult clients will know which exercise to perform when you simply call out its name. The exercise descriptions also identify the muscle group or groups that are targeted by each exercise.

It is important to emphasize appropriate breathing technique as well as correct form. As a general rule, clients should inhale just before each stretch, exhale during the stretch, and breathe evenly while holding the end position in the case of static stretches. A focus on breathing during flexibility training is particularly important in light of older adults' tendency to hold their breath when exercising. Remember that flexibility exercises should be selected on the basis of which muscle groups are to be targeted later in the class. The selected flexibility exercises can also be performed one after the other with no need to rest after each exercise. Occasional rest periods may be incorporated for more frail clients, but there should be very little need for recovery. Above all, activities should be challenging, efficacious, and enjoyable. There is no pain for gain in this approach.

The following exercises are presented in top-to-bottom order: upper body, trunk, and lower body.

You should also present flexibility exercises systematically, starting with the upper-body stretches and ending with the lower-body stretches (i.e., head to toe). The recommended readings at the end of the chapter offer additional flexibility exercises.

Upper-Body Flexibility Exercises

Exercises to improve older adults' upper-body flexibility are provided in this section, including exercises that can be done while seated or while standing. The dynamic flexibility exercises can be performed during the warm-up, while the static stretches can be integrated into the cool-down. A stand-alone flexibility-training component can also be added to any exercise session.

Seated or Standing Position

Rotating Neck Stretch

Target muscles: side of neck, upper back

Sit tall against the back of a chair or stand upright with the eyes directed forward. Gently turn the head to the left, keeping the chin parallel to the floor and the shoulders down and back. Rotate the head back to a centered position, pause briefly, and then rotate the head to the right. Try to increase the range of motion with each repetition. Encourage clients to perform each head turn slowly and to focus on a visual target at eye level to reduce the possibility of dizziness. Increase the time each turn is held if the client reports any dizziness or discomfort in the neck.

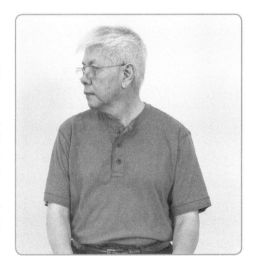

Assisted Side Neck Stretch

Target muscles: side of neck

In a seated or standing position, slowly tilt the head to the right side (ear toward the shoulder) while keeping the eyes directed forward and the shoulders down and back. At the same time, gently place the right hand on the opposite side of the head so that the weight of the hand increases the stretch. Do not force the stretch by pulling on the head. Repeat to the left side. As flexibility improves, the stretch can be performed unassisted.

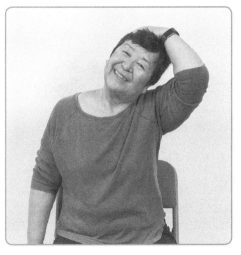

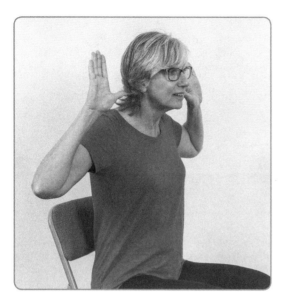

Turtle Stretch

Target muscles: front and back of neck, upper back

Sit tall in center of chair or stand with upright posture. Place the thumb side of the hands next to the ears, palms facing forward. Gently bring the head straight back behind the thumbs while keeping the chin parallel to the floor. Pause briefly in that position before slowly moving the head back to an extended position in front of the thumbs. Breathe evenly throughout the exercise and keep the eyes directed forward.

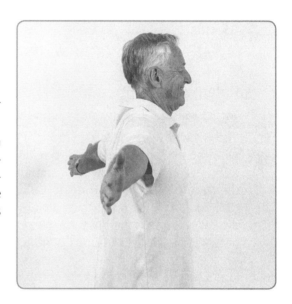

Backward Arm Stretch

Target muscles: shoulder adductors, internal rotators

Raise the arms out to the sides of the body with the palms facing forward. Slowly move the extended arms directly backward as far as possible. Tell your clients to sit or stand tall with the ears directly above the shoulders and the eyes focused on a visual target at eye level.

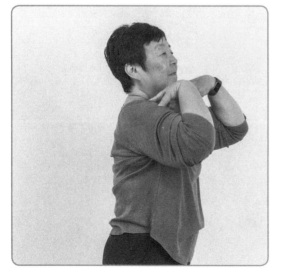

Alternating Arm Swings

Target muscles: all scapular and shoulder muscles

Place the hands on the shoulders. Circle both arms in a wide arc, first backward and then forward.

Triceps Stretch

Target muscles: back of the upper arms, chest, and shoulders

Sit tall against the back of a chair or stand tall with relaxed shoulders and arms loosely hanging by the sides of the body. Position one hand behind the head with the upper arm close to the ear and the elbow pointed to the ceiling. Reach with the fingers of the bent arm down toward the middle of the back while gently pushing the upper arm back and down with the opposite hand. Keep the back straight during the stretch and the stomach and chin tucked in.

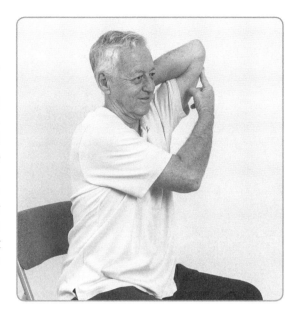

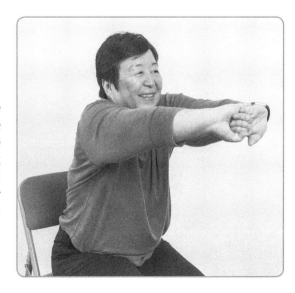

Cross Body Shoulder Stretch

Target muscles: back of the shoulders and upper back between shoulder blades

Sit tall against the back of a chair or stand tall. Bend the right arm up until the elbow is at 90 degrees. Bring the left arm up under the bent right arm and cradle it with the left elbow. Fingers are pointing up towards the ceiling and the eyes are directed forward. Gently bring the right arm across the body until a stretch is felt in the upper arm, shoulder, and upper back. Breathe evenly throughout the stretch.

Upper-Back Stretch

Target muscles: upper back and shoulders

Sit upright in a chair or stand erect, and raise the arms forward to shoulder level. Place one hand on top of the other so that the palms are facing away from the body; round the back and push the hands away from the body until a stretch is felt across the muscles of the upper back. Breathe evenly throughout the stretch and keep the eyes directed forward.

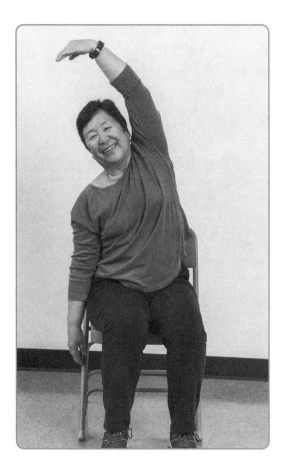

Side Stretch

Target muscles: side of trunk and shoulders, also the outer thighs and hips when performed in a standing position

Sit tall against the back of a chair or stand tall with feet shoulder-width apart or wider. Gently bend the trunk to one side as the opposite arm reaches up above and then across the head to form an arc. Keep the head, chest, and hips facing forward throughout the stretch and breathe evenly. Hold the position for 5 to 15 seconds, and then slowly return to the starting position. Repeat on the opposite side.

Alternating Hip Lifts

Target muscles: oblique muscles of trunk, hip flexors, knee flexors

Place both hands on either side of a chair. Slowly raise one hip off the chair. Hold raised position for 10 to 20 seconds before lowering hip back down. Repeat on the opposite side.

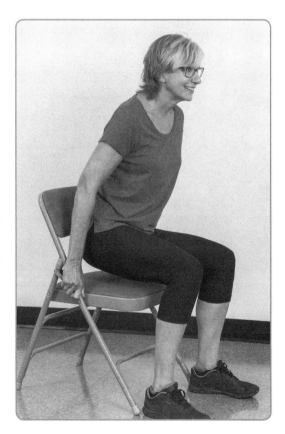

Standing Position

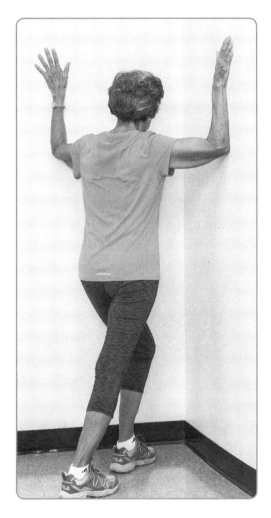

Chest Stretch

Target muscles: pectorals

Stand facing a corner or open doorway with one foot in front of the other. Raise the elbows to shoulder level and place the palms against the walls or door jam. Lean the body forward until the stretch is felt across the upper chest muscles.

Front Wall Crawl

Target muscles: scapular retractors and rotators, shoulder adductors and internal rotators

Stand facing a wall, approximately six inches (15 cm) away from the wall. Place both hands on the wall directly in front of the body. "Crawl" the fingers up the wall, bringing the arms up as high as possible with each repetition.

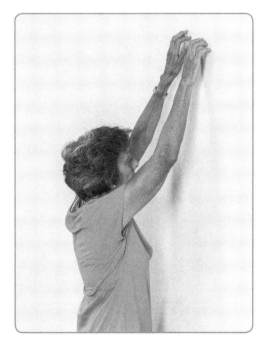

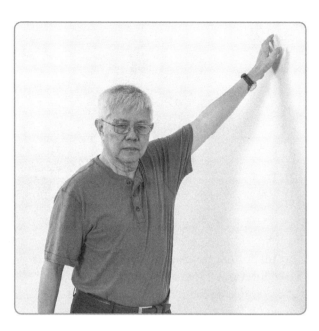

Side Wall Crawl

Target muscles: shoulders, oblique muscles of trunk

Stand with your side to the wall, feet approximately two feet (0.6 m) away. Stand tall with the stomach tucked in, chest up, chin back, eyes directed forward. Walk the fingertips up the wall until a comfortable stretch is felt in the shoulder and along the side of the body. Move closer to the wall as the fingers move upward. Walk the fingers slowly back down to the starting position. Repeat on the opposite side.

Lower-Body Flexibility Exercises

The flexibility exercises described in this section primarily target the muscles of the hip, buttocks, and lower body. Many of these exercises can be performed in multiple positions for greater variety. Most of these activities can also be modified to make them easier or more complex and demanding, thus expanding the basic repertoire of exercises presented here.

Lying or Kneeling Position

Side Leg Raises

Target muscles: hip abductors

Lie on your side on a mat, and place the palm of the uppermost hand on the floor at chest level to stabilize the body. Extend the lower arm above the head. Abduct the top leg up into the air, raising it higher and higher with each repetition. Point the toes away from the body as the leg is lifted.

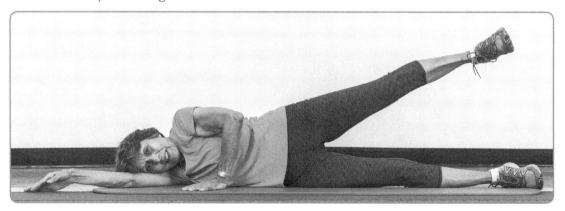

Alternating Leg Raises

Target muscles: hip flexors, trunk flexors

Kneel with the knees directly under the hips and the hands on the floor directly beneath the shoulders. Keep the head and eyes directed forward. Raise one leg off the ground; extend it and lift it toward the ceiling. Repeat with the opposite leg.

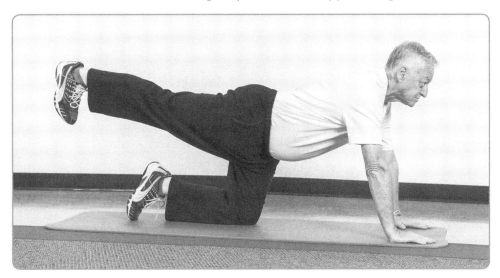

Single or Double Knee-to-Chest Stretch

Target muscles: lower back, buttocks, and hamstrings

Lie in a supine position on the floor with the knees bent and feet flat on the floor. Keep the neck extended and chin tucked in to chest. Slowly lift one or both feet off the floor and grasp the raised leg(s) below the knee(s). Gently hug the knee(s) in toward the chest. Release the hands and return one or both legs to the floor. Repeat with the other leg if performing the single knee-to-chest stretch. Less stress is placed on the lower back in the single-leg stretch and is therefore recommended for older adults with a history of lower back pain.

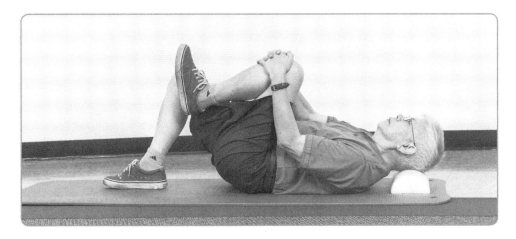

Cat and Camel

Target muscles: abdominals and upper, middle, and lower back

Start in a kneeling position with the hands on the floor and directly below the shoulders. Knees are directly under the hips and the eyes are looking at the floor. Lower the stomach, arch the back, lift the head, and look forward, keeping both hands and knees in contact with the ground. Reverse the movement by rounding the back and lowering the head until it is between the arms. A floor mat under the knees increases comfort.

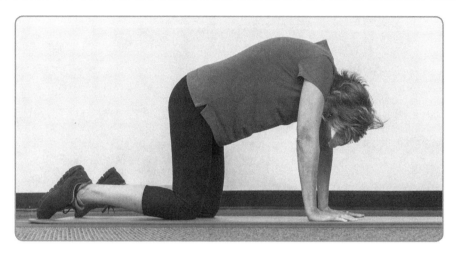

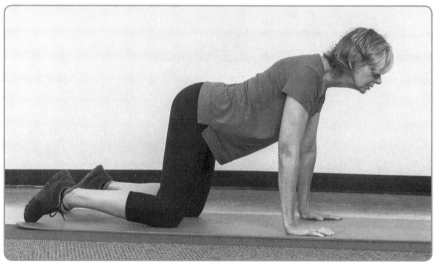

Spine Stretch

Target muscles: upper and lower back, front of the ankles, lower legs

Kneel on all fours as in the previous exercise. Moving the buttocks backward, sink down so that the forehead touches the floor. Keep the hands on the floor with arms extended.

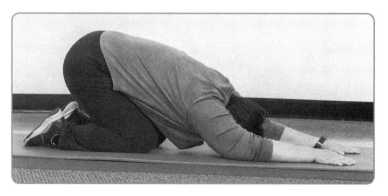

Concentrate on lengthening the spine during the stretch. Return to the starting position.

Hip Rolls

Target muscles: gluteals, hips, trunk

Lie supine on the floor with the arms extended to each side and the knees flexed. Slowly lower both legs to the floor on the same side of the body while keeping the elbows, shoulders, and head flat against the floor. Return the legs to the starting position. Repeat to the opposite side.

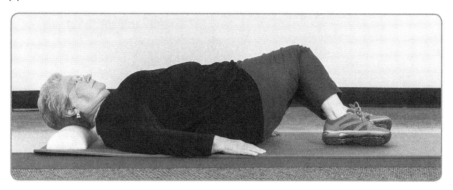

Hamstrings Stretch, Extended Leg

Target muscles: buttocks, back of the upper thighs, calves

Lie on the back with knees bent and feet flat on the floor. The abdominal muscles should be contracted, and the lower back in contact with the floor. The neck is extended and the chin tucked in. The hands are placed on the lower abdomen. Lift and extend one leg up to the level of the opposite knee. Hold the leg in an extended position, flex the ankle, and point the toes toward the ceiling. Continue raising the extended leg, feeling the stretch in the back of the leg. Return the leg to the starting position, and repeat with the opposite leg. *Note:* This exercise can also be performed with a rolled towel looped under the foot of the extended leg to help guide it through the stretch if the hamstrings muscles are tight.

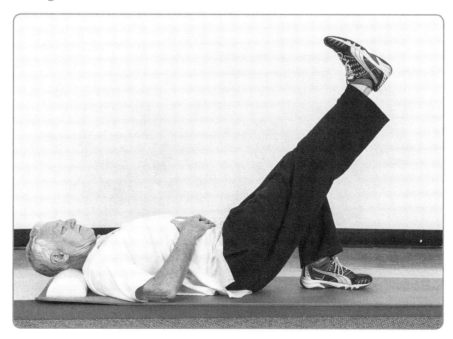

Seated Position

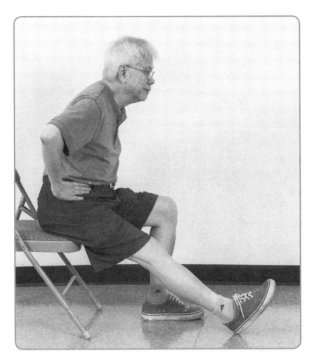

Seated Hamstrings Stretch

Target muscles: hamstrings, hip flexors, ankle dorsiflexors

Place a chair against the wall. Sit at the edge of the chair with one leg extended and the toes of that foot pointed toward the ceiling. Place both hands on the hips or on the thigh of the flexed leg. Slowly lean forward at the hips while keeping the trunk extended and chest lifted. The eyes are directed forward.

Hip Extensions

Target muscles: front of thigh and hips

Sit sideways on a chair close to the front edge. Hold on to the back of the chair with the closest hand for added support. Flex the knee of the opposite leg until it is pointing down to the floor. Reach back with that leg as far as possible, then let the toes of the foot touch the floor. Maintain an upright posture.

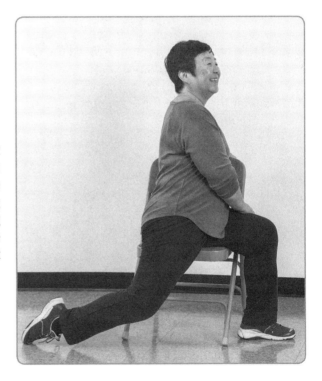

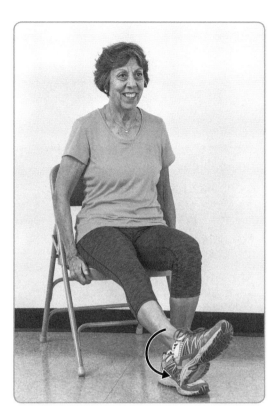

Ankle Circles

Target muscles: ankle and foot

Sit at the edge of a chair. Raise one leg off the floor and circle the foot at the ankle, first clockwise and then counterclockwise. Repeat with the other foot. This exercise can also be performed in a standing position, with or without support. Performing this exercise while standing unsupported adds a balance challenge.

Standing Position

Standing Side Lunge

Target muscles: hip adductors

Stand tall with feet wider than shoulder-width apart and toes pointed forward. Slowly bend one knee and shift the weight directly over the bent knee. The other leg remains extended. Place both hands on the thigh of the bent leg and hold the position until a stretch is felt along the inside thigh of the extended leg. Breathe evenly throughout the stretch. Return to a standing position and repeat the stretch on the other side.

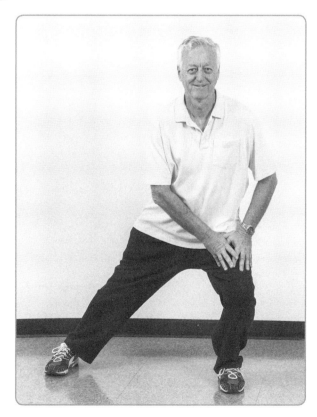

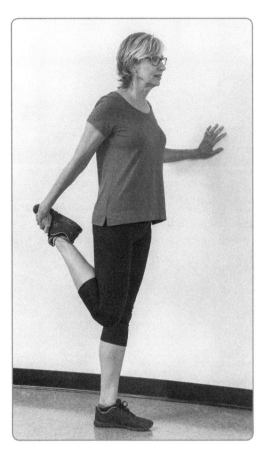

Quad Stretch

Target muscles: front of thigh

Stand upright with one hand against a supporting surface for balance. Flex one knee and raise the heel toward the buttocks. Slightly bend the knee of the stance leg. Reach behind and grasp the foot of the raised leg with one hand. Pull the heel gently toward the buttocks while keeping the thigh of the raised leg close to the stance leg. Relax and lower the leg to the floor. Repeat with the opposite leg.

Side Wall Stretch

Target muscles: hip abductors, oblique muscles of trunk

Stand upright close to a wall. Raise the arm closest to the wall above the head and rest it against the wall. Position the foot closest to the wall behind the ankle of the opposite leg. Slowly lean into the wall until a stretch can be felt along the outside of the thigh closest to the wall. Relax, and repeat on the opposite side.

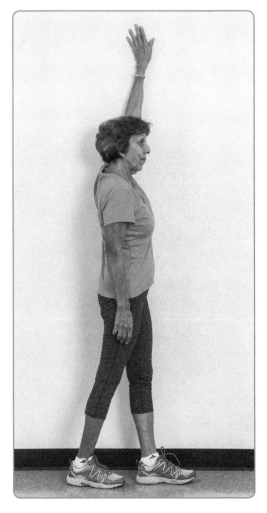

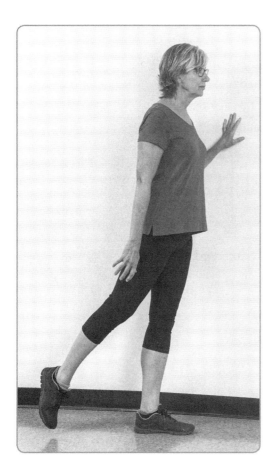

Backward Leg Extension

Target muscles: hip and trunk flexors

With one hand on a wall or chair for support, extend one leg backward and away from the body while maintaining an upright trunk. Repeat with the opposite leg.

Summary

This chapter provided an overview of the age-associated changes in the joints and muscles that contribute to reduced flexibility. The critical ranges of joint motion needed for the successful performance of daily activities were identified. The functional consequences of reduced flexibility and the functional and psychological benefits of regular flexibility training were summarized. Age-associated changes in the joints and muscles that contribute to reduced flexibility include an increase in connective tissue, changes in connective tissue matrix and collagen, and breakdown of articular cartilage.

Two types of stretching techniques were then described. The first of these techniques, static stretching, involves moving the joint through a single movement plane and then holding it at an end position for a period of time. The other technique, dynamic stretching, involves moving the joint through single or multiple planes of motion without holding the end position for any length of time. Dynamic stretching techniques should be introduced during the warm-up section of the class, while static stretches should be used later (e.g., after the aerobics component or during the cool-down) when the body is at its warmest and the muscles and joints are more receptive to being stretched.

In the final section of the chapter, a number of flexibility exercises were described. These can be performed in a variety of different positions (e.g., seated in a chair or on the floor, standing, kneeling on all fours) and can be modified to accommodate different functional abilities and medical conditions that may limit available range of motion (e.g., osteoarthritis, joint replacement, chronic pain). Experiencing improved flexibility and understanding how flexibility can positively affect the performance of daily, recreational, and sporting activities can motivate older adults to make flexibility training a part of their daily routine.

Key Terms

active range of motion   range of motion (ROM)

critical ranges   sarcopenia

dynamic stretching   static stretching

end range   stiffness

flexibility

Recommended Readings

Armiger, P., & Martyn, M.A. (2010). *Stretching for functional flexibility*. Philadelphia, PA: Lippincott Williams & Wilkins.

Nelson, A.G., & Kokkonen, J. (2014). *Stretching anatomy* (2nd ed.). Champaign, IL: Human Kinetics.

Study Questions

1. The greatest decline in range of motion with age is observed in

   a. hip extension

   b. spinal extension

   c. ankle dorsiflexion

   d. hip abduction

2. Range-of-motion changes in which of the following movements has been shown to be a significant factor in predicting the incidence of disability in community-residing older women?

   a. hip flexion

   b. ankle dorsiflexion

   c. knee extension

   d. ankle plantarflexion

3. The active range of motion refers to

   a. the minimum range of joint motion required to perform a certain activity

   b. the maximum distance a joint can be moved without any discomfort

   c. the range of movement through which a person can actively (without assistance) move a joint using the adjacent muscles

   d. the maximum distance a joint can be actively moved to a point of discomfort

4. Older adults with hip joint replacements are typically unable to bend the hip

   a. more than 110 degrees

   b. more than 70 degrees

   c. farther than 90 degrees

   d. beyond 60 degrees

5. The following types of exercise have been shown to improve flexibility in older adults with range-of-motion deficits:

   a. tai chi

   b. dance

   c. proprioceptive neuromuscular facilitation (PNF)

   d. all of the above

6. The primary difference between static and dynamic stretching is that

   a. once the joint is moved to a given end point, the position is held without additional movement for a period of time during a static stretch

   b. the end position is held for a shorter period of time during dynamic stretching

   c. the joint is not moved at all during a static stretch

   d. static stretching is the more functionally relevant stretching technique

7. At what point should static stretching techniques be used in an exercise session?

   a. as soon as the class begins

   b. during the cool-down portion of the class only

   c. when the body is at its warmest and the muscles and joints are receptive to being stretched

   d. at any point during an exercise session

8. All of the following flexibility exercises would be suited to improving the flexibility of the muscles in the lower back *except*

   a. cat and camel

   b. spine stretch

   c. alternating hip lifts

   d. single or double knee-to-chest stretch

9. The recommended range for holding a static stretch position is

   a. 10 to 20 seconds

   b. at least 90 seconds

   c. 10 to 90 seconds

   d. for as long as can be tolerated

10. Which of the following flexibility exercises is most appropriate for an older adult who can no longer fasten a dress with a zipper in the back?

   a. alternating arm swings in a seated position

   b. seated upper-back stretch

   c. alternating arm swings in a standing position

   d. front wall crawl

Application Activities

1. Your client is a fairly typical, community-dwelling, 78-year-old woman who reports having some difficulty with bending and stooping. She cannot roll onto her stomach or get up from and down onto the floor. She cannot get her hands behind her back to fasten a bra or pull up a zipper. This woman also has difficulty getting up from low furniture. She has come to you for an activity program to make her feel better and enable her to perform basic activities of daily living more easily. Identify six flexibility exercises for this client to perform regularly.

2. Design a warm-up that includes a number of flexibility exercises to prepare a class of older adults to engage in (a) upper-body strength exercises or (b) step aerobics later in the class.

Resistance Training

Joseph Signorile

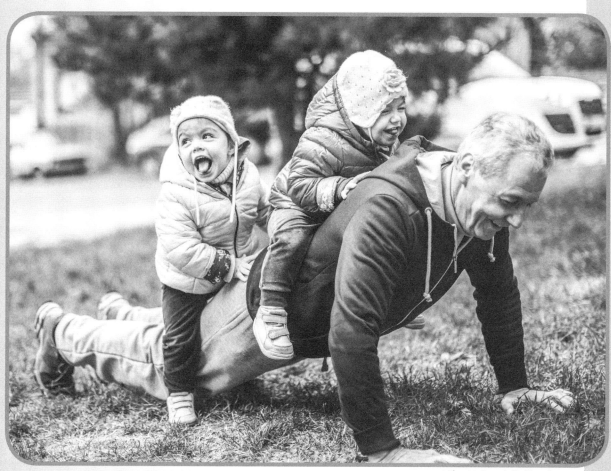

Objectives

After completing this chapter, you will be able to

1. describe the health- and performance-related benefits of resistance training for older adults;
2. describe the effectiveness and safety of resistance training for older adults;
3. manipulate the program variables that govern the development of muscle strength, power, and endurance;
4. explain the role and application of periodization and its value in meeting training goals;
5. evaluate and manipulate program design to accommodate the needs and training goals of older adults; and
6. design safe, effective resistance-training programs for older adults.

Advancing age is associated with a number of physiological changes that can be detrimental to both health and functional capacity. As a consequence of aging, individuals experience a well-documented loss of bone, muscle, and physical function that not only makes the activities of daily living (e.g., getting out of a chair, sweeping the floor, opening the window) more difficult but can also lead to injury and long-term disability (Baechle & Earle, 2016). The physiological consequences of aging are discussed in chapter 4, and an understanding of these changes is fundamental for developing strategies to counteract the physical decline associated with advancing age.

Benefits of Resistance Training

Traditionally, athletes seeking to improve strength, muscle hypertrophy, power, and sport-specific fitness have used resistance training. The use of resistance training as an intervention to improve health and performance in older persons has flourished since the breakthrough studies published over two decades ago (Fiatarone et al., 1990; Frontera, Meredith, O'Reilly, Knuttgen, & Evans, 1998). Today, resistance training is understood in a more multidimensional context than it was in the past. Scientists, clinicians, and practitioners are becom-

ing aware of its diverse benefits and ability to target specific health and fitness goals through variations in programming. Therefore, resistance training is considered to be one of the most cost efficient and effective interventions for preserving independence, improving health, and reducing injury in our aging population (Liu & Latham, 2011). The following sections discuss the health- and performance-related benefits of resistance training.

Health-Related Benefits

As noted above, researchers have elucidated the potential health-related benefits of resistance training, and resistance training is now recommended by national health organizations—including the American College of Sports Medicine (ACSM), American Heart Association, and the American Association for Cardiovascular and Pulmonary Rehabilitation—in conjunction with other exercise modalities (e.g., aerobic, flexibility, and balance exercise) for the maintenance and improvement of health and performance (Kraemer, Adams, et al., 2002). In a comprehensive health and fitness program, resistance training can reduce risk factors associated with many diseases and physical ailments and can preserve and improve functional capacity. Such benefits have been shown to improve the quality of life for a wide range of fitness levels and health conditions in older adults, including those with lower-back pain, osteoarthritis, cardiovascular disease, neuromuscular disease, renal failure, and type 2 diabetes, and those recovering from a stroke (Clyman, 2001; Hurley & Roth, 2000; Kraemer, Ratamess, & French, 2002; Pollock et al., 2000). Regular resistance exercise results in a remarkable number of positive health changes in elderly men and women. A number of these health benefits are described in table 12.1.

Physical Fitness and Performance-Related Benefits

As people age, declines in strength, power, and muscle endurance decrease functional capacity and reduce quality of life (Gersten, 1991). A substantial proportion of this reduction is not a direct result of the aging process but rather a consequence of the sedentary lifestyle frequently associated with aging. Not only can resistance training improve many health-related components of physical fitness, it can also have significant effects on performance-related fitness, including speed, strength, agility, flexibility, power, balance, and muscle endurance. Such motor performance skills are required for a variety of recreational (e.g., walking, bowling, hiking, biking, gardening) and sport (e.g., softball, tennis, basketball, racquetball) activities, and, more important, for nearly every activity of daily living.

Many studies have demonstrated large increases in maximal loads lifted and an accompanying enlargement of whole-muscle and muscle-fiber area in older adults who complete a resistance training program (Charette, McEvoy, Pyka, Snow-Harter, Guido, Wiswell, & Marcus, 1991; Häkkinen et al., 1998; Sipila, Elorinne, Alen, Suominen, & Kovanen, 1997). From such studies it has been determined that high-intensity resistance training can induce large increases in **muscle strength** in frail men and women up to 96 years of age (Fiatarone et al., 1990). Gains in strength of between 32 and 227 percent have been reported following eight or more weeks of training; older adults respond to weight training in a manner relatively similar to younger adults.

The production of muscle force and power are perhaps the most important factors in sport performance and maintaining an active lifestyle. All sporting and recreational activities involve some degree of power development (e.g., hitting, striking, carrying, kicking, cycling, throwing, lifting, running, jumping). In older men and women, walking speed relates positively with calf strength and hours spent in active leisure and relates negatively to age and the presence of health problems (Bassey et al., 1992; Bendall, Bassey, & Pearson, 1989). The increases in muscle strength, power, endurance, and hypertrophy (enlargement of muscle fibers) that accompany

Table 12.1   Wellness and Health Benefits of Resistance Exercise

Physical characteristic	Benefit
Body composition	Increased lean tissue mass, metabolic rate, and daily energy expenditure result in body fat reductions of up to 9%.
Blood pressure	Small reductions in resting systolic and diastolic blood pressure reduce the risk of stroke and coronary heart disease.
Bone mass	The weight-bearing activity in resistance training improves bone health and reduces the risk of osteoporosis.
Glucose tolerance	Favorable changes in glucose tolerance and insulin resistance are observed after physical activity, including resistance training.
Lower-back pain	Increased strength and cross-sectional area of the vertebral muscles reduce lower-back pain by maintaining muscle balance.
Blood lipids	Resistance training has beneficial effects on blood lipid profiles, including lower total cholesterol and triglyceride concentrations.
Balance and mobility	Increased strength and power have been shown to increase balance and improve gait characteristics in older adults with a history of falls or other medical conditions (e.g., Parkinson's disease, stroke).

resistance training can therefore improve motor skills. For older adults who participate in regular sporting and recreational activities, resistance training can improve performance. Maintaining adequate levels of muscle strength, endurance, and power is also important for reducing older adults' risk of falls and improving performance of their daily activities.

Today, **resistance training** is recognized as an intervention that can significantly impact quality of life, physical function, and injury prevention in older adults. Resistance training can ameliorate and even reverse the loss of muscle tissue and function, improve muscle quality, and improve neuromuscular performance as it relates to daily function and reduced probability of physical disability (Kraemer, Ratamess, & French, 2002; Liu & Latham, 2011). Through safe and correctly prescribed resistance training, older adults experience a variety of health and lifestyle benefits that include longevity, reduced fall probability, and the maintenance of long-term independence (Beebe, Hines, McDaniel, & Shelden, 2013; Kelley & Kelley, 2000).

During the course of this chapter we will examine the basic principles underlying resistance training so that as physical activity instructors of older adults you will better understand how this training component can produce positive structural and functional changes in the systems of the body. At a practical level it is also important that you (a) better understand how variables such as training load, intensity, and volume impact the responses to and effective application of resistance-training programs; (b) become familiar with the varied modalities and environments conducive to effective resistance training; and (c) recognize the importance of recovery as an acute and long-term component of any resistance-training program.

Principles of Resistance Training

The terms *strength training, weight training,* and *resistance training* all describe a type of exercise that requires the body's musculature to move (or attempt to move) against an opposing force or resistance (Fleck & Kraemer, 2014). This simple definition, however, belies the adaptability of resistance training as a method to address the diverse needs associated with the physiological, biomechanical, and psychological needs that may present themselves throughout the aging process. We will begin by first describing the basic training principles of overload, variation and periodization, and specificity and then proceed to discussing the training variables that can be adjusted to achieve targeted goals.

Overload

Fundamental to all resistance training is the principle of **overload**. The overload principle states that for improvements in any system of the body to occur, the demands placed upon that system must increase over time to stress it beyond its current capacities. The response to the application of a controlled pattern of overload is adaptation. Adaptation is the body restructuring or re-engineering itself in response to an overload, so that it may more effectively meet the challenge when it is again presented. For this re-engineering process to continue, the system being targeted must be provided with a new stimulus that is greater than that to which the body has already adapted. In resistance-training terms this is commonly called **progressive overload** and has been traditionally considered as a method for increasing muscle size and strength (Haff & Triplett, 2016).

It is perfectly logical that muscle size and strength should be the two factors most commonly considered in the earliest applications of resistance training with older individuals, since the most obvious consequences of the aging process are declines in muscle mass and associated losses in strength. However, given the realizations that other neuromuscular factors, such as power and endurance are critical factors affecting the aging process, the relationship between muscle size and strength is not linear, and many health-related variables such as body composition, metabolic syndrome, and bone health can be affected by resistance training (Clark & Manini, 2012; Cruz-Jentoft et al., 2010). For example, the capacity of the muscle cells to exert force increases and decreases relative to the demands placed on the muscular system. When the demands on muscle decrease, as is the case with the sedentary lifestyle that often accompanies old age, the cells decrease in size (atrophy), and the muscles lose strength or the ability to exert mechanical force. However, if the muscle cells are overloaded beyond normal daily use, as can occur in resistance-training programs, the cells increase in size (hypertrophy), which in turn increases strength, endurance, and muscle power.

Variation and Periodization

The systematic alteration of progressive overload over time creates **variation** in the physiological stresses placed on the body and optimizes the training stimulus. Variations in training volume and intensity are extremely important for optimal gains in strength, power, and endurance. A popular term for changing program variables is **periodization** (Fleck & Kraemer, 2014; Haff & Triplett, 2016). Periodization is the planned cycling of training variables, including volume (number of sets) and intensity, to minimize the risk of injury and other symptoms of overtraining. For older adults, precautionary measures to avoid overexertion and inappropriate stress should be taken. In the periodization of training for older adults, the program should begin with a gradual increase in both volume and intensity to allow the muscle and connective tissues to gradually restructure in response to the increased overload associated with training. During this time, volume would be increased at a faster rate than intensity. This adaptation period also provides an opportunity to gradually increase loads until the appropriate resistance is determined depending on the goal of the training cycle. This avoids the necessity of having to use either maximal testing or predictive equations to determine appropriate loading. As training progresses, the increases in volume will be superseded by increases in load, as intensity becomes a more dominant factor prior to active recovery or modifications of training goals.

Specificity

Specificity refers to the body's responses and subsequent adaptations to particular program variables. The principle of specificity dictates that the nature of the adaptations observed with a resistance-training program will be specific to the characteristics of load, velocity, movements, muscles exercised, and metabolic demands created by the exercise protocol (Haff & Triplett, 2016). In addition to the variables (e.g., load, volume, frequency, and rest periods) to be discussed in the next section of this chapter, there are a number of other program variables that can affect the nature of the overload provided and therefore the training response (specific adaptation). When developing suitable resistance-training programs for special populations (e.g., older adults), knowing how to adjust these acute variables is critical. The most effective resistance-training programs are individually designed to bring about specific adaptations while accommodating the needs and medical concerns of each individual.

Training Variables

A resistance-training program is designed using a variety of acute program variables, or training components. Altering one or several of these variables changes the training stimulus and ultimately affects the specific adaptations to the program (Kraemer & Ratamess, 2000). Simply manipulating the program variables can create an almost infinite number of workout protocols; however, the choices for each variable determine the effectiveness and benefits of the training program.

The Resistance Training Continua

There are two continua that are commonly associated with resistance training. The first is the repetition continuum, which is presented in table 12.2.

This continuum provides the correspondences between the load lifted relative to a maximum

Table 12.2   The Repetition Continuum

% 1RM	Repetitions
65%	14-15
70%	12-13
75%	10-11
80%	8-9
85%	6-7
90%	4-5
95%	2-3
100%	1 rep

effort (called the one-repetition maximum or 1RM) and the maximal number of repetitions that can be expected using that load. Figure 12.1 presents a second type of resistance-training continuum that provides a summary of how four of the major variables associated with any resistance-training program (load or resistance, number of repetitions, recovery time, and movement speed) can be varied in order to target specific goals. As can be seen in the figure, there are discernable patterns associated with the goals presented that will be explained in more detail as we examine program design for specific needs. However, some general statements can be made as you examine figure 12.1.

1. There is an interaction among some of the variables, notably number of repetitions, load, and recovery.

2. The application of high-speed work to target muscle power is possible across a wide range of loads and repetitions.

3. Body composition has been included within this classic continuum in association with hypertrophy given the combined impacts of lean body mass and body fat mass as contributing factors.

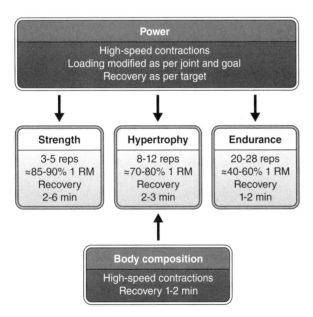

FIGURE 12.1   A modified resistance-training continuum.

Reprinted by permission from J.F. Signorile, "Resistance Training for Older Adults: Targeting Muscular Strength, Power and Endurance," *ACSM's Health & Fitness Journal* 17, no 5 (2013): 24-32.

Resistance

Often referred to as the most critical aspect of a resistance-training program, **resistance**, or **load**, represents the amount of force exerted against the working muscles and is expressed in absolute (i.e., weight in pounds or kilograms) or relative (i.e., as a percentage of maximal force or 1RM) terms (Haff & Triplett, 2016). Generally, loads corresponding to 85 to 90 percent of a person's 1RM are considered heavy; 70 to 85 percent of 1RM, moderate; and less than 70 percent, light. As seen in figure 12.1, the recommended resistance depends on the program's goal and is therefore presented as a major component of the resistance-training continuum.

Loads are commonly presented as percentages of the individual's 1RM or by the number of repetitions (reps) possible before failure (inability to complete the repetition using acceptable form). Heavier loads are commonly used for strength development, as can be seen by the 85 to 90 percent 1RM and 3 to 5 reps values presented in figure 12.1. In contrast, an intermediate load (70%-80% 1RM, 8-12 reps), designed to maximize volume of training (load, sets, and repetitions), appears more suitable for hypertrophy training. Finally, reducing the load to 40 to 60 percent 1RM substantially increases the number of reps (20-28) possible, thereby increasing local muscle endurance.

While these loads provide general guidelines for targeting specific goals, the appropriate loads to address any of these neuromuscular factors in a resistance-training program depend on a number of factors. These include the following:

1. The individual's training status: This is particularly important for beginners, where the potential for both acute and overuse injuries are greatest.

2. The training patterns: For example, concentration on eccentric work may cause damage even in a person who regularly engages in traditional resistance training.

3. The goals of the program: For example, the loads used to increase walking speed may vary considerably from those used to address activities like rising from a chair or climbing stairs (Cuoco et al., 2004).

4. The patterns of change within the periodization scheme: For example, planned cycling of

training variables (e.g., volume, intensity) are designed to minimize risk of injury and other symptoms of overtraining.

5. The expected pattern of adaptation based on age and gender.

6. The resistance training protocol adopted: For example, the loads used during typical multiple set programs may vary considerably from those used for a circuit-training program.

Number of Repetitions

The number of repetitions is closely related to load and also has an impact on training adaptations. As noted earlier, the specific goals of the program dictate both the load and the number of repetitions. The relationship between these two variables is, however, dependent on the assumption that there are a maximum number of repetitions that can be performed at a set percentage of an individual's 1RM. The practice of performing this maximal number of repetitions has been called into question for a number of reasons. First, performance of the maximal number of repetitions during a set, or so-called training to failure, may not be required to optimize improvement. Second, training to failure may not be effective unless performed at high intensities (i.e., lower repetition numbers) (Willardson, 2007). Third, training to failure, rather than maximizing improvements, will most likely lead to overtraining syndrome and ultimately to overuse injury. This is one reason that periodized training, which incorporates changes in intensity and volume of training, is so important. Finally, given the prevalence of orthopedic, neuromuscular, and cardiovascular issues in older adults, training to failure may be contraindicated (Willoughby, 2014).

Sets

Resistance training is performed in **sets**. For example, lifting a weight eight times with no rest between lifts constitutes one set of eight repetitions. As the number of sets increases, so does the level of fatigue and the amount of recovery time required. The volume of exercise that can be tolerated is initially low, but will increase as training continues. Fortunately, the use of single-set programs does

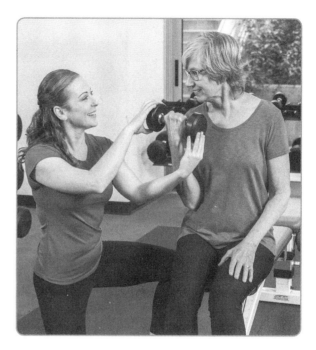

This participant is doing a warm-up set of biceps curls before increasing the resistance.

appear to provide an effective overload for persons beginning a training program; however, multiple-set programs are necessary once individuals are able to tolerate a greater volume of exercise. In an ACSM Current Comment, Willoughby (2014) summarizes these concepts by stating that older adults should "start with one set of each exercise and, depending on individual need, possibly progress up to no more than three sets when the fitness professional deems it appropriate. It should be noted, however, that an average of two sets of each exercise would be beneficial for most individuals." Additionally, many programs for older adults include a low-resistance warm-up set before the heavier sets are performed. If the target muscle group needs more stimulation, another exercise for that muscle group can be added.

Recovery Periods

The **metabolic (energy) demand** of a workout is determined by the interaction between the amount of work done during an active exercise interval (such as a set or the number of sets of a particular exercise) and the amount of recovery provided (times between sets or exercises). The length of a recovery period depends on four important considerations:

the intensity of the work interval, the fitness level of the individual, the goals of the training, and the proportional use of the aerobic and anaerobic systems as they relate to the specific fitness or performance goals.

The length of a recovery period depends on four important considerations:

1. The intensity of the work interval
2. The fitness level of the individual
3. The goals of the training
4. The proportional use of the aerobic and anaerobic systems as they relate to the specific fitness or performance goals

---

Activation of muscle tissue is related to the resistance and the total amount of work performed, and so rest period lengths should be consistent with the program goals. There is considerable research and empirical knowledge related to how each of the considerations listed above influences patterns of recovery. Concerning the intensity of the work to be performed, it is no mere coincidence that when looking at the resistance-training continuum presented in figure 12.1, the length of the recovery period increases with the load. Greater loads are synonymous with higher training intensities, which result in greater rates of energy utilization. The rapid reductions in high-energy phosphates and increases in waste products associated with these efforts dictate that similar efforts cannot be repeated unless sufficient recovery is provided.

Concerning the fitness level of the participant, it has been recognized for decades that recovery from high-intensity exercise is associated with aerobic fitness levels and age (Kosek, Kim, Petrella, Cross, & Bamman, 2006; Tomlin, 2001). Finally, when relating the length of a recovery period to the targeting of specific energy systems, the association may seem somewhat counterintuitive. While it may seem that short recovery periods would increase the contribution of the anaerobic systems during successive work bouts, quite the opposite is true. Studies examining multiple bouts of high-intensity training show that the shorter the duration of the

recovery relative to the work interval, the greater the contribution of the aerobic systems to the exercise bout (Barnett et al., 2004; Linossier et al., 1997). In fact this is quite logical, as pointed out by Kraemer and Ratamess (2004) in their review of the fundamentals of resistance training. They noted that a two-minute recovery was insufficient to allow completion of a 10-repetition set at 70 percent of participants' 1RMs. In other words, the rate of work performed declined across subsequent sets, which by definition indicates that the less metabolically powerful aerobic systems were required to contribute proportionally more energy during each subsequent set. This concept is especially important when designing programs targeting weight loss and muscle endurance.

One final caveat: the amount of rest is also dictated by an individual's medical conditions. For some older adults with type 1 diabetes, for whom gains in strength are the major goal, care must be taken to control the rest period between sets and exercises to avoid too great a metabolic stress.

Frequency

Training frequency refers to the number of training sessions completed in a given period of time, such as a week (Haff & Triplett, 2016). The frequency with which an individual performs resistance exercises needs to progressively increase during the early phases of a training program as the body becomes more tolerant to exercise stress. Resistance training can be performed as either a total-body workout or a split routine (e.g., upper body one day and lower body the next). Ultimately, the nature of the workout (total-body vs. split routine) determines the frequency with which each exercise is performed. Initially, total-body workouts performed two to three times per week are most appropriate for older adults. For individuals with more training experience, a split routine that requires more frequent exercise sessions (three to five per week) is recommended. It is important, however, that the training frequency allow sufficient recovery between exercise days. A general guideline is to schedule training sessions so that individuals with experience in resistance training have at least one recovery day between sessions that stress the same muscle group, and those just beginning training recover for at least two to three days between sessions.

When scheduling resistance-training sessions that stress the same muscle groups, it is recommended that beginners have at least two to three days of recovery, while experienced individuals need only one day.

Resistance Training Conditions and Modalities

Besides basic variables such as load, number of sets, frequency of training, and work/recovery cycles, other programming variables such as the type of resistance applied, the muscles and movements being targeted, the type of muscle action, and the exercise order should be employed. Given the number of interactions possible between training and program variables, an almost infinite number of protocols can be designed to address each person's specific needs and goals.

Type of Resistance

Traditionally, when we think of resistance training three modalities come to mind: **free weights** (e.g., barbells or dumbbells that are not attached to a machine or other apparatus); stack-loaded machines (e.g., machines with a stack of weights where resistance is chosen by inserting a pin); and, body-weight based resistance, commonly called calisthenics. Thanks to the driving forces of the marketplace and technology, as well as the knowledge and creativity of practitioners, scientists, and engineers, the training modalities available have increased exponentially, and many offer unique forms of resistance that will maximize responses for specific goals. For example, pneumatic machines, which use air pressure to provide resistance, all but eliminate inertia during exercise performance, making them a good choice for the higher-speed training programs often used to increase power. The new lines of pulley machines developed by a number of companies provide the individual with a better opportunity to perform multiple-joint exercises that simulate movement patterns used in daily living. Resistance bands and rubber tubing also allow the user to move in more varied patterns than typical machine-based modalities. With any of these modalities, the individual should be able to safely control the resistance throughout the full range of motion. On some fixed-weight machines, for example, even the minimal resistance is too high for older adults, who often experience difficulty producing the initial force required to start the movement. Also, on some machines the increments in resistance, especially at the lighter resistances, are too large to allow smooth progressions. Modalities such as pneumatic machines and resistance bands overcome these problems, allowing easier initiation of the movement as a result of being able to set the loads at a very low level or by the development of resistance throughout the ascending strength curve. It should be noted, however, that resistance levels are often limited and the amount of resistance increases throughout the range of motion when performing exercises with resistance bands.

Single- and Multiple-Joint Exercises

Another training variable to consider when examining program design is the number of joints engaged during an exercise. The simplest classification scheme is to divide exercises into two basic types: single-joint and multiple-joint exercises. During **single-joint exercises**, one specific muscle group or joint action is targeted (e.g., biceps curl). Conversely, **multiple-joint exercises** target more than one muscle group or involve multiple joint actions or interactions (e.g., squat). It is recommended that both single- and multiple-joint exercises be included in a resistance-training program; both have been found to be effective for increasing muscle strength and hypertrophy. The inclusion of multiple-joint exercises, especially those that simulate movement patterns employed during the performance of activities of daily living (ADLs) and many sport and recreational activities (e.g., golf, tennis, skiing) are important for translating strength, power, and endurance gains into relevant improvements in function and performance enhancement.

Muscle Action

Three contractile conditions can be imposed on a muscle during training: **isometric**; **isokinetic**; and **isoinertial**. The term isometric (same length) indicates that the muscle is contracting but there is no observable or overt movement of the body segment. During the two dynamic conditions (isokinetic and isoinertial) the muscle can shorten (called a **concentric contraction**) or lengthen (called an **eccentric contraction**). Isokinetic (same speed) is a unique contractile state produced by a specialized dynamometer that accommodates resistance to maintain a constant speed setting. Finally, isoinertial (also called isotonic or constant weight dynamic) contractions are dynamic contractions that are performed against a constant external load; this is the most common type of contractile condition created for resistance training.

The choice of isometric, dynamic concentric, dynamic eccentric, and isokinetic exercises is important when designing a resistance-training program. For example, eccentric muscle actions generate greater force (Hedayatpour & Falla, 2015), are most conducive to hypertrophy (enlargement of the muscle cell; Hather, Tesch, Buchanan, & Dudley, 1991), and are less metabolically demanding. Eccentric muscle actions, however, are most likely to produce delayed-onset muscle soreness (Ebbeling & Clarkson, 1989), particularly in individuals with little training history. Isometric (i.e., no change in muscle length as force is applied) muscle actions are more metabolically demanding than eccentric contractions yet less demanding than concentric muscle actions. Moreover, such contractions mostly increase strength at the specific joint angle at which they are performed. Unless the training you are providing is limited to a very specialized improvement, such as increasing isometric grip strength, the majority of the training programs you design will utilize alternating concentric and eccentric isoinertial contractions through the full range of motion.

> When designing resistance-training programs, be sure to select exercises that stress all major muscle groups so that muscular-system balance can be maintained.

Exercise Order

The sequence in which exercises are performed during a training session can significantly affect performance and subsequent adaptation. The sequence of exercises depends on the goals of the training program and on energy metabolism and threshold of fatigue, particularly for older adults. Exercises that use larger muscle groups are typically performed at the beginning of a workout (Haff & Triplett, 2016), while isolated muscle actions and single-joint movements are performed toward the end of the session. This order reduces muscle fatigue, allowing for higher intensity or greater resistance to be applied during performance of the large-muscle-group exercises. Typically, optimal stimulation of the large muscle groups in the legs (e.g., leg press) and the upper body (e.g., bench press, seated row) should be a priority in a training program designed for older adults; however, it has been suggested that this traditional concept should be modified and that exercises that address the specific goals of a program be performed first regardless of muscle size (Simão et al., 2010).

Resistance Training for Older Adults

The principles of developing a resistance-training program are very similar regardless of an individual's age. There are, however, a number of concerns that physical activity instructors should be aware of when working with older adults. First, it is very important to individualize the program, as older adults vary in their functional capacity and medical concerns. Existing medical conditions, exercise history, and nutritional status should be evaluated before a client starts a resistance-training program (Haff & Triplett, 2016). Even though older adults retain the capacity to adapt to increased levels of physical activity (e.g., resistance training), guidelines for safe and effective exercise should be followed.

Proper breathing technique, posture, and biomechanics during resistance training are critical to help prevent medical incidents. Another major concern is that the correct progression be used for older adults to avoid injury or acute overuse. Data indicate that intensity must be carefully adjusted so as not to cause overtraining syndrome in older adults (Hunter & Treuth, 1995). It is likely that older adults will take longer to recover from a training session, so varying work intensities in a periodized pattern may allow for better adaptation. The resistance-training programs investigated in many research studies involving older adults have been quite fundamental in design, and have still yielded positive results. Therefore, early in training, advanced program design may not be essential. Recommendations for progression have been developed by the American College of Sports Medicine, the key points of which are presented in table 12.3 (Kraemer, Adams, et al., 2002). It is important to remember, however, that these recommendations constitute general guidelines and will require specific modifications depending on the fitness level of the individual, the specific metabolic and biomechanical declines, existing injury or disease states identified in each person, and the goals of the program.

When working with older adults, it is important that the physical activity instructor understand that more frail older adults may initially possess minimal strength and be capable of producing a maximal force of only a few pounds. Therefore, in a progressive resistance-training program an older individual may lift only 0.5 pound (0.2 kg) during a set. Choosing the correct equipment capable of producing such low resistance increments and employing an adaptation phase where resistance is gradually increased to allow tissue adaptations is essential.

Table 12.3   ACSM's Models of Progression for Resistance Training

Training component	Recommendation
Muscle action	For novice, intermediate, and advanced participants, both concentric and eccentric muscle actions are recommended.
Loading	Novice to intermediate participants should train with loads corresponding to 60%-70% 1RM for 8-12 repetitions, and advanced exercisers should use loads of 80%-100% 1RM in a periodized fashion. For progression, a 2%-10% increase is recommended.
Volume	Novices should follow a general resistance-training program (consisting of either single or multiple sets). Multiple-set programs with systematic variation in training volume and intensity over time are best for intermediate and advanced participants.
Exercise selection	Both single- and multiple-joint exercises, with an emphasis on multiple-joint exercises, are recommended for novice, intermediate, and advanced exercisers.
Free weights and machines	A novice- to intermediate-level training program should include both free-weight and machine exercises. An emphasis on free-weight exercises is recommended for advanced strength training.
Exercise order	Large muscle groups should be worked before small muscle groups, and multiple-joint exercises should precede single-joint exercises.
Rest periods	For novice, intermediate, and advanced training levels, rest periods of at least two to three minutes should be used between multiple-joint exercises using heavy loads. For other exercises, a rest period of one to two minutes may suffice.
Velocity of muscle action	Novices should use slow and moderate velocities initially. For intermediate strength training, moderate velocities should be used. For advanced strength training, a continuum of velocities from slow to fast is recommended.
Frequency	It is recommended that novices train the entire body two to three days per week. A similar frequency is recommended for intermediate participants, but those using a split routine should train three to four days per week so that each muscle group is trained one to two days per week. Advanced participants should work out four to six days per week.

Data from Kraemer et al. (2002).

Design Considerations and Needs Analysis

The development of a resistance-training program for older adults consists of a preactivity screening, choosing and applying an appropriate physical assessment battery, setting individualized goals based on the results of that battery, designing a targeted program, and implementing the program within the guidelines previously provided. Appropriate preactivity screening and assessment tools have already been described in chapters 5 and 6. For older adults, resistance training should be an ongoing part of their lifestyles, so continual reevaluation and assessment of program goals and program design are necessary for optimal results and adherence. As noted in chapter 5, the American College of Sports Medicine adopted a new evidence-informed model to guide the conduct of exercise preparticipation health screenings (Pescatello, 2015). Unlike previous recommendations, risk-factor profiling is no longer included in the preexercise screening process.

After the individual's medical history and physical activity status have been determined, a preprogram evaluation to document baseline measurements and evaluate responses to specific exercise modalities should be performed. Strength tests or exercise protocols are commonly used as an exercise test to evaluate EKG and clinical symptoms specific to resistance exercise modality. One-repetition-maximum strength testing and resistance exercise workouts using as much as 75 percent of 1RM have been shown to cause fewer cardiopulmonary symptoms than graded treadmill exercise tests in cardiac patients with good left ventricular function (Faigenbaum, Skrinar, Cesare, Kraemer, & Thomas, 1990). One-repetition-maximum (1RM) testing is a safe and effective means of assessing older adults, provided that the client and the tester are adequately familiar with the test procedure and the appropriate testing guidelines are followed (Shaw, McCully, & Posner, 1995). Although 1RM testing is considered safe by most clinicians and researchers, due to the potential risks, ACSM recommends the use of submaximal tests and predictive equations. The tests most commonly used are the leg press, the leg extension, and the chest press. Knutzen, Brilla, and Caine (1999) examined the validity of six different repetitions-to-fatigue predictive equations for 11 machine-based resistance exercises for older adults and found a moderate to strong relationship between the actual and predicted 1RM values for all upper- and lower-body exercises evaluated. The authors concluded that the "use of a prediction equation for older adults appears to be a valid measure of 1RM within a range of 1 to 10 kilogram, depending on the machine lift" (p. 244).

A third, more conservative, option is to employ field tests such as the 30-second chair stand or 30-second arm curl tests to assess initial neuromuscular performance and subsequent training-related changes (see chapter 6). While the results of these tests will not allow computation of training loads, they can be compared to age- and gender-matched performance standards, and initial training loads can always be determined as the individual progresses through the tissue adaptation phase during the early stage of training. Although some older men and women may be able to tolerate high levels of resistance, this early tissue adaptation phase can be used to teach your clients proper exercise techniques and thereby minimize the potential for injury and muscle soreness. For healthy older adults, continual manipulation of acute program variables is recommended for long-term progression during resistance training. Caution must be taken with the rate of progression, as inappropriate increases in intensity or volume may lead to acute or overuse injury.

Older adults often have orthopedic problems that contraindicate the resistance training of affected joints. Recovery from a training session also takes longer for older adults, and care is needed not to exceed their physiological ability to repair tissues after a workout. Each individual responds differently to a given resistance-training program, based on his or her current training status, past training experience, and individual response to the training stress. A resistance-training program should aim to improve quality of life by enhancing muscle fitness, which includes muscle hypertrophy, strength, power, and **local muscle endurance**. Programs that include variation, gradual progressive overload, specificity, and careful attention to recovery are recommended (Kraemer, Adams, et al., 2002). Assessment of training progress should include the periodic testing of strength (on the equipment used in training if possible), body composition, and functional abilities (e.g., getting out of a chair) and tracking existing medical conditions. Once participants master basic exercises, standing exercises with free weights (e.g., barbells and dumbbells), multidirectional medicine ball exercises and other translational exercises can be incorporated into a program (Signorile, 2011).

Strength Training

The considerations when training strength in older persons should include the following: their training status, location in the training cycle, and individual needs. Concerning strength training status, especially in the case of the beginner who may not have formally exercised for decades, the tissue adaptation phase previously mentioned is imperative. The length of this period can range from two to three weeks for the active older person to eight weeks or more for more frail older adults residing in nursing homes who have never engaged in resistance training. Fortunately, this period allows time for form corrections since it employs relatively low loads. Periodized cycling of intensity and volume to maximize response and reduce overuse injuries should then follow this initial period

Biomechanically, poor chair stand performance or poor arm curl performance establishes the need for strength training of the lower body, upper body, or both. How to perform these tests is described in greater detail in the *Senior Fitness Test Manual* (Rikli & Jones, 2013). The typical lower-body muscle groups targeted for improving function and lowering fall risk would be the quadriceps, hamstrings, and triceps surae; however, critical muscles such as the dorsiflexors and hip abductor/adductors must also be addressed for maximum benefit (Rogers & Mille, 2003; Whipple, Wolfson, & Amerman, 1987). Finally, when addressing ADLs, recognize that most use sequential movement patterns (kinetic chains) that transfer forces from the lower to the upper body through the core, so simulating functional movement patterns using bands, functional trainers, or pulley, strap, or rod systems should be considered.

The ACSM recommendation that older adults begin with one set of repetitions and progress to no more than three sets seems appropriate for resistance-training programs; however, four or more sets have produced the best results in untrained younger and trained individuals. Additionally, most studies have utilized two to three sessions per week; a training frequency that is consistent with the current ACSM guidelines of two to four sessions per week (Rhea, Alvar, Burkett, & Ball, 2003).

Hypertrophy Training

Although the prevalence of sarcopenia, as it is classically defined, in the older adult population is low, declines in muscle size with age remains an important research topic and explains why hypertrophy training dominated early resistance-training studies. The loads commonly used in these studies were 70 to 80 percent 1RM (8-12 repetitions). To maximize results it appears that multiple-set programs offered three to four days per week are best. This recommendation is consistent with both the ACSM position stand on progressive resistance and the current comment on resistance training for the older adult by Willoughby (2014), suggesting that three sets of 10-12 exercises performed four times per week is safe and effective (Ratamess et al., 2009).

Muscle Power Training

Muscle power is arguably the most important neuromuscular factor affecting independence (Foldvari et al., 2000) and fall probability (Whipple et al., 1987). Muscle power also declines nearly twice as quickly as strength as we age (Metter, Conwitt, Tobin, & Fozard, 1997). Given that power training typically incorporates higher movement speeds, specific considerations must be applied when designing this component of a resistance-training program, such as the following:

1. Carefully choose the equipment to be used. Momentum is a problem during the initial breaking of inertia at the beginning and end (deceleration) of the concentric phase and during an eccentric contraction when momentum is increased by gravity. Therefore, stack-loaded machines with hard stops will require that deceleration begin early in the concentric phase and high-speed eccentric movements should be avoided. Free weights are an option, but are not recommended by ACSM for the older adult population. The most feasible choices are pneumatic machines, cable machines with multiple pulleys, tubes, bands, and aquatic exercises, especially those including drag devices.

2. The high-speed component should only be applied during the concentric phase of the lift because high-speed eccentric movements have the potential to cause muscle damage both acutely and on days following the training (delayed onset muscle soreness or DOMS).

Some other important caveats when implementing power training are listed here:

1. When providing power training, an important topic is optimal loading, defined as the load that will provide the greatest power output (product of load and velocity). Bear in mind that the load that produces the highest power will differ due to biomechanical differences in the joints. The longer lever systems such as those at the knee and elbow will show greater power at the velocity end of the load-velocity curve (less resistance) and the shorter levers such as the ankle and wrist will favor the load end of the curve (greater resistance) (Signorile et al., 2002).

2. The load used during power training should be dictated by the improvement in daily activities being targeted. For example, increases in gait speed are best addressed using lower loads (≈40% 1RM), while chair rises and stair climbs, where more of the individual's body weight is being moved against gravity, would benefit from loads of 70 to 80 percent 1RM (Cuoco et al., 2004).

3. Next, power training should not be restricted to the gym. During recovery periods in a periodization cycle, multidirectional and multijoint "translational" exercises can be used to increase movement velocity during activities of daily living and reduce power asymmetries that have been associated with falls (Signorile, 2011).

4. Finally, although the number of sets and training frequency are similar to values for strength and hypertrophy training, training durations plateau in three to four weeks (Signorile, Carmel, Lai, & Roos, 2005).

The available research evidence suggests that it is prudent to include high-velocity (nonballistic), low-intensity movements in the resistance-training program to maintain the structure and function of the neuromuscular system. Both single- and multiple-joint exercises are recommended for increasing power in healthy older adults. One to three sets per exercise using light to moderate loading (40%-60% 1RM) should be performed, and 6 to 10 repetitions at a high velocity promote the development of muscle power.

Muscle Endurance Training

Muscle endurance should not be confused with cardiovascular endurance. Muscle endurance is best described as a muscle's ability to maintain a power output. It can be increased through strength training because the trained muscle will use a lower percentage of its maximal strength to perform a task than before it was trained. However, programs using high-repetition (20 or more reps) protocols with short rest intervals (≈1 min) improve endurance more than low-repetition programs (3-5 reps) with longer rest periods (approximately 3 minutes) or intermediate programs (9-12 reps) with moderate rest periods (2 minutes). The most effective protocols list two to three sets at 40 to 60 percent 1RM (20-28 reps) with one- to two-minute rest periods.

Resistance-Training Activities

As discussed earlier in this chapter, resistance-training programs for older adults should be individualized. Specificity of training is necessary to meet the particular needs of each individual and a critical component is biomechanical specificity. This means that when designing a resistance-training program for older adults, you must consider which muscle groups are most important to address the specific needs of each individual and are therefore the most important to target. For example, calf strength is significantly correlated with walking speed and mobility, power in the hip abductors and adductors can reduce lateral instability during gait, and muscle endurance in the biceps and triceps is important for many of the manual tasks performed each day (see table 12.4).

A variety of exercises can be used to stimulate muscle development, from body-weight-only exercises that require no equipment to machine-based circuit programs, free-weight exercises, and exercises that can be performed at home using cans of food and other common objects of various weights. Examples of total-body workouts suitable for older adults are described in the sidebar.

Table 12.4 Important Muscle Groups for Functional Activities

Muscle group	Relevance for functional activities
Dorsiflexors and plantar flexors	Important for walking and functional mobility (e.g., getting up from a chair) Reduce fall probability
Knee extensors and flexors	Required for all mobility activities Reduce fall probability
Hip abductors and adductors	Required for lateral stability Increase stability when walking Used for movements around static and moving objects
Abdominals	Needed for the core stability vital to posture, balance, and mobility Transfer force and power from lower to upper body as in transfers and sweeping
Chest	Important for pushing and carrying Controls the upper body during gait Used for initial rise from prone position
Back	Required for all pulling activities Required for reaching objects on a shelf Controls posture in the spine
Biceps and triceps	Used for many activities of daily living (e.g., carrying groceries, dusting, drinking, and eating)
Shoulders	Needed for carrying objects Help to reduce the impact of a fall

Sample Resistance-Training Programs for Older Adults

Beginner's Home Strength Program

- For upper-body exercises, use food cans, wrist cuffs, rubber bands or tubing, or some other form of light resistance (2-5 lbs., 0.9-2.3 kg).
- Perform 1-3 sets of 8-10 repetitions.
- Rest between 1-2 minutes between sets and exercises.
- Be sure to perform all exercises through a full range of motion.
- Use a heavy chair or other immoveable piece of furniture as an anchor to improve stability if needed.
- Appropriate exercises include front shoulder raises, wall push-aways, standing knee lifts, toe and heel raises, arm curls, good-morning exercise, side bends, standing knee curls, single-arm shoulder press, quarter squats, single-arm bent-over rows, and side shoulder raises.

Program note: This light-resistance, callisthenic exercise-based program is designed to improve general muscular fitness and joint range of motion. To continue to make improvements, it is important to progress to using heavier resistances, especially for lower-body exercises.

(continued)

Sample Resistance-Training Programs for Older Adults *(continued)*

Beginner's Program in the Weight Room

- Arrange the sequence of the exercises to move from those that train large muscle groups to those that train small muscle groups. If an individual has specific biomechanical needs, arrange the exercises in a sequence that addresses the individual's needs first.
- Begin with a resistance that is 60-75% of the individual's 1RM for each exercise and gradually add resistance over time up to 80% of the 1RM, or the equivalent of a 10RM-15RM resistance.
- Start by performing one set and gradually progress to three sets over a 12-week program.
- Allow 2-3 minutes of rest between sets and exercises.
- Appropriate exercises include leg presses, knee extensions, knee curls, calf raises, bench presses, seated rows, upright rows, arm curls, and shoulder presses.

Long-Term Periodized Program in the Weight Room

Complete a 12-week cycle consisting of three nonconsecutive training days per week that is followed by a 2-week active rest period. Make any needed variations in the program based on the individual's training goals, and then repeat the cycle.

- Perform the exercises that train the large muscle groups first, followed by the exercises that train the small muscle groups.
- Vary the resistance throughout the week; use 60-75% of the 1RM for each exercise on day 1, 80-85% of the 1RM on day 2, and 40-60% of the 1RM on day 3.
- Start by performing one set and gradually progress to three sets over the 12-week cycle.
- Allow 2-3 minutes between sets and exercises on day 1, 3-4 minutes on day 2, and 1-2 minutes on day 3.
- Appropriate exercises include leg presses or squats, knee extensions, knee curls, calf raises, bench presses, seated rows, upright rows, arm curls, shoulder presses, and select Pilates exercises.
- Exercises can use free weights (e.g., barbell, dumbbells), fixed machine weights, resistance bands, stability balls, weighted cuffs (ankle, wrist), medicine balls, manual resistance, body-weight resistance, or water resistance (for aquatic exercises).

Adapted by permission from S.J. Fleck and W.J. Kraemer, *Designing Resistance Training Programs,* 3rd ed. (Champaign, IL: Human Kinetics, 2004), 323.

Functional Training

The use of only linear movements does not address some of the more common functional movement patterns of everyday life (e.g., twisting the trunk, circling the arms). **Functional training**, that is, performing exercises that train muscles in coordinated, multiplanar movement patterns requiring consistent changes in the base of support, can improve muscle balance, strength, and ADL disability (Heitkamp, Horstmann, Mayer, Weller, & Dickhuth, 2001; Liu, Shiroy, Jones, & Clark, 2014). Functional training means training in a manner that optimally carries over to real-life situations. Basically, this means training to improve strength in functional movement patterns rather than training simply to increase muscle strength or size. Functional movements are those that occur in all three planes of movement and involve acceleration, deceleration, and stabilization of the joint structures. Functional resistance-training exercises are executed in a variety of body positions, on a variety of surfaces, using a variety of resistance devices (e.g., resistance bands, weighted balls, specialized cable systems). The stabilizer muscles and not the mobilizing muscles limit functional strength. Development of the core muscles, which lie deep within the torso (i.e., the spine and pelvic muscles and muscles that support the scapula) and are used for stabilization, has a significant impact on the daily activities of older adults and reduces the incidence of injury as a result of falling.

While not as effective for developing strength and muscle hypertrophy as traditional weight-training methods, functional training promotes core stability and functional capacity, is simple to perform, and is cost-effective. Some standard exercises suitable for functional training for older adults include:

- Supine single-bent-leg raise
- Stability-ball single-leg raise
- Seated static contractions
- Supine pelvic tilts
- Pelvic tilts on all fours
- Abdominal curls (Progress from hands on thighs, to hands across chest, to fingers on temples.)

Functional training and core stability exercises can develop abdominal muscles (transversus abdominis, internal and external obliques, and rectus abdominis) and consequently help to protect the lower back (lumbar spine), stabilize the pelvis,

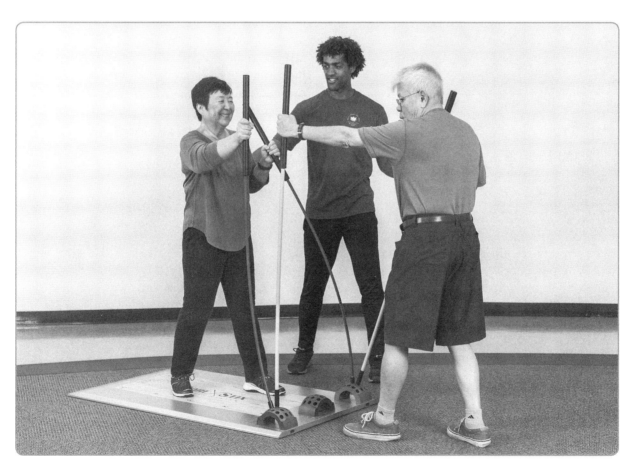

The inclusion of multiple-joint resistance exercises that simulate movement patterns performed during daily activities (e.g., pushing and pulling) are important to include in any resistance training program designed for older adults.

and aid in performing exercises more efficiently and with less likelihood of injury. Functional training and core stability should be considered when designing a resistance-training program for older adults. Whether carried out using free weights, resistance bands, stability balls, or other forms of resistance, functional training should simulate muscle actions performed daily (twisting, bending, leaning). Most important for core stability are the stabilizing muscles of the trunk, and exercises to promote strength and muscle tone in this region should be included in the program. Abdominal movements should be performed through the full range of motion. Movements should be controlled, and steady breathing maintained. Progression is similar to other exercise modes (beginner: one set of 12-15 repetitions; advanced: three sets of 15-20 repetitions). Examples of abdominal exercises suitable for older adults follow:

- Stability-ball chop-and-lift
- Supine heel slide
- Supine single-straight-leg raise
- Supine bent-knee fallout and return

The following are examples of Pilates exercises suitable for older adults:

- Roll-ups
- Hundreds exercise
- Oblique curl-ups

Pilates is an exercise mode that focuses on improving balance, proprioception, and postural alignment by exercising the core postural muscles. Pilates promotes muscle recruitment and motor control by requiring that stability be maintained. Core stability can also be promoted through the use of stability balls and appropriate exercises on an uneven base (e.g., wobble board, foam). For example, performing a shoulder press while sitting on a stability ball works not only the prime movers in the shoulder but also the stabilizers in the trunk (the abdominals) required to prevent a loss of balance. Refer to chapter 14 for information about other types of balance activities that can be combined with the resistance-training component of a program.

Exercise performed in the water is an alternative mode of resistance training and provides well-balanced resistance over the entire body. Because of the effects of buoyancy and the movement of the limbs and trunk against the resistance of the water, all muscle actions in the water are concentric. The level of resistance can be progressively increased by using hand and foot paddles to increase the surface area against which the resistance is applied. Aquatic exercise is a particularly good option for older adults with medical conditions that make it difficult or uncomfortable to exercise on land.

Safety Precautions

Resistance training can be a safe and effective exercise modality for older adults if appropriate training guidelines are followed (Kraemer, Adams, et al., 2002). However, if program design is poor, resistance training can be hazardous. Without the correct instruction and supervision, participants' risk of injury as a consequence of inappropriate resistance training increases. The risk of injury can be minimized with well-trained instructors, adequate recovery, and sound instruction (Baechle & Earle, 2016). As with any type of exercise or physical activity, resistance training requires that suitable safety precautions be employed. The risk of injury and infirmity must be minimized, particularly for older adults who are frail and may have special medical concerns. These are some safety recommendations that should be followed during resistance training for older adults:

1. Warm up muscles for at least 10 minutes before training.
2. Start with low resistance, and gradually add repetitions, intensity (resistance), and sets.
3. Conduct exercises through a full, pain-free range of motion.
4. Discontinue any exercise that causes pain. Then lower the resistance and see if the exercise can be resumed pain-free.
5. Never hold your breath; exhale during the exertion phase and inhale during the release phase.
6. Avoid hyperextending or locking joints.
7. Allow at least 48 hours between resistance-training sessions that use the same muscle groups.

Summary

Research indicates that resistance training can be a safe and effective method of exercise for men and women of all ages and abilities. The benefits for older adults include increased strength, power, endurance, muscle capacity, flexibility, and energy; improved self-image; and greater confidence. Enhancements of muscle and bone mass also have important implications for an individual's health. Moreover, improvements in neuromuscular performance enhance the performance of everyday activities, which in turn improves a person's overall health and well-being. Even for frailer older adults, research indicates that resistance training is beneficial. It is never too late to start a resistance-training program; of course, the proper design and progression of a resistance-training program are vital to optimize benefits for older adults.

Key Terms

concentric contraction	muscle strength
eccentric contraction	overload
free weights	periodization
functional training	progressive overload
isoinertial	resistance
isokinetic	resistance training
isometric	sets
load	single-joint exercises
local muscle endurance	specificity
metabolic (energy) demand	variation
multiple-joint exercises	

Recommended Readings

Haff, G.G., & Triplett, N.T. (2016). *Essentials of strength training and conditioning* (4th ed.). Champaign, IL: Human Kinetics.

Signorile, J.F. (2011). *Bending the aging curve: The complete exercise guide for older adults*. Champaign, IL: Human Kinetics.

Study Questions

1. To translate improvement in a weight-room task into improvement in a real-life task, what resistance-training principle is most important to consider?

   a. specificity

   b. intensity

   c. conversion

   d. periodization

2. A multiple-joint exercise

   a. stresses all muscles in the body

   b. uses muscles that cross more than one joint

   c. isolates the resistance to one muscle group

   d. can be done only with free weights

3. Which of the following muscle groups are most important for maintaining lateral stability during walking?

    a. dorsiflexor and plantar flexor muscle groups

    b. knee extensors and flexors

    c. hip abductors and adductors

    d. abdominals

4. One of the most important physical capabilities needed for everyday lifting tasks is

    a. flexibility

    b. coordination

    c. power

    d. endurance

5. Which age group can benefit from resistance training?

    a. 40- to 50-year-old men

    b. 100-year-old women

    c. 70-year-old men

    d. all of the above

6. Periodization is best defined as

    a. planned rest cycles to minimize the risk of injury and other symptoms associated with overtraining

    b. the use of heavy weights with long rest periods to minimize the risk of injury and other symptoms associated with overtraining

    c. the planned cycling of training intensity to minimize the risk of injury and other symptoms associated with overtraining

    d. the planned cycling of training variables, including volume and intensity, to minimize the risk of injury and other symptoms associated with overtraining

7. Which of the following range of loads and repetitions are recommended when the goal is to increase muscle power in healthy older adults?

    a. 40 to 60 percent 1RM, 6 to 10 repetitions

    b. 70 to 80 percent 1RM, 8 to 12 repetitions

    c. 85 to 90 percent 1RM, 3 to 5 repetitions

    d. none of the above

8. The length of a recovery period depends on the following considerations *except*

    a. intensity of the work interval

    b. age of the individual

    c. goals of the training

    d. proportional involvement of the aerobic and anaerobic systems during the training session

Application Activities

1. Develop a one-minute talk to motivate a group of sedentary older adults to participate in resistance training.

2. Design a periodized training program for a group of healthy 70-year-old and older men and women, and delineate any gender differences you think are important in the program. Be sure to discuss various training variables.

3. You are training three clients. Your first client, an 85-year-old man, wants to be able to develop strength to climb stairs and get up from sitting down. Your second client, a 76-year-old woman, wants to improve her posture. Your third client, a 61-year-old woman, wants to improve her golf game. Which resistance exercises would you recommend for each client?

Aerobic Endurance Training

Susie Dinan-Young
Dawn A. Skelton

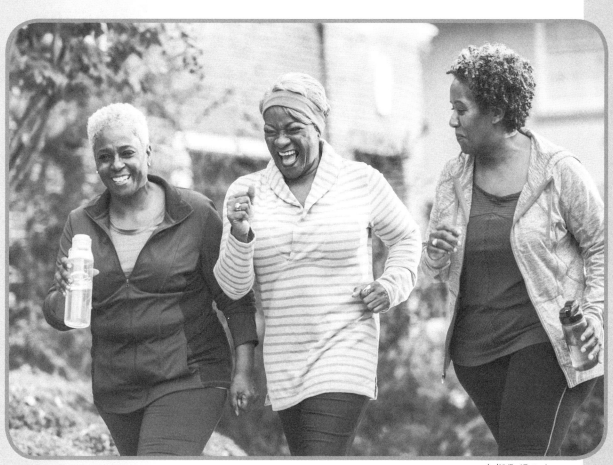

Objectives

After completing this chapter, you will be able to

1. explain the evidence related to aerobic endurance training in older participants,
2. describe the physiological and psychological benefits of aerobic endurance training for older adults,
3. apply exercise principles and variables to the design and implementation of the aerobic endurance training component of a physical activity program designed for older adults,
4. lead aerobic endurance training activities for individuals and groups of older adults, and
5. modify your instructional and leadership skills when you lead aerobic endurance training activities for older adults with different levels of fitness and different functional abilities.

As discussed in chapter 4, the decline in maximal aerobic power ($\dot{V}O_2$max) with advancing age can have a devastating effect on the quality of life of the oldest-old. Everyday tasks and activities require a greater proportion of $\dot{V}O_2$max for older adults, particularly those who are frail. In fact, older adults whose maximal oxygen intake declines to as low as 12 to 15 milliliters per kilogram per minute find it very difficult to complete the simplest of daily activities (e.g., dressing, rising from a chair) independently (Shephard, 2009). Such declines in aerobic capacity threaten their functional independence and should be addressed in any physical activity program designed for older adults. Successfully delivering the aerobic endurance component of your program can not only transform your clients' lives but also provide you with a high level of professional satisfaction.

In this chapter the evidence related to the physiological and psychological benefits of aerobic endurance training for older adults is described first, followed by a discussion of the important exercise principles and variables that need to be considered when developing the aerobic endurance component of any physical activity program for older adults. You will then learn how to manipulate each of these variables appropriately.

Benefits of Aerobic Endurance Training for Older Adults

Aerobic activity is a central part of public health guidelines for physical activity to maintain or improve **health** and **everyday function** in older adults (Nelson et al., 2007; PAGAC, 2018). Aerobic endurance training is important for older adults as even light housework and carrying groceries can require 40 to 50 percent of peak oxygen consumption (Arnett, Laity, Agrawal, & Cress, 2008). The good news is that older adults maintain their ability to respond to aerobic endurance training even into their eighth and ninth decades (Malbut-Shennan, Greig, & Young, 2000; Cho et al., 2017). Even women in their 80s and 90s can improve their $\dot{V}O_2$max by as much as 15 to 17 percent after 24 to 32 weeks of exercise training (Malbut, Dinan, & Young, 2002; Puggaard, Larsen, Stovring, & Jeune, 2000). Well-designed aerobic endurance training also improves older adults' ability to sustain exercise at a fixed, submaximal level of energy expenditure. This can have a positive impact on **functional ability**, particularly for frailer older women, because everyday activities then represent a lower proportion of their $\dot{V}O_2$max and can therefore be performed for longer durations and with greater ease. Aerobic endurance training can improve muscle strength, mass, and power in older adults, but gains in strength and aerobic capacity are quickly lost once training stops (Lovell, Cuneo, & Gass, 2010). Even older adults recently discharged from the hospital benefit from training, showing significant improvements in functional fitness, physical activity, and health-related quality of life (Brovold, Skelton & Bergland, 2013). **Quality of life** in general can also be improved with aerobic endurance training (Hill, Storandt, & Malley, 1993; Lavie & Milani, 1995); however, it remains unclear whether it is the exercise itself or the social contact during training that contributes more to improvements in mood and overall well-being (Brown et al., 1995; Hassmen & Koivula, 1997; Williams & Lord, 1995). What is known is that aerobic endurance training preserves or increases both gray and white brain matter volume and hippocampus volume in older adults, enhancing central nervous system health, memory, and cognitive functioning (Colcombe et al., 2006; Erickson et al., 2009).

Most of the benefits of preventing or managing coronary heart disease, stroke, hypertension, diabetes, and osteoporosis experienced by younger physically active people can also be achieved by those who are physically active in later life (American College of Sports Medicine [ACSM], 2009; Skelton & Dinan, 2008; Young & Dinan, 2005; PAGAC, 2018). Indeed, it is a challenge for exercise scientists to differentiate between how the natural aging process contributes to health and functional decline and what changes would be avoidable if it were not for inactivity (Taylor et al., 2004). However, aerobic endurance training can improve the metabolic profiles of even previously sedentary older adults (Alves et al., 2012). In frailer older adults, however, aerobic endurance training takes on a role less of **disease prevention** and more of **symptom alleviation**. Aerobic endurance training counters some of the well-known age-related physiological changes, reverses **disuse syndrome**, helps to control chronic diseases, maximizes psychological health, and preserves the ability to perform activities of daily living (ACSM, 2009; Young, 2001; Young & Dinan, 2005). Even those with chronic conditions such as stroke and Alzheimer's disease benefit from safely applied aerobic endurance training (Globas et al., 2012; Yu et al., 2011).

Principles and Considerations for Aerobic Endurance Training

In this section we describe how each of the exercise principles first introduced in chapter 8 (i.e., specificity, overload, functional relevance, challenge, and adaptation/tailoring) is specifically applied to the aerobic endurance component of an activity program for older adults. We will also discuss interindividual variability and rest and recovery, two programming considerations of particular importance for meeting the diverse needs encountered when instructing older adults.

Specificity and Interval Conditioning

Specificity is the foundation on which the successful application and manipulation of the other exercise principles and variables depends. Specific types of exercises elicit specific metabolic and physiological adaptations. For example, to improve a client's aerobic capacity, you must select physical activities that are aerobic in nature and are performed at an appropriate intensity to allow a training effect to occur (e.g., walking on a treadmill at an intensity rated light to somewhat hard on Borg's rating of perceived exertion [RPE] scale). For maximum effectiveness, instructors should select exercises and exercise modes for each individual, or a group of individuals, based on the results of the preactivity health screening (see chapter 5) and functional assessments (see chapter 6), and then target the physical fitness parameters that need improvement. The exercises selected must also be specific to both the energy system being targeted (aerobic or anaerobic; Bompa & Buzzichelli, 2018) and, importantly, to functional tasks performed in everyday life (Skelton, Young, Greig, & Malbut, 1995).

Everyday tasks such as hurrying to catch a bus or to avoid heavy rain, climbing a hill during a walk to the store, washing windows, and other recreational and leisure activities such as tennis, swimming, bicycling, and walking, all demand intermittent bursts of energy over time.

This alternating effort–recovery pattern forms the basis of the **interval training** method. Classic interval training alternates periods of maximal or near-maximal effort with short periods of complete rest, while **interval conditioning** alternates short periods (one to six minutes) of higher-intensity exercise with an equal or longer recovery period. In other words, in interval conditioning, the effort expended is a little greater than is comfortable for a certain amount of time, and then the effort returns to an easy, comfortable, and sustainable level for about the same amount of time (Brooks, 1997). Interval conditioning is recommended for use with older participants because it provides a flexible, systematic framework for progressing aerobic endurance training for older adults with a broad range of functional and fitness levels (Dinan, 2002; Masuki, Morikawa & Nose, 2017).

In addition to its greater adaptability, research suggests that the physiological benefits of interval conditioning versus **continuous training** (six minutes or longer of uninterrupted activity, usually performed at a constant submaximal intensity) are similar if not superior in older participants (Shephard, 1991; Whitehurst, 2012). The main reason is that in interval conditioning, regardless of age, the **total volume of work** is higher than when the submaximal intensity of exercise is constant. Alternating controlled fluctuations in intensity or duration with active recovery periods enables the older adult to work harder for a longer time and with greater comfort. It also mirrors real-life energy demands more closely than continuous training does. Therefore, interval conditioning is recommended as the safest, most effective tool for improving both cardiorespiratory and functional aerobic fitness in older adults.

To use interval conditioning skillfully when instructing older adults requires a more thorough understanding of the adapted interval training method. Brooks (1997) identifies three types of interval conditioning: **spontaneous**, **fitness**, and **performance**. When introduced sequentially, they form a logical and progressive continuum of train-

ing. All three types of interval conditioning tap into aerobic and anaerobic energy sources during the higher-effort intervals and have **active**, aerobic, lower-effort recovery intervals. In each type of interval conditioning, the client periodically increases the intensity and then recovers actively before initiating another higher-intensity bout. Intervals can also vary in the durations of the effort and recovery phases; this allows physical activity instructors greater flexibility in prescribing exercise based on their observation of each client's performance and rating of effort. An important feature of interval conditioning is that the client, armed with specific information about monitoring exercise, largely controls the intensity of the exercise. Specific guidelines for manipulating the different exercise variables for the three types of interval conditioning are provided in table 13.1. However, it is important to note that the performance end of the continuum is appropriate only for the more physically fit older adult exercisers. More recently, there has been interest in the use of High Intensity Interval Training (HIIT) in younger adults (PAGAC, 2018), particularly with the publication of systematic reviews suggesting that it improves cardiometabolic health (Batacan, Duncan, Dalbo, Tucker, & Fenning, 2017). HIIT is a form of interval training consisting of alternating short periods of intense anaerobic exercise with less intense aerobic recovery periods. There are currently no universally accepted lengths for either the anaerobic period, the recovery period, or the ratio of the two; no universally accepted number of cycles for any HIIT session or the entire duration of the training bout; and no universally accepted relative intensity at which the intense anaerobic component should be performed. Unfortunately, to date there has been little systematic research conducted with older adults participating in this form of training and there are concerns as to its overall safety for older adults (PAGAC, 2018).

The ultimate goal is to design an aerobic endurance component that combines both continuous- and interval-conditioning approaches. In the initial stages of training aerobic fitness, however, interval conditioning is recommended because it is more flexible and it yields rapid, specific aerobic endurance gains that enhance the performance of everyday activities. After a period of interval conditioning (approximately 12-16 weeks), participants should be encouraged to progress by extending the duration

Table 13.1 Interval Conditioning Training Continuum for Older Adults

	Spontaneous conditioning	Fitness conditioning		Performance conditioning	
Goal	"Get me started"	"Train me"		"Challenge me!"	
	Getting skilled up: feeling fitter	Getting trained up: getting fitter; gaining the training gains		Getting even fitter: maintaining the training gains and beyond	
	Fitter moments	Fit for life		Fit for sport or performance	
	"I want to reduce breathlessness enough to get to the store and back without stopping and without feeling so exhausted that I have to rest for the whole day to recover."	"I want to be able to increase my walking time to 30 minutes, increase my pace, and include uphill walking."		"I want to enter (or improve my time in) the super veteran category in my local triathlon."	
Fitness level	Deconditioned	Moderate to high (for anaerobic intervals)		High	
Intensity	Instructor programmed, participant controlled RPE guidelines 1-3	Instructor programmed, participant controlled RPE guidelines:		Set by instructor RPE guidelines:	
		Effort interval 2-4 progress to: 5-7	Recovery interval 1-3 remains: 1-3	Effort interval 5-7 progress to: 7-9	Recovery interval 1-3 remains: 1-3
	METS guidelines 2-4	METS guidelines 4-6 Progress to: 6-8		METS guidelines 6-10 Progress to: 10-12	
Time:					
*Work/ Rest: Effort/Recovery ratio	Instructor programmed, participant controlled Aerobic effort recovery	Set by instructor Aerobic effort 1: recovery 1 Anaerobic effort 1: recovery 3		Set by instructor Aerobic effort 1: recovery 1 Anaerobic effort 1: recovery 3	
*Duration/Time	Instructor programmed, participant controlled Effort interval: 10 seconds to 5 minutes Recovery interval: 10 seconds to 5 minutes	Set by instructor Aerobic: 3-5 minutes Anaerobic: 80-90 and progress to 90-270 seconds Recovery: 3-5 minutes		Set by instructor Aerobic: 3-5 minutes Anaerobic: 80-90 and progress to 90-270 seconds Recovery: 3-5 minutes	
Frequency	Participant controlled within fitness level and length of aerobic endurance component	Number of cycles depends on fitness level and type		Number of cycles depends on fitness level and length of aerobic endurance component	
*Type	Walking, stationary cycling, and stair climbing and descending	Walking, jogging, cycling, rowing, swimming, exercise to music, circuit training		Timed or race walks, runs, swims; triathlons; mini-marathons	

(continued)

237

Table 13.1 *(continued)*

	Spontaneous conditioning	Fitness conditioning	Performance conditioning
Time:			
Approach	Individualized "easy-does-it" 'speed play'-Fartlek. No or minimal structure "Speed up a little until you reach the next tree and you are breathing a little harder but are not breathless, then ease off a little and recover."	Comfortably challenged More structured "Work a little harder than you usually do."	Improved sports performance, going beyond improved fitness; only for better-conditioned clients Highly structured

*See table 13.4 for appropriate activities and modalities. All interval conditioning programming must be tailored to the client's health and functional needs, physical fitness levels, personal goals, and interests.

Based on Brooks (1997). Dinan and Skelton (2008).

of their workout to include continuous training using cardiovascular equipment (e.g., treadmill, stationary cycle, or cross trainer).

> The key to interval conditioning is to alternate short periods of exercise in which the effort expended is just a little greater than is comfortable with equal, or longer, recovery periods of easier, comfortable, sustainable exercise.

Overload

As first defined in chapter 8, the exercise principle of progressive overload states that for continued improvement in fitness, the cardiopulmonary and musculoskeletal systems must be progressively overloaded by periodically increasing the frequency, intensity, time (duration), or challenge of an exercise (Heyward & Gibson, 2014). Prevention of injury and overtraining is a priority at all ages. The instructor must strike a balance between ensuring sufficient progressive overload and preventing exhaustion and subsequent loss of coordination, muscle soreness, injury, and possible dropout (Skelton & Beyer, 2003). While it is true that cardiorespiratory overtraining is rarely a problem for noncompetitive older exercisers, maintaining this balance is even more critical for older adults because the safety margins are narrower, the consequences of overtraining are greater, and recovery takes longer. Manipulating the variable of intensity (speed, load) appears to be more stressful for the older adult exerciser than manipulating training volume (repetitions, time, frequency). In frailer older participants, whose bone strength, muscle force, and speed are already compromised, inappropriate programming can increase the risk of falls, injuries, and overtraining.

These are some helpful guidelines for applying the overload principle to the aerobic endurance component of your activity program:

- Increase only one variable at a time.
- Increase duration before intensity.
- Increase duration in one-minute increments as tolerated (Fiatarone Singh, 2011).
- Increase intensity by first using the arms in a more challenging way (e.g., raising arms above waist level) or by increasing resistance (e.g., walking with backpack, Nordic walking, using light hand weights during land- and water-based exercise) before increasing the speed of the movement (Fiatarone Singh, 2011).
- Allow a minimum of two weeks for adaptation before considering increasing the overload (Skelton & Dinan, 2008).

Functional Relevance

One of the unique principles for exercise programs for older adults, first described in chapter 8, is functional relevance. Examples of aerobic exercises that have functional relevance include activities such as stair climbing and descending, picking up objects and carrying them across the room, and certain line or ballroom dancing moves. Integrating specific functional tasks into your aerobic endurance component and overall physical activity program can help your clients realize additional improvements in both muscle strength and functional ability (Dinan, Lenihan, Tenn, & Iliffe, 2006; Skelton & Dinan, 2008). Although there is little evidence on specificity of aerobic training for older adults, it is likely that similar findings would apply. Therefore, it is best to select activities that are more functional in nature not only to improve physiological parameters but also to improve the performance of basic, intermediate, and advanced activities of daily living and to reduce the risk of falls.

Challenge

A second exercise principle critical to programs for older adults first introduced in chapter 8 is the challenge principle. This principle is similar to the overload principle, but it focuses on increasing the demands placed on multiple body systems rather than just manipulating the exercise variables (frequency, intensity, type, and time). The challenge of an aerobic exercise can be altered by increasing the complexity of the task, such as walking to different tempos of music, or by adding a second task, such as walking to a certain tempo in a particular direction and then using marching to turn and then walking in the opposite direction. For those older adults who prefer exercising in the water and for those with impaired movement (e.g., arthritis, injury), water-based endurance training activities can be more challenging and provide greater benefits than equivalent land-based training (Bocalini, Serra, Murad, & Levy, 2008; Skelton & Dinan, 2008).

Accommodation or Adaptation

Another important exercise principle to consider when designing the aerobic endurance component for older adults is the principle of accommodation or adaptation of exercise (Skelton & Dinan, 2008; Wilcox et al., 2006). Because many of your older clients may be taking multiple medications for various medical conditions, it is important to recognize that adverse side effects may influence their ability to exercise at the same intensity and for the same

duration each week. It is important for the instructor to know these possible associated adverse effects in order to ensure the aerobic component design is adapted not only to accommodate for the aging process, but also by tailoring it to each individual's response to exercise (Skelton & Dinan 2008; Wilcox et al., 2006). Possible adverse effects of medications during exercise are discussed in chapter 17. It is important to remember that even physically independent older adults are more likely to have one or more chronic conditions (Akushevich, Kravchenko, Ukraintseva, & Arbeev, 2013; Taylor et al., 2004) and that it is not unusual for people with arthritic conditions to feel fine one day but then be experiencing considerable pain the next day. Teaching clients to monitor their own exertion level, discomfort and pain levels, and personal safety limits, and to adapt their exercise accordingly, reduces exercise-related musculoskeletal injury rates and risk of cardiac events. These instructor and client skills are of particular importance for the successful implementation and progression of the aerobic endurance training component (see chapter 16 for a more in-depth discussion of these instructional skills).

Accommodation through monitoring, adaptation, and tailoring is the key to meeting the greater fluctuations in health, functional capacity, and fitness found in older adults.

Interindividual Variability

Some of your older clients will progress very slowly and need a lot of encouragement because of their medical conditions, sedentary lifestyle, previous physical activity history, or personality. For your program to be effective, exercises must be individualized on the basis of the information derived from the preactivity screening, your functional assessment results, and the behavioral goals you have established in consultation with your client. It is also important to understand the unique personalities of your clients in order to communicate effectively with them. Refer to chapter 16 for a more detailed discussion of developing your communication and leadership skills with older adults.

When educating clients about cardiorespiratory fitness, you can enhance their motivation by emphasizing the difference fitness can make in performing daily activities that they currently find difficult (e.g., breathlessness when sweeping the floors, having to stop multiple times to rest on the stairs). Engaging clients also means reassuring them that what they are experiencing is completely normal if they have not been active for a while; that progress will be slow; that they will receive individual attention; that there is no rush; that safety is the priority; that they will soon feel and see the difference; and that well-structured, free-moving endurance exercise also helps to prevent falls and improve balance, makes for a healthier heart, and can put a spring back in their step.

Rest and Recovery

It is crucial that you systematically plan for adequate rest and recovery periods in aerobic endurance training for older adult clients. Adequate, active rest and sufficient recovery help (1) prevent adverse events (cardiorespiratory, overuse, undue fatigue, injuries, and falls), (2) optimize the function of the cardiorespiratory system, (3) improve aerobic and functional performance, and (4) promote exercise adherence. Residual fatigue or muscle soreness that interferes with a client's performance during the next set of repetitions of a particular exercise, or the next exercise session, is a good indicator that the recovery period was inadequate. **Muscle acidosis**, a physiological condition that is characterized by low pH in the body tissues and blood and a buildup of lactate, is the primary performance-limiting factor in endurance exercise. Rest and recovery are essential preventive strategies and are most effectively achieved through careful exercise selection.

Yessis (1987) identified three phases of recovery following aerobic exercise: ongoing recovery within a session, quick recovery immediately after a session (through removal of metabolic wastes), and deep recovery during and between sessions (through training adaptation that enhances the body's ability to recover quickly and efficiently). Effective aerobic endurance program design for all ages must therefore consider the recovery period required for each of the following: between effort intervals; between the cycles (sets) of effort and recovery intervals; between specific exercises; between the compo-

nents of a session; between consecutive aerobic endurance sessions performed on the same day (e.g., in circuit training and swimming); and between specific endurance sessions over days, weeks, and months. The amount of recovery between workouts depends on the ability and fitness level of the participant and the intensity, frequency, and duration of the activity. Deep recovery improves as cardiorespiratory fitness is achieved.

Therefore, the key to older adults' recovery during and following endurance activities is ensuring *active* rest. Interval conditioning, with its lower-intensity active rest and recovery intervals, is most effective at clearing lactate from the muscles and facilitating quick recovery phases for older adult exercisers. Advise your clients to come a little early to rest and refresh before the session and to allow 20 minutes to relax and refresh after the session in order to be thoroughly alert and coordinated on leaving the exercise setting and to derive the greatest benefit from the session.

The key to older adults' recovery during endurance activities is best achieved through active rest and recovery periods of interval conditioning.

Variables for Aerobic Endurance Training

In addition to skillfully and mindfully applying the exercise principles and exercise considerations discussed in the previous section, it is also important to understand how to manipulate each of the relevant exercise variables: frequency, intensity, time (duration), and type (mode). In this chapter we prefer the terms *time* rather than *duration* and *type* rather than *mode* because the acronym FITT (frequency, intensity, time, type) serves as a useful mnemonic for remembering these variables for the aerobic endurance component of the program.

Frequency and Time

The variables that have the most direct bearing on aerobic training volume are frequency and time. All adults should avoid inactivity; even a small amount of physical activity will provide some health benefit (U.S. Department of Health and Human Services, 2008). However, these 2008 guidelines clarify that to gain substantial health benefits, the older participant must aim to engage in 150 minutes (2hr 30 min) of moderate aerobic exercise on most days of the week. For older adults who are already regularly active and physically fit, 75 minutes (1hr 15 min) of vigorous physical activity will bring equivalent benefits. Moreover, there is evidence that cardiorespiratory gains are similar whether the exercise occurs in several short bouts (e.g., at least 10 min) or in longer (e.g., 30 min) bouts. However, at all ages, health and disease prevention benefits are more extensive with longer time periods (300 minutes of moderate or 150 minutes of vigorous physical activity) (Fiatarone Singh, 2011). For frailer older participants, ACSM (2009) recommends a preparatory period of strength and balance training before beginning aerobic training to minimize injuries and falls among older adults. The United States (PAGAC, 2018), United Kingdom (U.K. Department of Health, 2011) and New Zealand (Ministry of Health, New Zealand, 2013) guidelines emphasize the importance, with older adults, of building up aerobic training gradually and of matching training to current fitness levels to allow for age and health-related fluctuations. The recommendation is to "start low and go slow" and to progress by first increasing the time and then increasing the intensity. It may be necessary to start with as little as three minutes a day for frailer or less healthy and more deconditioned clients (Skelton & Dinan 2008; U.K. Department of Health, 2011).

Intensity

The intensity of physical activity determines the physiological and metabolic changes in the body. There are three common methods of measuring and monitoring the intensity of aerobic exercise: (1) heart rate, (2) Borg's RPE scale, and (3) metabolic equivalent (MET) values.

Heart Rate

The most common method of prescribing and monitoring exercise intensity is by establishing a training heart rate that is based on a percentage of either **maximal heart rate (HRmax)** or **heart rate**

reserve (**HRR**). HRR is calculated by subtracting resting heart rate from HRmax. Unfortunately, both of these methods have certain disadvantages. First, unless a true measure of HRmax has been obtained, it must be estimated. Such estimates are particularly unreliable when applied to older adults (Tanaka, Monahan, & Seals, 2001). Second, clients must slow down or stop exercising to take their heart rate. Third, heart rates that are self-measured by palpation have been shown to be inaccurate (Bell & Bassey, 1996; Kobayashi, 2013). Finally, percentage of HRR may represent a higher than expected percentage of $\dot{V}O_2$max (Scharff-Olsen, Williford, & Smith, 1992), so using HRR percentage to prescribe or monitor exercise intensity may result in the older adult's working at an intensity that is higher than desired (Fitzsimons et al., 2005; Kohrt, Spina, Holloszy, & Ehsani, 1998).

When designing your aerobic endurance component, use the acronym FITT as an easy way to remember the variables:

Frequency

Intensity

Time (duration)

Type

Rating of Perceived Exertion

As first introduced in chapter 4, an alternative to using target heart rate to obtain the desired training intensity is using **Borg's rating of perceived exertion (RPE) scale**. This scale of self-perceived effort takes into account both central (e.g., heart rate and breathing) and local (e.g., muscle fatigue) sensations, so it does not rely on cardiovascular response alone to determine workload (Borg, 1982). It also does not require slowing down or stopping exercise to obtain a value, and it is effective for prescribing and monitoring exercise intensity for both younger and older adults (Ilarraza, Myers, Kottman, Rickli, & Dubach, 2004; Malbut et al., 2002).

According to the ACSM (2017) guidelines, exercise intensity for older adults should be at an RPE of 5 to 6 (CR10 scale) for moderately strong intensity and 7 to 8 for vigorous intensity. For sedentary older adults, walking at a moderate RPE of 3 to 5

(CR10 scale) does lead to a beneficial physiological response during endurance training and a weekly energy expenditure of nearly 1,200 kcal when exercising 5 times per week for 30 minutes (Donath et al., 2013). For a frail older adult, it is recommended that exercise intensity start at very light to light (1-2 on the CR10 scale and 9-11 on the RPE scale) and be increased slowly and cautiously.

However, whether you are using the 0 to 10 CR10 scale or the 6 to 20 RPE scale, Borg makes it clear that it is essential that the instructor and the participant understand what they are assessing and that the participant receives clear instructions on using the scale (Borg & Hassmen, 1999).

Metabolic Equivalent Values

The intensity of an exercise can also be regulated by selecting activities based on known metabolic equivalent (MET) values. It is important to know the MET value of specific aerobic activities so that any risk posed to certain older individuals by the activities can be eliminated. Some activities have a wide range of MET values (e.g., ballroom dancing, 4-6 METs; aerobic dance, 6-9 METs; and skipping, 8-12 METs), while others vary little (e.g., walking at 3 miles per hour, 3-8 METs; cycling at 10 miles per hour, 5-6 METs), because less-structured movements can be performed in a variety of ways (Ministry of Health, New Zealand, 2013; Skelton & Dinan, 2008; Warburton, Whitney, Shannon, & Bredin, 2006).

Type of Physical Activity

In addition to careful manipulation of the frequency, time, and intensity that will determine the cardiorespiratory overload, identifying the right type (mode) of physical activity is very important. Aerobic endurance exercise is defined as any activity that uses the large muscle groups, can be maintained for a prolonged period, and is rhythmic and continuous (Bell, 1996). When you select the type of aerobic endurance activity or exercise for your program, you should once again be guided by the results of the preactivity screening (chapter 5), physical and mobility functional assessments (chapters 6), and the behavioral goals (chapter 7) of your clients. Aerobic activities popular with older adults include walking, stationary cycling, treadmill walking or jogging, dancing, swimming,

aquatic exercise, and exercise to music. A balanced combination of physical activities is as important as the selection of each individual activity in ensuring your clients' safety, improved performance, and adherence.

The key recommendations for applying each of the exercise variables are as follows:

- Frequency: Exercise most days of the week; start with three days per week for frail and sedentary clients.
- Intensity: Remember the phrases "start low, go slow" and "moderate." Intensity is most easily estimated using METs and most easily and effectively monitored using Borg's RPE. Start with a RPE between 3 and 4 (moderate to somewhat hard; CR10 scale) for active, healthy older adults and between 1 and 2 (very light to light; CR10 scale) for frail and sedentary older adults.
- Time: Healthy older adults should exercise for 150 minutes per week at a moderate intensity or 75 minutes at a vigorous intensity in 30 minute bouts. For frail and sedentary older adults, exercise for 30 minutes most days; start with three periods of 3 to 5 minutes and build to three periods of 10 minutes per day.
- Type: Choose activities that involve the large muscle groups, can be maintained for a prolonged period, and are rhythmic and continuous. Walking is a great mainstay.

Types of Aerobic Endurance Exercises

Aerobic endurance exercise offers a wider range of potential modalities than any other fitness component and the largest number of activities that, with a little effort, can become part of your clients' everyday lives. Incorporating a variety of different aerobic endurance activities in a weekly exercise program minimizes overuse injuries, maximizes peripheral adaptation, and increases long-term motivation and adherence (King, Rejeski, & Buchner, 1998). This is particularly true of cross-training combinations that involve the large muscle groups of both the upper body and lower body (e.g., using a cross trainer, an elliptical trainer with arm handles, a crossover trainer, a recumbent stepper or doing circuit training exercises, Nordic walking, exercising to music). The dilemma of choosing the best type of aerobic endurance activity for a particular older adult client is solved by evaluating each activity from three distinct, yet related, perspectives: its health benefits and training effects, its risks, and its programming advantages, which include basing the selection on specific criteria or prompts.

First, the physical activity instructor needs to consider the health benefits and physical fitness training effects specific to each exercise or mode of exercise in relation to his or her client's unique needs, goals, preferences, and lifestyle. For example, determine whether the exercise preference lowers the risk of falls to a minimum, restores or preserves the client's functional ability, and increases the client's opportunities for socializing, working, being independent, and so on (see table 13.2).

Second, the instructor must analyze each aerobic endurance exercise or exercise mode carefully to ensure that its risks never outweigh its potential benefits to the client. Using the prompts in the risk-to-benefit analysis tool (see table 13.3) will assist both the instructor and the client in deciding whether the exercise preference is an appropriate goal for the client or whether it needs to be permanently excluded for health and safety reasons, such as jumping jacks for complete beginners, crossover steps (i.e., a grapevine) for groups of older exercisers with balance and mobility problems, or a cross-trainer for a client with knee problems.

Finally, the physical activity instructor should know the specific programming advantages of the different exercise modes (see table 13.4). For example, knowing which activities score highest (not only on physiological and psychosocial criteria but also on a cost–benefit basis and on how easily each activity can be integrated into everyday life) is important information to have at your fingertips when developing tailored recommendations for older clients. The modality-specific programming advantages are highlighted in table 13.4.

As can be seen in table 13.4, walking quite simply has more programming advantages at any age than any other type of aerobic endurance activity. For this reason alone, walking should be the mainstay for any aerobic endurance component designed for older adults. As we age, participation drops in all types of physical activities, except walking. Walk-

ing appeals to a wide range of people, is easily adapted to different fitness and functional levels and environments (indoors or out), and facilitates social interactions, particularly intergenerational ones. Of all aerobic endurance activities, walking is the most functionally relevant; it has the most natural relationship to the environment and is the easiest to integrate into activities of daily living. By teaching correct walking technique and incorporating more complex skills, routes, and intensity for those who wish to progress (e.g., power walking), this everyday activity becomes more interesting, challenging, effective, and inclusive. It makes good programming sense, therefore, to promote walking as the foundation of aerobic endurance programs and active lifestyle approaches for older adults. Although higher-intensity interval walk training provides greater benefits than low- or moderate-intensity walk training (Nemoto, Gen-no, Masuki, Okazaki, & Nose, 2007), care must be taken to ensure that the older adult has sufficiently good balance and fitness that the intensity does not put them at high risk for falls (Sherrington et al., 2008). Applying the interval conditioning approach described earlier is a sound basis for design.

Training Precautions and Considerations

There are a range of programming precautions and considerations that must be applied to the design and delivery of aerobic endurance training for older adults. While the authors support the exceptional potential of aerobic endurance training to achieve functionally relevant fitness outcomes in even the oldest old, it is important to stress that injury prevention must be the highest priority for this segment of the older adult population; this will require the dedicated, ongoing application of the following precautions and considerations to every aspect of the aerobic endurance component by the physical activity instructor of older adults. As we have seen, aerobic endurance training has potentially higher risks and involves a wider range of activities and environments than any other fitness component. It is therefore important to review the risks associated with inappropriate aerobic endurance training before moving on to a review of the risk-reducing

Table 13.2 Health Benefits and Physical Fitness Training Effects of Different Modes of Exercise for Older Adults

	Walking	Aerobic dance	Circuit training	Step training/ Stair climbing	Cardiovascular equipment		Water training		Active lifestyle
					Cycle	Treadmill	Swimming	Aquatics	
Health benefits									
Prevents disease	++	++	++	++	++	++	+	+	—
Counteracts the effects of disease and reduces disability	+	++	++	+	+	+	+	++	+
Improves or maintains bone density	+	++	+	++	—	+	—	+	+
Reduces fall risk factors	+	++	+	—	—	+	—	+	+
Improves mental health or mood	++	+	+	+	+	+	+	+	+
Increases social opportunities	++	++	++	+	—	—	+	++	+
Preserves functional capacity in old age	++	++	++	+	+	+	+	+	+
Physical fitness training effects									
Improves submaximal $\dot{V}O_2$max	++	++	++	++	++	++	++	++	+
Improves $\dot{V}O_2$max	+	++	++	++	++	++	++	++	+
Improves ability to perform specific functional IADL moves, e.g., sit to stand	+	++	++	++	—	+	+	+	++
Improves ability to sustain IADL endurance activities, e.g., walking, and reduces fatigue	++	+	++	+	+	+	+	+	+
Improves reaction time	—	++	++	+	—	—	—	+	+
Improves balance and coordination	+	++	++	+	—	+	+	+	+
Improves (leg) strength	+	+	+	++	++	+	++	++	++
Improves flexibility	—	+	+	—	—	—	++	++	+
Improves posture and body control	+	++	++	+	—	+	+	+	+
Improves body and spatial awareness	+	++	++	—	—	—	++	++	+

Note: The best exercise choices for each benefit are highlighted. All modes are assumed to be performed at a moderate (not vigorous or low) intensity and intermediate (not elite or low) skill level, with correct technique and alignment for a minimum of 30 minutes at a time on a regular basis. The "Active Lifestyle" mode assumes a combination of instrumental activities of daily living (IADLs) such as gardening, shopping, stair climbing, and recreational or sport activities. The social opportunities category is viewed with respect to its potential to increase opportunities to socialize both within and outside the activity. The aerobic dance, circuit training, and step training modes are assumed to be supervised groups. The status of each activity is graded on the bases of a combination of research evidence, consensus, recommendations, and our opinion as recognized experts in exercise and aging and instructor training.

Key: Significant improvements ++; Noticeable improvements +; Little or no change —

Table 13.3 Exercise Risk-to-Benefit Analysis Prompt Tool

Effectiveness specific prompts. Ask yourself:	Safety specific prompts. Ask yourself:	Additional exercise prescription prompts. Ask yourself:	Personal considerations
• Is it health or performance related? Is it specific to everyday activities? • Will it accommodate an interval conditioning approach? • Will it allow small incremental progressions? • Does it improve bone density? • Does it prevent or reduce falls and injuries? • Does it protect joints? • Does it improve performance and posture? • Will it increase confidence, enjoyment, social opportunity? • Will it improve long-term commitment? • Does it suit the client's lifestyle?	• Is it biomechanically and ergonomically sound according to current best practices? For example, short treadmills and drop-handle cycles are contraindicated for older adults. • Is it biomechanically and energetically sound when performed by the individual? For example, treadmill walking is contraindicated for a beginning exerciser who is frail. • Is it stable and symmetrical? Do the muscles pull in the correct line of force? • Does it allow a controlled, pain-free range of movement? For example, step training with inappropriate step height and inadequate support could create an unsafe exercise with little benefit. • Is the speed, resistance, body position, and length of levers appropriate, effective, and safe? (For example, exercising to music with too fast a tempo is inappropriate.) • Can it be done in a controlled manner, with a linear heart rate response, easily maintained work rate, and standardized progression in small increments?	• Is it adjustable? Can it be adapted to meet the needs of the individual? • Is it comfortable for this individual client? • Is a safe setting available (at home or in the community)? For example, does the space have adequate access and sufficient space? Is it in good repair and well maintained? Does it allow safe transitions from one area or piece of equipment to another? • Does it require special equipment (e.g., hip protectors, wall or support railings, chair, saddle padding) for this individual to perform it? • Can it be part of a balanced, varied, cross-training fitness program? • Does this mode require further consultation with a physician or therapist or both?	• Will the client perceive it as a safe exercise mode? • Does it match the client's level of training or stage of behavioral change? • Does it match the client's perceived levels of skill and fitness? • Does it meet the client's perceived functional capacity and health needs? • Is it enjoyable? • Is it motivating? • Is it realistic?

Table 13.4 Specific Programming Advantages of Different Exercise Modes for Older Adults

	Walking	Aerobic dance	Circuit training	Step training/Stair climbing	Cardiovascular equipment		Water training		Active lifestyle
					Cycle (station only)	Treadmill	Swimming	Aqua	
Low cardiac risk with high cardiorespiratory and functional endurance gains	✓✓	✓	✓✓	✓	✓✓	✓	✓✓	✓	✓
Accommodates interval conditioning approach	✓✓	✓	✓✓	✓	✓	✓	✓✓	✓	*
Linear heart rate response	✓	*	*	*	✓✓	✓✓	✓	*	*
Standardized progression increments, easily controlled	✓	✓	✓✓	*	✓✓	✓✓	✓	✓	*
Low to medium skill level	✓	✓	✓	*	✓✓	✓	*	*	✓
Low impact	✓✓	✓	✓	✓	✓✓	✓✓	✓✓	✓✓	✓✓
Low injury risk	✓	*	*	*	✓✓	✓	✓✓	✓	✓
Multilevel (i.e., a range of intensity levels to meet older individual's needs and goals)	✓✓	✓	✓	*	✓	*	*	*	✓✓
Mixes well with other modes	✓✓	✓	✓	✓	✓	✓	✓	✓	✓
Client's satisfaction with progress	✓✓	✓	✓✓	✓	✓✓	✓✓	✓✓	✓	✓
No or low cost (fees, equipment, clothing)	✓✓	✓	✓	✓	*	*	*	*	✓
Can be integrated into life safely	✓✓	✓	✓	*	*	*	✓✓	*	✓✓
Autonomous (unsupervised)	✓✓	✓	✓	✓	✓	✓	✓✓	✓	✓✓

Note: The best exercise choices for each programming advantage are clearly highlighted. The chart assumes that all modes are performed regularly at a moderate (not low or vigorous) intensity for a minimum of 30 minutes at a time, using correct technique, form, and alignment. The active lifestyle mode assumes a combination of instrumental activities of daily living (IADLs) and recreational/sports activities. The aerobic dance, circuit training, and step training modes are assumed to be supervised groups.

Key: Very good = ✓✓; Good = ✓; Little or not at all = *

precautions. Table 13.5 summarizes the musculoskeletal, cardiovascular, and metabolic risks associated with inappropriate aerobic exercise in older adults (Fiatarone Singh, 2011).

The number of injuries and medical emergencies can be reduced for older adults by following a few simple rules. The sidebar summarizes the key precautions and considerations for optimizing the benefits of aerobic endurance training in older adults.

The final precautionary strategies listed in the

Table 13.5 Risks of Inappropriate Aerobic Endurance Exercise for the Older Adult

Musculoskeletal	Cardiovascular	Metabolic
Falls (excess fatigue, loss of coordination, unsafe exercises)	Arrhythmia	Dehydration
	Myocardial infarction (MI)	Electrolyte imbalance
Fracture	Hypertension	Energy imbalance
Joint or bursa inflammation, exacerbation of arthritis	Hypotension	Hyperglycemia
	Ischemia	Hypoglycemia
Ligament or tendon strain	Pulmonary embolism	Hypothermia (in cold weather)
Muscle rupture or tear	Retinal hemorrhage or detachment, lens detachment (exercising too soon after surgery)	Heat stroke
Skin tears		Seizures
Muscle soreness		
Hemorrhoids	Ruptured cerebral or other aneurysm	
Hernia	Syncope or postural instability symptoms	
Stress incontinence		

Adapted by permission from M.A. Fiatarone Singh, The Exercise Prescription. In *Exercise, Nutrition, and the Older Woman: Wellness for Women Over Fifty*, edited by M.A. Fiatarone Singh (Boca Raton: CRC Press, 2002), 84.

Precautions and Considerations
for Aerobic Endurance Training in Older Adults

General Exercise Guidelines for Older Adults

- Outdoor exercise should be avoided in extremes of heat or cold or in icy conditions.
- Prescribed exercise should progress slowly and cautiously.
- Exercise should never leave the participant more than pleasantly tired the following day.
- There should be an adequate warm-up and cool-down.
- Sudden twisting or turning movements and forms of exercise that adversely affect balance should be avoided (e.g., turns of more than 90°).
- Activity should be halted temporarily for angina, premature ventricular contractions, or excessive breathlessness.
- Vigorous exercise should be prohibited during acute viral infections.
- Avoid exercising indoors where the air conditioning is inadequate
- Avoid unsupported exercise if balance problems are worse than usual.
- Aerobic endurance activity should be eased off and halted temporarily if the legs or arms feel so tired and heavy that coordination or quality of movement is impaired (e.g., uncharacteristic clumsiness or slight tripping).

(continued)

General Exercise Guidelines for Older Adults *(continued)*

- Ensure adequate hydration before, during, and after aerobic endurance exercise.
- Toileting should occur before the activity to avoid interruption and minimize stress incontinence. (Dinan & Skelton, 2008)

When Exercise Should Not Be Performed

Contraindications to exercise are covered in chapter 5. These include acute and uncontrolled or unstable health conditions. Participants and instructors must strictly adhere to those criteria. Instructors and participants should also consider the following additional intrinsic contraindications prior to aerobic endurance training:

- Older adults should not exercise if they are feeling unwell or have a fever or acute systemic illness (e.g., bronchitis, respiratory infection, rheumatoid arthritis).
- Older adults should not exercise if they have new or worsened symptoms (e.g., pain, dizziness, breathlessness, unsteadiness).
- Older adults should not exercise after a recent injurious fall until they have undergone a medical consultation.

The instructor must also consider extrinsic factors that might cause an unsafe exercise environment:

- Paint or dust fumes
- Damaged or slippery flooring
- Unacceptable lighting, heating, or ventilation
- Objects such as pillars in the middle of the working area
- Unsafe footwear (e.g., high-heeled, open-toed or sling-back shoes, untied laces)
- Unsafe clothing (e.g., wide-legged trousers, tight belts)
- A ratio of more than 25 participants to one instructor
- A temporary or substitute instructor who is not a specialist in physical activity for older adults

When Exercise Can Be Continued

Instructors of older adults must be aware of when exercise should be stopped, but they also need to know when it can be resumed.

- Exercise can be continued when breathlessness resolves by reducing the intensity of the exercise as gauged by the Borg RPE scale or by taking an active cardiorespiratory rest.
- Exercise can be continued when loss of coordination, loss of concentration, or aching or burning sensations in the muscles resolve by reducing the intensity, using a seated alternative activity, or changing the task.
- Exercise can be continued when joint pain resolves on realigning the joint or improving exercise technique.

All the above physical signs are normal responses to exercise.

When Exercise Should Be Stopped

Once exercise is under way, it should be stopped if any of the following symptoms occur:

- Severe dyspnea
- Dizziness
- Angina (chest pain)
- Extra pulse beats or abnormal heart rhythms
- Nausea
- Confusion
- Extreme fatigue
- Near syncope
- Intermittent calf pain (Shephard, 1990)
- New joint or muscle pain or increased pain that is unresolved by adapting the exercise (Dinan & Skelton, 2008)
- General or local muscle fatigue resulting in unresolved loss of coordination in the lower limbs, tripping over own feet, bumping into others or objects, or severe loss of concentration
- Unresolved loss of concentration
- Consistently refusing or being unable to follow instructions or perform exercises and thus putting the exerciser or others at risk (due to the chance of injury to others, this consideration is of significant concern to the instructor)

Caution should be taken particularly by participants with a history of arrhythmia, chest pain, congestive heart failure, hypertension, or a history of falls. Medical management must be sought and symptoms controlled before resuming participation.

Note: Learning to listen to, interpret, and respond appropriately to the body's messages is an important life skill and the key to safer, more effective exercise and greater autonomy for the exerciser. The preactivity screening, physical performance assessment and orientation, individualized program planning, tailoring, and ongoing review are all ideal opportunities for the physical activity instructor to educate each older participant about listening and responding to her or his body before, during, and after exercise.

sidebar footnote—preactivity screening, physical performance assessment, adapted program planning and individualized tailoring (in particular, effective teaching of motor skills), and the ongoing monitoring of signs and symptoms of overexertion—cannot be overemphasized in the ongoing safety responsibilities of the physical activity instructor when preparing, supervising, adapting, and evaluating aerobic exercise for older adults. Successful strategies rely on highly competent leadership and instructor skills. (See chapter 16 for a more detailed discussion of the importance of progressing your leadership and instructional skills and chapter 15 for an in-depth discussion of important motor learning principles that can be applied to the teaching of motor skills.)

Observation of, and communication with, your clients is particularly important before beginning any exercise session. Simple eye contact can help you better assess how a client is feeling, physically and psychologically, and guide your decisions about how best to deliver the activities you have planned for each client. Advice to a client to "take it easy" should be explicit (e.g., "Do the exercises without the arm movements" or "Do the exercises sitting down today"). Establishing your expertise and authority is important for client and peer confidence and is all part of integrating leadership skills into your teaching. In assisted-living settings, requesting a daily health update or additional staff assistance are ways of meeting the fluctuating health needs of your frailer clients. Staff training also helps to raise awareness and ensure that assistance to clients is administered safely (this leadership aspect of the instructor role is explored in chapter16). The risks and benefits of any type of exercise ultimately depend on many factors; following the precautionary training guidelines is a crucial best practice and should come first in your design considerations. Part of all good program design must also include how well the exercise is taught (Young & Dinan, 2005).

Implications for Program Design and Management

Whatever the exercise type, it is important to apply the training principles (i.e., specificity, overload, functional relevance, challenge, accommodation, interindividual variability, progression, and rest and recovery) and adjust the variables (frequency, intensity, time, and type) as recommended earlier, paying particular attention to the progressive overload guidelines and to progressing slowly and cautiously while accommodating individual functional limitations. Regular reevaluation of the aerobic endurance component of the program is necessary to respond to clients' changing needs and preferences.

Tailoring the exercises to suit the individual needs of your clients is particularly important in group exercise settings, where clients are likely to have a wide range of fitness levels, pathologies, disabilities, and preferences, and where socializing and competition, while likely to increase enjoyment, can also decrease concentration and caution.

Meeting Clients' Individual Needs and Goals

When deciding how best to adapt the exercise program to address the needs and personal goals of the clients, it is important that you consider the questions "fitness for what?" and "fitness for whom?" For example, are your clients interested in improving their level of fitness so they can more easily perform the instrumental activities of daily living, or is their aim to maintain their active lifestyles or even take part in athletic competitions? Once you have identified each client's interests, you can design a multilevel aerobic endurance program in which the levels of intensity are graded and the exercise choice(s) meet group goals as well as each participant's personal goals. Moreover, these goals need to be specific, measurable, realistic, and behavioral, and they need to be determined through negotiation and discussion and agreed on by the whole group. When promoting aerobic endurance training, the messages you convey must be adapted to address the benefits (and goals) that older participants find sufficiently motivating. For the majority of older clients, the more personal, functional, and social the goal, the more motivating it will be for them (Dinan et al., 2006).

Adapting Session Structure and Content

Adaptation is the key to overall program design and the creation of safe and effective aerobic endurance sessions. The changes are subtle but crucial. The safety margins are narrower for *all* older adults, and, without sufficient instructor skill, some older adults may experience unnecessary falls. To be safe, particularly during free-moving group exercise (including circuit training), certain exercises need to be adapted or excluded altogether.

Exercise Selection

Factors such as speed, intensity, the structure of the warm-up and the cool-down, and exercise selection, combination, and repetition can independently, or collectively, transform a safe aerobic endurance exercise into a potentially high-risk activity for particular older individuals. The risks of certain exercises outweigh the benefits for *all* older participants. The following expert guidelines are examples of aerobic endurance activities and exercises that should be avoided or carefully adapted (Skelton & Dinan, 1999) when working with older adults:

- No turns of more than 90 degrees; even 90-degree turns may need to be altered to three- or even five-point turns for frailer individuals.
- No exercises involving lateral movement of one

leg across the other, in front or behind (e.g., the grapevine). Although some controlled lateral movement is necessary to master compensatory stepping to regain balance (see chapter 14), this is very different from traveling across a room at a quicker pace and in a group. The client can simply bring the feet together rather than crossing them over to retain all the proprioceptive and aerobic endurance benefits while significantly reducing the risk of an adverse event.

- No sudden changes of step, speed, direction, or level. Many instructors working with older participants fail to invite or listen to their clients' feedback and then modify activities based on that feedback. As a consequence, some aerobic endurance components remain too difficult for clients to perform confidently. For example, a frequent instructor error is to move too quickly or to incorporate too many complex step patterns into an aerobic routine that requires a higher skill level that ultimately leads to high-risk aerobic endurance training. Instructors must recognize that even the fittest older adult is at greater risk on days when he or she is tired or has poor concentration.

Instruction

Good physical activity instruction of older adults is teaching at its very best. This sums up the specialized, consistent, and exceptional level of skill, attention, and application to individuals you must provide when supervising aerobic endurance training for older adults. The importance of technical, administrative, communication, observation, mentoring, negotiation, teaching, and leadership skills cannot be overemphasized for ensuring safer, more comfortable, more enjoyable sessions and, more important, enhancing effectiveness and long-term commitment (Dinan et al., 2006).

To provide a safe and enjoyable physical activity environment, the following additional guidelines are recommended:

- Demonstrate each exercise and transition using correct technique and at an appropriate speed (neither too fast nor too slow).

- Ensure that participants can hear and understand you by projecting your voice louder and lower, making sure your lips can be seen and that your lips move normally, and adjusting the volume of music with participants' feedback.

- Use body language and timely, larger-than-life hand signals for ample warning of directional changes; this also improves clarity and safety for those with hearing or vision problems.

- Ensure that, if using circuit cards, lettering and numbers are in a thick, large, plain font on a light reflective color (yellow or white) and feature simple, accurate, single-line drawings or clear photographs of an older adult exercise model.

- Perform all levels of an exercise initially then return to perform the least challenging option yourself rather than the most difficult to validate and support working "at your own level."

- Avoid phrases that provoke competitiveness such as "Ready, steady, go" or "See how quickly you can get from here to the wall." Instead, use phrases such as "When you're ready, off you go," "Walk to the wall with as much energy and efficiency as you can," "Work at your own pace; avoid slowing down or speeding up to keep pace with your neighbor."

- Observe each participant by truly seeing, not just looking at, him or her. Then analyze movement needs and provide not just a correction but a tailored solution, discreetly and effectively. Continue to monitor the participant until the movement is accomplished correctly.

- Emphasize body awareness skills. Regularly remind clients that we all have different body sizes, leg lengths, and health and fitness levels, and we all have different amounts of energy on different days. Emphasize that listening to your body is an important exercise skill.

- Encourage clients to take active rest periods and to adjust their pace to accommodate fluctuations in health and energy levels. For example, the following phrases are all empathetic, encouraging, commonsense reminders: "If it's one of those days when you're feeling a bit sluggish, even after the warm-up, then today isn't the day for an endurance challenge"; "Take it easy"; "Stay comfortable"; and "You can work harder next week."

- Encourage and motivate your participants by using specific praises and a gentle sense of humor.

Instructor checklists also work well to keep your teaching standards high. The instructional techniques checklist provided here includes a number of important questions you should ask yourself regularly:

- Am I working hard enough on my teaching technique?

- How is my teaching position? Am I moving around the room and demonstrating from different angles?

- Are my verbal cues effective? Are they precise, plentiful, accurate, and constantly reinforced?

- Am I using advanced cueing (visual and verbal) effectively?

- Am I constantly and consistently providing multilevel adaptations of the aerobic endurance exercises and then performing at the lower level myself?

- Am I really seeing what my clients are doing so that I can analyze their movements and provide tailored solutions for each individual? Am I communicating these effectively and positively?

- Am I educating my clients about the purpose and benefits of different exercises and refining their use of the Borg RPE scale?

- Am I relating my feedback to their day-to-day performance, progress, and personal goals? Do I notice and praise improvement?

- Am I reviewing the program regularly, seeing where change or progression is needed for individual clients, and setting new goals?

- Am I encouraging and implementing client feedback about the content of my sessions, the exercise environment, or my teaching?

- Am I encouraging good posture and technique (the participants' and my own) on a regular basis?

- Am I patient, polished in my teaching approach, and punctual, and do I look like I am having fun while teaching?

- Am I making time before and after each exercise session to answer clients' questions and socialize and to follow up on any absences?

Summary

Aerobic endurance training has a central role in maintaining health and function as we age, yet its' potential is often underestimated and underutilized. Even the oldest old can improve their $\dot{V}O_2$max, functional ability, and quality of life with aerobic endurance training. For optimal benefits, the aerobic exercise prescription for older adults must tailor exercises to suit individual needs. This is essential in older groups where there is a wider range of initial fitness levels, pathologies, disabilities, and preferences than in any other participant group.

For all ages, effective exercise prescription involves the skillful, mindful application of the exercise training principles (i.e., specificity, overload, functional relevance, challenge, and accommodation) and variables (i.e., frequency, intensity, time, and type). With older adults these must be applied according to the best practice guidelines for older adults. Older adults need multilevel, multiactivity, multipurpose aerobic endurance programs that use interval conditioning approaches to achieve life-related cardiorespiratory gains. Injury prevention should be your highest priority as an instructor. Structured, thoroughly adapted programs tailored for individuals and led by a knowledgeable, skilled, empathetic, motivating, and committed physical activity instructor can greatly minimize the risks for the older participant.

The ultimate challenge for a physical activity instructor of older adults is to follow the aerobic endurance guidelines discussed in this chapter while accommodating the heterogeneity of your clients. Your goal is to encourage long-term participation in aerobic endurance activities by ensuring that all the important exercise principles are applied while creating a training atmosphere that is safe, effective, purposeful, sociable, and fun. Adaptation and tailoring are key to safer, more effective, and more enjoyable aerobic endurance training for older adults.

Key Terms

active

Borg's rating of perceived exertion (RPE) scale

continuous training

disease prevention

disuse syndrome

fitness interval conditioning

functional ability

everyday function

health

heart rate reserve (HRR)

interval conditioning

interval training

maximal heart rate (HRmax)

muscle acidosis

performance interval conditioning

quality of life

spontaneous interval conditioning

symptom alleviation

total volume of work

Recommended Reading

Skelton, D.A. & Dinan, S.M. (2008). Ageing and older people. In J.P. Buckley (Ed.), *Exercise physiology in special populations: Advances in sport and exercise science* (pp. 161-223). Edinburgh, UK: Elsevier Books.

Study Questions

1. Which of the following statements is *not* true?

   a. Exercise intensity for older adults should be set at an RPE of 5 to 6 (CR10 scale) for moderate intensity.

   b. An RPE of 7 to 8 is appropriate for older adults engaged in vigorous intensity exercise.

   c. Frail older adults should start an aerobic training program at an exercise intensity set at an RPE of 2-3 (CR10 scale).

   d. Walking at a moderate RPE of 3-5 (CR10 scale) can elicit a beneficial physiological response for sedentary older adults.

2. Which of the following statements is true?

   a. For older people, interval conditioning is not effective for achieving the energy gains needed for everyday activities.

   b. Interval conditioning is inappropriate for older people.

   c. The three types of interval conditioning are spontaneous, fitness, and performance.

   d. Interval training and interval conditioning are equally appropriate for older participants.

3. Manipulating which variable appears to be most stressful for older adult exercisers?

   a. intensity

   b. duration

   c. frequency

   d. type

4. It is recommended that continuous aerobic training should be added to an older adult's aerobic training program after _____ weeks of interval conditioning.

   a. 12 to 16

   b. 8

   c. 4

   d. 4 to 8

5. Which of the following is not a recommended way to apply the principle of overload to aerobic endurance training?

   a. Increase only one element at a time.

   b. Increase duration before intensity.

   c. Increase intensity before duration.

   d. Allow a minimum of two weeks for adaptation before increasing the overload again.

6. Which exercise adaptation is not recommended?

   a. standardized, minimal, incremental progressions

   b. instructor demonstrates all levels and then selects the most challenging level

   c. alternatives for every exercise

   d. simpler, fewer moves

7. Which aerobic endurance exercise or movement is contraindicated for older adult exercisers?

   a. stepping

   b. hill walking

   c. exercises involving lateral movement of one leg across the other such as the grapevine

   d. turns of less than 90 degrees

Application Activities

1. An older adult client asks for your assistance to improve her stamina so that she can play tennis at a more competitive level. Describe the types of aerobic endurance activities you would include during her first four weeks in your physical activity program.

2. Design a 30-minute aerobic endurance component that is suitable for a group of older adults who are generally healthy and have been regular participants in your class for at least 16 weeks. List the specific activities you would include, identify exercises you would exclude, and describe any adaptations you might consider to accommodate the different functional needs of your clients. Practice teaching this component to a group of older adults, and solicit their feedback.

3. If you are currently teaching a physical activity class for older adults, have someone videotape your session so that you can evaluate your performance. On the teaching techniques checklist provided in this chapter, check off each question you were able to answer in the affirmative. Make note of the questions you did not check, and think of ways to improve these teaching techniques. Make an action plan to implement these improvements in your next few physical activity classes.

Balance and Mobility Training

Debra J. Rose

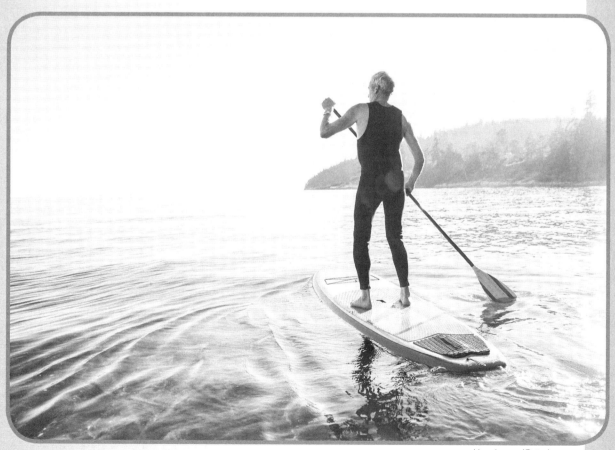

Objectives

After completing this chapter, you will be able to

1. describe how age-associated changes in multiple body systems affect balance and mobility,

2. identify the essential skills needed for good balance and mobility,

3. teach a set of progressive exercises that address each of the essential skills needed for good balance and mobility,

4. manipulate the level of challenge of balance exercises, and

5. organize the instructional setting to accommodate older adults with different levels of balance and mobility skills.

Good balance and mobility are essential to the successful performance of most activities of daily living as well as a number of recreational pursuits. According to the Centers for Disease Control and Prevention (CDC, 2016), "Every second of every day in the United States an older adult falls, making falls the number one cause of injuries and deaths from injury among older Americans." Falls are also costly for the health care system with an estimated $31 billion in annual Medicare costs being spent on fall-related injuries sustained by older Americans (29 million falls resulting in seven million injuries) in 2014. In light of these alarming statistics, it is critical that any exercise program designed for older adults include activities specifically designed to improve their balance and mobility.

As a result of age-associated declines in multiple physiological systems that lead to reduced muscle strength and flexibility, slower central processing of sensory information, and slowed motor responses, even a relatively mild fall could be potentially dangerous for an older adult (Panel on Prevention of Falls in Older Persons, American Geriatrics Society, and British Geriatrics Society, 2011). The good news is that activities to improve balance and mobility have become increasingly evident in physical activity classes designed for older adults. What is less evident, however, is whether the chosen activities adequately target the multiple dimensions of balance and mobility in a systematic and progressive manner. Unlike other parameters of fitness such as strength, flexibility, and aerobic endurance, it is often not until the first fall that older adults realize that their balance is significantly impaired.

Before describing the age-associated changes in balance and mobility, it is important to first define some terms in the context of this chapter. **Balance** can be defined as the process by which we control the body's **center of mass** (**COM;** i.e., the balance point or location about which all the segments of the body are evenly distributed) with respect to the base of support, whether it is stationary or moving (Rose, 2010). For example, when standing upright in space, our primary goal is to maintain the COM within the confines of the base of support. This aspect of balance is often referred to as **static balance**, even though the body is still moving. This movement is necessary to counteract the pull of the gravito-inertial environment in which we live. Conversely, when we are walking, the COM is continuously moved beyond the base of support and a new support base reestablished with each step taken. Maintaining balance while purposefully leaning or moving through space is often referred to as **dynamic balance**.

Another term used frequently throughout this chapter is **mobility**. This term describes our ability to independently and safely move from one place to another (Shumway-Cook & Woollacott, 2017). Adequate mobility is required for many different activities we perform during our daily lives, including transferring from the bed to a chair, climbing or descending stairs, walking or running, and a variety of sport and recreational activities.

The primary goals of this chapter are first to briefly describe the important age-associated changes in multiple body systems that affect balance and mobility and then to provide examples of the different types of balance activities that best address each of these age-related changes. The final section of the chapter presents instructional strategies for manipulating the challenge offered by a balance activity in a way that matches but does not exceed the intrinsic capabilities of the older adult client.

Age-Associated Changes in Balance and Mobility

Irrespective of how physically active we are throughout the course of our lives, certain inevitable age-associated changes occur in the multiple body systems (i.e., sensory, motor, and cognitive) that contribute to balance and mobility. While some of these changes have no observable effect on how well certain balance- and mobility-related tasks are performed in different environments, other changes adversely affect dimensions of balance and mobility. For example, changes that affect multiple systems

simultaneously (e.g., sensory, cognitive, and motor) or are compounded by existing medical conditions such as diabetes or arthritis can be expected to affect not only the strategy older adults use to perform a certain balance task but whether they choose to perform it at all.

Although a number of age-associated physiological changes are described in chapter 4, it is important that you understand how changes in the sensory, motor, and cognitive systems are likely to specifically affect the balance and mobility of your older adult clients. You will then be better able to decide which types of balance and mobility activities are most appropriate for your older adult clients. In general, age-associated changes in the peripheral and central components of the sensory and motor systems and changes in various cognitive functions (i.e., attention, memory, and executive processing), have all been shown to alter the quality and speed with which tasks are performed, even by healthy older adults. The peripheral and central components of the sensory and motor systems are illustrated in figure 14.1.

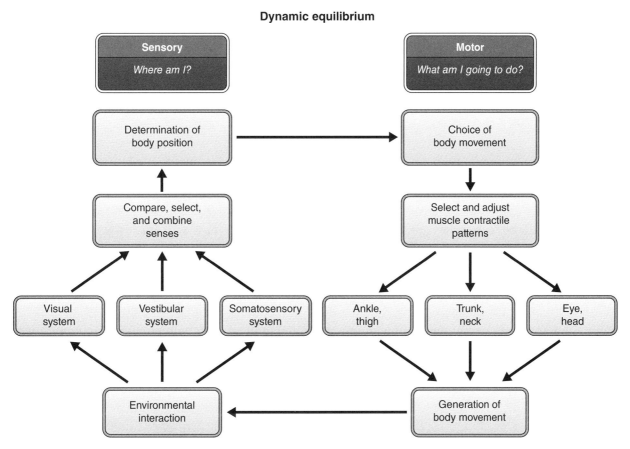

FIGURE 14.1 Dynamic equilibrium model.

Reprinted by permission from NeuroCom International Publications, 1990, "Illustration of Dynamic Equilibrium Model."

Sensory System Changes

The sensory systems that contribute to balance are the visual, somatosensory, vestibular, and auditory systems. Any changes in the peripheral or central components of each of these systems will affect balance and mobility to some degree. For example, the age-associated changes in the visual system that adversely affect an older adult's ability to perform a variety of balance and mobility activities include reduced visual acuity, narrowing of the field of vision, decreased depth perception, and loss of contrast sensitivity. Reduced visual acuity can also result from certain eye diseases, such as macular degeneration or cataracts. Any narrowing or blurring of the visual field makes it increasingly difficult to clearly discern the edges and shapes of objects in the environment. Any reduction in the peripheral visual field can also be expected to affect dynamic balance and mobility in particular because of the greater head and trunk rotation needed to see the missing information.

A decline in the ability to see depth affects an older adult's ability to safely negotiate obstacles, climb and descend stairs, and participate in sporting activities that require the accurate estimation of an object's position in space (e.g., tennis, golf, softball, or baseball). Changes in contrast sensitivity make it more difficult to detect objects against a background or rapidly adjust to changes in lighting when moving from a brightly lit room into a dark corridor.

Age-associated changes in the somatosensory (i.e., touch and proprioception) system have a direct impact on postural stability and the ability to quickly restore upright control after an unexpected loss of balance (Ribeiro & Oliveira, 2007). In addition, age-associated changes in **kinesthetic sensibility** (i.e., the conscious awareness of limb position and movement) also affect an older adult's ability to perform certain balance activities, particularly when vision is not available or is distorted (e.g., in busy or moving visual environments). A decline in the number of **cutaneous receptors** in the skin that detect pressure and vibratory sensations (i.e., Pacinian corpuscles) also affects both the speed and efficiency of different types of postural responses and is cited as an important contributor to balance problems among older adults (Perry, 2006). In addition to receptor loss, a decline of as much as 30

percent in the number of sensory fibers innervating the peripheral receptors has been observed with increasing age (Shaffer & Harrison, 2007). These changes result in reduced somatosensation and greater reliance on the visual and vestibular systems for sensory information.

Age-associated reductions in the density of vestibular hair and nerve cells and a moderate reduction in the gain of the **vestibular-ocular reflex (VOR)** in the inner ear or vestibular system can also be expected to negatively affect postural control (Arshad & Seemungal, 2016). Because the VOR helps stabilize vision when the head is moved quickly, any reduction in the gain of this reflex affects older adults' ability to accurately determine whether it is the world or they who are moving in certain situations. In addition to assisting with the correct positioning of the head and body with respect to gravity, the vestibular system becomes critical for balance when sensory information is not available from one or both of the other two sensory systems or when the information being provided by one or both of the other systems is not congruent (not in agreement) with the information coming from the vestibular system. This is called **sensory conflict** and can lead to a momentary loss of balance or even a fall in some cases. We often experience moments of sensory conflict during our daily lives when an object, usually moving through the peripheral visual field, leads us to believe that we are moving instead of the object. Sitting in a car at a traffic light and suddenly thinking that our car is rolling when it is the car next to us that is moving is an example of this type of sensory conflict.

Finally, increasing research evidence shows that age-associated changes in the auditory system can also affect balance and gait speed (Li, Simonsick, Ferucci, & Lin, 2013; Lin & Ferucci, 2012). Even a mild degree of hearing loss (i.e., 10 decibels) has been shown to increase the risk of falling in older adults 65 years and older by as much as 40 percent. Significant reductions in gait speed (i.e., −0.05 m/sec per 25 dB of hearing loss) have also been associated with hearing loss in older adults. While no definitive explanation has yet been advanced to explain this relationship, researchers have suggested that the heightened fall risk might be due to the fact that older adults with hearing loss are less aware of events occurring in the environment around them. Others theorize that older adults experience increased cognitive load as a result of their hearing loss. Simply stated, as a result of having to compensate for hearing loss, the older adult expends more cognitive energy on analyzing the environment and may not be able to allocate enough cognitive resources to maintaining balance or gait speed. Because the auditory and vestibular systems are also closely connected to each other anatomically, any dysfunction occurring concurrently in the cochlear or vestibular sense organs may also adversely affect balance and gait.

Collectively, changes in one or more of these sensory systems result in slower processing and integration of sensory inputs and an inability to control the level of body sway when the amount of available sensory information is reduced. Among healthy older adults, the amount of body sway is most affected when somatosensory and visual inputs are distorted or absent (Shumway-Cook & Woollacott, 2017). The encouraging news is that the sensory systems are very adaptable, and if older adults are presented with progressively more challenging physical activities and greater exposure to these types of altered sensory conditions, they can learn to adapt their postural responses appropriately (Hu & Woollacott, 1994; O'Connor, Loughlin, Redfern, & Sparto, 2008). In the case of audition, the gradual introduction of amplification devices (e.g., hearing aids) may also benefit balance and mobility in numerous ways.

One example of an appropriate activity is to have an older adult practice standing on an altered surface (e.g., foam pad, foam roller) with the eyes closed or while reading a poem. Standing on an altered surface makes it more difficult to use somatosensory inputs, while engaging vision in the performance of a second task or removing it altogether effectively negates its use for maintaining upright balance. Additional balance and mobility activities that are designed to systematically manipulate the sensory systems are presented in a later section of this chapter.

> Older adults can improve their ability to balance and move in altered sensory environments because the sensory systems are very adaptable, or amenable, to change.

Motor System Changes

An increase in the time required to plan and then execute an appropriate motor response appears to be the greatest consequence of the age-associated changes in the motor system (Spirduso, MacRae, & Francis, 2005; Stöckel, Wunsch, & Hughes, 2017). Stöckel et al. (2017) found that age-related declines were even more apparent for fine motor dexterity, processing speed, and cognitive flexibility. Many older adults also begin to experience difficulty selecting the appropriate movement strategy to use in a given movement situation. Inappropriate **scaling** (i.e., adjustment of movement parameters, such as force, to match the action plan to the demands of the task or environment) of the selected response strategy is also evident in many cases. That is, older adults exhibit a tendency to over- or underrespond, particularly when their balance is unexpectedly perturbed or disrupted (Mille, Johnson, Martinez, & Rogers, 2005; Shumway-Cook & Woollacott, 2017).

Electromyographic (EMG) studies have further shown significant age-related differences in the temporal sequencing and magnitude of muscle activation patterns in response to unexpected losses of balance. Unlike the stereotypical and symmetrical patterns of muscle activation observed in younger adults, apparently healthy older adults exhibit considerably more variable activation patterns and a decline in their ability to inhibit inappropriate responses (Shumway-Cook & Woollacott, 2017). Inappropriate postural responses are most evident when the functional base of support is reduced (e.g., standing sideways on a narrow beam), when the support surface is compliant or unstable (e.g., standing on a foam surface or rocker board), or when visual input is altered (e.g., visual environment moves so that vision no longer provides accurate information for balance; Alexander, 1994). Real-world equivalents of these experimental conditions include putting on a pair of trousers while standing on one leg (reduced base of support), walking across a grassy or slippery surface (standing on foam or a rocker board), or walking along a busy city street (moving visual environment).

Age-associated changes in the anticipatory component of **adaptive postural control** have also been documented (Kanekar & Aruin, 2014) and these changes may be important contributors to falls among older adults. Adaptive postural control describes our ability to modify the sensory and motor systems in response to changing task and environmental demands (Shumway-Cook & Woollacott, 2017). This type of control can be anticipatory (e.g., changing from one type of surface to another in good lighting, carrying objects while walking) or reactive (e.g., tripping over an undetected obstacle, being bumped in a crowd).

The research findings suggest that older adults become increasingly less able to activate the postural muscles required to stabilize the body before the muscles responsible for executing the movement are activated (e.g., activating the stabilizing muscle groups in the trunk and lower legs before pulling on the handle of a door). The reactive component of adaptive postural control is also affected with age (Maki & McIlroy, 2006). Specifically, healthy older adults are slower to execute a stepping response after an unpredictable loss of balance, even though their reaction to the loss of balance is not appreciably longer than that of young adults (Thelen, Wojcik, Schultz, Ashton-Miller, & Alexander, 1997).

Other researchers have also demonstrated that healthy older adults are more likely to take multiple steps following a perturbation (Maki & McIlroy, 2006; Mille et al., 2013). Coupled with the decline in absolute muscle strength and power described in chapter 4, these changes in the central and peripheral components of the motor system compromise an older adult's ability to make anticipatory and reactive postural adjustments quickly and efficiently. As is the case with the sensory systems, however, physical activities designed to challenge the motor system can significantly improve an older adult's ability to respond more quickly and appropriately when balance is compromised (Dijkstra, Horak, Kamsma, & Peterson, 2015; McCrum, Gerards, Karamanidis, Zijlstra, & Meijer, 2017).

Changes in Cognition

One of the most noticeable cognitive changes observed with aging is an inability to perform multiple tasks simultaneously without compromising postural stability (Shumway-Cook & Woollacott, 2017). Recovering balance after an unexpected perturbation also requires more attention for older adults than for young adults (Melzer, Liebermann, Krasovsky, & Oddsson, 2010). These research findings suggest that older adults can find it particularly

challenging to perform multiple tasks at once, especially if one of those tasks involves the maintenance of postural stability. This knowledge is important for selecting balance exercises that require attention to be distributed across multiple tasks or that involve a high cognitive component.

> Older adults find it particularly challenging to perform multiple tasks at once because of age-associated changes in attention.

Balance and Mobility Exercises

A wide variety of balance and mobility activities should be considered an essential component of any well-rounded physical activity program. At least 10 to 15 minutes during every class or personal training session should be allocated to balance and mobility activities. Balance and mobility activities can also be incorporated into the warm-up and cool-down sections (see chapter 10) in addition to the core component of the class. Another way for more advanced clients to incorporate balance activities is to perform selected strength and flexibility exercises in a balance-challenging environment. For example, clients can perform certain upper-body strength and flexibility exercises while sitting on a balance ball or standing on a foam pad. Remember that your primary goal when presenting balance and mobility activities to your older adult clients is to challenge but not exceed their intrinsic capabilities by systematically introducing increasingly complex balance and mobility tasks that can be performed in a variety of practice environments that simulate those encountered in daily life. A simple model of the factors that interact to affect mobility and balance is illustrated in figure 14.2.

You should vary either the task or environmental demands in a way that matches your client's individual capabilities. An additional guiding principle should be applied to decide which of the two variables to manipulate and when: determining whether the goal is to improve the motor system or to improve the sensory systems.

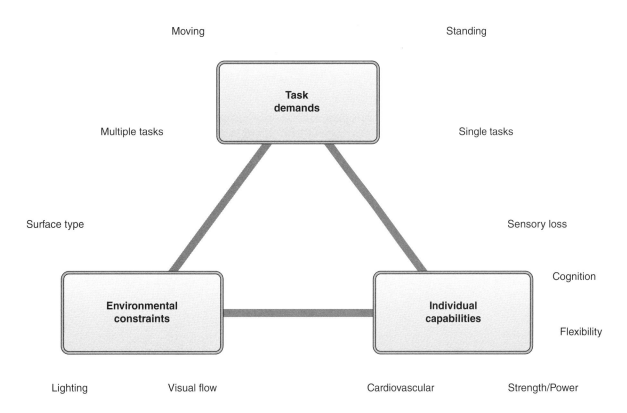

Moving

Standing

Multiple tasks

Single tasks

Surface type

Sensory loss

Cognition

Flexibility

Lighting

Visual flow

Cardiovascular

Strength/Power

FIGURE 14.2 Balance and mobility training triad. Systematically manipulate the task or environmental demands of a balance activity to challenge but not exceed the individual capabilities of your clients.

Reprinted by permission from D.J. Rose, "Promoting Functional Independence in Older Adults at Risk for Falls: The Need for a Multidimensional Programming Approach," *Journal of Aging and Physical Activity* 10, no. 2 (2002): 207-225.

If the goal is to tune up the motor system, it is most appropriate to alter the task demands of a particular balance and mobility activity. One easy way to manipulate the task demand is to perform a balance activity while standing or moving through space rather than sitting on a stability ball.

If the goal is to tune up each of the sensory systems that contribute to good balance and mobility, then your goal should be to manipulate the environment in which the task is performed. Our sensory systems are most receptive to changes in the environment. This manipulation can be done by having the client perform balance activities with reduced or no vision or while standing on a compliant or moving surface. Additional ways to manipulate the task or environmental demands and thereby alter the challenge of a particular balance or mobility activity are presented in table 14.1.

Four skills considered essential to good balance and mobility should be the focus of your efforts in this component of the program. These skills are (a) the voluntary and involuntary control of the center of mass (COM), (b) sensory integration and organization, (c) selection and scaling of postural strategies, and (d) development of a flexible and adaptable gait pattern. Let us now consider the types of balance and mobility activities you can use to train each of these skills and how you can manipulate the practice environment or demands of the task for systematic progression.

Voluntary and Involuntary Control of the Center of Mass

The balance and mobility activities presented here are designed to improve the ability to maintain a more upright and steady position in space (static balance) or to move the body through space with greater control, speed, and confidence (dynamic balance). In addition, these exercises are also designed to improve adaptive postural control abilities (anticipatory and reactive) through manipulation of the task and environmental demands. Calling these the "belly button control" exercises readily conjures up an image in clients' minds of the body part that must be manipulated to maintain postural control. A few examples of seated, standing, and moving activities suitable for this type of balance training are shown in the sidebar. Many more balance and mobility activities appropriate for training each of the four essential skills at multiple functional levels are presented in *FallProof! A Comprehensive Balance and Mobility Training Program* (Rose, 2010).

Involuntary control of the COM can also be practiced in a seated, standing, or moving environment. While the client is standing or seated on a ball, either you or a trusted assistant can deliver small, quick perturbations (pushes or pulls) to the individual. These can be applied at the level of the hips, shoulders, or hips and shoulders simultaneously to prompt a small amount of trunk rotation during the perturbation. Quickly pushing the ball on which the client is seated is also an effective method of causing

Table 14.1   Manipulating Task and Environmental Demands

	Easy	More difficult	Most difficult
Task demand			
Arm position	In contact with seat surface	Resting on thigh	Folded across chest
Base of support	Feet together	Feet in tandem stance	Single-leg stance
Pacing of exercise	Self-paced (own speed)		Externally paced
Length of movement sequence	Single activity	3-4 sequential movements	6-8 sequential movements
Additional task	Cognitive (e.g., counting backward)	Self-paced manual task (e.g., reaching)	Externally paced manual task (e.g., catching)
Environmental demand			
Lighting	Dim room lights	Dark glasses	Closed eyes
Support surface (seated)	Balance disk on chair	Stability ball (with holder)	Stability ball (no holder)
Support surface (standing)	Thin foam (0.25 in., 0.6 cm)	Dense foam (2-4 in., 5-10 cm)	Balance disk(s)

Balance challenge can be further increased by combining two or more task or environmental demands.

Seated, Standing, and Moving Balance Activities

Seated Balance Activities (With Eyes Open and Closed)

Equipment needed: Chair with or without backrest and arms, balance disks, stability balls

1. Sitting upright in space, first with eyes focused on a target and then with eyes closed, visualizing same target

2. Voluntary arm movements through space (single arm or both arms moving horizontally, vertically, and diagonally)

3. Voluntary trunk movements through space (leaning forward, backward, and diagonally from hips, rotating trunk to right and left)

4. Voluntary leg movements (heel and toe raises, marching, single-leg raises)

5. Dynamic weight shifts through space (shifting COM away from and back to midline in multiple directions, shifting to multiple positions in space without pausing at midline)

6. Dynamic body movements against gravity (bouncing up and down, front to back, and side to side)

7. Perturbations (push or pull at hips or at hips and shoulders) applied with varying force, with altered support surface to increase balance challenge

Standing Balance Activities

Equipment needed: Foam pads of different thicknesses, balls, benches of different heights, colored spots

1. Standing upright with changing base of support (feet together, tandem stance, single-leg stance), first with eyes open then with eyes closed

2. Dynamic weight shifts through space (leaning away from midline in multiple directions; shifting weight from side to side, forward and back, and diagonally)

3. Dynamic weight transfers through space (marching in place and while turning the head or body, forward and backward stepping, lunging in multiple directions, stepping up onto and off benches of different heights)

4. Kicking stationary and moving balls toward a target

5. Perturbations (push or pull at hips or at hips and shoulders) applied with varying force, with altered support surface to increase balance challenge

Moving Balance Activities

Equipment needed: Masking tape, colored spots, balance disks, small objects, various pieces of equipment to create obstacle courses, resistance bands

1. Walking with altered base of support: Tandem walking on a line or narrow beam, toe walking, heel walking

2. "Crossing the river." Lunge across an area marked by two lines that are spaced increasingly farther apart, then return to starting position. Alternatively, attempt to step or jump across area.

3. "Rock hopping." Place colored spots at different distances apart within same area as in previous activity. Each client moves "down the creek" stepping only on spots. To increase challenge, (a) replace spots with balance disks for more instability, or (b) place small objects on floor within the area that clients must retrieve as they progress along the creek.

4. Navigating obstacles. Design obstacle courses that require participants to control the COM during static activities (e.g., stepping up onto foam and standing with feet together for 10 seconds before moving to next obstacle) and dynamic activities (e.g., do tandem walking on a narrow beam in the obstacle course). To increase the balance challenge, you can place objects on the floor or at other levels that clients must place in a basket that they carry through the course.

5. Resistance-band walking. While client walks, partner or instructor increases and releases tension on a band wrapped around the hips.

a perturbation. To force clients to involuntarily or reactively control the COM, it is important that they be unaware that the perturbation is about to occur. Applying different amounts of force to the body or ball also keeps the client guessing.

Resistance bands can also be used to perturb balance in a moving environment. As the client attempts to walk around the room, the instructor first applies tension to a resistance band that is wrapped around the client's waist and then unexpectedly releases the tension, forcing the client to make a rapid postural adjustment. Because these activities pose a great challenge to older adults' balance abilities, it is very important to pay careful attention to creating a safe practice environment. Spotting less balanced clients during each activity and positioning clients close to a wall or sturdy chair for additional support are effective ways to promote safety.

Be sure to observe how quickly and efficiently participants are able to respond to unexpected perturbations. Individuals with good reactive balance control will respond quickly to an unexpected loss of balance and in a direction that is opposite to the direction of the push or pull. Unfortunately, this type of activity can be performed only once or twice before the client begins to change his or her postural set to one that is prepared for the perturbation. Once this happens, your participants are now demonstrating their ability to anticipate rather than to react to an unexpected perturbation. While this is also an important aspect of balance to practice, recognize that their postural control has shifted from reactive to anticipatory. Teaching your class participants how to respond to an unexpected or even an expected perturbation better prepares them for opening doors, being jostled in crowds, or tripping on uneven sidewalks.

Sensory Integration and Organization Activities

The instructional ideas presented in this section are designed to optimize the use of each of the three sensory systems that contribute most to balance (research is limited regarding the auditory system, so it is not included in this section). If there is no indication in the client's medical history of any impairments in the sensory system that you want to challenge, then the primary goal for this set of balance activities is to construct a practice environment that encourages the older adult to use one particular sensory system more than another to maintain balance. Medical conditions that indicate impairment in a specific sensory system include macular degeneration and cataracts (visual system), peripheral sensory neuropathy (somatosensory system), and Ménière's disease (vestibular system). If there is evidence of impairment in a particular sensory system, your goal is helping the client to compensate for that loss.

For example, eye diseases such as macular degeneration or glaucoma seriously impair an older adult's use of vision to control balance. In this case, your goal would be to help the client learn how to better use somatosensory and vestibular inputs to compensate for the losses in the visual system. As another example, if an older adult client has a history of diabetes that has adversely affected his or her ability to sense touch and pressure beneath the feet (i.e., peripheral neuropathy), you would have that client practice balance activities to learn how to better use the unimpaired visual and vestibular systems.

When working on improving your older adult clients' sensory organization and integration skills, you should follow the second guiding principle presented earlier in the chapter: manipulate the environment rather than the task demands initially. Most of the balance activities presented in the sidebar "Seated, Standing, and Moving Balance Activities" can be used to improve your clients' sensory organization and integration skills.

In addition to reviewing each client's health and activity questionnaire and the results of any balance testing you conducted at the outset of the program (see chapter 6 for a discussion of appropriate balance tests), you are well advised to observe your clients' behavior while they stand on a firm surface with their eyes closed and then on a foam surface with eyes open and closed. Of course, if the functional level of your clients made it possible for you to administer the Fullerton Advanced Balance Scale described in chapter 6, you will already have a good idea of their performance in each of these different sensory conditions. Being able to stand steady on a firm surface with the eyes closed requires good use of somatosensory inputs, while standing on foam with eyes open and then closed requires the effective use of vision when the eyes are open and the vestibular system when the eyes are closed. If any of your clients perform any of these activities poorly, you should make sure that they begin multisensory activities in a seated position or with additional manual support (assistant, wall, or sturdy chair).

Somatosensory System Activities

If your goal is to increase clients' reliance on somatosensory inputs for controlling balance, you should have them practice progressive balance activities both on a firm, broad surface *and* with reduced or absent vision. These exercises can be performed while seated, standing, or moving, depending on each individual's intrinsic capabilities. While some clients find it challenging enough to perform certain seated exercises with vision reduced (e.g., wearing sunglasses), others have no difficulty performing standing or moving balance activities with their eyes closed. The important thing is that the surface be firm so that they can derive as much sensory information from the surface as possible. Teaching clients to better use the somatosensory system for controlling balance can measurably increase their safety when performing activities in dark or poorly lit environments (e.g., going to the bathroom in the middle of the night, entering movie theaters after the lights have been lowered, walking outside at night).

Visual System Activities

Although it is a commonly held belief that adults rely on vision more than any other sensory system, many older adults do not use it very efficiently for controlling their balance and mobility. To help your older adult clients better use vision for balance, it is important to teach them how to fixate their eyes on specific targets in space. While they are performing a balance activity in a seated or standing position, they should be verbally cued to fixate on a target directly in front of them and at eye level. A vertical target, such as a door jam or line on the wall, is a particularly good target to choose.

In addition to actively coaching older adults to fixate on a target, it is also important to alter the surface under the feet to distort the information provided to the somatosensory system (see figure 14.3). Have clients perform balance activities while seated with their feet on a compliant or moving surface (rocker board, balance disk) or while standing on the same types of surfaces. Begin to increase the balance challenge by introducing head movements

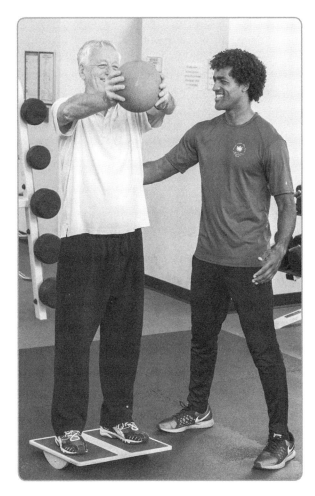

FIGURE 14.3 Performing balance activities while standing on a moving surface increases both the task and environmental demands.

to a particular balance activity. It is still important to verbally cue clients to fixate their gaze, but now they must fixate for a shorter period of time as the head or body turns during an activity. Using vision more effectively helps older adults perform a number of daily activities with greater efficiency. Examples include walking with greater confidence and stability when they are out in the community, maintaining their balance more effectively when the head or body is turned to greet a friend, or watching for approaching cars as they cross a two-way street.

Vestibular System Activities

The third sensory system important for balance is the vestibular system. Unfortunately, many older adults experience balance problems that are related to changes in this system. These changes are caused not only by advancing age or the medical conditions described earlier but also by the tendency for older adults to engage less frequently in physical activities that require high-velocity head movements (e.g., spinning, jumping, certain sports) as they grow older. This reduced head movement likely compounds the age-associated changes in the peripheral and central components of the vestibular system.

To tune up the vestibular system, it is necessary to practice activities that make it difficult to get the information needed for balance from either the visual or somatosensory systems. Have your older adult clients perform various balance activities while their feet are in contact with a compliant or moving surface (foam, rocker board) and their eyes are either closed or involved in a second, non-balance-related task (e.g., reading aloud, tossing and catching objects). Because it is now difficult to use two of the three sensory systems for balance, you will observe higher levels of sway during these activities. It is therefore important both to know your clients' abilities before they try any of these more challenging activities and to provide a safe practice environment in which to perform them. Start with less-challenging seated activities, or position clients close to a wall or behind a chair for additional support when performing standing exercises.

Improved use of the vestibular system positively affects the performance of a number of daily activities, including walking on uneven surfaces at night, maintaining balance when the head is tilted back in the shower, and maintaining balance when turning the head quickly. In some cases, repeating vestibular system activities can result in less susceptibility to dizziness during activities that require fast head or body turns.

Each of the three sensory systems can be improved by manipulating the environmental demands associated with a balance activity. Ways to do this are summarized in table 14.2. Because several of the activities described may be challenging for older adults who have medical conditions that affect one or more sensory systems (e.g., macular degeneration, diabetes, Ménière's disease), extra safety precautions are needed to ensure the safety of your clients. In this section of your balance and mobility component, it is particularly important to apply the principles of challenge and adaptation/ tailoring discussed in chapter 8.

Selecting and Scaling Postural Strategies

At least three clearly defined postural strategies have been described in the research literature (Rose, 2010). These are referred to as the ankle, hip, and step strategies and are used either to control sway in a forward and backward direction or to reestablish a new base of support when the limits of stability have been exceeded (see figure 14.4). These postural strategies are used individually and in combination to help maintain or control balance while performing a variety of tasks. For example, the ankle strategy controls sway while standing, the hip strategy is used to maintain balance when leaning into a cupboard or dishwasher to retrieve an item, and the step strategy reestablishes a new base of support after tripping over a pet or a child's toy.

Manipulating either the task or the environment in at least four different ways enables your older adult clients to practice each of these strategies: (a) maintaining balance while standing on different support surfaces (e.g., firm, compliant, moving, narrow), (b) voluntarily swaying farther away from midline in different directions and while standing on different support surfaces, (c) trying to minimize

Table 14.2   Environmental Manipulations for Sensory Systems

Sensory system	Environmental manipulation
Visual	Verbally encourage gaze fixation (i.e., keep eyes on a target at eye level); alter surface under buttocks and feet in seated activities and under feet during standing and moving activities
Somatosensory	Reduce or remove vision (e.g., dim the room lights, wear dark glasses, close eyes) or engage vision in a second task (e.g., read, reach for objects); perform all activities on a firm, broad support surface
Vestibular	Reduce or remove vision or engage vision in a second task (e.g., read, toss and catch objects); perform all activities on a compliant or moving support surface

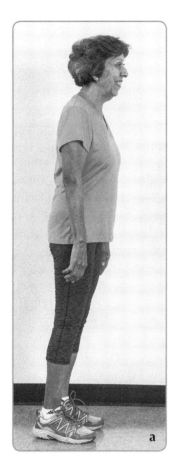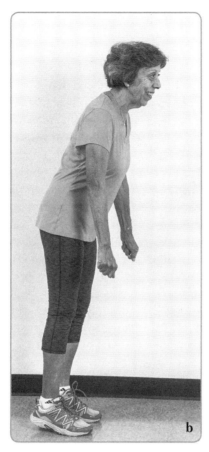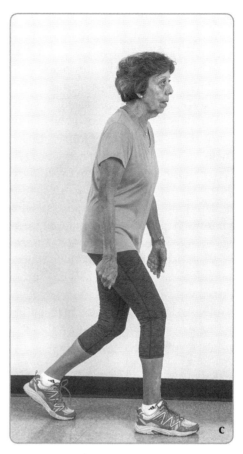

FIGURE 14.4   Three postural strategies have been identified: *(a)* ankle, *(b)* hip, and *(c)* step.

the amount of sway when the body is externally perturbed, and (d) making adjustments in body position in anticipation of a destabilizing limb movement (e.g., stepping over an obstacle).

Ankle Strategy

Voluntarily swaying in a forward and backward direction is one way to practice the ankle strategy. To ensure that the ankle joints are controlling the sway, the speed of the sway must be slow and the distance leaned in either direction small. Check that the upper body and lower body are moving in the same direction during this activity and that the heels do not lift off the floor. This is a nice activity to include in a cool-down segment. It is also an excellent means of reinforcing somatosensation or kinesthetic sensibility by verbally cuing clients to focus on the changing pressure under the feet as they sway forward and backward. Chairs can be placed in front of and behind the client so that he or she can focus on touching the chair in front with the hips on the forward lean and the chair behind with

the buttocks on the backward lean. This reinforces moving the upper body and lower body together during the activity. Place the chairs close enough to ensure the client can accomplish this movement.

This activity can be combined with another one called the "honey pot." Clients are asked to imagine that their bodies are stirring sticks and their job is to stir the honey forward and backward, side to side, and then in a circular motion, first clockwise and then counterclockwise. The application of small, unexpected perturbations (pushing or pulling action) at the level of the hips is another way to practice using the ankle strategy more subconsciously. A person with good balance can respond to the perturbation with a quick countermovement initiated at the ankles.

Hip Strategy

The hip strategy can be practiced by simply swaying in a forward and backward direction at a faster speed and over a larger distance than for the ankle strategy. Manipulating the task demands in this way necessitates the use of the larger hip muscles to control the sway. Unlike the coupled movement of the upper body and lower body that characterizes a movement controlled by the ankles, the upper body and lower body become uncoupled during the hip strategy and move in opposite directions: The upper body moves forward as the lower body moves backward. This is an excellent follow-up activity to the ankle strategy activity just described. You can clap your hands or use a metronome to pace the sway.

You can also force a more subconscious use of the hip strategy by having clients stand sideways on a narrow beam or on top of a half foam roller (see figure 14.5). Because the support surface is now narrower than the length of the feet, it becomes more difficult to use the ankle strategy to control sway. You can elicit the use of a hip strategy in your more stable clients by having them reach for an object held at various distances at or above eye level. A progressively larger perturbation at the hips also forces the client to counter the loss of balance using the hip rather than ankle muscles.

Step Strategy

Finally, activities that force your clients to exceed their **limits of stability** (i.e., the maximum distance a person can lean away from a centered position in any direction without moving the feet) require the use of the important step strategy to prevent falls. Simply increasing the challenge of balance activities performed on different surface types is usually sufficient to stimulate the use of this strategy. You can also apply progressively larger external perturbations at the hips to force a step.

No matter which postural strategy your clients practice in a session, carefully observe whether they select the appropriate strategy and scale it appropriately for the task demands. For example, watch to see if a client begins to use a hip strategy even when swaying at a slow speed over a small distance.

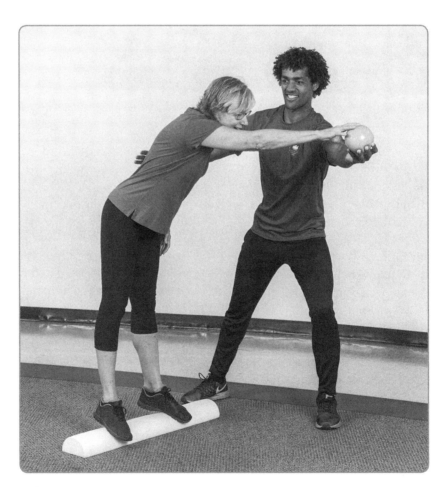

FIGURE 14.5   Reaching for objects while standing on top of a half foam roller encourages the use of a hip strategy to control balance.

Watch also to see if the size and type of postural response match the amount of force you applied in an external perturbation. Many older adults, even healthy ones, often choose to take multiple steps in response to a perturbation, even though the force applied could have been managed using a hip or ankle strategy.

With sufficient practice and increased confidence in their balance abilities, your older adult clients likely will require fewer steps to restore balance or will resort to a step strategy less often. Given that very few older adults voluntarily practice losing their balance on a daily basis, it will likely take some time for them to reacquire an efficient step strategy. The more often you present activities that require them to lose their balance, the more quickly they are likely to learn how to restore it. Just be sure to provide a safe and confidence-building practice environment, and do not increase the difficulty of balance activities too quickly. A summary of how to manipulate the task or environmental demands to elicit each of the movement strategies described is provided in table 14.3.

Gait Pattern Activities

Perhaps the best way to help your older adult clients achieve a flexible and adaptable gait pattern and also improve their overall coordination and agility is through activities that require them to walk at different speeds using a variety of different gait patterns. For example, have them walk around the room on their toes or on their heels; have them walk using a sidestep, braid, or a longer and wider than normal stride; or have them stop quickly or change directions on command or even walk backward. You can use the music tempo very effectively here to set different gait speeds, and pause it periodically to see how quickly the clients stop walking. These are wonderful activities for the warm-up routine, and if they are performed long enough, they can also improve aerobic endurance.

Manipulating the Challenge in a Group Setting

By carefully manipulating the balance challenge for each client during the balance and mobility component of the program, you can have a group of older adult clients perform the same balance activities at the level that best matches their individual abilities. For example, a group can perform the same set of seated weight-shift activities but at different levels of task difficulty; simply manipulate the task or environmental demands appropriately for each individual. For example, to make it easier for some clients to perform seated dynamic weight shifts, they can perform the activity while sitting on a balance disk placed on a chair and holding on to the chair (a stable support surface). At the same time, more advanced clients can perform their set of dynamic weight shifts while sitting on a stability ball with arms folded across the chest. This illustrates applying the exercise principle of challenge by matching the task demands to the individual's current capabilities (see figure 14.6). You can also

Table 14.3 Manipulations to Elicit the Ankle, Hip, or Step Strategy

Strategy	Manipulation of task or environment
Ankle	Forward-backward sway over short distance at slow speed (voluntary control)
	Small external perturbations (involuntary control)
Hip	Forward-backward sway over large distance at fast speed (voluntary control)
	Standing sideways on narrow beam or half foam roller
	Forward reaching if standing position is stable (voluntary control)
	Medium-sized external perturbations (involuntary)
Step	Leaning forward, backward, or to the side until limits of stability are exceeded (voluntary control)
	Large external perturbations in standing position (involuntary control)
	Walking against resistance band that is unexpectedly released (involuntary control)

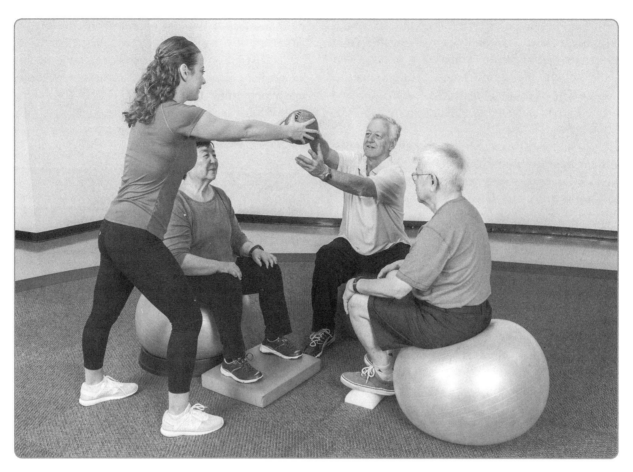

FIGURE 14.6 Different levels of challenge can be achieved in a group setting by having clients sit on different support surfaces.

manipulate the challenge of this group activity by manipulating the environmental demands of the activity. Some clients in the group may only be ready to perform the dynamic weight shifts with their eyes open and feet in a wide base of support on a firm surface, while others may be able to do the same activities with their eyes closed and their feet in a narrow base of support or with foam under their feet. Through careful manipulation of the task and environmental demands, you can accommodate many different functional levels of most of the activities in the balance and mobility component of the program.

Summary

Given that balance abilities are critical to safe mobility and the prevention of falls, it is essential that specific activities targeting the multiple dimensions

of balance and mobility be an integral component of a well-rounded physical activity program. These activities should address four essential skills needed for good balance and mobility: the voluntary and involuntary control of the center of mass, sensory integration and organization, selection and scaling of postural strategies, and development of a flexible and adaptable gait pattern. Two guiding principles for the effective implementation of activities designed to improve each of these essential skills were presented in this chapter: To tune up the motor system, alter the task demands, and to tune up the sensory systems, alter environmental demands. By progressively increasing the balance challenge for each essential skill by adding non-balance-related tasks (e.g., counting backward, reading aloud, catching objects), the cognitive contributions to balance (i.e., attention, memory, and executive control) are also enhanced.

The aim of this chapter was to expand your

knowledge about balance and mobility and provide you with a good rationale for choosing balance activities for an exercise program for older adults. Of course, to become really proficient in this specific area of exercise programming requires more specialized knowledge and practical training. Reviewing the recommended readings and completing additional training to become a certified balance and mobility specialist can help you obtain this additional expertise.

Key Terms

adaptive postural control

balance

center of mass (COM)

cutaneous receptors

dynamic balance

kinesthetic sensibility

limits of stability

mobility

scaling

sensory conflict

static balance

vestibular-ocular reflex (VOR)

Recommended Readings

Rose, D.J. (2010). *FallProof! A comprehensive balance and mobility training program (2nd ed.)*. Champaign, IL: Human Kinetics.

Sherrington, C., Michalef, Z.A., Fairhall, N., Paul, S.S., Tiedemann, A., Whitney, J., . . . Lord, S.R. (2017). Exercise to prevent falls in older adults: An updated systematic review and meta-analysis. *British Journal of Sports Medicine, 24,* 1750-1758.

Study Questions

1. In which of the following situations is adaptive postural control most likely to be needed?

   a. during an unexpected loss of balance

   b. when changing from a nonslippery to an icy surface

   c. when carrying a load of laundry up a flight of stairs

   d. b and c

2. The combined role of the sensory systems is to

   a. determine the visual layout of the environment

   b. assist in the planning of actions

   c. create sensory conflict that must be resolved by the CNS

   d. determine where our body is in space

3. Sensory conflict occurs when

   a. the sensory information provided by one or more of the three sensory systems is not congruent

   b. the sensory systems become overloaded with sensory inputs

   c. the vestibular system provides inaccurate information

   d. vision has been reduced or removed

4. Healthy older adults tend to sway most when
   a. vision is reduced or absent
   b. vestibular information is distorted
   c. somatosensory inputs are distorted
   d. vision is not available and somatosensory inputs are distorted

5. If your goal is to improve the motor system's contribution to balance and mobility, which of the following variables should you manipulate first?
   a. environmental demands
   b. task demands
   c. the individual's capabilities
   d. a and b

6. Which of the following is *not* an example of manipulating a task demand?
   a. altering the position of the arms during an exercise
   b. reducing the base of support
   c. adding a second non-balance-related task
   d. altering the support surface

7. To improve the use of the somatosensory system for balance, you should
   a. remove vision and alter the support surface
   b. alter the support surface only
   c. remove vision and distort vestibular inputs
   d. reduce or remove vision only

8. Which of the following activities will encourage the older adult to use a hip strategy to control balance?
   a. reaching for objects while standing sideways on a narrow balance beam
   b. a perturbation of large intensity
   c. swaying forward and back over a large distance at a fast speed
   d. a and c

Application Activities

1. Describe *one set of progressive* balance activities you would use to improve the use of the (a) somatosensory system, (b) visual system, and (c) vestibular system. Develop a seated, standing, and moving version of each activity.

2. Design a four-week balance and mobility program component for a class of community-residing older adults. Describe how you would manipulate the challenge of each exercise to accommodate the different functional levels of your clients.

PART

IV

Program Design, Leadership, and Risk Management

Training Module 1:
Overview of Aging and Physical Activity

Training Module 9:
Ethics and Professional Conduct

Training Module 2:
Psychological, Sociocultural, and Physiological Aspects of Physical Activity and Older Adults

Training Module 8:
Client Safety and First Aid

International Curriculum Guidelines for Preparing Physical Activity Instructors of Older Adults

Training Module 3:
Screening, Assessment, and Goal Setting

Training Module 7:
Leadership, Communication, and Marketing Skills

Training Module 4:
Program Design and Management

Training Module 6:
Teaching Skills

Training Module 5:
Program Design for Older Adults With Stable Medical Conditions

The final section of the book provides you with additional knowledge and skills needed to become an effective instructor of physical activity programs for older adults. The four remaining chapters focus on understanding motor learning principles and the skills for teaching and leadership, knowing how to develop a risk management plan, and understanding the legal standards and professional ethics of this field. Chapter 15 addresses specific topics included in training modules 4 and 6 of the *International Curriculum Guidelines for Preparing Physical Activity Instructors of Older Adults*—applying movement analysis and motor learning principles to the selection and implementation of specific activities designed to enhance the skill-related components of functional fitness. Chapter 16 addresses recommended areas of study from training modules 6 and 7—developing effective motivational, communication, and leadership skills for teaching individual and group classes. Chapter 17 addresses training modules 5 and 8 of the international guidelines, including information on how to prevent injury by adapting or tailoring exercises to suit the fitness levels and medical conditions of your older adult clients and information on the physiological and psychological effects of common medications. Another recommended area of study from training module 8, knowing how to give first aid and to respond appropriately to emergencies, is covered in chapter 18. The knowledge recommended in training module 9—legal, ethical, and professional conduct—is also addressed in chapter 18.

- Chapter 15 provides an overview of the important tasks associated with a qualitative analysis of movement skills and how to prioritize the methods used to correct errors in performance. Several important motor learning principles you can use to decide how best to create an optimal learning environment for your older adult clients are presented. You will learn how to use demonstrations and verbal cues effectively to introduce new movement skills, how to structure the practice environment to maximize learning, and how to provide augmented feedback to older adults as they learn movement skills.

- Building on the skills presented in chapter 15, chapter 16 presents ways to develop your leadership skills and thereby enhance your teaching effectiveness. A variety of techniques and strategies are presented, including how to motivate and effectively communicate with clients in both individual and group settings, how to create a positive learning environment, and how to analyze your effectiveness as an instructor.

- Chapter 17 discusses disabling conditions and specific medical issues that can affect older adults, and presents ways to adapt or tailor exercises to prevent injury and ensure the safety of your older adult clients. Also discussed are the effects of commonly prescribed medications and how they can influence client safety during exercise. Furthermore, you will learn how to recognize the signs and symptoms of overexertion and other physiological risks and what to do if they occur while your older adult client is exercising.

- Chapter 18 is devoted to a discussion of legal and ethical standards that will minimize your liability as a physical activity instructor. Legal case studies, legal concepts and definitions, and many issues related to lawsuits are introduced, including negligence, types of applicable insurance coverage, and how to develop a risk management plan.

This information is provided to help you better recognize the boundaries of your professional competence and know when it is appropriate to refer older adult clients to physicians or other qualified health professionals. The last section of chapter 18 presents the professional ethics of the field today. This information can help you establish an exemplary reputation as a physical activity instructor of older adults and also help you elevate the reputation of the profession in general.

Applying Movement Analysis and Motor Learning Principles to Program Design

Debra J. Rose

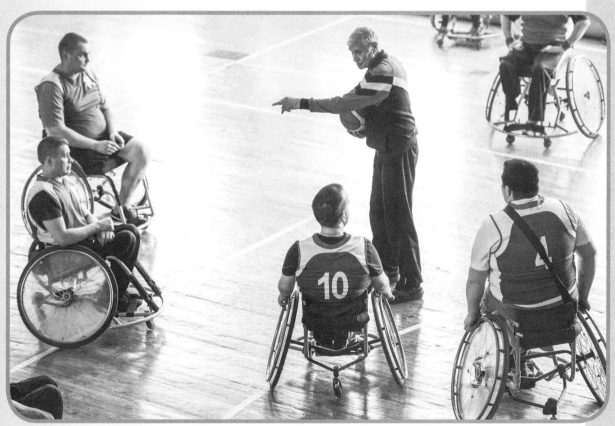

Objectives

After completing this chapter, you will be able to

1. systematically evaluate the movement patterns of older adults so that effective instructional and practice techniques are employed when introducing movement skills to older adults,

2. understand how the Later Life Training guide to common functional movement problems can be used to individually tailor exercises to optimize motor performance across a range of functional abilities,

3. describe specific behavioral changes that are typically associated with the learning of new motor skills,

4. structure the learning environment to facilitate optimal learning of motor skills,

5. explain the factors that determine when skills should be practiced in their entirety or in parts, and

6. vary the practice of different movement skills and appropriately allocate time to the practice of each skill.

Although physical activity instructors of older adults are taught how to lead group exercise classes, the skill of effectively *teaching* movement skills to older adults is often overlooked in instructor training programs. An essential goal of instruction is to enable class participants to successfully learn new motor skills or further refine existing skills. Although any instructional environment presents challenges, instructing older adults poses a unique set of challenges. Over the course of this chapter you will learn how to (1) systematically evaluate the movement patterns of older adults so that the most appropriate instructional and practice techniques are employed to facilitate learning; (2) adapt or tailor movement patterns in order to optimize motor performance using the Functional Movement Solutions (FMS) guide; and (3) apply fundamental motor learning concepts when teaching older adults in group-based settings. These concepts include how to introduce new movement skills, provide augmented feedback to class participants, and structure the practice environment for optimal learning and transfer of movement skills.

Nervous and Musculoskeletal System Changes and Motor Skill Learning

Changes within the nervous system influence how well older adults are able to learn and perform movement skills. For example, age-associated changes in cognitive, perceptual, and sensorimotor functions deserve special consideration by the physical activity instructor because of their possible effects on motor skill learning (Rodrigue, Kennedy, & Raz, 2005; Voelcker-Rehage, 2008). Because many of the age-associated changes in neurological function are discussed in greater detail in chapter 4, changes that are likely to influence how the exercise setting should be structured for optimal performance and learning are only briefly highlighted here.

Declines in cognitive functioning may have the greatest impact on motor skill learning for older adults. For example, older adults often perform complex motor skills (fine and gross motor tasks) more slowly and with less accuracy when compared to younger adults (Voelcker-Rehage, 2008). However, both performance and learning differences appear to be related to the structure, complexity, and difficulty of the task and to the level of familiarity with the task. Also, the capacity to acquire new concepts or to apply existing concepts quickly and accurately to complex movement situations declines. The older adult's capacity to quickly adapt movement patterns in response to environmental conditions also declines (Spirduso, Francis, & MacRae, 2005). In addition, older adults typically demonstrate slower **simple reaction times** (i.e., to a single event) and even slower **choice reaction times** (i.e., to multiple events), which are measures of how quickly they react to changes in task demands or the environment (Woods, Wyma, Yund, Herron, & Reed, 2015a; Woods, Wyma, Yund, Herron, & Reed, 2015b). What is especially noteworthy for the physical activity instructor is that physically active older adults do not exhibit a reduction in reaction times to the same extent as their inactive peers (Spirduso et al., 2005).

Aging effects on memory and attention are also relevant for motor skill learning. Deficits in memory functioning, especially short-term memory, can reveal themselves in difficulty remembering instructions and feedback and can lead to difficulty learning new movement patterns. Attention, attending to multiple environmental events at a given time, also declines with age. Older adults experience increased problems with tasks that require them to maintain their attentional focus for a period of time (e.g., reading a book), to selectively attend to certain events in the environment while tuning out all others (e.g., the movements of the instructor and rather than those of the other participants in the class), or to divide their attention between two or more different tasks (e.g., performing a cognitive or manual task while balancing or walking while conversing with a friend). Changes in the musculoskeletal system will also influence how well an older adult is able to perform different motor skills. As discussed in chapter 4, significant changes in muscle (e.g., strength, power, and endurance) and bone (e.g., mass and density) have been documented and will influence how well an older adult performs and learns movement skills.

Movement Analysis of Skills

How does an instructor decide how much to try to accomplish in a teaching session? A comprehensive model of the qualitative analysis of skills proposed by Knudson and Morrison (2002; Knudson, 2013) suggests that these decisions should depend on the results of four tasks for the instructor. As can be seen in figure 15.1, these tasks are sequential and cyclic.

The first task in the model is *preparation,* when the physical activity instructor acquires the prerequisite knowledge about the activities to be taught and the population (i.e., older adults) to be taught. This knowledge is essential for the physical activity instructor to become an effective analyzer of movement skills performed by older adults. The instructor's second task is the *observation* of the class participants' performance of the skill or activity. This should be done from several different vantage points and should include several observations of each class participant. From these multiple observations comes the instructor's third task: the *evaluation* and *diagnosis* of each participant's performance. This task requires that the instructor first assess how correctly the critical features of the skill or activity are being performed (i.e., identifying and prioritizing the critical errors involved in the performance of the skill) and then determine the strengths and weaknesses of the participant's task performance.

Finally, on the basis of the information accumulated from multiple observations and evaluation of the participants, the instructor then determines the appropriate *intervention* strategies to improve performance of the skill or activity. Because of the cyclic nature of the model, the instructor further observes and evaluates the results of the intervention strategies on the participants' performance and then continues with the same intervention strategies or alters them accordingly.

It is important to note that the evaluation, or assessment, of movement skills immediately precedes the selection of appropriate instructional techniques and practice condition characteristics. How does an instructor analyze movement skills? In the Knudson and Morrison model, the instructor

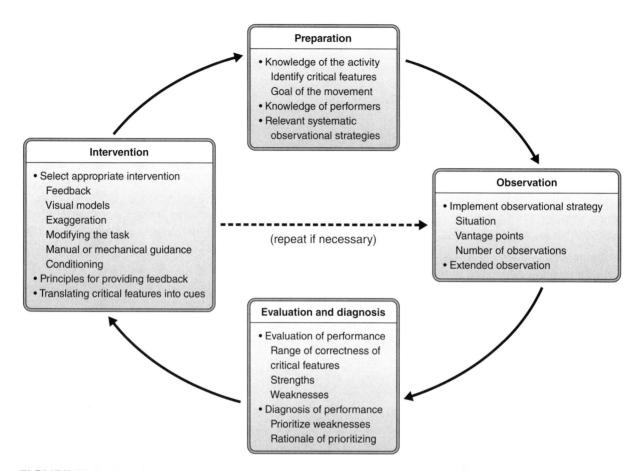

FIGURE 15.1 This four-step model provides a systematic approach to the qualitative analysis of movement skills.

Reprinted by permission from D.V. Knudson, *Qualitative Analysis of Human Movement: Improving Performance in Sport and Exercise,* 3rd ed. (Champaign, IL: Human Kinetics, (2013), 10.

primarily uses **qualitative analysis**, which means the "non-numerical analysis of movement . . . or a judgment on the quality of an aspect of movement" (Knudson, 2013; Knudson & Morrison, 2002). To engage in this type of movement analysis, the instructor must have an adequate knowledge of the skill being evaluated. This knowledge is an important part of your preparation as a physical activity instructor. Being able to identify the critical features (i.e., characteristics that a person must perform correctly to achieve the goal of the skill) is particularly important.

Identification of the performance characteristics that are most important for successful performance of the skill results from an analysis of the skill. For example, an analysis of a chest press performed on a weight machine results in the identification of five critical features, which are described in table 15.1.

The instructor also should establish an acceptable range of correctness when evaluating a person's performance of a skill or activity. Although the critical features of a skill need to be performed correctly, a certain amount of performance error is acceptable for any given critical feature. Some flexibility is necessary to accommodate for medical conditions your clients may have, such as structural deviations that affect postural alignment (e.g., scoliosis, kyphosis), back pain, joint surgery, or osteoporosis. However, performance error that is greater than this acceptable range needs to be corrected. The width of the acceptable range of correctness for any critical feature depends on the performance context. For example, a wider range of error is acceptable for an activity that involves sitting than for one that involves standing, especially if loss of balance is of concern. Because the safety of the participants is

Table 15.1 Critical Features of the Chest Press and Associated Verbal Cues

Critical features	Verbal cues
1. Five-point body contact position (left and right feet on floor, upper back and shoulders, lower back and buttocks, and back of head against seat and backrest)	Five points of body contact
2. Grasp handles with closed grip; wrists pronated	Firm hold, palms down, wrists extended not flexed
3. Push handles away from chest (at chest height) to fully extended position	Push using a 1-2 count, fully extended arms
4. Exhale on concentric phase and inhale during the eccentric phase of movement	Blow out as you push away, inhale as you pull back, four-second count
5. Maintain five-point body contact position during both movement phases	Press down and back against seat with body

the number one priority for all activities, the acceptable range of correctness for any activity should be determined according to the risk of injury that could result from a performance error.

The intervention task that follows performance evaluation and diagnosis should be based on the prioritizing of weaknesses identified during the diagnosis. Knudson (2013) describes six approaches to determining priorities for correcting errors: (1) relating errors to previous actions, (2) maximizing improvement, (3) correcting errors in order of difficulty, (4) sequential error correction, (5) correcting errors starting from the base of support, and (6) correcting the most critical error first. Each of these six approaches is briefly summarized in table 15.2. No single approach should be considered the best. The approach you select depends on the goal and type of skill presented and the learning stage of your client.

Table 15.2 Approaches to Determining Priorities for Performance Correction

Approaches to determining error-correction priorities	Description of approaches
Relationship to previous actions	Correct errors that are symptoms of previous movement problems; e.g., contacting a step with the lead leg because of not looking at the step rather than because of a leg movement error
Maximizing improvement	Correct errors that can lead to the most skill improvement during the practice time available
In order of difficulty	Correct errors that are the easiest to correct first, and then progress to errors that are more difficult to correct; this is an effective approach for older adults who exhibit low self-confidence in their ability to perform skills
In temporal sequence	Correct errors in the sequence of affected skill components; an error in the performance of the first component of a skill (e.g., backswing of forehand tennis stroke) should be corrected first
Base of support	Correct errors from the base of support up; e.g., for golf swing errors, begin error correction with stance errors
Most critical first	Correct errors in the component that is most important for the successful performance of the skill first

(For a more detailed discussion of this movement analysis model, see Knudson, 2013.)

Functional Solutions to Movement Problems

To further assist the physical activity instructor optimize motor performance during classes, particularly for those older adults experiencing functional limitations for various reasons (e.g., chronic medical conditions, medications, injury, sedentary behavior), Townley and Dinan (2003) created the Functional Analysis and Solutions model (see figure 15.2). This model is currently used in all Later Life Training (LLT) courses (see chapter 1 for a detailed description of the LLT continuum). The Functional Movement Solutions (FMS) guide that is based on this model helps physical activity instructors identify potential functional movement problems (i.e., physical, sensory, cognitive) that might be observed among older adult clients and then provides guidance as to what to observe and communicate to clients and how best to adapt or tailor movement patterns in order to optimize motor performance. Exercise contraindications or precautions are also provided to ensure the safety of older adults when exercising.

Definition of Motor Skill Learning

How do you know when the client you are teaching has learned the skill or activity? To answer this question, it is important to have a working definition of the term **motor skill learning**. Most textbook authors (e.g., Magill & Anderson, 2014; Rose & Christina, 2006; Schmidt & Lee, 2014) agree that motor skill learning involves several distinct characteristics, as follows: (1) Learning results from practice or experience that takes place over a period of time, (2) during this period of time there is an observable

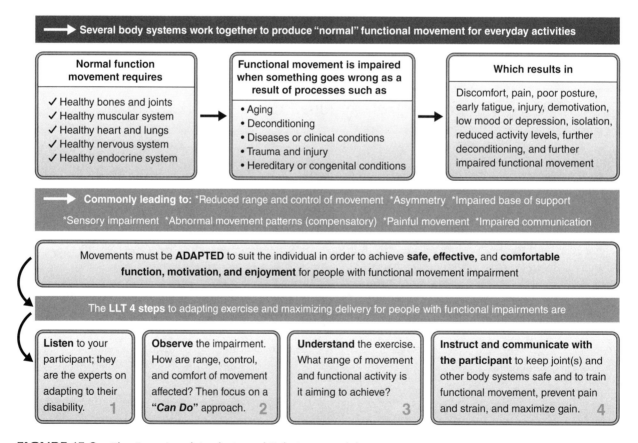

FIGURE 15.2   The Functional Analysis and Solutions model.

Reprinted by permission from R. Townley S. Dinan, (Eds.), *'Sit tall, stand strong' - The Chair-Based Exercise Programme for Frailer, Older Adults & Disabled Adults*, 2nd edition (London, UK: Later Life Training. 2013).

improvement in the performance of the skill, (3) as performance improves, it becomes increasingly more consistent from one attempt to the next, (4) the performance improvement remains relatively permanent over time, and (5) the learner can perform the skill in a variety of contexts in which the skill needs to be performed. Most of these characteristics are addressed by this working definition of motor skill learning: "a change in the capability of a person to perform a skill; it must be inferred from a relatively permanent improvement in performance as a result of practice or experience" (Magill & Anderson, 2014, p. 257). Although the ability to perform the skill in a variety of situations is not explicitly stated in this definition, it is implied in the phrase "a relatively permanent improvement in performance." This transfer capability is discussed next.

Transfer of Motor Skill Learning

People perform many skills in contexts and situations that differ from those in which they learned them. An important reason that many of the older adults in your class participate is to acquire skills that will enhance their performance of activities of daily living as well as sport or recreational activities. For example, older adults may engage in aerobic and resistance exercises to help them better perform the activities they need or want to do every day, such as go up and down stairs or have better stamina when they play sports such as tennis or golf. In motor learning terms, this application of skills from one performance context to another is known as the **transfer of learning**.

Transfer of learning is typically judged by the degree to which the performance of a skill in one context influences the performance of the same skill in a different context or the performance of a different skill. For example, physical activity instructors are often interested in knowing how well the skill they taught in class influences their clients' abilities to perform the same skill in their everyday lives. The transfer of learning can be *positive,* when the previous skill experience is beneficial, or it can be *negative,* when the previous skill experience hinders performance of either the practiced skill in a different context or a new but similar skill. In general, the greater the similarity between the practiced skill or practice environment and the new skill or

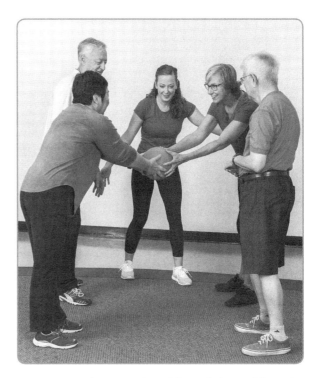

Activities that require older adults to lift and lower balls of different weights will transfer to the performance of daily activities that involve lifting and lowering heavy objects such as wet laundry or bags of groceries.

performance environment, the greater the amount of positive transfer. This principle of transfer provides a good rationale for the inclusion of aerobic, resistance, and balance activities that mimic real-life skills in any class designed for older adults.

Applying the four steps of movement analysis described earlier is especially important to ensure positive transfer of skills. For example, suppose that a client wants to participate in an exercise class to help his or her tennis game. The instructor needs to determine the characteristics of playing tennis that could be enhanced through exercises and activities presented in the class. Positive transfer to playing tennis can be expected if the class activities help the client increase relevant aspects of physical fitness such as aerobic endurance and strength of the specific muscles involved in playing tennis as well as the relevant motor skills, or performance-related components, such as balance and agility. As a second example, consider a client who wants to participate in an exercise class to improve his or her ability to go up and down stairs safely and without feeling undue fatigue. Again, the instructor needs to first evaluate the movement requirements of stair climbing in combination with the physical capabilities of the client before developing exercises and class activities to optimize the client's performance of this activity. The bottom line is that the instructor needs to provide practice experiences that are as specific as possible to the types of activities that clients need or want to be able to perform outside of the classroom environment.

> It is important that the physical activity instructor provide practice experiences that are as specific as possible to the types of activities that clients need or want to be able to perform outside of the classroom environment.

Assessment of Motor Skill Learning

Three important characteristics of motor skill learning should be taken into account when assessing how well a person has learned a skill. One is that learning involves a change in a person's capability to perform a skill at a certain level. Of course, factors in the performance may still influence the person in such a way that his or her performance is worse than he or she is capable of producing. For example, an older adult may be able to perform an aerobic dance sequence without music but may find it more difficult to remember the steps or perform them to the beat once music is added. Second, because learning involves internal processes within the central and peripheral nervous systems that we cannot directly observe, the assessment of learning requires an *inference*. This means that we must depend on repeated observations of a person's motor performance to evaluate learning. It is from these observations that we infer the extent to which learning has occurred. Third, it is essential to assess *adaptability* because people typically must perform a movement skill in contexts and situations that differ from those in which the skill was practiced.

The most relevant method for the physical activity instructor to assess movement skill learning is via a transfer test. A **transfer test** primarily assesses how

well the learner adapts to contexts and situations that differ from those in which the skill was practiced. Because transfer of learning is commonly the underlying reason to participate in an exercise class, the physical activity instructor should use some form of transfer test to assess the participants' abilities to perform learned activities outside the exercise class.

One practical and easy way to administer a transfer test is to ask participants in your class to write short anecdotes about changes they have experienced in their daily activities over the course of the exercise program. For example, a client writing that she can walk more regularly again because she feels more steady when moving about the neighborhood or another writing that he is now able to walk down a flight of stairs without fear of falling can serve as evidence of the positive impact of the class on motor skill development. Clients may write that their tennis or golf performance has improved. Or, you could have your clients complete the Composite Physical Function (CPF) scale introduced in chapter 5 when you conduct your regular screening and assessments. As you may recall, this questionnaire is used to evaluate how well clients believe that they can perform basic, instrumental, and advanced activities of daily living.

Why is it worth the instructor's time and effort to develop or use learning assessments? An important reason is *instructor accountability*. If people spend money and time with you to acquire capabilities they did not have previously or to improve their present capabilities, you need to be accountable by providing evidence to them that their time and money have been well spent. Keeping daily records of class performance and asking clients to write short anecdotes about changes they have experienced in their daily activities over the course of the physical activity class are ways to collect this type of evidence. If these records show improvement, you and your clients can have confidence that the exercise program you have designed is effective and that their time and money have been well spent.

Stages of Motor Skill Learning

The improvement in performance a person makes when learning a motor skill typically progresses through distinct stages. Although motor learning scholars have proposed several models to identify and describe these stages, one developed by Ann Gentile (1972, 2000) nicely captures the essence of these stages for the practitioner. Gentile described two stages that characterize the learner's progression from being a novice to being a highly skilled performer. During the initial stage of learning, the primary goal is to acquire a movement coordination pattern that enables the person to experience some degree of success at performing the skill. Some common characteristics of the beginner's performance include the following:

- The movement coordination pattern is not well developed and requires much refinement. This movement pattern is sometimes referred to as "in the ballpark."

- Performance of the skill is inconsistent from one attempt to another, which means the person may be reasonably successful on some but not all attempts.

- The errors the learner makes tend to be obvious errors that are easy for the instructor to observe.

- The learner is aware of making errors but typically does not know what the errors are or how to correct them.

- The learner's attention is devoted almost exclusively to what to do and how to perform the skill. As a result, the learner has difficulty engaging in another activity at the same time, such as listening to instructions or carrying on a conversation.

- Performance of the skill involves an excessive amount of movement because more muscles are activated than necessary, which results in the person using more than an optimal amount of energy to perform the skill.

Based on Gentile (1972); Gentile (2000)

In the second stage, the learner's goal depends on the type of skill being learned. If the skill is a **closed skill**, which means that nothing in the environment is changing and the person can initiate the skill at a time of his or her own choosing (e.g., riding a stationary bicycle or walking in an empty hallway), then the goal is to refine the movement pattern acquired during the first stage so that the skill can consistently be performed successfully. Gentile refers to this process as *fixating the skill*. But, if the skill is an **open skill**, which means that the person must perform the skill in a changing environment (e.g., playing a competitive game of tennis or walking in a crowded mall), then the goal is to be able to modify the movement pattern acquired in the first stage so that it successfully meets the changing demands of a performance situation. Gentile refers to this process as *diversifying the skill*. In this second stage of learning, the person makes fewer and smaller errors, which might be more difficult for you to detect, depending on your knowledge of the skill. Some implications of Gentile's two learning stages for instruction are presented in table 15.3.

Table 15.3 Implications of Gentile's Learning Stages Model for Instructional Settings

During the initial stage of learning	During the second stage of learning	
	Closed skills	Open skills
- Emphasize the development of the basic movement coordination pattern for both open and closed skills. This can be accomplished by promoting the achievement of the goal of the skill rather than the correct performance of the critical movement features of the skill. - Expect inconsistent performance of both open and closed skills. - Focus correction on flaws that cause the greatest performance errors.	- Emphasize successful and consistent achievement of the goal of the skill. - Establish practice situations that are as similar as possible to situations in which a test will occur.	- Vary the situations in which the skill must be performed so that the client must adapt to conditions not previously experienced. This improves the ability to adapt movements to the demands of unique situations.

Motor Learning Principles for the Physical Activity Instructor

The following sections describe specific ways to present a new skill, provide augmented feedback, determine whether a skill should be practiced as a whole or in parts, schedule the activities presented during class sessions, and determine how long participants will be engaged in performing those skills or activities during class sessions. Of course, the best way to acquire expertise in teaching new skills is to practice teaching motor learning skills and solicit evaluative feedback from your clients and peer instructors.

Demonstration

The most commonly used strategy for communicating how to perform a new movement skill is to demonstrate the skill. Research indicates that in certain situations a demonstration is likely to be more effective than other forms of conveying a skill (e.g., verbal instructions, physical guidance). One of these situations is when the skill requires the production of a new movement coordination pattern, which involves a combination of limb and body movements that is unique to each individual (Magill & Anderson, 2014; Rose & Christina, 2006). For example, if a physical activity is new and different from any activity the client has previously performed, the client needs to produce a new coordination pattern and a demonstration can effectively communicate how the skill should be performed.

Demonstrations are effective in part because of the relationship between vision and the motor system. When we watch a person perform a skill, our visual system detects the relative motions of the body and limbs (Ashford, Bennett, & Davids, 2006). This visually detected information is used by the motor system to enable the observer to move in a way similar to the observed movement. Because of this sensorimotor relationship, the most effective type of demonstration usually is of the correct performance of the skill.

An interesting alternative to a correct demonstration is to have beginners observe other beginners as they practice. Research has shown that beginners can benefit from observing other beginners practice a skill, especially when they can hear the instructor's correct evaluation of the observed person's performance (McCullagh, Law, & Ste-Marie, 2012; McCullagh & Weiss, 2001). This strategy can be especially useful in a large class where it is difficult for the instructor to provide evaluative comments on each participant's performance. Whatever type of demonstration you decide to use, these guidelines should be helpful to you:

- Be certain that the class participants observe the demonstration from a location that allows them to see the most critical parts of the skill performed. Everyone should be able to see the skill performed from the same vantage point.
- Demonstrate the correct way to perform a skill several times.
- Demonstrate the skill at a speed that is similar to its actual performance speed.
- Do not provide a lot of verbal feedback during the demonstration.
- If verbal feedback is necessary, use verbal cues before the demonstration to direct the participants' attention to key features of the skill.
- Allow beginners to observe other beginners practicing a skill but make sure that the observers can also hear the instructor's corrective feedback.

Verbal Instructions

Verbal instructions are often used to communicate how to perform a movement skill. One important function of verbal instructions is to focus learners' attention on the critical features of the movement skill or the environmental context that will enhance their performance of the skill. It is particularly important when teaching older adults, however, that the number of instructions provided does not exceed older adults' limited capacity to attend to or retain the information provided.

Several important factors influence the effectiveness of verbal instructions. These factors include characteristics of the instructions and of the learners:

- Compared with younger adults, older adults typically can pay attention to less information at one time and can remember that information for a shorter amount of time.

- People to whom instructions are directed must be able to interpret the meaning of the instructions. The meaning of a term to the instructor may not match its meaning to the client.

- Instructions influence how and where participants focus their attention as they learn and perform a skill or activity. This is important because a person's focus of attention while performing a skill influences how well he or she learns the skill.

- Instructions can help simplify what may appear to the learner to be a complex sequence of movements. When verbal instructions provide a strong visual image that the learner can associate with performing a skill, learning the complex coordination required by the skill becomes much easier. For example, the coordination between the arms during the sidestroke in swimming can be better visualized with the instruction, "Reach above your head with your lower arm and pick an apple off the tree, put the apple in your other hand at the level of your waist, and then put the apple in a basket by your hip."

Verbal Cues

A useful technique to help people remember how to perform a skill or activity is to have them repeat **verbal cues** while they perform the skill. Verbal cues are single words or short, concise phrases. When teaching new movement skills, these cues can serve two functions. First, verbal cues can direct people's attention to specific features of their own movements, an object they must do something with to perform the skill, or the environment in which the skill is performed. For example, when you introduce step aerobics exercises, it is important that the class participants look directly at the step prior to stepping on it. The verbal cue "look at the step" tells them where to direct their visual attention.

Second, verbal cues can serve as reminders about critical features or parts of the skill. For example, if the activity involves several parts that must be performed in a specific sequence (e.g., an aerobic dance sequence), one or two words can be assigned to each part as a verbal reminder of what to do in that part of the sequence (e.g., step-kicks,

knee lifts). You can use verbal cues to reinforce the critical features of an exercise while the client performs the exercise. A set of appropriate verbal cues associated with the critical features of the vertical chest press is listed in table 15.1. For example, you might present the first two verbal cues as the client prepares to perform the first repetition and each of the subsequent cues prior to the next few repetitions.

The verbal instructions you provide are the first method by which you introduce a new movement skill to learners. It is therefore important that you choose your words carefully and avoid saying too much before demonstrating the skill or before the learner has had an opportunity to practice the skill. These guidelines can help you effectively use verbal instructions:

- Include no more than one or two points about how to perform a skill or activity.

- Use terminology that all the participants understand; avoid jargon that is commonly used among physical activity professionals but will probably not be understood by the people in your exercise class.

- Give instructions that conjure up well-known visual images that help the learner think about moving in such a way as to produce the image rather than about the many parts of a complicated skill.

- Use verbal cues to direct the participants' attention to the aspects that are critical to performing the skill successfully, such as how high the foot is lifted when stepping onto exercise equipment, the position of a limb at a key part of the backswing in golf or tennis, or what to look at or for when catching a ball.

Verbal Cues and Demonstration

In some situations it is helpful to combine a demonstration with verbal cues. This strategy can be especially beneficial for teaching older adults a skill that requires performing a series of movements in a specified sequence. Research shows that older adults' reduced short-term memory makes remembering a verbally presented sequence difficult (Landin, 1994; Voelcker-Rehage, 2008). To help older adults overcome this potential problem, you can supplement a demonstration with verbal cues. These cues can be especially helpful for remembering the sequence if they form a sentence or if their first letters spell out a word or phrase. For example, to help participants remember the transitional sequence for moving from one step to another in a step aerobics class, the verbal cue "MOON" can be a signal to "Move Over Onto the Next step."

Augmented Feedback

Learners obtain sensory information from the various sensory systems (e.g., vision, somatosensory, vestibular) while they perform a skill. The instructor can provide additional feedback that supplements, or augments, this internal sensory feedback. This additional feedback is commonly referred to in the motor learning research literature as **augmented feedback**. For example, if you putt a golf ball that misses the hole, your own sensory systems allow you to feel the direction and distance of the putter movement during the backswing and the force used to hit the ball, to hear the club and ball make contact, and to see the direction and distance of the ball and by how much it missed the cup. A golf instructor who watched your putt could provide augmented feedback by telling you that the ball did not go in the hole because of the way you initiated the backswing.

Role of Augmented Feedback in Skill Learning

When working with beginners, an instructor should describe the critical error and what should be done to correct the problem. When used in this way, augmented feedback facilitates the learning of the movement skill by not only identifying the error but also clarifying how to correct it on the next attempt. Another role that augmented feedback serves is to motivate the learner to continue striving toward a goal. For example, when an instructor tells a participant in a physical activity class about the amount of progress he or she has made toward achieving a personal performance goal, this augmented feedback motivates the participant to continue to pursue that goal. Finally, augmented feedback can be used to facilitate learning by reinforcing the components of a movement skill that are being performed correctly or simply acknowledging the effort being made. Providing praise or compliments such as "Good effort" or "Your form is improving. Keep up the good work." is particularly helpful when teaching new movement skills or when working with older adults

who have low levels of self-confidence. Nonverbal types of communication, such as a smile or nod of approval, can also reinforce correct movement and strengthen the learner's desire to improve during the early stages of learning.

Types of Augmented Feedback

Instructors can provide augmented feedback about the outcome, or result, of a skill performance. This type of information is known as **knowledge of results**; for example, telling a participant the amount of time he or she took to complete an activity. Augmented feedback can also provide information about the quality of the movement pattern produced that led to a particular performance outcome. The term used to describe this type of information is **knowledge of performance**. For example, knowledge of performance can be information about what a participant is doing that facilitates or hinders his or her achievement of a performance goal, such as completing an activity in a specific amount of time. Providing meaningful augmented feedback during practice is one of the most important responsibilities of a physical activity instructor, particularly when working with older adults who may have little pre-

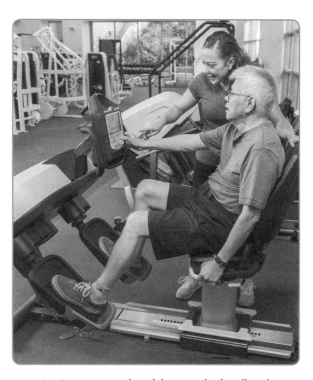

An instructor should provide feedback to a client to assist him in performing the exercise correctly.

vious motor skill experience or may have difficulty learning due to age-associated changes in cognitive or perceptual-motor processing.

Frequency of Feedback

How frequently should an instructor provide augmented feedback to a learner? A common misconception is that the more often an instructor provides augmented feedback, especially to a client in the initial stage of learning, the more effective it is in helping the client learn a skill. However, research has shown that augmented feedback presented less frequently than on every practice attempt is more beneficial for beginners than feedback during or after every attempt (Magill & Anderson, 2014). One reason for this is that beginners in the initial stage of learning who receive augmented feedback every time they perform a skill can become dependent on that feedback. This means that receiving augmented feedback becomes a necessary part of performing the skill. When required to perform the skill without the augmented feedback, the learner's performance is worse than with it. Acquiring the capability to perform skills without augmented feedback is important because most motor skills are performed in situations in which the performer cannot receive augmented feedback from an instructor. It should be noted, however, that reducing the frequency of augmented feedback as learning progresses does not hold the same learning benefits for older adults as it does for younger adults (Behrman, Vander Linden, & Cauraugh, 1992; Wishart & Lee, 1997). The optimal frequency of providing knowledge of results appears to be influenced by the type of skill being learned and the skill level of the learner (Guadagnoli & Lee, 2004). Reducing the frequency of augmented feedback makes the practice environment more difficult and may therefore not be as beneficial for older adults, depending on the skill being learned and their level of motor expertise.

There is also some evidence that providing learners with feedback after relatively good as opposed to poor practice trials leads to more effective learning in both younger and older adults (Chiviacowsky & Wulf, 2007; Chiviacowsky, Wulf, Wally, & Borges, 2009). While this method of feedback delivery contradicts traditional views of providing feedback after poor practice trials so that the learner can use the informational properties of feedback to guide them to the correct response, it is argued that pro-

viding augmented feedback after good trials serves to both reinforce correct movement and motivate the learner by creating a more successful practice experience. Given that a lack of motivation is a primary reason why older adults do not participate in or remain engaged in physical activity (see chapter 7), manipulating feedback in this way may be particularly beneficial when working with older adults in physical activity environments.

Augmented feedback

- is additional feedback that supplements, or augments, sensory feedback;
- can facilitate skill learning, reinforce correct movement, and motivate class participants to continue striving toward a performance goal or participating in the exercise class;
- can provide information about the outcome of performing a skill (knowledge of results) or the characteristics of performing the movement that led to the outcome (knowledge of performance); and
- should be provided less frequently as learning progresses and following relatively good practice trials.

Structuring the Practice Environment

Three issues that are especially relevant for determining the best way to practice skills to facilitate learning are discussed in this section: how to decide when to practice a skill as a whole or in parts, how to organize the practice schedule for optimal learning and transfer, and how to allocate practice time, particularly when working with older adults.

Skill Practice

An important decision that physical activity instructors face when introducing a new skill to clients is whether they should practice the skill in its entirety or in parts. Motor learning research indicates that this decision should be based on two characteristics of the motor skill. One is the **complexity** of the skill, which refers to the number of component parts in a skill. A highly complex skill has more parts than a less complex skill. For example, an aerobic dance routine is a more complex skill than putting a golf ball. The other characteristic is the **organization** of the parts of the skill, which refers to the temporal and spatial relationship among the parts. A highly organized skill is one in which the performance of any one part depends on the performance of the previous and succeeding parts. The golf putt is thus more highly organized than the aerobic dance routine. For skills and activities that are low in complexity and high in organization, practicing the whole skill is recommended. For example, a bench press in weight training has only two component parts (pushing the bar above the chest and returning the bar to the chest), which depend on each other to be performed properly. For skills that are high in complexity, the best decision is to practice them in parts.

A problem inherent in making the decision to practice a skill in parts is determining what constitutes a part for practice purposes. The organization of the skill helps solve this problem. You should first analyze the skill by identifying its component parts and then evaluating the extent to which the performance of any one part depends on the performance of the preceding or succeeding part. One common method used to identify the different components of a skill is on the basis of certain spatial or temporal characteristics (e.g., leg kick and arm action used in front crawl swimming stroke). Parts that are dependent on each other should be practiced together (e.g., putting a golf ball). Parts that are independent of other parts can be practiced individually (e.g., aerobic dance routine).

An effective way to engage beginners in practicing skill components is to use a strategy known as **progressive-part practice**. Participants practice the first part, then the second part, then the combination of the first and second parts, then the third part, and then the combination of the first three parts. This progression continues until all the parts have been practiced individually and then in sequence with all the previous parts. Eventually, the whole skill is practiced. This strategy works particularly well when teaching older adults an aerobic dance sequence or certain swimming strokes.

Class Schedule

Physical activity classes typically involve learning and performing several variations of a skill. For example, swimming involves the learning of different strokes; stair climbing includes going up a set of stairs, going down a set of stairs, and going up and down stairs of different heights; step aerobics requires a variety of different movements such as stepping up, stepping down, and side-stepping on and off steps of different heights. You must decide whether class participants practice the variations in the same class session or individually over a series of sessions.

Motor learning research has examined this practice schedule issue from the perspective of a learning phenomenon known as the contextual interference effect (Magill & Anderson, 2014). This effect is relevant in situations when multiple movement skills need to be learned. Research has shown that people learn skill variations better when they practice all the variations in each practice session rather than practicing each variation independently over a series of sessions. For example, if class participants must learn three different swimming strokes, they will learn them better if they practice all three strokes in every session than if they practice only one stroke for several sessions, then only the second for several sessions, and finally the third for several sessions.

The two types of practice schedules create different amounts of **contextual interference**, which refers to the memory-related interference that results from practicing variations of a skill within the same practice session. The greatest amount of contextual interference occurs when all the skills are practiced in a random order in each practice session, which is referred to as **random practice**. The least amount of contextual interference occurs when each skill is practiced independently in its own block of practice trials, which is referred to as a **blocked practice** schedule. Because the amount of memory-related interference is lower when skill variations are practiced according to a blocked schedule, performance of the skills during the initial practice session often improves more rapidly and to a higher level than when multiple skill variations are practiced according to a random schedule. However, performance on transfer tests, used to assess how well the skill has been learned, is typically better for those who experience random practice. Researchers interested in this motor learning phenomenon believe that when learners practice skills according to random practice schedules the practice is more cognitively effortful and the learning of each skill variation more distinctive and memorable as a result (Magill & Anderson, 2014).

Blocked and random practice schedules are the extremes of a continuum of possible ways to organize the skill practice within and across class sessions. For example, a third practice schedule called serial practice introduces a moderate level of contextual interference and involves practicing each of the skill variations in a nonrepeating manner but in a predictable order. As such, this practice schedule combines the predictability of a blocked practice schedule because the learner knows which skill will be practiced next, but still requires more cognitive effort because the same skill variation is not practiced repeatedly for a set number of trials. Figure 15.3 presents three different schedules for practicing three different bench-stepping skills.

As beneficial as random practice schedules appear to be for learning multiple movement skills, especially in controlled laboratory settings, it is important that the physical activity instructor of older adults consider learner characteristics before deciding how best to schedule practice during a given class. Research has demonstrated that the age

and skill level of the learner may limit the degree to which random practice is effective. For example, introducing lower levels of contextual interference into the practice environment has been shown to result in better learning in children while low-skilled learners have also been shown to benefit more from practicing different movement skills according to a blocked versus random practice schedule (Rose & Christina, 2006). Similarly, the complexity of the skills being learned must also be considered when deciding how best to schedule the practice environment (Guadagnoli & Lee, 2004). Even though practicing skills that are lower in complexity in practice conditions with greater contextual interference (i.e., serial, random) may benefit learning, the opposite may be true when the skills to be learned are higher in complexity. Practicing each higher-complexity movement skill according to a blocked practice schedule may produce better learning.

Practice Time

In addition to deciding how best to organize the practice of different skills within a class session, the instructor needs to determine the amount of

Practice schedule	Practice time	Day					
		1	2	3	4	5	6
Blocked practice	24 min	A	A	B	B	C	C
Serial practice	4 min	A	A	A	A	A	A
	4 min	B	B	B	B	B	B
	4 min	C	C	C	C	C	C
	4 min	A	A	A	A	A	A
	4 min	B	B	B	B	B	B
	4 min	C	C	C	C	C	C
Random practice	4 min	B	B	C	B	A	C
	4 min	A	C	A	C	B	B
	4 min	C	A	B	A	A	C
	4 min	A	C	A	C	C	A
	4 min	C	B	B	B	A	B
	4 min	B	A	C	A	B	A

Skill A: Step onto and off low benches

Skill B: Step onto and off benches of medium height

Skill C: Step onto and off high benches

FIGURE 15.3   Sample blocked, serial, and random practice schedules for three different skills, A, B, and C. Each schedule consists of six 4-minute sessions.

Adapted from Magill and Anderson (2014).

time to devote to practicing each skill or activity. In the motor learning literature, this decision is called **practice distribution**. Because there is only a certain amount of time available in which to carry out planned activities, the available time must be distributed to allow each of the activities to be carried out and also to provide an optimal learning opportunity for all participants.

The research literature indicates that shorter and more frequent practice periods are better for skill learning than longer and less frequent periods (Magill & Anderson, 2014; Rose & Christina, 2006). This means that if you determine that participants in your activity class need about two hours to learn to perform an activity properly, the two hours should be distributed across several practice sessions rather than getting it over with quickly in the fewest possible sessions. It is important to keep in mind that the issue of practice distribution relates specifically to the learning of motor skills and not to the physical fitness–related benefits of performing skills. The amount of time that is optimal for learning is specific to the skill or activity. As a rule of thumb, shorter and more frequent practice periods are better for skill learning than longer and less frequent periods. Your experience teaching a particular skill or activity will help you determine the total amount of time participants need to learn it.

How well the practice environment is organized strongly influences how much is learned. You have to decide how best to schedule the practicing of each skill or variation, whether the skill should be practiced in parts or as a whole, and how best to distribute the practice time based on the skill you are teaching and the skill level of your clients. The following guidelines will assist you in making these decisions:

- Determine whether class participants should initially practice a skill or activity in its entirety or in parts on the basis of an analysis that identifies its complexity (i.e., number of component parts) and degree of organization (i.e., temporal and spatial relationships among the parts). In general, skills that are high in complexity but low in organization can be practiced in parts, while skills that are low in complexity but high in organization should be practiced in their entirety.
- When class participants must learn several variations of a skill or activity, organize practice

sessions in a way that creates more as opposed to less contextual interference. Practicing each skill variation in each session creates more contextual interference than practicing only one variation in each session.
- Shorter and more frequent practice periods are better for skill learning than longer and less frequent periods.

Applying Motor Learning Principles in Group Settings

Your challenge as a physical activity instructor is to provide effective instruction for older adults with diverse characteristics. Older adults vary in both physical and cognitive abilities as well as stage of learning. The guidelines in the preceding sections provide suggestions for applying each of the five motor learning principles in group-exercise settings. However, because of the heterogeneous nature of the groups you will work with, be prepared to adapt each suggestion to the individual characteristics and needs of the older adults in the group.

Instructional techniques also should be adapted to individual needs. Do not take a "one-size-fits-all" approach to instructing a class; be prepared to individualize your instruction so that learning is optimized for each client. Use the guidelines for each of the five motor learning principles as starting points. Experiment with each suggestion, and then carefully observe the performance of each individual client to determine whether the demonstration or practice method you are using or the feedback you are providing need to be adapted for clients at a different stage of learning or less physically capable of performing the skill being taught. With ongoing conscientious application of the motor learning principles presented in this chapter, you will soon learn how to adapt your teaching methods to meet the individual needs of your clients at different stages of the learning process.

Summary

The motor learning principles described in this chapter are the basis on which physical activity instructors can determine how to use demonstrations or verbal instructions and cues to convey a new skill, how to present augmented feedback, whether clients should practice a new skill or activity as a whole or in parts, how the practice of different skills should be varied, and how to distribute the time available to the practice of different skills or activities. It is important to design a physical activity program with content that addresses the individual needs of your clients, but it is equally important for optimal learning that you apply each of the motor learning principles described in this chapter. The most successful physical activity instructors are those who combine strong leadership skills with effective teaching strategies.

Key Terms

augmented feedback

blocked practice

choice reaction times

closed skill

complexity

contextual interference

knowledge of performance

knowledge of results

motor skill learning

open skill

organization

practice distribution

progressive-part practice

qualitative analysis

random practice

simple reaction times

transfer of learning

transfer test

verbal cues

Recommended Readings

Knudson, D.V. (2013). *Qualitative analysis of human movement* (3rd ed.). Champaign, IL: Human Kinetics.

Magill, R.A., & Anderson, D. (2014). *Motor learning: Concepts and applications* (10th ed., units 4, 5, and 6). New York: McGraw-Hill.

Study Questions

1. According to the Knudson and Morrison model that describes the qualitative analysis of skills, identifying and prioritizing critical errors in the performance of a skill would be a component of which of the four analysis tasks?

   a. preparation

   b. observation

   c. evaluation or diagnosis

   d. intervention

2. Which of the following is an essential part of the definition of motor skill learning?

   a. can be observed during practice

   b. can occur without practice

   c. results in correct performance

   d. results in relatively permanent improvement

3. The greatest amount of positive transfer of learning between two skills can be expected to occur when

   a. the number of component parts of the two skills are equal

   b. a similar amount of practice occurs for each skill

   c. there is a small amount of similarity between the performance contexts of the two skills

   d. there is a high degree of similarity between the component parts of the two skills

4. A transfer test assesses primarily which of the following characteristics of motor skill learning?

   a. relatively permanent improvement

   b. adaptability to a variety of situations

   c. increased performance consistency

   d. the degree of correctness of performance of the skill

5. According to Gentile's model of the stages of motor skill learning, which of the following skills is an example of one for which the goal of a learner in the second stage should be to perform the movement pattern consistently each time?

   a. throwing a dart at a target that is mounted on a wall

   b. passing a soccer ball to a teammate who is running down the field

   c. stepping onto a step of a moving escalator

   d. any of these skills

6. For which of the following skills is a demonstration by a skilled performer most likely to benefit someone in the initial stage of learning?

   a. all motor skills

   b. all motor skills when verbal cues are given also

   c. motor skills that require learning a new coordination pattern

   d. motor skills that can be performed at different speeds

7. Verbal instructions can help simplify the initial stage of learning of a complex skill by

   a. describing how to perform each movement component of the skill in detail

   b. providing a strong visual image that the learner's movement should imitate

   c. describing all the critical features of the skill before the learner practices the skill

   d. directing the learner to think about each movement component as it is performed

8. Which of the following is an example of augmented feedback?

   a. seeing one's golf ball go into a sand trap

   b. being told by the golf instructor what was incorrect about a swing

   c. hearing the sound of the golf club hitting the ball

   d. feeling the position of the golf club at the top of the backswing

9. Practice of a motor skill in its entirety is recommended when the skill is

   a. high in complexity and low in organization

   b. low in complexity and high in organization

   c. high in complexity and high in organization

   d. low in complexity and low in organization

10. Which of the following practice schedules involves the least amount of contextual interference?

   a. repetition of short blocks of each of three skill variations

   b. random trials of three skill variations

   c. serial trials of three skill variations

   d. serial repetition of short blocks of each of three skill variations

Application Activities

1. Movement analysis. With a partner, select a specific skill or activity to teach to older adults in an exercise class.

   a. Analyze the critical features of the selected skill; that is, the parts that must be performed correctly to be successful in the skill or activity.

   b. For each critical feature, describe the range of correctness that you would rate as satisfactory when an elderly participant first attempts to perform the skill or activity.

   c. For each critical feature, propose a statement that would provide appropriate knowledge of performance to a class participant whose performance is outside your permitted range of correctness. Explain why this statement would be appropriate.

2. Structuring the practice environment: Variability of practice.

   a. Which of the following activities have high complexity and low organization, and which have low complexity and high organization? Why?

   - A tennis serve
   - The sidestroke in swimming
   - A six-part tai chi sequence
   - An aerobic dance combination
   - A chip shot in golf

   b. Which of the preceding physical activities can be practiced in parts and which should be practiced as a whole? For the activities that you decide can be practiced in parts, how would you organize that practice?

3. Verbal cues. Materials needed: Videotape or voice recorder. With a partner, take turns as instructor and learner in this exercise. Select one physical activity that your partner is not skilled at performing. Determine the critical features of the skill. Record yourself as you provide verbal instructions to your partner for performing those critical features of the skill. Listen to or watch the recording and evaluate the following:

   a. Which verbal cues were best to remind your partner of the critical features of the movement?

   b. Was the timing of the verbal cues appropriate for the component of the skill being performed?

Teaching and Leadership Skills

Helen Hawley-Hague
Susie Dinan-Young

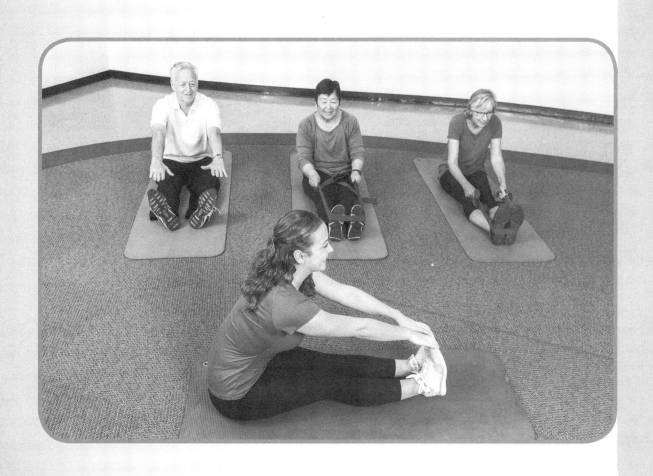

Objectives

After completing this chapter, you will be able to

1. explain the evidence related to teaching and leadership instructional styles for older adults,

2. compare and contrast the specialized teaching and leadership skills required to instruct exercise for independently active older adults with those required for younger participants,

3. apply evidence-based approaches and recommended techniques to sustaining positive communication with older adults (one-to-one or within a group) to ensure their needs are met and positive behaviors and social connections are reinforced,

4. adapt and tailor functionally relevant movement solutions for a range of older adults,

5. demonstrate advanced teaching and leadership skills when delivering exercise training activities, and

6. conduct a self-evaluation of the effectiveness of your teaching and leadership skills.

While the principles of teaching and leadership presented in this chapter are applicable to the full functional range of older adults, the practical approaches described are aimed at independently active older adults (as opposed to the frailer older adult with frequent fluctuations in health and disability who requires highly specific, evidence-based content and additional specialized instructor skills as part of a multidisciplinary, goal directed, exercise/rehabilitation care pathway). We define an **independently active older adult (IAOA)** as an individual who is community-dwelling, independently mobile (with or without an assistive device), and does not require the assistance of another person.

Teaching and *leadership* need to be defined because they are separate competencies requiring slightly different but complementary skill sets. To learn well in any subject, students need access to high-quality instruction and well-crafted, well-communicated programs that are tailored to meet individual needs. This requires well-developed teaching *and* leadership skills. It is important to acknowledge that not all leaders are good teachers, but all teachers must have competent leadership skills (Marzano, 2007).

Teaching skills are the competencies required to teach exercise safely and effectively. It is well recognized that there is both an art and a science dimension to effective teaching (Marzano, 2007). The science dimension entails a comprehensive knowledge of the discipline (i.e., research-based exercise science and aging approaches). The art dimension involves the translation and application of knowledge to practice (i.e., planning, delivering, and managing complex learning activities) in terms that are readily understandable to each student. Because of the physical dimension, this is particularly true of the art and science of teaching exercise and therefore to the education of physical activity instructors. Teaching exercise involves utilizing this technical knowledge base (including anatomy and physiology; evidence-based exercise science guidelines; **communication** and behavioral theory; and specific instructional, teaching, and leadership theory) to deliver skillfully adapted and tailored programs to safely and effectively meet the needs of the specific group or individual participants.

Leadership affects the interaction with participants while teaching exercise programs. Leadership in a group environment can be defined as "a process of social influence in which one person is able to enlist the aid and support of others in the accomplishment of a common task" (Chemers, Watson, & May, 2000). However, even in a one-to-one situation, leaders must appear competent and trustworthy. They must coach, guide, and support their "followers" in a way that allows them to satisfy their participants' personal needs and goals. In a group setting leaders also need to enable all participants to contribute to achieving the group goal. To accomplish this, leaders must understand the abilities, values, and personalities of those they are working with (exercise participants) so that they can provide the most effective support. Creating a sense of group confidence and empowerment through successful leadership encourages each group member to participate (Chemers, Watson, & May, 2000; Marzano, 2007; Hawley-Hague, Laventure, & Skelton, 2018). A growing body of research documents the positive effects and importance of the teacher's leadership role in the success of physical activity programs for older adults (Hawley-Hague et al., 2014; Hawley-Hague, Horne, Skelton, & Todd, 2016; Scott et al., 2008; Stigglebout, Hopman-Rock, Crone, Lecher, & Van Mechelen, 2006).

Although becoming competent in teaching one type of exercise class for the general population is an accomplishment, developing the competencies necessary to teach fitness classes to older adults (e.g., gym/circuit, exercise to music, step, dance fitness, aqua, walking, Nordic walking, Pilates, tai chi) is a highly specialized undertaking. Regardless of the age and functional capacity of your older participants, the type of training session, or your goal of being a personal trainer or a group instructor, the art of teaching is central to the successful application of knowledge to practice. It is a well-established, worldwide view of experts that teaching exercise to older adults is a specialized skill (American College of Sports Medicine, 2009; Department of Health [UK], 2011; Ministry of Health [NZ], 2013; Nelson et al., 2007; PAGAC, 2018). To ensure safety and success, teaching exercise to older adults requires a higher level of teaching, leadership, and communication skills than that required for the younger adult population (Buchner & Coleman, 1994; Ecclestone & Jones, 2004; Young & Dinan, 2005). These skills must align with an internationally agreed-upon set of curricula (Ecclestone & Jones, 2004), and

a quality assurance framework of occupational standards (Craig, Dinan, Smith, Taylor, & Webborn, 2001; Dinan, Buckley, Lister, Gittus, & Webborn, 2001-2009). Therefore, an advanced instructor qualification should be required to ensure a minimum practical competence when working with older adults in exercise environments (Ecclestone & Jones, 2004; Young & Dinan, 2005). The evidence is clear, as we have seen in earlier chapters, that safety margins narrow with age (Young, 2001). Even independently active older adults are at higher risk of an exercise-related event (e.g., an injurious fall, earlier onset of fatigue, cardiac arrhythmia, fracture, tendon injury,) and have a higher likelihood of vision, hearing, or other sensory impairments or one or more managed, chronic diseases (e.g., osteoporosis, arthritis, cardiovascular disease, diabetes) or a combination of these risks and impairments (Akushevich, Kravchenko, Ukraintseva, & Arbeev, 2013; Taylor et al., 2004; Young, 2001). Despite these age-associated factors, a broad range of older adults can be safely accommodated with properly trained and experienced instructors.

> It is a well-established worldwide view of experts that teaching exercise to older adults is a specialized skill that, to ensure safety and success, requires a higher level of teaching, leadership, and communication skills than that required for the younger adult population.

Earlier chapters have focused on the best practice adaptations to content, structure, and programming required to assist older participants achieve fitness and restore function safely, effectively, and enjoyably. The focus of this chapter is the instructor competencies required to teach older adults. The aim is to identify the essential teaching and leadership qualities and skills and explore how to become a gold-standard level, respected instructor of older adults. If successful, both you and your physical activity classes will be in high demand and you will keep your older adult clients coming back; like you they will be in it for the long haul! This chapter will help you develop and excel in both the art and the science of teaching, including the understanding and mastery of your leadership skills. Once you have understood and mastered the specialized teaching and leadership skills required, you will be fit for purpose with older participants. Moreover, your abilities as a physical activity instructor of all ages and abilities will transform from the ordinary to the extraordinary. In addition, your ability to provide a positive, personal, safe, effective, varied, and fun exercise environment for your participants, will, in turn, increase their long-term commitment to your program and motivate them to be more physically active in their daily lives (Hawley-Hague et al., 2014; Hawley-Hague et al., 2016; Scott et al., 2008).

Developing Your Leadership Style

Leadership has been described as "the most important determinant of participation in physical activity groups" (Estabrooks et al., 2004, p. 233). However, there is limited evidence about which particular leadership aspects are important to older adults. In a study with younger adults (Fox, Stathi, McKenna,

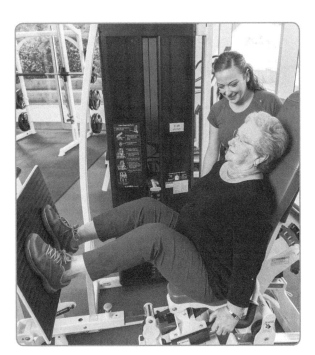

Providing encouragement and positive feedback can be very motivating to your clients because it can help to build their self-esteem.

& Davis, 2007) where an exercise class conducted using an enriched style of leadership (described as including encouragement, social interaction, and positive performance) coupled with a more enriched social environment (relaxed and interactive, motivating) was compared to a class that combined a bland environment (lack of warmth and interaction) with a bland leadership style (the instructor provided technical teaching corrections but, while not acting negatively, did not show supportive behaviors), the level of enjoyment was significantly higher for the group exposed to the enriched social environment and leadership style.

Person-Centered Qualities

Being responsive to individuals, having certain personal qualities, and making time are highly valued leadership attributes. Being sensitive, patient, and caring have been cited by older adults as important qualities they value in an instructor (Dinan, Lenihan, Tenn, & Iliffe, 2006; Stathi, McKenna, & Fox, 2010). Commitment to the class and to the quality of delivery (i.e., being well prepared, organized, punctual) and interaction with the task (i.e., ensuring it is tailored and giving task-specific reinforcement) are additional qualities that have been linked to both satisfaction with involvement in the exercise and also to client satisfaction with service (Dinan et al., 2006; Loughead & Carron, 2004).

Using appropriate music at an appropriate volume, having an instructional voice (clear, steady in pace, and loud enough to be easily heard), showing a confident manner, and being good at facilitating social interaction are all deemed to be important older adult instructor skills and qualities (Dinan et al., 2006; Estabrooks et al., 2004). Schutzer and Graves (2004) found that incorporating music into exercise programs added interest and facilitated exercise participation, socialization, and adherence. Selecting the correct style of music (e.g., instrumental) and playing it at an appropriate speed and volume is also considered to be important (Kennedy-Armbruster & Yoke, 2014). From the instructor perspective, respect for participants, a person-centered approach, and consideration of the social impact of the class were cited as important to participants (Hawley-Hague et al., 2014; Hawley-Hague et al., 2016; Stathi et al., 2010).

Expertise

Studies with exercise instructors and older adults who attend exercise classes have shown that participants needed to feel that the instructor was appropriately qualified and a good role model (Dinan et al., 2006; Hawley-Hague et al., 2016). They also suggest that the instructor should consider each individual class member and her or his needs, provide personalized feedback and individual encouragement, create an appropriate learning environment, facilitate group integration, vary the pattern of activities, and monitor group progress. We suggest that education and training are important means to gain these desired qualities. Instructor education, training, and qualifications in physical activity and aging have been found to correlate with instructors' attitudes about their older adults' participation in exercise classes (Hawley, Skelton, Campbell, & Todd, 2012). Instructors with specialist, condition-specific qualifications (e.g., balance and strength training for frailer older participants at risk of falls, cardiac rehabilitation training for those recovering from heart surgery) tended to express more positive attitudes about exercise that was predominantly standing (i.e., weight-bearing) and greater acknowledgment of the benefits of more challenging exercise for older adults. Thus, advanced education and training appears to link to increased confidence not only in participants but in instructor delivery. Hawley-Hague et al. (2016) found that qualified instructors believed that advanced practical training was essential, as was exercise-teaching experience. However, more work needs to be done to establish an evidence base that demonstrates how instructor training influences the success of instructor delivery with older adults (Hawley, 2011; Hawley et al., 2012; Hawley-Hague et al., 2014; Hawley-Hague et al., 2016; Scott et al., 2008). For example, evidence is needed to establish whether a successful instructor of older adults requires two separate qualifications based on their target audience; one for independent older adults and a more specialized one for frailer older adults with multiple comorbidities.

There is some evidence that instructors undertaking motivational training (understanding motivation and supervised practice in the specialized skills of motivating older participants to exercise) appear to have more successful classes. In one study,

instructors who completed a motivational training program (Hawley-Hague et al., 2014) were shown to be more likely to have participants who attend more frequently and, significantly, more frequently in the first three months. Instructors have suggested that this is the stage when there is the most explicit encouragement of participants to keep attending. This three-month period also is when the instructor's motivational function appears to be key to assisting older adults make the transition to becoming habitually active (Hawley-Hague et al., 2014).

Experience

There is emerging evidence to suggest that the experience of the instructor is important to session attendance and adherence in older adults (Dinan et al., 2006; Hawley-Hague et al., 2014; Seguin et al., 2010). In these studies, instructor experience tends to have been measured by self-report on how long the instructor has been delivering exercise classes to older adults. Besides duration, however, it is helpful to know what aspects of experience define an "experienced instructor" so that you can ensure you have these aspects in your older adult toolbox. Although this has not yet been explored specifically in research, expert consensus is that age-adapted exercises that are then individually tailored to each participant are more likely to achieve the agreed participant goals because this individualized approach has been shown to increase the likelihood of good attendance and improve adherence to the specifics of the exercise program (Estabrooks et al., 2004). Therefore, experience is likely to be about being aware of, and meeting, older adults' expectations and having the teaching skills and qualities to be able to assist them in achieving their desired outcomes.

Participant self-efficacy in terms of health improvement and restoration of function has been demonstrated routinely to relate to older adults' adherence to classes (Lachman, 2006; Sjösten et al., 2007). If older adults feel empowered to improve their own functional performance in both everyday life and the exercise session, they are more likely to continue (Stathi et al, 2010). Prioritizing safety and injury prevention and reducing the chances of pain and discomfort to a minimum can also decrease the chances of participant drop-out (De Groot & Fagerstrom, 2011). Qualitative work with instructors has shown that having confidence in their own skills of delivery results in a positive impact on their participants (Hawley-Hague et al., 2016). These skills and associated confidence are not necessarily or automatically immediate after qualifying, but can be developed and refined consciously over time through practice and observation of others.

Older Adult Instructor Evidence-Based Toolkit

- Be sensitive, patient, and caring
- Be well organized, well prepared, and punctual
- Present varied content and opportunities for socialization
- Use music and voice volume skillfully and give audible instructions
- Be qualified, experienced, and a good role model
- Be person-centered and tailor instruction to individuals
- Be respectful, patient, committed, and confident

Personality

When interviewing instructors who teach older adults, they report that they believe it is their personality and enthusiasm for what they are doing that can make a difference to the success of the class (Hawley-Hague, Horne, Skelton, & Todd, 2015). Although little has been done to explore which personality factors are important in this specialized field, practical pointers can be gained from the psychosocial literature. Personality scales are often based on what are considered to be the "big five" personality traits (see table 16.1). These originated from a series of studies and statistical analyses examining traits that tend to co-occur in people's descriptions of themselves or of other people (Digman, 1990). The five personality traits can be applied to assist the physical activity instructor in developing their people skills. The big five personality traits are described here:

Extroversion, which includes traits such as being talkative, energetic, and assertive

Agreeableness, which includes traits such as being sympathetic, kind, and affectionate

Conscientiousness, which includes being organized, thorough, and outcome oriented and using planning and goal setting

Emotional stability, which includes being calm and relaxed

Intellect, which includes being imaginative and insightful

A study of these big five personality traits enabled the researchers to confirm that there is a relationship between the instructors' personality and older adults' class attendance (weekly) and adherence (whether they dropped out) (Hawley-Hague et al., 2014). Instructors whose personality traits were stronger in extroversion, agreeableness, and intellect had poorer class attendance. On the other hand, instructors with a stronger conscientiousness trait were found to have better attendance and adherence to their older adult exercise classes. Factors associated with conscientiousness, such as goal setting and being organized, may be related to having a person-centered delivery style and therefore meeting the expectations of older participants (Hawley-Hague et al., 2014).

Ability to Foster Group Cohesion

Previous research has established the evidence for the considerable benefits of group sessions for older adults in relation to increased enjoyment and adherence (King, Haskell, Taylor, Kraemer, & Debusk, 1991; King, Rejeski, & Buchner, 1998; King, Taylor, & Haskell, 1993). Here we provide further insight into the reasons why groups work. The development of **group cohesion** has been found to be particularly important to success if you are delivering exercise classes for older adults (Estabrooks et al., 2004; Hawley-Hague et al., 2014; Hawley-Hague et al., 2015). In addition, Loughead and Carron (2004) found that participants were more likely to feel cohesion with the class as a group if the leader was interactive. Therefore, the physical activity instructor's role in fostering these bonds could be key. Recommendations for how to approach this are outlined in a later section of the chapter.

Evidence suggests that peer support is important to older adults when participating in exercise because this can increase self-efficacy and promote the social aspects of the class (Fox et al., 2007;

Table 16.1 Examples of Potential Advantages and Disadvantages of Strong Personality Traits in the Exercise Setting

	Instructor	Older adult (participant)
Extroversion	You are engaging and fun. However, you need to take care that you do not intimidate or alienate class members. Ensure that you are adjusting your approach to meet everyone's needs.	Your participants are the life and soul of the class and make new members feel welcome. However, ensure they don't dominate at others' expense.
Agreeableness	You are caring and considerate. However, you need to ensure you continue to challenge your class members so they can achieve their desired outcomes.	Your participants are warm and considerate and will help to ensure strong group bonds are forged, provided you ensure they are also encouraged.
Conscientiousness	You are organized and focused on outcomes and goal setting for your participants and work hard to support them in achieving their goals. Just remember that fun is still important!	Your participants are focused on outcomes and goals, and help facilitate shared successes between peers and other participants. However, it is important you support them in dealing with setbacks.
Emotional stability	You have a relaxed approach to delivering your classes. Although this can be great in terms of your adaptability to people and circumstances, ensure you don't forget to challenge your participants!	Your participants are easy going and can help to defuse tensions within the group. However, you need to ensure they continue to challenge themselves and progress their exercises.
Intellect	You make your classes more exciting because you impart information with ease, add variety and challenge, and perceive needs. However, be careful not to come across as too intellectual or this may intimidate your participants! Be concise, clear, and motivating so your participants will be participating, not listening!	Your participants are good to engage with because they may offer useful advice for adding variety to sessions or give you insights into group responses such as the intensity of the exercises. However, remember to facilitate class integration and group-wide feedback so that no one participant is seen as more important or superior.

Based on Hawley (2011); Hawley-Hague et al. (2014); Hawley-Hague et al. (2016).

Horne, Skelton, Speed, & Todd, 2010; Laventure, Dinan, & Skelton, 2008). However, in one study, instructors said that loss of specific peer support could lead an individual to lose confidence and self-efficacy, leading to drop-out from the class (Hawley-Hague et al., 2015). Previous studies suggest that group cohesion could be a barrier as well as a motivator for some older adults, with new participants finding an already-established exercise group intimidating (Costello, Kafchinski, Vrazel, & Sullivan, 2011). Therefore, the instructor must ensure facilitation of strong group cohesion, but ensure that it includes all participants. There is also evidence that if a health professional recommends your class and follows up with regular feedback and encouragement, this will help build the participant's confidence and reaffirm positive beliefs about the

importance and value of exercise (Hawley-Hague et al., 2015; Hawley-Hague et al., 2018).

This section has summarized what we know of the evidence base relating to the person-centered qualities of the instructor of exercise for older adults. The section that follows provides practical guidance and case-study examples to help you further develop the practical skills and qualities you will need to deliver safe, successful, and meaningful exercise programs for older adults.

Teaching and Leadership Competencies

Think of personal trainers, group instructors, and teachers you admire. What specific skills and qualities do you think contribute to their effectiveness?

Although at first glance the teaching of exercise may look relatively simple, it actually requires a complex and continuous orchestration of many skills, methods, techniques, and approaches used in ever-varying degrees (Jones & Rose, 2005; Rose, 2010; Skelton & Dinan, 2008; Young & Dinan, 2005). Instructors must consider factors such as clarity and timing in their teaching instructions (the *what, where, when,* and *how many* of exercise) and teaching points (the all-important *how* of exercise; i.e., using safe, effective exercise technique, which involves correct alignment, speed, plane, and quality of movement), as well as teaching and leadership style (being motivating and encouraging, having good class management skills, providing variety and fun), one-to-one and group observation and correction, problem solving, communication strategies, empathy, confidence, approachability, sense of humor, and environment. These factors have all been found to have an effect on participants' response to each session and each program and their long-term success (Dinan et al., 2006; Hawley-Hague et al., 2014; Hawley-Hague et al., 2015). Like orchestra conductors, exercise teachers, especially group instructors, have to learn the skills of integrating numerous complex movements occurring simultaneously or successively. Instructors require a greater mastery of their skills in order to undertake more challenging work. They have the additional responsibility of ensuring that physical risk is reduced to a minimum. When providing exercise opportunities for older adults, the instructor, the employer, and, where relevant, the health professional should be aware of the expert view that increased knowledge is not enough—there also needs to be a more advanced level of practical competency. In professional terms, in order to meet the higher duty of care, there must be evidence of more skilled execution and manipulation of the teaching and leadership methods and techniques and more conscious development of the personal attributes and communication strategies outlined in this chapter (Dinan & Skelton, 2008; Hawley-Hague et al., 2014; Rose, 2010).

The three **core competencies** identified by experts as key markers of these more highly developed practical exercise teaching and leadership skills are as follows:

1. *Listening.* **Listening** is not the same as hearing; it is not only hearing but also consciously paying attention to words and how they are spoken, the tone of voice, and the speaker's body language and then responding appropriately. Listen to your participants so you can make adaptations in your planning and tailor your delivery, teaching, and communication to accommodate group or individual needs (e.g., visual and hearing impairments, anxieties, or fluctuations in health); follow up any participant concerns, specific interests, or questions; and receive feedback from your peers and participants (peer and self-evaluation).

2. *Seeing.* **Seeing** is not the same as looking at or observing; it is not only observing but also actively seeing, perceiving, and analyzing what you are looking at and responding appropriately in practice. Actively seeing enables you to read each participant's typical everyday functional movement strengths and challenges by observing them closely before and during the session. It also allows you to note changes (i.e., improvement or deterioration) in a participant's functional movement, health, fitness, facial expression, posture, and mood, and respond appropriately with tailored exercise and communication solutions.

3. *Understanding movement and body language.* This entails not only analyzing movement from a musculoskeletal and functional point of view, but also, crucially, interpreting body gestures in order to design appropriate safe, culturally acceptable, functionally relevant, and realistic solutions to restore or maintain optimal function. It requires the ability to apply knowledge rapidly and continuously. For example, by understanding movement and body language the instructor can ascertain the nature and extent of the individual's postural and functional problems and particular strengths, what actions and ranges of movement are anatomically possible at major joints, which joints and muscles are used in everyday functional movements, and which everyday functional movements can be utilized to restore function as well as strength. Movement is an important form of nonverbal communication. The relationship between movement and emotion is well established; understanding posture, movement, and body language can give important insights into an individual's mood, confidence, and energy levels.

In order to become competent in mastering and applying these advanced core competencies to the practice of teaching of exercise to the older participant you must develop the following:

- *Sharper eye.* Use your eyes to see what is actually happening to, and for, each person in the group by observing and analyzing performance and concentrating on tailoring the exercises to individual participant needs. For example, watch for postural problems, incorrect technique such as unsafe joint alignment, poor concentration, loss of balance or stability, overexertion, anxiety, signs of pain, unwellness, and confusion. Injury prevention must be an even higher priority with this client group.

- *Keener ear.* Having a keen ear means actively listening to and engaging with your participants. You should not just hear what they are saying but take on board, and act on, unconscious clues and comments such as "I seem to be very out of breath today." Ensure that participants with hearing problems are positioned near the front so that volume is optimal and they can lip-read.

- *Greater sensitivity to, and control of, your participants.* Equally important to being heard by your participants is that you *can see everyone* in the room and *be seen by them* at all times. To prevent injuries, your class management or crowd control skills will need to be better than ever before. In order to be more sensitive to, and respond appropriately to, your participants' needs, you will need to be vigilant. Observe individuals constantly, conscientiously checking that they know what you want them to do. Don't stay in one spot during the session; change your teaching position frequently. Your teaching and leadership skills will need to be amplified and refined to meet these challenges.

Specific teaching methods and techniques for developing each of these core older adult teaching skills are discussed and illustrated with a variety of practical examples provided later in the chapter. In addition, three 10-step guides have been compiled to summarize the key points to focus on when developing your advanced listening, observation, movement analysis and problem solving, adaptation, tailoring, communication, leadership, and planning skills.

The evolution into a more advanced instructor takes time. Excellent physical activity instructors of older adults are not created in just a few days of training. Teaching exercise to older adults, perhaps more than any other client group, provides numerous, ongoing opportunities to apply, learn from, and hone these skills. Teaching and leadership skills and styles are learned in developmental stages and refined over time through continuing education, observation (of experienced peers and of participants), age-adapted planning, preparation, delivery with individualized tailoring and . . . practice, practice, and more practice . . . with regular self-evaluation and self-reflection. As we have seen from the evidence-based section, expertise and experience are important not only to experts but also to this discerning, life-experienced client group. Once bonds are built, older participants are honest, fair critics from whom physical activity instructors can learn a great deal about themselves and their teaching abilities. The following section provides you with a resource of best practice teaching methods and techniques and a 10-step guide to assist you in the development (or reevaluation) of your planning, teaching, and leadership skills and styles.

Preparation and Planning Skills

Being well-organized and prepared starts with planning. With older adults and other special populations, your planning needs to step up a gear to ensure every possible eventuality is covered. After reviewing the information, results, and insights obtained from your preactivity readiness screening (Young & Dinan, 2005), your functional performance assessments (British Heart Foundation, National Centre for Physical Activity & Health, Glasgow Caledonian University, & Later Life Training, 2014; Rikli & Jones, 2013a) (see chapters 5 and 6), and interviews with your participants about their expectations and exercise objectives (see chapter 7), the next step is to develop a lesson plan for each session that aligns with the goals of the overall program. Advance exercise planning is a best practice "must" to establish appropriate safety and counseling protocols for older individuals. In addition to meeting required professional responsibilities, a written lesson plan also ensures that cover or substitute instructors can immediately familiarize themselves with your group and proceed safely. The lesson plan must record the age-adapted exercise selections, combinations and progressions, and tailoring strategies or movement solutions provided to meet the needs of individual participants. The overall program and lesson planning should reflect the science and current evidence on exercise for older adults (see chapters 10 through 14) in terms of session content and exercise dose (intensity, duration, and so on) teaching, leadership, and person-centered communication approaches that have been shown to be most effective. Lesson and program plans must be updated regularly to record progress (e.g., adverse or positive reactions) and ensure they remain fit for purpose for that group or individual. Preparation goes beyond planning to include action.

Ten steps for older adult class preparation and planning follow to help you develop and deliver safe, successful lesson plans for older participants with tailored strategies for individuals.

1. *Know your participants.* Be clear about your group and individual participants and your goal for them as a group of individuals. Start by getting to know them, one by one, and their dynamics and scope as a group. Carry out a validated recommended preactivity screen (see chapter 5) with agreed safety and counseling protocols that are appropriate for older adults. This will also aid in your participants' transition from sedentary living to physically active lifestyles (Chodzko-Zajko & Resnick, 2004). Wherever possible, include a functional assessment of each individual's functional capacity, health status, preferences, and interests and agree on short and long-term goals (British Heart Foundation et al., 2014; Jones & Rose, 2005; Rikli & Jones, 2013a,b). Schedule in time at the beginning of each session to check each client's personal health, fitness and mobility status, safety precautions, and exercise adaptations.

2. *Use evidence-based and older adult–centered approaches.* Ensure your warm-up, workout, and cool-down exercises are adapted and align with current expert consensus and evidence-based guidelines for older adult exercise; examine the appropriateness of each exercise you select. Ask yourself questions such as, "Will this exercise session and overall program efficiently and effectively meet the needs, interests, and goals of my clients?" "Do the risks of this exercise outweigh the potential benefits?" "Can I adapt or replace these exercises

with others that are not only safer and more effective but are also more related to everyday life (e.g., replace supine abdominal curls with prone or box position curls, which are safer and more functionally relevant)?" Ensure you allow time for physiological adaptation (i.e., a minimum of two weeks prior to any progression), and progress training variables one at a time (see chapters 12 and 13). Embed multilevel activities, variety, and opportunities to socialize into the overall program and each session.

3. *Begin by setting functionally relevant fitness priorities.* Use the recommendations provided in chapters 5 and 6 to guide your decisions on which health-related and performance-related components and functionally relevant activities need to be prioritized. Planning for older adults must also address balance training effectively; see chapter 14 for evidence- and expert-based recommendations for primary and secondary falls prevention strategies that simulate the types of balance challenges encountered in everyday life. As we have seen in chapters 11 through 13, although all the components of fitness should be included in your program for life-related results, training and supervised practice of functional activities and varied approaches to strength, power, and balance training become even higher priorities with older adult participants in order to facilitate safer and improved performance of everyday tasks (getting into and out of a chair or car, walking, and so on). Doable, win-win task training designed to bring your participants personal success, satisfaction at seeing and feeling benefits, and enjoyment of exercise are key to engagement.

4. *Know your best practice exercise adaptations and individual tailoring strategies.* Determine and record how, based on the guidance provided in chapters 11 through 14, you will adapt not only the structure of the session but also each of the selected exercises to accommodate the aging process, specific health conditions common in older populations, and the wider range of fitness levels and motor abilities you will encounter (e.g., using a longer, more gradually graded warm-up and cool down; see chapter 10). Ensure your plan includes a graded range of adapted options (e.g., legs only, low arm swings). You can then establish the safety precautions needed, such as monitoring effort, watching for signs of adverse effects of exercise, and providing individual assistance or equipment.

Writing down the specific teaching techniques and skills that you will use for each exercise is an investment that will pay dividends in advancing your teaching skills with all age groups. Examples of techniques and skills include using clear, concise cues; knowing the specifics of demonstrations and teaching position(s); explaining the purpose of the exercise (understanding the functional relevance of an exercise is known to motivate older participants). Being prepared to offer and demonstrate three different levels of the exercise, three different tailoring strategies, and at least one alternative exercise will help to ensure that you are, and appear to be, well prepared and committed to your group which are qualities and skills older adults want in their instructor (Hawley-Hague et al., 2014; Hawley-Hague et al., 2015).

5. *Be more economical and considerate when planning transitions for older adults*. Group similar types of exercises together (e.g., strength and power exercises, standing and floor exercises) so that your program begins to develop a logical and efficient sequence. Transitions (moving from one circuit or fixed equipment station to the next or from one exercise to the next) with older adults can be a steep learning curve and demand your full attention because they are often where accidents happen. Transitions must be carefully planned and observed because individuals will often need assistance.

6. *Be guided by expert recommendations when choosing the appropriate environment and types of equipment*. Consider the venue, space, access (including transport, building and room entries and exits, toileting, and showering facilities), lighting, and temperature as well as the style and tempo of music, acoustics, and session format (e.g., lines, semicircle, circuit stations). Also consider what equipment (including exercise mats and chairs) or props are needed for greater effectiveness of certain exercises or for variety to enhance the enjoyment of your session (e.g., resistance balls and bands, weights). A word of warning if using music (older adults have identified music as important to enjoyment and adherence): music can increase participant risk and detract from enjoyment. A surprisingly common mistake made by instructors of older adults is selecting a tempo that is so fast the participants cannot keep up. Be considerate of your participants and only use music that enhances the experience (Karageorghis, Terry, Lane, Bishop, & Priest, 2012).

7. *Practice, practice, practice teaching your session plan*. Nothing takes the place of practicing what you have planned. It will help you deliver all the previous steps confidently, resulting in a more fluid and relaxed session.

8. *Self-evaluate regularly using peer- and participant-provided feedback*. Self-evaluation, in combination with informed external evaluation, is invaluable in stimulating, maintaining, and measuring your development as a teacher (Marzano, 2007). Take time to conduct critical self-evaluation before seeking participant feedback. Reflect on the similarities and differences between your own and their feedback to gain insights into your strengths and make an action plan for the skills or qualities needing further work. Even when you are feeling more confident and teaching regularly, continue to ask your participants for their thoughts on what they liked or improved. While keeping this informal, it is worth remembering that specific questions help to elicit specific feedback. Ask "Was the music too loud? Could you hear and follow my instructions throughout the session? Did you feel I was paying attention to you? Did you ever feel an exercise or part of the class was not effective?" Based on the evaluations, refine your delivery of the exercises by adjusting factors such as speed, music and voice volume, choice of music, transitions, program content, and teaching skills and leadership style as appropriate for each group of individuals.

Older adults have untapped resources of life experience and, in the authors' experiences, once mutual trust has been gained, not only appreciate being asked for their input but also provide insightful, balanced feedback that can really make a difference to your professional and personal development if you listen and act on it. In addition, find a critical **friend** or two! You cannot beat working with informed peers to assist each other in developing advanced teaching and leadership skills. Videotaping your teaching of an older adult class can be valuable, providing you take care not to change the way you normally teach.

9. *Become an outstanding instructor of older adults*. In addition to the higher level of planning competency required in the preceding steps 1 through 9, there is also a need for evidence of a higher level of commitment to your professional codes of conduct and responsibilities when working

with any special population (see appendixes B and C). The following specific recommendations made by experts, older adults, and health professionals are considered to be important to participant and peer confidence in you as an instructor and in the safety of your exercise sessions:

- Update and practice all safety and emergency procedures regularly with staff members and with older clients. Agree and record additional specific procedures and protocols to follow if there is an adverse event.

- Conduct re-activity screening (when participants are rejoining after a relapse or enforced break) and also group-wide periodic functional assessments and provide client feedback.

- Keep, and regularly review, confidential, up-to-date client records (e.g., participant attendance, health records, emergency contacts). Keep individual tailoring strategies up to date, and record any notable improvement or deterioration, unusual reactions, or any atypical behaviors or responses as well as your action plan. Recording individualized baselines, tailoring strategies, and progressions in the session record reinforces the importance of individual programs. Organizing relaxed review sessions for each individual and referring to her or his record communicates a professional integrity and interest in the progress of all your participants. Where appropriate, encourage participants to make their own record of their progress and milestones. These can become the basis for a monthly postsession question and answer session.

- At the beginning of each session schedule in time to check each client's personal health, fitness, and mobility status, safety precautions, and exercise adaptations.

- Be accurate about what improvements can be achieved. This is where realistic goal setting begins.

- Keep your Continued Professional Development (CPD) up to date and aim to keep abreast of evidence-based guidance to ensure your delivery continues to achieve the best outcomes for your participants. Ideas for continuing your education include attending specialist exercise and aging workshops and conferences, reading related journal articles and books, observing expert older adult and other special population instructors, and completing specialist vocational or academic physical activity and aging certifications.

10. *Ensure the program and each class meet the needs and interests of your older adults.* An annual program of work for older adults will benefit from multidisciplinary, multiagency collaboration. Involve exercise, sports, dance, health care, and social care colleagues and older participants to ensure consistency of delivery and teaching standards and a long-term commitment to a mixture of adapted exercise, physical activity, and sports activities in accessible venues. Regular, widely promoted, physical activity–related educational and social events with information that older adults can apply to their everyday lives (e.g., talks on healthy aging that include nutrition tips) have been shown to improve participant retention and recruitment. Planning should be an interactive, dynamic, and ongoing process that is the foundation of effective teaching and education about the benefits of exercise.

Developing Your Instructional Methods, Techniques, and Strategies

The preparation and planning, no matter how thorough and aligned with a standardized curriculum, is only as sound as the practical competence of the instructor delivering it. It is at the point of action—the delivery of the plan to one or more older participants—that the true test of the planning and preparation begins. Being a competent exercise instructor begins with an understanding of universally recognized instructional methods and techniques and continues with the successful matching of these to the conceptual and practical issues found in the delivery of a teaching session (Kennedy-Armbruster & Yoke, 2014). Properly trained, experienced instructors of older adults can meet the higher standard of care because they have learned, with supervised practice, to apply the recommended teaching methods and techniques to the delivery of exercise to older participants and then to evaluate and review their practice accordingly.

This section will provide useful practical recommendations, examples, and ideas to help you to develop, or sharpen, your teaching methods and techniques to an advanced level. The exercise teaching skills to be developed include: teaching instructions/cues, teaching points, teaching position and exercise demonstration, observation, analysis, and importantly, functionally relevant movement solutions and individualized tailoring and communication strategies.

A distinctive marker of advanced instructional skills for older adults is greater frequency of, and competence in, the conscious integration and manipulation of recognized teaching methods and techniques than is required with younger adults. The heterogeneity observed in older adults means that there is a wider range of learning styles than in any other population group. Competent teaching includes using a range of methods, techniques, and strategies to ensure there is a style to suit everyone (Young & Dinan, 2005).

As with any art taken to a higher level, there must be greater knowledge of, and mastery in, the application of all the practical teaching skills. These practical teaching competencies can be added to a toolkit of various instructional methods and techniques. The exploration of best practice teaching methods, techniques, and strategies that follows illustrates this complex and continuous integration associated with advanced teaching skills.

Other chapters (e.g., 8 and 17) have discussed how the diverse range of function and chronic disease found in older populations increase exercise risk; here we examine how the teaching skills, such as layering and **cuing**, can mediate these risks.

Cuing

To learn an exercise, participants need brief, simple, and clear instructions or cues. Cues also prepare a participant for what is coming next in the sequence of movements or in the transition between movements. When timed correctly, signals or cues not only help clients to follow with greater safety, efficiency, and confidence but also facilitate both the learning and the performing of exercise (Kennedy-

Armbruster & Yoke, 2014; Rose, 2010). Cuing can also increase effectiveness by being used to enhance teaching points (e.g., using body language to clarify or emphasize which part of the body or muscle should be feeling the effort). While teaching points (how) and cuing (what, where, when) remain distinct skills, in advanced practice there is a need to expand your cuing vocabulary and its application. Mastering the art of integrating and manipulating the different cuing methods and techniques and doing this continuously will not only improve your ability to teach participants *how* to do an exercise correctly, it will also transform your overall teaching, leadership, and communications skills. Once mastered, the cuing skills become a versatile resource that will enable you to accommodate the diverse functional changes and learning styles observed in older adults.

Three cuing methods have been identified: *visual, verbal, and physical* (Dinan & Skelton, 2008; Kennedy & Yoke, 2014; Rose, 2010). Although cuing tends to be associated primarily with group management skills, each of the following methods is equally valid, with modification, when working with individual clients. Keep in mind that mastering the art of advanced cuing requires lots of practice.

1. A **visual cue** signals or indicates a change and can be used with verbal cuing. For example, an overhead hand and arm signal to indicate a change of step pattern or direction, with the correct number of fingers up to indicate the number of steps to come, visually reinforces the verbal cuing. It can take the form of a visual preview such as a clear physical demonstration of the upcoming exercise. Visual previews are most effective between exercises and during rest, or active rest, periods. All visual cues should be larger than life to allow for visual, hearing, and physical impairments and, it is important to remember, they rely heavily on the instructor's teaching position for maximum effect (e.g., turning sideways to the class to demonstrate posture and extensor exercises). The value of visual cuing is highest among clients with diminished hearing or diminished visual acuity, poor body awareness, poor concentration, and language or cognitive difficulties. When combined with skillful verbal cuing, visual cues are more effective than either alone.

2. A **verbal cue** can be either a specific informative instruction for the upcoming directional change, exercise, or sequence. It communicates the *what*, *where*, *how many*, and *when* of exercise: "We are going to take four side steps toward the window and then four back toward the door. Get ready; and start . . . now." Verbal cues can be used as a verbal preview to accompany a demonstration. Combined verbal and visual cues (i.e., "show and tell" cues) often are presented together to increase sensory input and impact in order to improve clarity and to optimize learning.

3. A **physical cue** (kinesthetic cue) is recognized as an extremely effective way of helping participants to learn (Kennedy-Armbruster & Yoke, 2014; Rose, 2010). Physical cuing uses body language or touch, as necessary and appropriate, to guide the participant to a safer, more comfortable or effective execution of a movement pattern they are finding hard to achieve. Physical cues can be employed to direct attention to a specific body part to assist understanding. For example, when introducing a calf stretch, instructors should first indicate, on their own calf muscle, the exact position where the effort should be felt. Physical cuing can be the most effective method where visual and verbal correction alone has been ineffective. Since this method is usually performed one-to-one, it can take your attention away from the rest of the group, so ensure you also involve the rest of the class in a meaningful way such as having them all check that their own calf stretch position is correct.

For older adults, applying these combined cuing skills to ensure that each participant is clear about what's coming next can transform not only their performance but also their confidence and enjoyment of the session. It truly prepares older participants for the next change of direction, speed, or exercise and is an important safety tool and a challenging and specialized teaching competency. The more freely moving the exercise (e.g., step patterns) or the more change of level is involved (e.g., getting down to and up from floor work), the more comprehensive and competently delivered the cuing skills must be in order to ensure the risks never outweigh the benefits

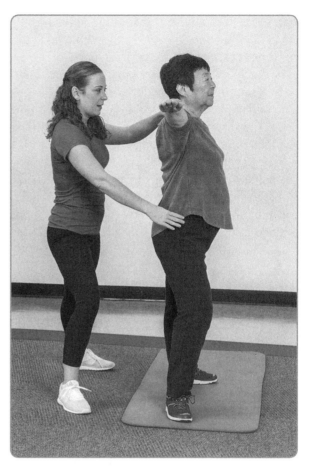

An instructor provides a physical cue to a participant to direct her attention to a specific body part during an exercise.

for the older participant (Skelton, Dinan, Campbell, & Rutherford, 2005).

Techniques using **process-oriented cues** and **goal-oriented cues** combine well to sustain effort, quality, and engagement in older participants. American College of Sports Medicine (ACSM, 2009) guidelines on the progression of resistance training are more effective if you ask your participants to do the following:

1. Make a note of their current maximum number of repetitions and sets for a particular strength training exercise and any changes they think they could make to this baseline over the next two weeks. Then you can discuss their goals and how best to progress.

2. Keep reminding themselves that quality, not quantity, is most important. Six well-performed repetitions will be more effective toward gain-

ing strength than ten reps performed with poor technique. Remember that it's important not to compete with anyone but yourselves.

3. Learn to listen to his or her body for cues about such things as when to rest and recover and when to rejoin the activity. Think about their strong points and the ones they need to work on most.

Layering

The next stage in developing your advanced teachings skills is to learn the technique of layering information. Layering is the organizing of important complex information into separate components that interact in a sequential and hierarchical order. You start by breaking information down into bite-sized chunks (which become your layers), begin instruction with the most important layer, then add layers when the time is right. In exercise teaching, layering must start with key exercise safety essentials and maybe one exercise technique pointer, then, once the exercise is underway, more technique tips or layers can be added in order of importance to increase effectiveness of performance (Dinan & Skelton, 2008). By adding layer upon layer in this way, the older participant is not overwhelmed by information but can work on each point as they arise. It also ensures that they get active as soon as possible rather than enduring long periods of instructor information with no action. Layering using the different cuing methods and techniques is an advanced skill and particularly important with older adults. It not only accommodates age-related changes such as poorer visual or auditory acuity or slower processing, but also ensures that by adding on technique points and information as performance improves, even the simplest exercise can remain interesting and motivating over long periods of time.

Adapting and Tailoring

Perhaps the teaching skills that define a skilled practitioner more than any others are the adaptation and tailoring of exercise. Adapting and tailoring are recognized as core teaching competencies regardless of the subject and age group being taught (Marzano, 2007). With special and patient populations, they are considered to be crucial to optimize individual learning, safety, and progress in the delivery of physical activity programs. The development of these two distinct, yet linked, teaching competencies requires a deeper understanding of their function; the techniques by which they are achieved; and their importance in minimizing risk and achieving safe, functionally relevant, individualized fitness outcomes and satisfied, committed clients.

Although the instructor must ensure each adaptation and tailoring strategy is first and foremost based on evidence or expert recommendation, it is central to the strategy's efficacy that it is a functionally relevant solution that addresses the specific functional movement problems of the individual and enables her or him to participate more safely and effectively in the session, the program, and everyday life.

Communicating

To communicate effectively with older participants, we must first understand what communication really is. As with the highly specific physical teaching skills, this understanding first requires studying, learning, and practicing the recognized methods, techniques, and expert tips by which effective communication can be achieved. Then you can progress to learning how these skills must be further adapted for older people. Again, as with the development of all the teaching skills, communication takes time and practice to master. You can constantly refine and advance your skills until thoughtful, positive, purposeful communication becomes second nature.

Advanced communication skills are particularly important when working with older people because many have some degree of hearing, speech, or cognitive loss (including memory loss), all of which complicate communication and interpersonal relationships if not handled competently. If the functional movement solutions and cuing techniques are not communicated in words, and with a tone, manner, and body language that is appropriate for that individual and that setting, the point will, at best, be lost. Worse, ineffective communication may not only alienate the individual from further interactions with you and the group but also put them off exercise altogether.

Although we have explored nonverbal cues in detail in relation to enhancing the effectiveness of our teaching skills, here we consider how the cuing skills can be combined with other nonverbal and

Definitions of *Adaptation* and *Tailoring* in the Context of Designing Exercise and Fitness Training Programs for Older People

Adaptation: the life-process modifications (e.g., aging) and clinical condition–specific process modifications (e.g., arthritis) to program and session aims, to structure, to content, and to teaching methods that need to be made to accommodate the specified processes, ensure optimal safety and effectiveness for all participants, and minimize risk.

Tailoring: the highly individualized, prescriptive solutions that are required for individual participants in order to ensure the age-adapted exercise or session ensures optimal outcomes by meeting each participant's individual functional needs (e.g., health, fitness, movement, psychosocial/emotional).

Adaptations can be accomplished in the following ways:

- Include longer, more carefully graded, warm-up and cool-down components and maintain a steadier overall pace to accommodate age-related changes in the cardiovascular, musculoskeletal, and nervous systems (see chapter 10). Common medical conditions observed in older adults are described in greater detail in chapter 17.

- Provide a longer, more gradual build up and cool down in the aerobic training component to accommodate the slower redistribution of blood to the skeletal muscles and slower increase in coronary supply to meet the increasing demands. This is particularly important to reduce risk in inactive beginners and those with cardiovascular disease (see chapter 13).

- Select appropriate seated options for specific standing exercises for older individuals who are feeling a little tired or unsteady on that day (see chapters 11 through 14).

Examples of tailoring strategies are listed below:

- Use two chairs, one on either side, to provide sufficient additional support for an individual.

- Identify the depth of cushion that a particular individual needs on his chair seat to ensure pain-free movement in knee joints during sit-to-stand exercises.

- Make small individual adjustments in exercises that involve gripping (i.e., where hand and finger coordination or range of joint motion make gripping difficult).

- Set out the session exercise stations in a particular order, position, or height to suit an individual with visual field, height loss, or attention difficulties.

- Use specified techniques for safe methods of mounting/dismounting particular pieces of equipment (e.g., bike or step) for an individual with coordination or memory problems.

Based on Dinan and Skelton (2008); Dennis et al. (2013).

verbal methods to enhance the interpersonal relationship between the older student and the teacher. Nonverbal communication includes eye contact; facial expressions; gestures (displayed through body language and posture); physiological changes (e.g., blushing, pallor); the tone, pitch, and volume of the voice (known as para-language); and personal space or physical distance between the communicators. These subsets of nonverbal signals can provide clues and additional information and meaning over and above the spoken word.

Be Aware of the Person You Are Communicating With

Because interpersonal communication involves a sender (or senders) and receiver (or receivers), the first thing to establish is knowing whom you are speaking to and what his or her communication-related functional problems might be (e.g., hearing loss, sight loss, speech problems, memory difficulties). Communication experts emphasize the importance of preparation (in particular, paying attention to differences in culture, past exercise experiences, beliefs and attitudes, and interpersonal relationships) before deciding which techniques to use to convey your message. By considering how your message may be received by the other person and by communicating clearly, you can help to avoid misunderstandings and potential conflict or distress (Arnold & Underman Boggs, 2016; Marzano, 2007). Think through the meaning of what you want to communicate, pay close attention to what you are going to say and how you are going to say it, and take note of how it is received. It is important to present information as clearly and simply as possible and take time after the class to chat with individuals to check for understanding.

Be Aware of the Power of Words

Use simple words and short sentences. Keep to key, inclusive take-home messages such as "this exercise strengthens your bones." Complicated physiological explanations are not appropriate in the participants' practical session; they can be exclusive, convey a sense of being talked at rather than talked to, and take up exercise time! Eliminate words such as *don't, stop doing,* and *please* because they are negative in tone and indicate something is wrong. Select positive words to convey your message: "avoid leaning forward as you . . . ," "make sure you are safe

by . . . ." It may take months to change old habits, but positive words communicate a positive and empowering teaching style. Learning to use positive language is also a key leadership skill. Other words to avoid when teaching are *try* and *it*. "Try to lift and lower your leg with control" tends to disempower rather than inspire. Instructions need positive action verbs. "Lift and lower your leg with equal control" is more likely to inspire a more effortful outcome. Similarly, "Feel *it* in the muscle" is not helpful and leaves most participants wondering what *it* is (feel what? in which muscle?) Compare that with "As you ease slowly into the hamstrings stretch, you should feel a slight tension along the back of the thigh; wait till this tension eases or disappears. Then breathe in and, on the outbreath, move slowly and further into the stretch until you can feel the slight tension in the thigh again."

Older participants are keen students from diverse backgrounds and will often look up information on the health benefits of, and contraindications to, exercise. If you're not sure of the meaning of a word or how to pronounce it, it is better not to use it. This accuracy is also important for authority in your role as an **educator** and **mentor**. Many of the points made here on the use of words are equally pertinent to the leadership, as well as the teaching, function.

Be Aware of the Power of Your Voice

Your voice is a powerful tool in ensuring effective communication with older adults. Mastery of the range, pitch, tone, speed, volume, and articulation of your voice can make all the difference to delivery of your communications and the enjoyment and learning experience of your participants. These aspects of your voice, together with phrasing and the use of pauses between words or sentences, are known collectively as *para-language* (Arnold & Underman Boggs, 2016). Being able to project your voice at the correct pitch and with the appropriate intonation (e.g., when cuing the group to slow their pace before a direction change during a lively aerobic endurance section and then, as contrast, praising them for having accomplished it safely) is an advanced skill. Projecting the voice is different from shouting (a fault often committed just because the person is older). Avoid shouting and instead experiment with your pitch. It is well known that a lower, well-projected pitch is easier to hear than a high, shrill pitch that does not project well and is not helpful for people with hearing problems. An added bonus is that a lower pitch is also thought to convey more authority (Arnold & Underman Boggs, 2016; Marzano, 2009).

Practice combining lower pitch and projecting your voice by giving instructions in the middle of a field, investing in some voice coaching, or joining a choir! Your pitch should lift and lower periodically to animate your voice. Arnold and Underman Boggs (2016) recommend listening to a radio presenter or disk jockey to focus on how to do this as naturally as possible. As discussed briefly in the core competency of developing sensitivity to hearing problems, it is important to take time to find a pitch and volume that will work for both you and your older participants. As recommended earlier in this chapter, always check the volume of your voice with your participants both in relation to the exercise setting acoustics and, if being used, to the simultaneous volume of the music. You may need to convince some participants that hearing your safety instructions is more important than hearing the music. Adjust your voice to suit the exercise component (e.g., speaking more softly during the relaxation and stretching sections or when you are delivering individual praise). Skilled intonation is something that will emerge as you think about the meaning of the words you are using, what you are saying, and to whom. Be aware that pitch and intonation can also convey emotion or mood (e.g., anger, disappointment, pleasure, or satisfaction with what is being said).

Speed of delivery is very important and a key challenge for many physical activity instructors working with older adults for the first time. Consciously slow down your speech a little. This means speaking *slower*, not *slowly*. Speaking slowly distorts the natural rhythm of language and makes it harder to recognize the words and decipher the meaning; slow speech can also appear patronizing. Speak clearly by taking the time to articulate your words. Avoid mumbling; instead, pronounce your words precisely. Do not, however, change your lip pattern as this reduces people's innate skill to lip read, which is often developed to a high level in people with hearing or visual impairments. Emphasizing one word in a phrase (e.g., "one, two, three, STAND") is another communication technique that works particularly well in the exercise setting to initiate concerted action and therefore assists with

group management (Dinan & Skelton, 2013). Two more practical communication strategies for older adults who may have hearing loss are to direct your words toward the individual's face and to position him or her as close to you as possible during the session to ensure that your face and body can be clearly seen.

Making sure that the exercise area is calm and distraction free is important with older groups because it affords better acoustics and improves concentration and, therefore, assists with communication. Any aspect that may affect hearing, speech, or concentration (e.g., disturbing background noise, music, traffic, talking, poor classroom acoustics, physical closeness of other participants) can usually be dealt with by using good communication skills. If communication problems persist, discreetly ask participants if they would prefer a quieter space or a different time.

As with all the communication elements, these practical and organizational aspects demonstrate the close relationship between the teaching and leadership skills. Teachers who understand and master the full spectrum of communication techniques are well on the way to developing the leadership qualities and skills that will lift their teaching style out of the ordinary. Nonverbal communication is perhaps the most vivid example of the integral nature of the teaching and leadership functions.

Be Aware of the Influence of Nonverbal Methods of Communication

Nonverbal communication is an extremely complex yet integral part of overall communication skills. Consider adopting these techniques:

- *Understand body language; that is, what your body (and your participant's) is saying.* Be aware of the nonverbal messages you are sending if you display impatient body language or allow your eyes to wander rather than maintaining eye contact when speaking. Learn to spot and preempt these communication barriers in yourself and detect and explore signs in your participants and adjust your delivery. An example is nodding the head vigorously when saying "yes" to emphasize agreement with the other person. Another example is that a shrug of the shoulders and a sad expression when saying "I'm fine, thanks" usually indicates that things are not really fine.

• *Maintain eye contact.* Eye contact is particularly useful to the exercise instructor because it is a clear indicator of loss of concentration, lack of comprehension, distress, or boredom! Eye contact can be used to reinforce verbal communication when giving or receiving feedback. Looking at a participant tells you that the participant is focusing on you and hopefully on the meaning of what you are saying. Listeners who avert their eyes frequently may be indicating a lack of confidence, anxiety, or dislike, all of which make effective communication more difficult.

For example, eye contact can be used as a signal to alert a particular participant to listen to the next safety point. Adding other nonverbal cues to eye contact, such as a smile or hand gesture, helps to clarify the message, creates a friendly atmosphere, and encourages questions and interaction.

• *Be aware of posture.* As well as offering insight into an individual's health and functional capacity, posture communicates volumes about an individual's emotions, attitudes, and intentions. Research has identified a wide range of postural signals and their meanings, such as "open" and "closed" postures (Norris, 2011; Winters, 2005). Someone seated in a closed position might have his or her arms folded or legs crossed or be positioned at a slight angle from the person with whom they are interacting. In an open posture you might expect to see someone directly facing you with hands apart on the arms of the chair. An open posture can be used to communicate openness or interest in someone and a readiness to listen, whereas the closed posture might imply discomfort or disinterest. Subtly mirroring another person's gestures or facial expression (e.g., nodding or smiling) indicates interest and approval between people and serves to reassure others of interest in them and what they are saying. Postural signals are generally well adopted by the exercise instructor; however, further understanding will ensure that the postural signals can be even more consciously applied to improve your reading of a participant's state of mind, health, and mood and your selection of verbal and nonverbal techniques to assist in communicating your message.

• *Communicate with touch.* Touch was discussed earlier in the context of physical cuing. Here, the focus is on its potential as a nonverbal communication strategy. The appropriateness of using this communication strategy can only be decided once insight has been gained into an individual's preferences, background, and health and a relationship has been established. It can be a subtle way of showing, or responding to, empathy and affection. The need for touch will vary on a day-by-day basis, and an understanding of personal space is important to using touch effectively.

• *Develop a feel for proximity and personal space.* Every culture has different levels of physical closeness appropriate to different types of relationships, and individuals learn these distances from the society in which they grew up. For an instructor in today's multicultural society, it is important to consider the range of nonverbal codes as expressed in different ethnic groups. Individuals may feel uncomfortable or defensive if their appropriate personal space is intruded upon and their reactions may well be open to misinterpretation. In Western society, specific distances have been defined according to the relationship between the people involved. Although instructors are fairly expert at sensing whether or not, and how far, to enter an individual's personal space, learning more about **proximics**, the study of personal space, would provide further understanding of this craft.

• *Evaluate your personal presentation.* Instructors are generally more aware of the influence of personal presentation than are many other professions. However, there is a strong case to be made for reviewing our personal presentation skills based on what older people have identified as important in their exercise instructor's personal attributes. Personal presentation is about positioning yourself in as positive a light as possible—at all times conveying appropriate signals for the situation and for the other individuals involved. Instructors who do not dress appropriately, cannot be heard, or lack confidence (older participants appear to particularly appreciate these personal presentation aspects) may fail to convey their message effectively or fully utilize their skills and abilities. Everyone presents himself or herself differently, and most of us can improve our personal presentation if we look at ourselves objectively.

• *Be aware of your personal appearance.* Note not only the way you dress and take care of your general grooming but also your body language, gestures, and other nonverbal messages that you use. Being aware of this can help you identify a dress and appearance code that is appropriate for the setting and group.

• *Practice time management.* This is part of presentation and has strong links to leadership. Persistently running late (getting to, starting, or finishing the session) or being disorganized (not having the equipment or room prepared in advance) has a negative effect on how you are perceived by older participants and means they lose part of their exercise time. Prepare equipment in advance, allow more time, and avoid being late.

• *Inventory your personal qualities.* Being a good listener is perhaps the most important personal quality. Learn to listen not only to the words being spoken but *how* they are being spoken and the nonverbal messages sent with them. Use verbal and nonverbal communication techniques, but also use clarification and reflection to confirm exactly what the other person has said to try to avoid any confusion. Closely linked to listening is being sympathetic, empathetic, respectful and kind. This will give you the edge as a teacher and a leader.

• *Be sympathetic, empathetic, respectful, and kind.* Most of us have a memory of a teacher who had an impact on our lives; in most cases this will have been someone who was not only passionate about her or his subject but who was also someone who listened and was kind, empathetic, or respectful to us in some way. To develop these qualities you need to become aware of other peoples' misfortunes, anxieties, and achievements; in other words, what is going on in other people's lives and emotions. Keeping confidences, as well as being clear about professional boundaries, is crucial to building trust. Remembering and using first names and getting to know participants' health and personal circumstances are natural features of the exercise environment. The earlier recommended preexercise health screen can also be used to read participants' nonverbal signals. To empathize with the participants, you will also need to try to understand and respect their points of view even if those views are different from your own. To avoid confusion, you may need to offer your viewpoint honestly. Do not be afraid to ask your participants for their opinions, as this will help to make them feel valued. Acting on this information will show participants that they are also respected. Always consider the emotional effect

of what you are saying and communicate within the norms of behavior acceptable to the other person. In the context of teaching and of leadership within the teaching role, these qualities demonstrate a humanity that is essential for the success of both functions. This aspect of leadership is explored further in the next section.

• *Provide encouragement and praise.* Offer words and gestures of encouragement as well as praise. Making older participants feel welcome, wanted, valued, and appreciated in your communications means they are much more likely to give you their best. Each week, ensure that each person you teach has been included in an interaction or communication with you; this may be direct or through effective body language and other nonverbal, one-to-one communication. Also use open questions (where a simple *yes* or *no* answer is not possible) to encourage participants to interact. For example ask, "Which part of the sit to stand exercise do you find most challenging to do?"

• *Treat people equally.* Treating people as your equal and also equal to each other is important to your effectiveness as an educator, mentor, and friend because it will build trust and respect. It is also crucial to your leadership role. The particular challenge with older participants is balancing the time you give participants: frailer individuals, where fluctuations in health and function are more frequent and significant, need more of your time, but you also need to give ample time and attention to more able participants. Instructors who strike this delicate balance gain respect because, on the whole, older people are supportive of their less fortunate peers. However, it is important to be clear with the group about confidentiality and its boundaries and remain impartial, discreet, and loyal to all participants. This is explored further in the leadership section, as trust and respect is hard-earned and will be easily lost if you do not observe this. The key yet again is to use your listening skills and nonverbal reading skills to detect potentially stressful situations and, without taking sides, remain calm and focused, resolving or delaying the discussion until after the session.

• *Have a sense of humor.* Humor is a great communication tool, and a strong positive correlation has been found between humor and good attendance and student performance (Arnold & Underman Boggs, 2016). Humor enhances the atmosphere not only by breaking the ice and lowering barriers but also by providing a physiologically and psychologically beneficial experience and a way of dispelling negative comments and resolving conflict at an early stage. We all enjoy having fun, and laughing has been shown to increase muscle relaxation, circulation, respiration, and endorphin production; reduce stress and anxiety in most situations; and improve self-esteem. It is important to be clear that in the teaching and leadership context we are talking about having a good sense of humor, not about being good at telling jokes. Humor is a strategy to improve learning. The only guideline is to ensure that your humor is appropriate to the situation and the participants, includes a humorous look at yourself on occasion, and is never cruel. Instructors also report there is more fun and laughter with their older participants than with any other group.

- *Keep a positive attitude and smile.* A final tip on the importance of nonverbal signals to effective teaching and leadership is to be aware that you are a communication role model. Your words, tone, movements, gestures, demeanor, expressions, and appearance all send signals that make an impression. However, perhaps the two most important aspects of your personal presentation are a positive, friendly attitude and a genuine smile. When things do not go as planned, stay optimistic, remain calm, take responsibility for your mistakes ("Oh! I've got it wrong; let's start again," rather than "You've got it wrong so we will have to start again."), put the mistake right competently, and laugh at, and learn from, your mistakes.

Advancing Your Instructional Skills and Strategies

The essence of education is the close relationship between a knowledgeable, competent, caring instructor and a motivated participant (Marzano, 2007). The physical activity instructor is uniquely placed to communicate important safety messages in a positive way. Older participants welcome and benefit from hearing new messages such as "there is a difference between discomfort and pain" and "where there is pain and strain, there is no gain."

The 10 steps that follow will guide you in prioritizing the ongoing development of your instructional skills and strategies. These key steps are designed to help you review your core teaching competencies and further develop them. Achievement of these advanced skills will not only ensure you are fit for purpose with older populations but will also ensure you have the necessary practical skills to teach patient populations.

1. *Master the art of combining cuing methods and techniques.* Become an instructor who all older participants can follow easily and confidently; an instructor who can be seen, heard, and understood by every participant in your session. Master combining and delivering the verbal and nonverbal cuing methods and techniques to improve your ability to communicate exercises, information, tailored movement solutions, praise, and encouragement. Mastering methods and techniques also enhances the safety and effectiveness of the session and your interpersonal participant relationships. Expert advice also suggests that mastery requires study, practice, patience, and ongoing reflection.

2. *Layer your teaching points to enhance your teaching of exercise technique.* Become an instructor whose technique pointers and demonstrations can be easily understood, followed, learned, and applied by the full functional range of older participants. Master the art of layering your exercise technique points in order of priority to enable participants to focus on key safety points before you add the next layer of technique tips once the exercise is underway. Add each layer separately, accompanying each verbal instruction with a combination of non-verbal cues to assist with participant modeling. The inbuilt pauses also allow you to scan the room to see if your point has been understood and is reflected in participants' performance. This approach can also build trust in your teaching style and attention to detail with individuals. Be aware of the impact of well-positioned, well-modeled teaching demonstrations, particularly helpful with older adults to accommodate hearing and sight changes and impairments. Also, be aware that the satisfaction of being able to mirror exercise also increases participant enjoyment.

3. *Develop a sharper eye and a keener ear, and become more sensitive to and practice better*

management of your participants. The importance of listening and seeing skills and becoming more sensitive cannot be overestimated with this client group in respect to safety (the anticipation, detection, analysis, and management of risk), effectiveness, interpersonal communication, and motivation. Older participants appreciate knowing they will be praised if they have mastered the exercise and will be corrected, kindly but honestly, if they have not, while being supported until they achieve their goal. Watching you be vigilant, conscientious, and competent with other participants builds trust and confidence in your skills among all the participants.

4. *Develop a storehouse of expert adaptation and individualized tailoring strategies*. Become an instructor who not only sees, listens, and observes, but also expertly analyzes and problem solves each participant's functional movement challenges in a way that is meaningful and helpful to that individual while simultaneously achieving the agreed upon fitness goals. Earlier in the chapter, a distinction was made between skillful, mindful adaptation (of structure and content to accommodate the aging process) and individualized tailoring (prescriptive, personalized, often subtle adjustments of adapted exercises to accommodate individual functional needs and ensure greater safety and comfort). Devote time to (1) establishing a process to help you make decisions about functional movement problems and (2) systematically building up a storehouse of evidence- and expert-based tailoring strategies and functional movement solutions. Identifying, recording, and updating individual baselines and strategies is essential to remaining organized and professional and keeps fresh in your mind each participant's progress.

5. *Think function! Become an expert in tailoring.* Become an instructor who expertly and consistently tailors individualized, evidence-based, functional movement solutions to meet the full range of functional needs encountered in older participants. Best practice requires that the instructor understand the basics underpinning aging and the effects of diseases and medications common in old age. The instructor also needs the ability to analyze how each individual's function is impaired by these processes, and to problem solve by developing simple and functionally relevant movement solutions.

While not every older participant has a medical condition, there is a greater likelihood that some will have certain medical conditions, use medications, be deconditioned, and experience functional decline and frailty, and, therefore, have increased risk during exercise. Being able to manage the potential impact of these fluctuations on general performance, postural stability, safety, comfort, and enjoyment during exercise is essential when designing and supervising exercise with this group. Highly competent communication strategies are recognized as crucial to achieving successful short- and long-term tailoring outcomes in participants with functional impairment.

6. *Know and develop advanced communication skills*. Become an instructor who is clear, concise, and informative as well as positive, respectful, encouraging, empathetic, and kind. These qualities are central to both the teaching and leadership roles even though the outcomes may be different. Therefore, they are covered slightly differently in this teaching skills 10-step guide and in the leadership 10-step guide later in the chapter.

A basic awareness of advanced communication strategies, over and above what is actually spoken, can help to improve interactions with others. Recommendations include gaining greater knowledge of and skill in these nonverbal signs so that they can be used to encourage people to talk about their concerns, which can lead to a greater shared understanding. The skills are identified as being aware of the person (or persons) you are communicating with, the power of words and your voice, the influence of the environment, and nonverbal methods of communication. Nonverbal communications include body language and movement, posture, eye contact, voice (tone, pitch, and volume, not the words spoken), physical distance or personal space, facial expressions, and physiological changes.

7. *Develop your role as an educator, mentor, and friend*. Become an instructor who is an interactive educator. Provide key, take-home physical activity messages to build participants' confidence, respect, and trust in you as an instructor, a professional, and a person. Emphasize the health and everyday functional fitness benefits of exercise and physical activity, the purpose of each exercise and the different fitness components, and why you are teaching exercises in stages. People tend to be more interested in performing an exercise if they understand *why* they are being asked to do it and if they can relate it to an activity of daily living or a specific aspect of maintaining independence. It is also

important to be concise, have a light touch, and be available. Schedule weekly time before and after the session to encourage participants to become more confident in sharing interests and ideas and in confiding concerns.

8. *Be organized, creative, flexible, and fun.* Become an instructor who is prepared for, and can deal calmly and resourcefully with, the unexpected. The recommendations for both the teaching and leadership functions agree on the importance of these qualities not only for safety and effectiveness but also for participant enjoyment. The different applications (i.e., in teaching and leading) determined their inclusion in both 10-step guides. Instructors are advised to learn (or refresh their learning of) how to prioritize safety through creative resourcefulness, because this takes experience and confidence in your teaching skills. Learning to be creative and sensitive in helping clients modify goals they are having trouble with assists with achieving the goal and avoids distress. Instructors need to look out for signs of boredom or inattention, such as chatting, as an indicator for action. Such action may be varying the activities, the dynamics of the specific activity, or your teaching leadership or communication style. Demonstrating flexibility by doing such things as altering your voice, the equipment, exercise, or program content can refocus and re-motivate the participants. Laughter has also been demonstrated to be a powerful communication strategy for enhancing enjoyment and assuring long-term engagement with older participants.

9. *Go that extra mile.* Become an instructor who is willing to provide further information when asked, such as sharing information about the latest evidence-based exercise. If the answer is outside of your expertise, then put your participants in touch with an expert or advise them where they can go to discuss any particular complex functional issues (e.g., a medical specialist or physical therapist).

10. *Be a highly competent teacher who is ethical and has a drive to improve her or his professional skills to reach a high standard of personal excellence.* Throughout the best practice recommendations, there have been implicit references to the importance of observing professional codes of practice and professional boundaries. Person-centered, informed, and responsive exercise sessions delivered in a professional manner require ongoing reflection and a constant dedication to refine and learn new teaching skills, both from formal courses and from your participants. This does not mean that you cannot approach your classes with humor and enthusiasm!

Developing Your Leadership Skills

Leadership is a crucial part of the teaching function of all subjects but is never more important than when applied to, and observed in, the teaching of physical activity and exercise. Older adults have considerable life experience and are adept at both being leaders or following leaders; therefore, effective leadership skills are at the core of success with this special population. Competency in leadership skills within the function of teaching exercise starts with understanding the leadership methods, techniques, and qualities. The introduction to this chapter acknowledged that while there is a great deal of overlap between the teaching and leadership skills, there are specific leadership markers that teachers can consciously employ to invigorate their teaching style.

A number of factors are related to, and predictive of, an older adult instructor's leadership effectiveness. These include client adherence, client satisfaction, and individual and program outcomes. The ability to cultivate positive relationships with participants and create group bonds (Loughead & Carron, 2004) is accomplished by having a genuine desire to help people, which is achieved by establishing trust with and inspiring your participants in order to improve their well-being. Based on the evidence and teaching methodological theory related to leadership, on many years of teaching group exercise to adults of all ages, on observing master instructors, and on interviewing research subjects and experts in aging and physical activity, the following 10 steps to good leadership are recommended for effective leadership function as part of the teaching skills.

1. *Establish your leadership style.* Be well organized and consistent from the start. Arrive early. Whenever possible, be at your facility before participants arrive. If using music, have it prepared, cued, and ready to go. Without adequate time, it is difficult to complete your preworkout tasks and you will look rushed, which diminishes your professionalism. Being prompt gives you time to screen new

participants and to interact with regular participants, noting anything of concern (or celebration!). First impressions will stay with your participants, and older adults will often drop out after the first class if you do not meet their expectations. Welcome each person by name as he or she enters the class. Taking a register or roll call in the weekly welcome process is recommended not only for audit purposes but also because it highlights missing participants so you can follow up with them.

Taking the initiative and demonstrating active concern is an important leadership skill. Control emotions by staying calm and clearheaded in times of high stress, crisis, or emergencies in the class. Manage your own personal stress, and leave negative moods outside the classroom. Genuine enthusiasm can be an instructor's greatest asset. Your passion carries the energy of excitement that can arouse enthusiasm in those you lead. You can instill a passion for physical activity through your words and behaviors. Enthusiasm is a powerful tool for inspiring others. Being enthusiastic and optimistic and helping others to see the positive side of life can be very motivational because clients connect with your enthusiasm.

Another important leadership skill is generating respect between the leader and participants. One of the best ways to show respect for your clients is by sincerely listening to them without passing judgment. Listen with both your ears and eyes. Listen for the message and the feeling behind the message; nonverbal gestures often speak louder than words. Respect is also expressed through your attention to details such as the selection of workout and background music, your interaction with other staff members, accommodating special requests, and remembering special occasions. A comfortable physical environment coupled with polite, cordial interactions and thoughtful anticipation of preferences sets the stage for mutual respect and positive experiences.

2. *Set the mood.* Before starting the exercise program, it is important for you to create a positive and supportive atmosphere. Many people believe that the single most important factor for health, happiness, success, and quality leadership is having a positive attitude. John Maxwell, the author of the best-selling book *The Winning Attitude* (1993), defined attitude as "inward thoughts and feelings expressed by our behaviors" (p. 20). As we saw

in the communication section, physical activity instructors with positive attitudes are likely to have more clients, have higher retention and compliance rates, and demonstrate more effective outcomes than instructors with negative attitudes. As you begin each session, influence the mood by projecting a positive attitude. Make a couple of statements or announcements such as the day's workout goals and specific safety reminders, ask a couple of open questions, and tell a brief, amusing story. Humor is an important communication strategy and spontaneous, situational humor has been demonstrated to improve your participants' enjoyment and learning experience. This is your opportunity to express the positive elements of your personality and your human relationship skills.

Maintaining a relaxed, nonthreatening atmosphere requires skillful communication, both verbal and nonverbal. Be aware of your facial expressions and body language. For example, if you look at participants without saying anything, they may become anxious. They may worry about your evaluation of their abilities. Your smile is rarely intimidating, but a blank face can feel unwelcoming. A nod of the head, a wink of the eye, or a positive comment such as, "I'm so glad to have you here today" helps to dissolve any tension instantly.

3. *Adopt a participant-centered approach.* Effective instructors do not just teach *exercise*; rather, they use leadership skills to teach *people* how to exercise by presenting various types of movements and activities and allowing participants to discover for themselves the physical exercise that is right for them. Exercise itself is important, yet more important is recognizing how a participant relates and responds to the exercise. One important characteristic of participant-centered teaching is to curtail using the word *it,* and replace *it* with *you* when appropriate in conversations. Also, simply referring to your participants by their names makes them feel they are important in your eyes.

Compassion involves being empathetic, or having the ability to appreciate another person's suffering. How do *you* feel about someone who is kind and compassionate toward you? Although you do not want to encourage long-term self-pity, you should listen to the worries, pains, concerns, and losses of your clients. Indicate concern through nonverbal gestures and expressions. Learn to be patient with difficult individuals and always stress the positive outcomes to be gained by doing the exercises. Allow beginners to be beginners and avoid any insinuation that beginner level is less prestigious than other levels. To help you be empathetic (sensing others' emotions and understanding their perspective) toward beginners, try a new activity yourself at which you are not naturally adept. This will help you to remember or learn what it is like to be a beginner. To show this sensitivity you have to become fully observant, which requires practice, and taking action on those observations is even more difficult. Effective leaders are emotionally self-aware; that is, they are attuned to their feelings and how those feelings affect them and their clients. They also have an accurate awareness of their limitations and strengths; they are not afraid to say, "I don't know," they welcome constructive evaluations from others, and they are willing to ask for help.

4. *Choose your language carefully.* What you say is as important as what you do. The importance of the words you choose when teaching is often underestimated, yet what you say and the way that you say it make a big difference in how your participants perceive you as a person and as an instructor. It is challenging to become conscious of the words that you habitually use while teaching. Do you use phrases such as "you guys," "good job," and "well done"? If you are serious about improving what you say, here are two suggestions for self-evaluation: (1) Ask your clients to write down (without signing their names) any irritating or annoying words or phrases that you use and put the names in a box. Read the words by yourself or as a class, and after you or your participants evaluate your word choices, write down key replacement words on an index card and place the card on the floor near you when teaching a class or in your pocket when training a client. (2) Videotape or audiotape yourself teaching a class, and have your peers, participants, or both critique your performance.

Sometimes you have to deal with your participants' word choices. Some people have had negative experiences with physical activity. Downplay self-defeating statements, and replace them with statements such as "It's never too late to improve" to promote the positive aspects of exercise. Emphasize how your class or delivery is different from their previous experiences and is tailored to meet their needs.

5. *Create a social connection.* Many older adults find it difficult to develop new friendships, especially after retirement. Exercise, particularly in a group setting, helps people connect with one another. Many participants have reported that the anticipation of seeing the instructor or their exercise buddies is the highlight of their week. This anticipation and feeling of inclusion can be particularly important when participants first start attending a class. Making them feel integrated (Hawley-Hague et al., 2014; Hawley-Hague et al., 2016) also has the potential to increase their self-efficacy (belief they can carry out the exercises). When you create a supportive environment that brings about socializing, a person's ethnic background and economic status are inconsequential. Your openness and acceptance of every individual create a bond that often becomes an integral part of your client's life. You can become the catalyst for social connections among your participants through creative programming. One way to create social connections is to keep moving around during the class and interacting with participants, being careful not to make some individuals nervous by invading their personal space. It is important to try to make everybody feel like "somebody." However, be careful of different personality types, because some extroverts can monopolize your time. Everyone in the class deserves your attention, not just the gregarious clients. Bestow generous amounts of attention, acknowledgment, and smiles on participants. You can chat to the quieter participants before or after the class to ensure that they feel involved. Inquire about your participants' activities or family life outside of the exercise sessions. As long as you feel comfortable doing so, share experiences about your own life with your participants. The interactions can continue for weeks afterward as everyone asks about certain aspects of your life that you have shared with them. Plan on staying after class to spend time with participants and get to know them. Create a designated area that is conducive for gathering and socializing before and after workouts. Providing refreshments will also encourage participants to stay and interact with you and the other participants. Create promotional events where the class can showcase their skills or provide opportunities for them to get together outside of the class. Such events as trips to the

cinema, Christmas parties, and other outings can help the class to bond.

6. *Discourage criticism, gossip, or comparisons with others.* Participants need to work within their own limits and the focus needs to be everyone's individual achievement with respect to their personal goals. Encouraging participants to share their own positive outcomes such as improved circulation, improved ankle mobility, or being able to use the stairs is more important than the number of repetitions they have managed to achieve. Provide corrective feedback with sensitivity. Addressing a few people or the class in general helps to draw attention away from any single person, which is especially important if that person is very sensitive. Simply considering a participant's suggestion can boost his or her self-esteem (the way a person feels about himself or herself) and his or her self-efficacy (a person's perception of his or her ability to do, learn, or master something). As a bonus, taking suggestions will also improve your class. Use positive affirmations. Offer encouragement before, during, and after each exercise session and specific exercise: "You can do it," "Believe in yourself," and "Look at how much you have progressed."

7. *Consider personalities.* Communicating effectively with different personality types requires skill and practice. Discretion is needed when approaching people because each individual has her or his own personality characteristics. Some people are outgoing whereas others are introverted. Some participants do not like you crowding their personal space but may feel uncomfortable telling you so. Some people prefer to keep to themselves or are highly sensitive to corrective comments. It is worth using different strategies to interact with your more introverted or sensitive participants, such as giving verbal cues rather than physical ones, communicating one-to-one, and providing lots of reassurance. Dealing with people who have very extroverted personalities and may be very talkative or attention seeking also requires a set of skills. You can engage people who are very extroverted by allowing them to assist you with teaching by giving them a specific task (e.g., they could be the person who counts how many times the exercise is performed while you focus on technique). While this can help with extroverts, making sure that you mediate in a firm but friendly way to enable other people to take part is also an important skill.

8. *Constantly reflect and improve.* Undertaking motivational training may help you improve your leadership skills and your engagement with your older adults, which can help to improve key skills such as individual goal setting. Constantly reflect on how you motivate your participants and what you can do to reach out to them.

9. *Provide consistency in your scheduled sessions.* Contact members of the class as far in advance as possible when there are changes to the schedule. If you are unable to teach the class due to sickness or holidays, then try to identify a suitable replacement. Ensure the participants are familiar with the substitute instructor. Breaks in delivery can cause participants to drop out or lose motivation or improvements they have gained (Hawley-Hague et al., 2014; Hawley-Hague, 2016).

10. *Be prepared to go the extra mile.* Working on behalf of your participants outside of class will help you to connect participants with the class. This can take the form of being actively supportive of your participants by contacting them before they first attend class or if they are ill or miss several weeks. You could also pair new participants with more experienced and compatible class members to encourage class attendance. One way to do this is by phoning them to suggest that they carpool to class if they live near each other. It is well known that the lack of transportation can be a barrier to participating in exercise programs (Newson & Kemps, 2007; Yardley et al., 2006). Providing feedback to health professionals who have encouraged their patients to enroll in your class is another example of going the extra mile. Staying in touch with this interdisciplinary liaison on behalf of your participants can help to build participant confidence and resolve. It also reaffirms their positive beliefs about what they have undertaken.

Summary

The field of gerokinesiology is a new, specialized, and rapidly changing area of study that focuses on the professional training in, and research on, physical activity and aging. Its rapid global growth is due to a number of service initiatives driven by the health, social care, and physical activity sectors (e.g., the increase in the provision of community programs for older adults, the increasing number of older adults living with multiple long-term conditions, and the demand for evidence-based programs and properly trained physical activity instructors of older adults). These initiatives give rise to important research questions about optimal programming and, crucially, optimal professional training for the specialized research, education and development, implementation, and practitioner professionals working in this field. Your choice to become a physical activity instructor of older adults carries with it many responsibilities and opportunities to influence the health and well-being of our aging population. Being part of the multidisciplinary, multi-agency network that is needed to support the physical activity opportunities for the full functional range of older adults is a lifelong learning curve and a privilege.

Effective teaching is both a science and an art. Factors such as mastery of advanced skill levels in the planning, teaching, and leading of an older adult class have been demonstrated to have an impact on program design, effectiveness, and long-term adherence. In addition to the steps described in this chapter, information obtained from the preexercise screening and assessments, as well as discussions that explore each client's expectations and exercise objectives, help you develop effective lesson plans that are targeted and meaningful to your clients.

The teaching and leadership skills described in this chapter are easy to understand, but require dedicated commitment to master in practice. They must be applied and practiced over time if you aim to become an excellent physical activity instructor of older adults. Remember to be participant-focused in your communication strategies. Also, learn and practice how to deal with the different personalities you will meet as an instructor of older adults. Most important, remember that your empathy and kindness along with your enthusiasm and positive attitude are key components of being a successful physical activity instructor of older adults.

Key Terms

communication

core competencies

cuing

educator

friend

goal-oriented cue

group cohesion

independently active older adult
(IAOA)

leadership

listening

mentor

physical cue

process-oriented cue

proxemics

seeing

teaching skills

verbal cue

visual cue

Recommended Readings

Kennedy-Armbruster, C., & Yoke, M.M. (2014). *Methods of group exercise instruction* (3rd ed.). Champaign, IL: Human Kinetics.

Kolb, D.A., & Fry, R. (1975). Toward an applied theory of experiential learning. In C. Cooper (Ed.), *Theories of group process*. London: John Wiley.

Rose, D.J. (2010). *FallProof! A comprehensive balance and mobility training program* (2nd ed.). Champaign, IL: Human Kinetics.

Skelton, D.A., & Dinan, S.M. (2008). Ageing and older people. In J.P. Buckley (Ed.), *Exercise physiology in special populations. Advances in sport and exercise science* (pp.161-223). Edinburgh: Elsevier Books.

Study Questions

1. Which of the following has not been identified in the evidence as being important when engaging older adults in exercise/physical activity?

    a. being sensitive and caring

    b. being appropriately qualified

    c. being well organized

    d. being very outgoing or extroverted

2. Which of the following is not a teaching skill?

    a. providing concise cuing

    b. adopting appropriate teaching positions

    c. facilitating group interaction

    d. offering alternative exercises

3. Which of the following types of cues relies heavily on teaching position for maximum effect?

    a. visual

    b. physical

    c. verbal

    d. none of the above

4. The big five personality traits identified by Digman (1990) include the following *except*

    a. extroversion

    b. emotional stability

    c. introversion

    d. conscientiousness

    e. intellect

5. The best strategy to respond to a client who is very extroverted and talks a lot during exercise classes is to

    a. suggest that the person move to the back of the room

    b. ask the person to leave the class

    c. ask the person to be quiet

    d. give that person a specific role, such as keeping count of the number of repetitions

6. Which of the following instructor personality traits are associated with poorer class attendance?

    a. extroversion

    b. conscientiousness

    c. agreeableness

    d. (a) and (c)

7. Which of the following voice pitches is easier for older adults to hear?

    a. a low voice pitch

    b. a high voice pitch

    c. a well-projected voice pitch

    d. (a) and (c)

8. Proxemics is the study of

   a. personal presentation

   b. personal space

   c. personal touch

   d. personal appearance

Application Activities

1. You are asked to take over an exercise class for older adults. It is held in a community center multipurpose room. The program has had mixed results since starting two years ago. There have been three interruptions of three to five weeks' duration when one instructor left and another was recruited and trained. You have been informed that the most recent instructor was popular and that participants were disappointed by her departure. The program is scheduled to restart in four weeks. It will be held twice a week at 10:00 a.m. There is a meeting held in the same room that ends at 9:30 a.m. on exercise days. You are informed that 12 participants are returning students, and 11 new participants are registered for the same class. No preactivity screening, testing, or evaluation has been conducted in the past.

   a. Describe what additional information about the history of the program would be helpful to you as the next instructor, and explain why.

   b. Discuss any obstacles you think you might encounter entering this new position.

   c. What elements of instruction do you think would help increase the likelihood of a successful program?

   d. What elements of leadership do you think you could use to engage with your participants?

2. Using the description in activity 1, describe how you would develop your exercise lesson plans. What types of activities would you include?

3. A participant in your class is a constant complainer. What strategies would you use to handle this person effectively before, during, and after class?

Exercise Considerations for Medical Conditions

Matthew J. Peterson

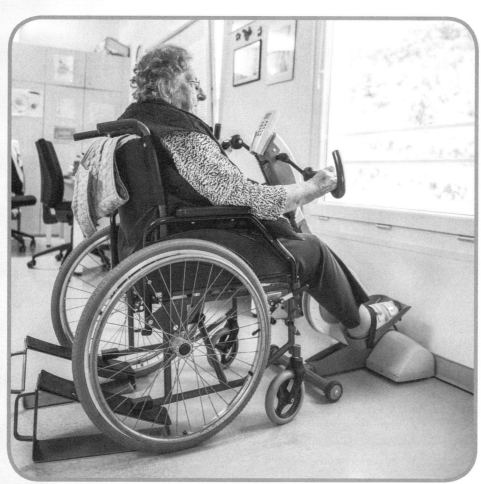

Objectives

After completing this chapter, you will be able to

1. identify the major disabling conditions that affect older adults,

2. recognize the major effects of each disabling condition on exercise tolerance or participation that may require modifications to the exercise program, and

3. modify exercises to enhance safe participation and reduce injury among older adults with specific medical conditions.

With advances in medicine, rehabilitation science and technology, public health, and consumer education, older people with disabilities and chronic health conditions are living longer (Kirkland, 2013). Bypass surgeries are becoming more common among older adults, replacement parts such as knees and hips are lasting longer, and portable breathing devices are allowing people with chronic lung diseases to lead more active lives. These and other technologies have resulted in a growing number of elderly people with disabilities who, in many instances, need physical activity more than their healthier older counterparts in order to maintain their narrower margin of health (Cadore, Pinto, Bottaro, & Izquierdo, 2014).

It is not uncommon for older adults with one or more disabilities to lose a significant amount of mobility and physical independence after a minor illness, injury, or exacerbation of their condition (Gill, 2014). Older adults with disabilities who are physically active are more likely to maintain their independence for a longer portion of their life and can often improve their health in a substantial way by engaging in low to moderate levels of physical activity (Fielding et al., 2017; Pahor et al., 2014).

The purpose of this chapter is to provide physical activity instructors with a general understanding of various exercise modifications and safety-related guidelines that can allow older adults with disabilities and chronic health conditions to participate successfully in various types of exercise programs. Common health conditions affecting older adults in their later years include coronary heart disease, hypertension, stroke, pulmonary disorders, diabetes, osteoporosis, arthritis, Parkinson's disease, and Alzheimer's disease, which are each discussed in this chapter. While it is difficult to ascertain the cumula-

tive toll on health care costs and personal burden, having one or more of these conditions significantly affects the lives of many older individuals. This chapter serves only as a primer for understanding how to work with people with these conditions. For a more complete overview of each disorder, refer to the recommended readings at the end of this chapter.

Cardiovascular Conditions

Cardiovascular disease is a major cause of death and disability in the United States. Older individuals with coronary heart disease have a high rate of functional limitations and disability (Xie et al., 2008). Exercise can have a substantial positive impact on cardiovascular health.

Coronary Heart Disease

Coronary heart disease (CHD) is a condition in which one or more of the coronary arteries are narrowed by atherosclerotic plaque or vascular spasm. The prevalence of CHD increases with age, and by the eighth decade, the prevalence of CHD is approximately 70 percent in men and 75 percent in women (Stolker & Rich, 2010). CHD is considered a multifaceted disorder with a great deal of heterogeneity (De Schutter, Lavie, & Milani, 2014). Some individuals with CHD are greatly limited physically, while others are able to maintain their usual daily activities. Approximately one quarter of individuals over the age of 65 have symptoms of CHD, and older adults in this age group account for approximately 80 percent of deaths caused by CHD (Go et al.,

2013). Symptoms often include shortness of breath, chest pain, confusion, dizziness, and palpitations (Stolker & Rich, 2010).

Since the purpose of this chapter is to discuss conditions that physical activity professionals are likely to encounter in an exercise facility such as a YMCA or private fitness center, advanced CHD is not discussed in this chapter. Cardiac rehabilitation or medically supervised exercise programs that are associated with many hospitals are more appropriate for individuals with advanced CHD.

Exercise is effective in maintaining the integrity of the cardiovascular system and should be prescribed to older individuals whether or not they have been diagnosed with CHD (Nelson et al., 2007). The physical activity instructor should initially avoid high-intensity exercise, which brings a greater likelihood of injury, with the goal of progressing the exercise program appropriately. Throughout the session, watch for the warning signs that indicate exercise should be stopped. The exercise program for people with known CHD should include a longer warm-up period consisting of low-intensity exercise such as light walking or riding a stationary bike with little or no resistance; several different stretching exercises, particularly of the chest region if a person has had open-heart surgery; and some mild breathing exercises, which could be part of a yoga or postural relaxation section of the class. A longer warm-up can reveal any chest discomfort or dizziness before initiating higher-intensity exercise. The longer warm-up can include various stretching exercises, done first while sitting in a chair, then while standing, then finally while down on the floor if the client is able to go down to and get up from the floor. Many excellent yoga and stretching videos developed for older adults can also be used during the warm-up.

Resistance training is a useful intervention strategy for older people with coronary heart disease (Liu & Latham, 2009). Since many older adults with CHD become increasingly sedentary, loss of skeletal muscle mass and strength can lead to a loss in physical function and can compromise

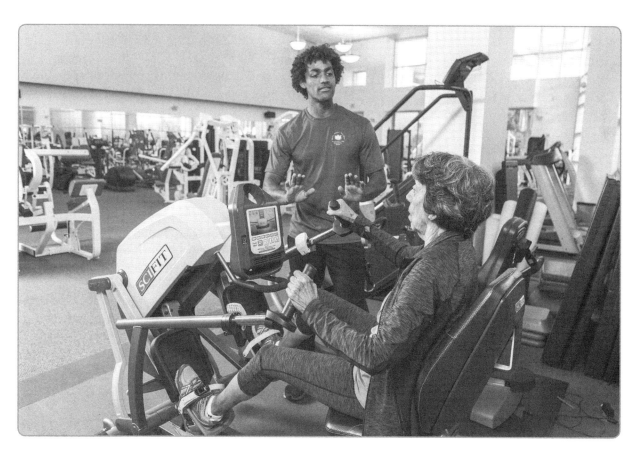

Avoid high-intensity exercises for people with cardiovascular disease, and be alert for warning signs for stopping exercise (e.g., breathlessness, chest discomfort, dizziness).

the person's ability to perform common activities such as walking up a flight of stairs or lifting a bag of groceries (Hamm et al., 2013). In medically unsupervised settings where there is no input or guidance from a physician, the physical activity professional should develop a gradually progressed resistance-training program based on current recommendations, taking into consideration the client's health and fitness status. For many clients, the initial intensity of the resistance training program may be low, with appropriate progression to moderate or high intensity, based on the client's fitness and experience, using the rating of perceived exertion (RPE) to monitor intensity levels. Verbal or visual signs of symptoms or discomfort should be ascertained and monitored carefully to ensure that the program is not unsafe for the individual. You should always consult with the client's physician if you become aware of any symptoms (e.g., breathlessness, chest discomfort, dizziness) related to the exercise program. Routine blood pressure and vital signs monitoring can assist in tracking client health status over time.

> Approximately three out of four adults 80 years and older have coronary heart disease.

Hypertension

Hypertension is a rise in systolic or diastolic blood pressure above normal values. Most research indicates that resting blood pressure increases with age and that elevated blood pressure is a major cardiovascular disease risk factor in the elderly (Stolker & Rich, 2010). The American Heart Association (2018) categorizes hypertension into the following stages:

1. *Elevated:* Systolic blood pressure of 120 to 129 mmHg and a diastolic blood pressure of less than 80 mmHg

2. *Stage 1:* Systolic blood pressure of 130 to 139 mmHg or a diastolic blood pressure of 80 to 89 mmHg

3. *Stage 2:* Systolic blood pressure of 140 mmHg or higher or a diastolic blood pressure of 90 mmHg or higher

Exercise training has been shown to have substantial benefits for older individuals with hypertension (Ehsani, 2001; Maniu, Flipse, Patton, & Fletcher, 2010).

The most important precaution is to ensure that the person's hypertension is being well controlled with medication and that the exercise program is not causing abnormal fluctuations in blood pressure. Monitor blood pressure more frequently in older clients with hypertension, particularly during the early stages of the program. You should invest in a good blood pressure monitor and stethoscope and take refresher courses on how to accurately measure blood pressure.

Medications used to treat hypertension include beta-blockers, calcium channel blockers, and diuretics. For people who are on beta-blockers, which are heart medications that blunt the heart rate response to exercise, rating of perceived exertion (RPE) is recommended for gauging exercise intensity. It may be necessary, however, to first teach the client how to measure RPE to ensure its accuracy (see chapter 13 for instructions on teaching your older adult clients how to rate their perceived exertion).

Thiazide diuretics are also used to treat hypertension. These drugs decrease blood pressure by increasing urine output. A complication that may arise in people taking these medications is that plasma lipids, with the exception of HDL cholesterol, can increase (Rosenstock, 2001). Clients taking diuretics may avoid drinking fluids so that they do not have to use the bathroom as often. This unfortunately increases the risk of dehydration. It is important to explain to the client that exercise causes a loss of body fluids through perspiration, and if the client does not ingest fluids during and after exercise to compensate for this loss, there is a greater likelihood of dehydration and other secondary complications.

Occasionally, antihypertensive medications may predispose a person to **postexercise hypotension** (a drop in blood pressure after exercise) resulting from the reduction of total peripheral resistance, which affects blood flow to the extremities (Gordon, 2009). To avoid this, you should conduct a longer cool-down period, gradually restoring heart rate and blood pressure to resting levels. It has also been noted that exercise training at lower intensities (i.e., 40 to 50 percent of maximal oxygen consumption) appears to lower blood pressure as much as exercise at higher intensities in people with hypertension (Gordon, 2009). Therefore, for older clients who have hypertension, lower-intensity exercises may be safer and yet achieve the same benefit as higher-intensity exercise in terms of reducing blood pressure.

Stroke

A **stroke** occurs as a result of a sudden, severe decrease in cerebral circulation caused by either a thrombus (blood clot) or a hemorrhage (leaking or ruptured blood vessel) that results in a cerebral infarction (interrupted blood flow in a cerebral artery). It is the fourth leading cause of death and a leading cause of disability and health resource use in the United States (Go et al., 2013). Strokes are classified as *hemorrhagic* or *ischemic* (reduced blood flow to brain). Hemorrhagic strokes constitute approximately 10 to 15 percent of all strokes, while ischemic strokes make up the vast remainder (Robinson, Brodie, & Manios, 2010). Most people who have had a stroke experience a significant improvement during the first six months after the stroke, while others take up to a year or longer to experience significant improvement (Kwakkel & Kollen, 2013). The goal of exercise training for those who have had a stroke is to maximize recovery and sustain and improve fitness and mobility throughout life. All types of activities should be used to improve health and function among individuals with stroke, including endurance activities, resistance training, flexibility exercises, and balance and mobility activities.

Aerobic endurance training for stroke survivors requires adequate supervision. Individuals who have survived a stroke often vary widely in age, severity of disability, motivational level, and number and severity of comorbidities, secondary conditions, and other associated conditions. Appropriate cardiovascular exercise may reduce these associated conditions and improve functional capacity. Aerobic exercise training can improve tolerance to activities of daily living and allow more physical activity to occur at a lower submaximal threshold, thus reducing myocardial oxygen demand (Gordon et al., 2004).

Examples of cardiovascular training modalities for stroke survivors include stationary cycling (recumbent and upright), over-ground walking or walking on a treadmill (provided that the clients have adequate balance and do not exhibit joint pain), and recumbent stepping (especially useful for clients with severe hemiplegia). Stair stepping in a vertical position may be at an intensity level that is too high for some stroke survivors, but if this activity is important to the client, it could become part of their long-term exercise goals with appropriate training and progression. Participants should be given the opportunity to select their own mode of exercise as long as it is considered safe and does not cause musculoskeletal pain or injury.

Resistance training is also very important for stroke survivors (Gordon et al., 2004). A major determinant of training volume is the amount of muscle mass that is still functional. People with **paralysis** (loss of sensory and motor control), **hemiplegia** (paralysis or weakness on the right or left side of the body), impaired motor control, or limited joint mobility have less **functional muscle mass** (muscle groups that contain nerve innervation and can respond to training) and therefore tolerate a lower training volume. For individuals who cannot lift the minimal weight on certain resistance machines, resistance bands or cuff weights are recommended. If bands and cuff weights are too difficult, the person's own body weight is used as the initial resistance. For example, lifting an arm or leg against gravity for 5 to 10 seconds may be the initial starting point for clients with very low strength levels. Another alternative for clients with very little strength is performing exercises that eliminate or minimize the resistance from gravity, such as horizontal movements, aquatic exercises, and isometrics (Nicola & Rimmer, 2010).

Participants who have survived a stroke should be taught a variety of stretching exercises targeting both upper- and lower-body muscle groups. Participants should stretch at the beginning of each exercise session, following the aerobic endurance section, between strength exercises, and during the cool-down. Stretches should be held for 15 to 30 seconds. Emphasize stretches for the tight (spastic) muscle groups on the hemiparetic side, which include the finger and wrist flexors, elbow flexors, shoulder adductors, hip flexors, knee flexors, and ankle plantar flexors.

Balance and mobility training is also important for clients who have had a stroke. The hemiparesis that often occurs after a stroke causes sensory loss on that side of the body along with a loss in strength and range of motion. Lack of sensation on one side of the body can result in a higher risk of falls because the person is unaware of where their center of mass is relative to the affected side. The loss in strength and flexibility may exacerbate the problem. Therefore, balance and mobility exercises are important for greater stability and function and to reduce the incidence of falls (see chapter 14 for specific balance exercises that can be performed in seated, standing, and moving environments). If you feel uncomfortable prescribing balance and mobility training exercises, consult with a physical therapist for specific recommendations for your client.

Pulmonary Disorders

Pulmonary disorders are increasing in prevalence in the United States and are now the third leading cause of death in the United States (Minino, 2013). These conditions manifest themselves as shortness of breath and, in severe cases, as major limitations in physical function and independence. The primary pulmonary disorders include asthma, chronic bronchitis, and emphysema.

Asthma

Asthma is a respiratory condition characterized by reversible (in most cases) airway obstruction, airway inflammation, and increased airway responsiveness to a variety of stimuli (McFadden & Gilbert, 1992). It appears to be a relatively common health condition in older adults (Interiano & Guntupalli, 1996). In the United States, approximately 19 million adults have asthma (Centers for Disease Control and Prevention, 2013). For people at an advanced age, asthma can be very disabling. The diagnosis and medical management of asthma in older adults is more difficult because the condition is often masked by other conditions that simulate asthma, such as emphysema or congestive heart failure (King & Hanania, 2010). The majority of people with asthma have a reduction in breathing capacity during and, more commonly, after exercise (Eves & Davidson, 2011). This is called **exercise-induced asthma**. In addition to exercise, other conditions that may trigger an asthma attack are cold, stress, and air pollution (Blakey et al., 2013). Use of a short-acting beta$_2$-agonist (e.g., Albuterol) 10 to 15 minutes

prior to exercise has demonstrated reduced risk of exercise-induced asthma (Clark & Cochrane, 2009). Low-intensity warm-ups may also be very helpful in reducing the risk of an asthma attack. The client should perform light cardiovascular activity below 50 percent of target heart rate for 5 to 10 minutes prior to exercise.

> A reduction in breathing capacity during and, more commonly, after exercise is common in people with exercise-induced asthma.

It is important that the timing of the administration of asthma medication be coordinated with the timing of the exercise session. Based on input from the client's physician, you must calculate when the medicine has to be taken to avoid an asthma episode during exercise. The timing depends on the type of medication that is prescribed. Medicines used in inhalers work within a few minutes, while medicines in oral form may take up to 30 minutes before they reach full effect.

Some older individuals may experience greater difficulty exercising at a moderate intensity because of the severity of their asthma. The appropriate intensity needs to be individually determined and should take into account the person's health status and aerobic capacity (Clark & Cochrane, 2009). It is important to use the RPE scale to monitor the intensity of the exercise.

People with exercise-induced asthma should *always* carry their inhalers with them. If asthma symptoms occur, a beta-adrenergic agent (used in inhalers) is the only way to reverse the symptoms of a full-blown attack. The physical activity instructor should make sure that a person with asthma has an inhaler at all times. Since cold air is a major trigger of asthma attacks, when exercising outdoors, it may be wise to advise the client to wear a scarf or surgical mask over the nose and mouth to warm the inspired air and reduce heat loss. After a cold or the flu, people with asthma are even more susceptible to breathing problems during exercise. These clients should be monitored closely after an illness and should be encouraged to start back slowly with exercise of reduced duration and intensity. Of most importance, however, is to reassure people with asthma that exercise is very beneficial for them, provided that the program is tailored to the individual's needs and severity of asthma (Carson et al., 2013).

Chronic Obstructive Pulmonary Disease

Chronic obstructive pulmonary disease (COPD) refers to a group of conditions characterized by airway obstruction. COPD usually refers to **bronchitis** (inflammation of the bronchial passageways in the lungs) or **emphysema** (destruction of alveoli, where the exchange of oxygen and carbon dioxide occurs) but can also include other respiratory conditions such as asthma and cystic fibrosis (O'Donnell, Laveneziana, Webb, & Neder, 2014). In this chapter, COPD refers to chronic bronchitis, emphysema, or both. Conditions that characterize COPD include impaired respiratory muscle function due to respiratory muscle weakness, more labored breathing due to pathologic changes in the lungs, and inefficiency of the inspiratory muscles due to hyperinflation. Approximately 14 percent of adults aged 65 and older are affected by COPD, and it is responsible for one out of five hospitalizations in older adults (Gooneratne, Patel, & Corcoran, 2010). Symptoms of COPD include **dyspnea** (difficulty breathing), coughing, sputum (mucus) production, weight loss, and fatigue (Cooper, 2009).

Exercise is considered an essential component of treatment for people with bronchitis and emphysema. The primary aim of the exercise program is to improve breathing efficiency and exercise tolerance. Exercise intensity should be based on RPE, which seems to be a more reliable indicator than heart rate in this clientele (Cooper, 2009). Individuals who are in the advanced stages of emphysema may require supplemental oxygen during exercise. If you do not feel comfortable working with these clients, you should refer them to a respiratory therapist or physical therapist. The more impaired an older adult with COPD is, the greater the emphasis should be on interval training techniques (see chapter 13 for a more in-depth discussion of interval training). Some individuals with very low exercise tolerance may find it necessary to exercise for 30 to 60 seconds and then rest for 30 to 60 seconds. As the person's fitness improves, the ratio of work to rest can be manipulated to achieve progressively higher intensity levels.

> Intensity of exercise for people with COPD should be based on RPE because it is a more reliable indicator than heart rate.

In addition to improving breathing efficiency and exercise tolerance, the exercise program for older adults with COPD should address their interests and capabilities with aerobic endurance activities that vary little in oxygen cost. A relatively constant intensity may help prevent dyspnea, which is the number one problem associated with exercise for adults with COPD. Examples of low-variability exercises include walking, recumbent stepping, and stationary cycling. High-variability exercises that should be avoided are calisthenics, dancing, and sports such as basketball and racket sports. Low-intensity weight training is also relatively safe and is generally recommended for people with COPD (Cooper, 2009). The client should feel comfortable lifting the weight and should not hyperventilate or become breathless. Avoid large increases in breathing rate by making sure that the weight is not too heavy and that the client is not holding his or her breath.

Although warm-up and cool-down activities are important components of exercise programs for all individuals, they are particularly important for people with COPD. The goal of the warm-up is to gradually increase heart rate so that the lungs can slowly adjust to the increased workload. If strenuous exercise is started too quickly, there is a higher likelihood of respiratory distress. In addition, make sure the cool-down includes exercises of decreasing intensity (e.g., walking or cycling at a progressively slower rate). The following are exercise guidelines when working with a client with COPD.

- Modify the program (e.g., use interval training or low-intensity activities) on days when the client has difficulty breathing.
- Emphasize good diaphragmatic and pursed-lip breathing during various exercise routines and during the warm-up and cool-down sessions.
- Emphasize strength training for improved muscular strength and increased lean muscle mass.
- Avoid activities that cause dyspnea or hyperventilation.

- Emphasize breathing exercises that target increased pulmonary function.
- Avoid excessively warm or cold environments that may trigger dyspnea.

Teach clients to decrease their breathing frequency and to increase the amount of air they take into their lungs with each breath. Many clients with COPD take shallow breaths and therefore do not get enough oxygen into the pulmonary system, which ultimately leads to increased breathlessness and fatigue. Yoga is an excellent activity for teaching clients appropriate breathing techniques.

Diabetes

Diabetes is a metabolic disorder that results in impaired glucose metabolism. It is a common disorder in older adults. Diabetes prevalence in adults older than 65 years is approximately twice that of younger adults. Additionally, it is estimated that about half of older adults with diabetes are undiagnosed (Kalyani & Egan, 2013). The condition can progressively worsen over time, leading to many other health problems, including loss of vision, heart disease, amputations, stroke, and renal failure. Approximately 56 percent of all medical costs related to diabetes are attributable to older adults (Caspersen, Thomas, Boseman, Beckles, & Albright, 2012).

The two major forms of diabetes, type 1 and type 2, have similar consequences, but people with type 1 diabetes usually experience an earlier onset. Type 1 diabetes is caused by a destruction of pancreatic cells that produce the body's insulin, whereas type 2 diabetes results from insulin resistance combined with defective insulin secretion.

Over 85 percent of people with type 2 diabetes are also overweight or obese (Carnethon, Rasmussen-Torvik, & Palaniappan, 2014). Exercise can have a significant effect on lowering blood glucose and is an essential component of treatment for people with type 1 or type 2 diabetes. Exercise is a central component of diabetes treatment and can have a significant positive impact on body weight, glycemic control, and cardiac risk reduction (Hornsby & Albright, 2009).

Glucose is needed to perform exercise; however, people with diabetes can begin to experience difficulties if their baseline blood glucose level is too high (over 300 milligrams per deciliter) or too low (under 100 milligrams per deciliter). Most diabetes experts recommend that blood glucose levels be lower than 300 milligrams per deciliter (or 250 milligrams per deciliter if ketonic) before exercise is initiated (Colberg et al., 2010). It is important for people with diabetes to maintain the proper balance of food and insulin. High blood glucose values often occur when a person forgets to take his or her oral diabetes medicine or insulin, or has eaten significantly more calories than usual. As a result, glucose is not sufficiently metabolized and controlled. In clients with poor glycemic control, participation in exercise can worsen **hyperglycemia** (high blood glucose) and increase ketosis, which is a by-product of fat metabolism (the lack of insulin needed to facilitate the use of glucose causes the body to metabolize fat instead). A key precaution for clients who have diabetes is to maintain blood glucose levels in a safe range (100 to 250 milligrams per deciliter). People with diabetes should carry a portable **glucometer** with them. This device is inexpensive and can be used to check blood glucose levels before and after exercise.

Another common problem in people with diabetes is hypoglycemia. **Hypoglycemia** is defined as having a blood glucose level less than 60 milligrams per deciliter. Most experts agree that this is an even more dangerous situation than hyperglycemia (high blood glucose) because it can happen very quickly and can lead to an insulin reaction (a medical complication resulting from too much circulating insulin or too little blood glucose). Signs of hypoglycemia are discussed a little later. Physical activity instructors should always keep rapidly absorbed carbohydrates (e.g., orange juice, fruit drinks, or sport gels) on hand in case of an emergency. Blood glucose should be measured after exercise to make sure that the client does not become hypoglycemic. People with recently diagnosed diabetes may need a few sessions to learn how to maintain a normal balance of glucose and insulin before and after exercise.

The intensity, frequency, and duration of exercise should be based on the client's medical history, taking into consideration other conditions that may affect the exercise prescription. Older adults with type 2 diabetes often have hypertension and joint pain as well, thus challenging the physical activity professional to find activities that are both beneficial and enjoyable but do not require intensities beyond the prescribed training zone.

Since it is difficult to maintain an optimal balance of glucose and insulin, clients with diabetes should exercise daily. This does not necessarily mean that the client has to come to the fitness center on a daily basis. There are many activities that can be performed at home. A client may decide to attend a community-based program three days a week and to walk, garden, or use a stationary cycle the remaining days of the week. The key factor is consistency and regular monitoring of blood glucose levels. General information and safety guidelines to follow when working with individuals who have diabetes include the following:

- Regulating blood glucose levels requires optimal timing of exercise periods in relation to meals and insulin dosage.

- Aim to keep blood glucose levels between 100 and 200 milligrams per deciliter when measured one to two hours after a meal.

- Exercise can have a significant effect on insulin reduction. Some experts note that insulin may need to be reduced by 10 to 50 percent when starting an exercise program.

- If blood glucose levels are lower than 100 milligrams per deciliter before exercise, have the person consume a rapidly absorbed carbohydrate to increase blood glucose.

- If blood glucose is greater than 300 milligrams per deciliter before exercise, make sure that insulin or the oral hypoglycemic agent has been taken. Some doctors recommend that exercise not be initiated when blood glucose is greater than 250 milligrams per deciliter.

- No client should be allowed to exercise if his or her blood glucose level is not within a safe range before exercise.

- Teach clients to examine their feet periodically for foot ulcers. If an ulcer is found, have the

Early Symptoms and Treatment of Hypoglycemia

Major Symptoms
- Anxiety, uneasiness
- Irritability
- Extreme hunger
- Confusion
- Headaches

Action to Be Taken
1. Stop the activity immediately.
2. Have the client sit down and check blood glucose level.
3. Have the client drink orange juice or ingest some other rapidly absorbed carbohydrate.
4. Allow the client to rest and wait for a response.
5. When the client feels better, check blood glucose level again.
6. If blood glucose level is above 100 milligrams per deciliter and the client feels better, resume activity. If not, either wait another 5 to 10 minutes and check blood glucose level again or provide additional food.
7. Check blood glucose level after 15 to 30 minutes to ensure that it is still within a safe range.
8. Check blood glucose at the end of the exercise session to make sure that it is greater than 100 milligrams per deciliter before the client leaves the facility.

client consult with a physician immediately for proper treatment. Foot ulcers can worsen and lead to other medical complications if left untreated.

- Check blood glucose at the end of each exercise session to make sure that the client does not become hypoglycemic. This can happen very quickly, particularly after high-intensity or long-duration activities or if the person does not yet understand how his or her body reacts to exercise.

Older people with diabetes usually have one or more coexisting conditions, including coronary artery disease, hyperlipidemia, or hypertension (Hornsby & Albright, 2009). The medications used to treat these conditions can have an adverse effect on blood glucose levels. Thiazide diuretics, used to control hypertension, may induce glucose intolerance by diminishing insulin sensitivity (Rosenstock, 2001).

It is important for older adults participating in exercise programs to maintain good glycemic control. Avoiding hypoglycemia is just as important as avoiding hyperglycemia. The risk for hypoglycemia is a major concern for all individuals with diabetes, but it is a particular concern among older adults and those beginning a new exercise program. Rates of hypoglycemic episodes increase as medication doses used to stabilize glycemic control are increased (Tseng, Soroka, Maney, Aron, & Pogach, 2014), and frail older individuals who use multiple medications are at the greatest risk of drug-associated hypoglycemia. The preceding sidebar lists the major symptoms of hypoglycemia and what to do if a person becomes hypoglycemic.

Musculoskeletal Conditions

The prevalence of arthritis and osteoporosis has increased dramatically in recent decades (Johnson & Hunter, 2014; Modi, Sajjan, & Ghandi, 2014). Because of this it is important that physical activity instructors develop exercise programs that allow individuals with these musculoskeletal conditions to maintain an active lifestyle.

Osteoporosis

Thirty percent of women over the age of 65 are diagnosed with osteoporosis (Dawson-Hughes, 2012). The most commonly cited risk factors are heredity and estrogen deficiency (either aging related or due to hysterectomy; Smith, Wang, & Bloomfield, 2009). The World Health Organization's criterion for a diagnosis of osteoporosis is a spine and hip bone mineral density (BMD) more than 2.5 standard deviations below the mean for young, normal adults of the same sex (also referred to as a T-score; Smith et al., 2009).

In the early stages of osteoporosis, there are often no symptoms. However, as a person reaches his or her 60s and 70s, signs of osteoporosis may develop. As the bones in the spine lose their mineral content, **kyphosis** (a vertebral disorder in the thoracic region of the spine that causes hunching of the spine) often occurs, accompanied by pain and psychological distress.

It is not entirely clear to what extent exercise can improve bone density in postmenopausal women and older individuals. A systematic review conducted by Howe and colleagues (2011) reported that modest but significant increases in bone mass can occur in older, postmenopausal women (Howe et al., 2011). Exercise has other significant benefits for older adults with osteoporosis, including improved balance and stability, which decreases the risk of falling. Postmenopausal women and older adults need to increase their physical activity levels to at least slow or delay the onset of osteoporosis and to possibly make modest improvements in bone mass.

Weight-bearing activities seem to be the most effective terms of preventing or slowing osteoporosis. Clients diagnosed with osteoporosis may benefit if their physical activity instructors obtain detailed recommendations from their physicians for a specific resistance exercise program that will be safe and effective for them. For safety, it is always best to progress slowly using light weights during the first month of the program. Have clients perform one to three sets of 8 to 12 repetitions, depending on their comfort level. Clients with significant osteoporosis (as indicated by their physician) may need to use resistance bands during the early stages of the program. Some weight machines start at too high a resistance and are difficult to get into and out of for some older clients who are frail. After two to three months, progress to heavier resistance bands or light weights. Individuals with advanced osteoporosis require more time to adapt to a resistance-training program and must progress at a much slower rate to avoid injury than do healthy older adults.

Resistance exercises should be performed two to three days a week. If the client has pain, avoid exercises near or over the spine such as back extension and flexion exercises, bent-over rowing, overhead presses, or using weight-training machines that require extensive spinal flexion (e.g., abdominal machines) or extension (e.g., back extension machines). If the client does not have pain, target the muscles in the back with shoulder retraction exercises and shoulder raises. Make sure that the client performs the movements slowly and does not feel pain. These exercises also improve posture (many older adults become round-shouldered as they age) and load the vertebrae, potentially maintaining or hypothetically increasing bone density.

Older people with osteoporosis may have difficulty performing repetitive exercises using the same muscle groups for extended periods of time. Therefore, circuit-training programs that require short periods of work using various muscle groups are recommended. In addition to circuit training, interval-training activities that require brief periods of work followed by a rest interval may also be beneficial for deconditioned clientele with advanced osteoporosis. For example, riding a stationary bike for one minute followed by a 30-second rest interval may delay fatigue and allow the client to sustain longer periods of activity.

Other cardiovascular activities can be used to improve functional performance, provided they do not lead to pain or result in premature fatigue. Although swimming and aquatic exercises are excellent modalities for improving cardiovascular endurance, they are not recommended for maintaining or improving bone density. Water is a non-weight-bearing environment and does not seem to place a sufficient stress load on bone tissue to increase its mass (Becker, 2009).

Flexibility exercises are safe for people with osteoporosis, unless they are experiencing pain in a region of the body that is prone to fracture (e.g., hip, spine, wrist). Avoid flexibility exercises that cause pain in any of these areas. Although flexibility exercises do not lead to improvements in bone mass, they are very important for improving posture,

relieving muscle tightness, and maintaining good mobility. People with osteoporosis often become very inflexible in the chest and neck muscles as a result of stooped posture. Avoid exercises such as the bench press that promote forward head and shoulder position and shorten chest musculature, and instead use exercises that open the chest by retracting the scapula (e.g., pectoral stretch performed on an exercise ball). Modifying the grip and exercise technique of certain exercises can also facilitate better posture and alignment (e.g., have the client adopt a supinated hand position and avoid front pull-down movements except for lat pull-downs on a machine). The hip flexors should also be stretched, since these muscles become tight in older adults from sitting for long periods and walking with a stooped posture. General information and guidelines for working with older adults with osteoporosis include the following:

- Know the visible signs of osteoporosis (e.g., kyphosis, recent fracture), and develop an appropriate strength and flexibility program for affected areas with physician input.

- Physician input is important when developing a new exercise program for a client in the advanced stages of osteoporosis.

- Avoid jarring and high-load exercises for clients with osteoporosis.

- When older clients who have a high risk of falls or fractures perform standing exercises, make sure they have something to hold on to at all times (e.g., ballet barre, parallel bars, chair).

- Reevaluate the program if the client experiences any pain or fatigue in the osteoporosis zones (hips, back, or wrists) during or after an exercise session.

Arthritis

The two major types of arthritis are osteoarthritis and rheumatoid arthritis. **Osteoarthritis (OA)**, previously referred to as degenerative joint disease, is the most prevalent form of arthritis in the United States (Johnson & Hunter, 2014). OA results in a thinning of the articular cartilage on the outside of bones in diarthrodial (freely moveable) joints. Symptoms of osteoarthritis include pain, morning stiffness, and decreased range of motion in the affected joints.

Many older adults have a hip or knee replacement after living with arthritis for several decades. Joint replacement is one option when the chronic pain cannot be controlled through medication, assistive aids, or exercise and when the pain and decreased range of motion in the affected joint interfere with the person's ability to ambulate (Stevens, Reininga, Bulstra, Wagenmakers, & van den Akker-Scheek, 2012). After the client completes physical therapy, exercises to improve strength and range of motion are important.

The post joint-replacement exercise protocol can follow a plan similar to that described for arthritis. The only difference is that more attention should be devoted to strength and range-of-motion exercises for strengthening and stretching the muscles supporting the affected joints, in accordance with the physical therapy plan prescribed for the individual. It is important that you maintain an active dialogue with the client's physical therapist or physician to ensure that the treatment plan is progressing smoothly.

Rheumatoid arthritis (RA) is more common in women than in men. It may begin early or later in life. Symptoms include chronic inflammation in the affected joints, pain, morning stiffness (lasting longer than with osteoarthritis), and swelling in the affected joints (Gibofsky, 2012). Osteoarthritis is a "wear and tear" disorder, while rheumatoid arthritis is a whole-body autoimmune disease, in which the body's own immune system attacks healthy tissue. Both disease types have joint-destroying properties and similar treatment strategies, including exercise (Knittle, De Gucht, & Maes, 2012). Most people with arthritis can benefit from an exercise program in a number of ways, including reduced pain and fatigue, improved fitness, and increased ability to perform various physical tasks independently (Bennell, Dobson, & Hinman, 2014; Iversen, Brawerman, & Iversen, 2012; Knittle et al., 2012).

A major emphasis of the exercise program for people with arthritis is to mitigate pain during activity. The program must not place excessive loads around damaged joints. For people who have been sedentary for a long time, starting slowly is very important. Low-impact, non-weight-bearing activities are recommended. The client may have to learn to tolerate some pain or discomfort.

However, pain should be minimized in every way possible, including using braces or straps, applying ice or heat before and after exercise, isolating the damaged joint during exercise, doing water-based exercises, and avoiding overuse of the damaged joint.

Exercise machines that allow the use of all four limbs simultaneously seem to have the most benefit for people with arthritis, since the load is evenly distributed across all the limbs. Examples of machines that involve all four limbs include certain brands of recumbent steppers, which are used in a seated position, stationary upright bikes, and elliptical or cross-trainer machines, which are used while standing. General exercise guidelines for people with arthritis include the following:

- Discontinue any exercise that causes pain during or after exercise.

- Find alternative ways to exercise muscles around painful joints. For example, straight-leg exercises are a good way to strengthen the leg muscles around a painful knee.

- Warm-ups and cool-downs are essential components of all exercise programs but are especially important for people with arthritis because of joint stiffness.

- Resistance training should be prescribed, but exercises that cause pain to a particular joint should be replaced with isometric strength exercises.

- For water-based exercise, try to maintain water temperature between 85 and 90 degrees Fahrenheit (29-32 °C).

- Encourage smooth, repetitive movements during all activities.

- Keep the exercise intensity below the discomfort threshold.

- Be aware that people with rheumatoid arthritis can experience acute flare-ups. Exercise may not be advisable until the flare-up subsides.

- Clients with osteoarthritis often perform better in the morning, whereas clients with rheumatoid arthritis may be better off exercising several hours after awakening.

- Use cross-training to avoid overuse of certain joints.

Neurological and Cognitive Conditions

Two of the most commonly observed neurological conditions in older adults are Parkinson's disease and Alzheimer's disease. Both of these conditions are progressive and often result in declining physical and cognitive function. The course and rate of progression of these disorders vary by individual.

Parkinson's Disease

Parkinson's disease is a progressive neurological disorder that in adults aged 65 and older is expected to increase in prevalence by over 70 percent by the year 2030 (Dorsey, George, Leff, & Willis, 2013). Individuals with Parkinson's disease often experience the following symptoms: **bradykinesia** (slowness of movement), muscle rigidity, resting tremor, postural instability, and impaired balance control (Stanley & Protas, 2002).

One of the hallmark signs of Parkinson's disease is an abnormal gait pattern that is characterized by increasingly short but quicker steps. This is sometimes referred to as *festinating gait* (Ebersbach, Moreau, Gandor, Defebvre, & Devos, 2013). The gait pattern makes it appear as if the person is trying to catch up with someone in front of him or her, but he or she does so by leaning forward at the waist first before taking any steps. Once movement does occur, short, shuffling steps are taken. This condition is associated with disequilibrium, which is the inability to readjust the center of mass quickly enough to prevent a fall. As a result, many individuals with Parkinson's disease are susceptible to falling, so it is important to protect these individuals from falls during class.

Ways to prevent falls include having the client perform exercises while seated in a chair, having the client lightly hold on to a ballet barre or wall rail during standing activities, and supervising the client closely during exercises that require him or her to move around the facility or transfer between different exercise machines. Activities for clients with Parkinson's disease should include slow, controlled movements through various ranges of motion while lying, sitting, standing, and walking. There is emerging evidence that tai chi is beneficial in improving balance and gait in persons with Parkinson's disease and many other patient populations (Gillespie et al., 2012; van der Kolk & King, 2013). Caution must be taken if aerobic exercise is performed on a treadmill. If a treadmill is prescribed for aerobic exercise, the client should be supervised at all times or wear a harness to prevent a fall due to loss of balance. Aerobic activities performed in a sitting position, such as stationary cycling, recumbent stepping, or arm cycling, are usually safer modalities for this clientele.

Alzheimer's Disease

Alzheimer's disease (AD) is a progressive neurological disorder resulting in impaired mental function. It is the most common cause of dementia among older adults. The number of adults diagnosed with AD is expected to increase fourfold by 2050. In the United States alone, AD is associated with over $170 billion in health care costs per year (Reitz & Mayeux, 2014). Individuals with AD often experience severe declines in cognition and moderate to severe balance impairments. AD is marked by progressive, irreversible declines in memory, performance of routine tasks, temporal and spatial orientation, language and communication skills, and abstract thinking accompanied by personality changes and impairment of judgment.

Implementing an exercise training program for individuals with AD poses three major challenges: (1) addressing problems arising from the declining physical and mental health of the participant, (2) accommodating behavioral changes that may cause the client to become agitated with the exercise program or in the exercise setting, and (3) dealing with a caregiver's unwillingness to continue bringing the client to the exercise program as the disease progresses.

The cornerstone of an exercise program for this population is consistency and patience. The physical activity professional must constantly provide verbal encouragement and support to maintain the client's interest in the program. Many people with Alzheimer's disease are uncomfortable participating in new activities; therefore, it is important for the exercise leader to use behavioral modification techniques to increase compliance. (See chapter 7 for a discussion of behavioral management techniques.) It may also be necessary to have the client's spouse or caregiver attend the program to provide a familiar face.

Summary

When designing exercise programs for older adults with medical conditions and disabilities, the same general guidelines for programs for healthy older adults apply. However, additional disease- or disability-specific exercise guidelines and precautions must be followed to ensure a safe and effective program. It is important to understand the general underlying mechanisms associated with each disabling condition and, when necessary, to consult with rehabilitation professionals, such as physical and occupational therapists, about concerns regarding specific disabling conditions. Moreover, do not hesitate to contact the client's physician if you have questions about the client's condition.

Perhaps your single most important task when working with clients with physical or cognitive disabilities is to thoroughly familiarize yourself with their specific functional abilities and limitations and understand how their health condition may limit their ability to perform certain exercises. Many older clients have multiple disabilities that often interact with each other (e.g., depression, osteoporosis, heart disease), and each of these conditions and their interactions must be taken into consideration when developing an exercise prescription.

Key Terms

Alzheimer's disease (AD)

bradykinesia

bronchitis

chronic obstructive pulmonary disease (COPD)

coronary heart disease (CHD)

dyspnea

emphysema

exercise-induced asthma

functional muscle mass

glucometer

hemiplegia

hyperglycemia

hypertension

hypoglycemia

kyphosis

osteoarthritis (OA)

paralysis

Parkinson's disease

postexercise hypotension

rheumatoid arthritis (RA)

stroke

Recommended Readings

American College of Sports Medicine. (2009). *ACSM's exercise management for persons with chronic diseases and disabilities* (3rd ed.). Champaign, IL: Human Kinetics.

American College of Sports Medicine. (2009). *ACSM's resources for clinical exercise physiology: Musculoskeletal, neuromuscular, neoplastic, immunologic, and hematologic conditions* (2nd ed.). Philadelphia: Lippincott Williams & Wilkins.

National Center on Health, Physical Activity and Disability. www.NCHPAD.org

Study Questions

1. Currently, the third leading cause of death in the United States is
   a. heart disease
   b. stroke
   c. multiple sclerosis
   d. pulmonary disorders

2. A primary symptom characteristic of Parkinson's disease is

   a. postural hypotension

   b. bradykinesia

   c. irregular breathing

   d. impaired vision

3. Hypoglycemia occurs when blood glucose falls below

   a. 60 milligrams per deciliter

   b. 80 milligrams per deciliter

   c. 100 milligrams per deciliter

   d. 120 milligrams per deciliter

4. A longer warm-up phase is recommended for clients who have

   a. Alzheimer's disease

   b. osteoporosis

   c. coronary heart disease

   d. Parkinson's disease

5. According to the World Health Organization, the criterion for a diagnosis of osteoporosis is a spinal bone mineral density of more than ___ standard deviations below the mean for young, normal adults of the same sex.

   a. 1.5

   b. 2.5

   c. 3.5

   d. 4

6. Clients who are taking _____ often avoid ingesting fluids during exercise because of the increased need to void their bladders.

   a. beta-blockers

   b. calcium channel blockers

   c. benzodiazepine

   d. diuretics

Application Activities

1. Diabetes is prevalent among older adults. Prepare a five-minute presentation that you will deliver in the community about the benefits of exercise for people with diabetes to recruit more participants into your program.

2. Clients with arthritis often have pain during movement. List specific activities you should prescribe to mitigate pain and help the client have a more successful exercise experience.

Legal Standards, Risk Management, and Professional Ethics

Debra J. Rose

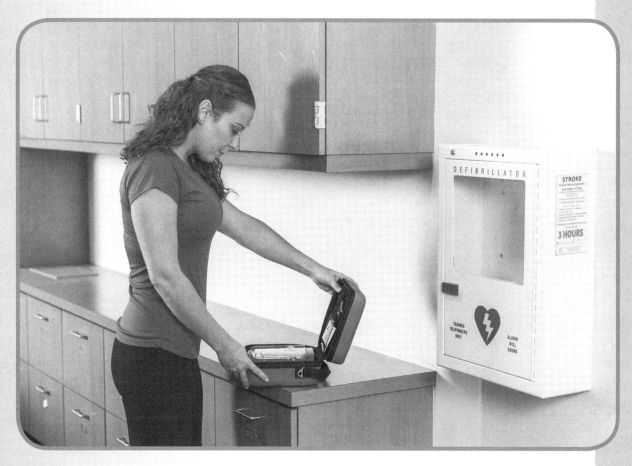

Objectives

After completing this chapter, you will be able to

1. differentiate between negligence and product liability legal cases and identify the parties involved in a lawsuit,
2. discuss the legal concept of standard of care as it applies to physical activity instructors,
3. understand and explain the difference between guidelines and standards,
4. articulate and apply professional standards to program design and management,
5. understand how to develop a risk management plan to promote a safe exercise environment and respond to emergency situations, and
6. understand and comply with ethical guidelines for personal trainers and group instructors.

In the 1980s, a lady named Ann sued a fitness club and one of its instructors for injuries suffered as a result of a training session. Ann was a private secretary and engaged in minimal physical activity. She joined the club because it advertised special expertise with adults over the age of 40 years and new to exercise. The first day, her instructor had her complete a series of strength-training exercises on various pieces of equipment. While working on one of the machines, she felt a pain in her neck and upper back. She told the instructor, who replied, "No pain, no gain," and had her continue exercising. When Ann got home, she was in great pain, to the point that she was unable to go to work the next day. Her doctor's examination revealed that she had suffered a significant injury to her neck and upper back, which he attributed to the incident at the club the day before. Ann was required to wear a cervical collar and was told to stay home from work for at least 10 days. Does Ann have grounds for a lawsuit against the fitness club and instructor?

The purpose of this chapter is to provide physical activity instructors of older adults with the necessary knowledge to minimize the risk of injuries to their clients and to help them avoid being part of a scenario like the one just described, thereby minimizing the risk of becoming involved in a lawsuit. The first section of this chapter defines a number of important legal terms associated with a lawsuit and the important elements of a negligence case. Other

topics covered in this chapter include the components of a risk management plan (facility standards and guidelines, injury and medical emergency prevention, responding to emergency situations) and professional ethics for personal trainers and group instructors.

The Law and the Physical Activity Instructor

In a lawsuit, the injured party bringing the action is the **plaintiff**, and the party accused of having caused the injury is the **defendant**. In the event of an injury resulting from fitness training, the most common case is brought by the client against the physical activity instructor, the fitness facility, or both for **negligence**. If a piece of equipment is involved, the client may also bring a case against the product manufacturer for product liability, alleging (claiming) that injury was caused by a defect in the manufacture or design of the equipment or a failure to warn of risks, which makes the equipment unreasonably dangerous. **Defenses** (legal reasons for limiting a defendant's liability) that may be viable include **assumption of risk** (the client knowingly and voluntarily assumed the risk inherent to the activity) and **comparative negligence** (the client's actions were part of the cause of the damages so that liability is distributed in proper shares to the parties to the action).

To win a negligence case, the plaintiff must prove four elements: The defendant owed a **duty** to the plaintiff to use reasonable care to avoid risk of injury, that duty was **breached**, the breach caused the injury (**causation**), and the breach resulted in legally recognized **damages** to the plaintiff. In Ann's case, the fitness facility and the instructor both owed Ann a duty to use reasonable care to avoid risk of injury. That duty was breached when they failed to meet the standard of care. The specific breaches of each defendant are discussed later in this chapter when we revisit Ann's case.

Standard of Care

As a physical activity instructor, your duty to use reasonable care is based on a legal **standard of care**. That standard is based on a reasonably prudent physical activity instructor, which means you must have the knowledge, training, skill, and education (ability and competence) of an ordinary member of your profession in good standing. That is, you must know what is expected of a physical activity instructor of older adults in good standing. It would not be appropriate, for example, to advise clients on such topics as family problems, nutrition, or medications unless you have additional credentials (e.g., licensed counselor, dietitian, physician).

A number of nationally published guidelines and standards are available and should be carefully reviewed by physical activity instructors (see the recommended readings at the end of the chapter). It is important to understand the difference between guidelines and standards. **Guidelines** are usually recommendations or suggestions, while **standards** are required procedures that may indicate a legal duty. In a lawsuit, nationally published standards may be introduced as evidence to establish the standard of care to which you or a fitness facility may be held.

Examples of a breach of a physical activity instructor's standard of care might include the following (American College of Sports Medicine, 2012):

- Designing a program that contains inappropriate exercises or an unsatisfactory progression of exercises

- Utilizing inappropriate equipment
- Providing inadequate instruction or supervision
- Neglecting to screen a client before he or she begins an exercise program
- Not having the required expertise to train a client

Examples of a breach of a health or fitness facility's standard of care include these:

- Allowing inadequate maintenance of equipment by the facility
- Allowing facility employees to take inadequate precautions to ensure client safety, such as not providing safe equipment layout and traffic patterns and not having sufficient security
- Not having a **risk management plan (RMP)**
- Not ensuring adequate staff training
- Employing unqualified staff
- Distributing false or misleading advertising
- Not having an emergency plan in place

If the plaintiff fails to prove that the breach of duty caused legally recognized damages, one of the essential elements of negligence is missing and the case will not be successful.

The *standard of care* to which you are held is that of a reasonably prudent physical activity instructor, which means that you must have the knowledge, training, skill, and education (ability and competence) of an ordinary member of your profession in good standing.

Minimizing Risk of Exposure to Legal Problems

To minimize your risk of exposure to legal problems, you must work within your personal bounds of competence. In other words, you must only offer or perform services that fall within the scope of your expertise. Therefore, your education, training, experience, and skill determine the standard of care to which you are held. You are responsible for knowing and adhering to the guidelines and standards established for your profession. Remember, the key in a negligence case is whether you acted *reasonably* to protect your client from risk of injury under the circumstances, based on your expertise. If you fail to follow procedures that you are reasonably expected to know and follow as a physical activity instructor, you are exposing yourself to the possibility of legal problems.

The following sections offer several suggestions to help physical activity instructors and personal trainers avoid litigation if a client sustains an injury or dies. These suggestions are largely based on published standards and guidelines from the American College of Sports Medicine (American College of Sports Medicine, 2012; Riebe et al., 2015) and the National Strength and Conditioning Association (National Strength and Conditioning Association Professional Standards and Guidelines Task Force, 2009), and my own experience as both a director of a university-based center that provides exercise programming for older adults and prepares students for careers working with older adults in physical activity and rehabilitation settings and a kinesiologist with more than 30 years' experience designing and delivering physical activity programs to older adults ranging from the very frail to the very fit. Several of these suggestions also help you provide a safe and effective environment for your clients. A more detailed discussion of injury and medical emergency prevention is discussed later in the chapter.

Facility and Equipment

Here are three suggestions to ensure your facility provides safe equipment:

1. Purchase equipment that is of commercial quality and includes older adult friendly features (e.g., longer handrails on treadmills, visible and easy to use adjustment features, easy entry and exit features).

2. Be sure that equipment is properly set up and regularly inspected and maintained and that safety signage is clearly visible where appropriate.

3. Develop a written risk management plan and make sure that it is readily available and posted in the facility. This topic is discussed in more detail later in the chapter.

Instructor

The following list contains several ways to reduce your risk of liability as an instructor of physical activity with older adults:

- Be sure you are adequately and properly educated, certified, and experienced to train within the sphere of expertise in which you are practicing. If you do not know something, acknowledge it and seek guidance from a more qualified professional or mentor, or do the necessary research to find the answers.

- Obtain or keep current your training and certification in cardiopulmonary resuscitation (CPR) and first aid.

- Continue your education. Regularly attend conferences or workshops related to your profession in order to update your knowledge, and keep any certifications current.

- Have a written emergency response plan readily available, and practice with your staff in responding to different types of emergency situations.

- Keep a written or electronic training record of each personal training or group session you conduct and a permanent file for each client. The file should contain the client's health history, signed medical release (where appropriate), a signed participant consent form, a copy of the client's training record, documentation of any changes in medical conditions or medications, and written notes of any conversations with the client or his or her physician. Any other client information should be included and treated as confidential unless you have written permission to share the information. This information may later be used as evidence in a lawsuit. It is important never to disclose a client's personal information without his or her written permission. Keep client files confidential at all times and filed in a locked cabinet or in an encrypted form on a secure laptop computer.

- Instruct your clients in the proper use of equipment or techniques for any exercise, warn them of inherent risks, and provide continuous supervision.

- Be aware of potential conflicts of interest. As a physical activity instructor, you are building a relationship of trust with your clients. Your recommendations regarding supplements, diet, and weight loss or gain may be seriously considered by your client. Using your position of trust to market or sell products or other services (insurance, financial planning, and so on) may be contrary to your responsibility to watch out for the best interests of your clients. If you engage in another activity resulting in financial gain to you or your employer, disclose the potential conflict in a written document and have your clients sign the document to show that they have been notified of the potential conflict.

- Avoid any appearance of sexual harassment. When teaching a new exercise, either demonstrate it yourself or ask permission first before touching the client. Also avoid saying anything that can be construed as inappropriate (such as jokes or innuendos). Do not assume because your client is the same sex as you that a risqué comment or joke is OK.

- Do not tolerate sexual harassment by a client. Never assume that age precludes sexual harassment. Reaching a certain chronological age does not necessarily mean that a person has lost interest in sex or an understanding of sexual overtones. You, as the instructor, must establish what is acceptable behavior for both you and your clients. If a client is acting or dressing inappropriately, first try talking with the client. If that fails, be prepared to withdraw as the instructor. If this occurs in a group situation in a facility and talking to the client does not help, discuss the matter with your supervisor before proceeding. You may also want to discuss it with your attorney. It may be necessary to ask the client, in private, to drop the class. A follow-up letter may also be needed. If so, keep a copy in the client file, along with a written record of the dates and circumstances of, and any witnesses to, the sexual harassment.

- Purchase malpractice insurance. Some organizations offer professional trainer liability policies. Ask your certifying agency for a recommendation. Carefully read the policy to understand what is covered and what is excluded. A policy may provide an *aggregate* coverage of $1.5 million, with *each occurrence* covered up to $500,000. Discuss these limits with your insurance agent so that you understand them.

- Consult with an attorney. If you have questions about potential liability related to training older adults, consult with an attorney before

a problem occurs. An ounce of prevention is definitely worth a pound of cure.

- Never photograph or videotape a client without first providing full disclosure of how the client's likeness will be used and obtaining his or her written consent.

- If you utilize music in your group classes make sure that it has been obtained legally through a licensed vendor or website (e.g., Dynamix, Power Beats, Fitbeatmusic).

- Exercise caution when posting anything to social media (Facebook, LinkedIn, and so on) related to advertising your class or services. It is much too easy to infringe on existing copyrights or trademarks if you are careless with your wording or post photographs of a client without first obtaining his or her permission.

Participant

As discussed in chapter 5, it is important that you interview your clients individually and have them complete a health history and consent form before the start of the program. Have the clients read, sign, and date the consent form, and make it part of the client's file. The health history should disclose any physical limitations, problems, illnesses, diseases, and medications. This information forms the basis of your program design. The consent form should include both an agreement that the client will immediately let you know if he or she is feeling any pain or discomfort and a warning about the potential risks inherent in an exercise program. If you need to talk to the client's physician, be sure to obtain written authorization from the client.

Negligence Case Example

Let us now return to the case study presented in the beginning of the chapter involving Ann and her lawsuit for negligence against the instructor and the fitness facility. Ann's case alleged negligence on the part of the fitness club for failing to meet the standard of care of a reasonably prudent fitness facility. This was evidenced by the following:

- Hiring unqualified staff
- Allowing inadequate staff instruction on using equipment and in working with special populations

- Not having a risk management plan
- Not having requirements for continuing education of staff
- Distributing false and misleading advertising

In this case, the instructor had no credentials to work as a fitness trainer. When hired, she claimed that she had previously taught group aerobics at a community college. On the basis of this knowledge the club provided her with only cursory instruction on the resistance-training equipment, provided no training on how to instruct special populations (i.e., sedentary adults over 40 years of age), failed to have a risk management plan in place or to provide instruction on how to respond to complaints of pain from a client, and had falsely advertised special expertise with adults over 40 and new to exercise.

The **allegations** (assertions or claims of a party to a lawsuit) against the fitness instructor evidencing her failure to meet the standard of care included the following:

- Not requiring the client to complete a health history questionnaire, waiver, and assumption of risk form before starting the training program
- Not being properly trained to work with this client
- Not being current in her education yet representing herself as a fully qualified strength and conditioning instructor
- Not recommending appropriate exercises for the age and physical condition of the client
- Not choosing appropriate exercise equipment

Before the case went to trial, it was settled. This was in the 1980s. The standard of care was not as clear as it is today because there were fewer published standards and guidelines, certifying agencies, and educational opportunities for professionals interested in working with adults in physical activity settings. Now there is virtually no excuse for a case like Ann's to happen. If you ignore the standards and guidelines that have been established for health and fitness facilities, forgo the education necessary, or work outside your personal bounds of competence, you may find yourself involved in legal action.

> Always operate within your personal bounds of competence, follow the standards and guidelines that have been established for health and fitness facilities, and pursue the education necessary within your field to avoid potential legal action being taken against you.

Risk Management Plans

No matter how well trained you are as a physical activity instructor of older adults, an injury or health-related emergency is bound to happen if you teach long enough, especially when your clients are frail older adults. Unfortunately, many fitness and wellness facilities do not have a comprehensive risk management plan. Such a plan can help you to promote a safer exercise environment for your clients, more effectively respond to emergency situations, and minimize your risk for legal ramifications. If the facility where you work does not have a risk management plan, you should recommend that the facility purchase the *ACSM's Health/Fitness Facility Standards and Guidelines, Fourth Edition* (American College of Sports Medicine, 2012). This section of the chapter provides some resources to help you develop your own risk management plan, including some basic injury and medical emergency prevention and response procedures.

Health and Fitness Facility Standards and Guidelines

The *ACSM's Health/Fitness Facility Standards and Guidelines, Fourth Edition* (American College of Sports Medicine, 2012) contains six standards that represent the standard of care that must be followed by all health and fitness facilities; it also contains more than 500 guidelines. It is important to meet five of the six standards that apply specifically to providing a safe exercise environment for your older adult clients; courts allow these standards to be introduced as evidence of the standard of care (i.e., legal duties) in negligence cases (Eickhoff-Shemek, Herbert, & Connaughton, 2009). Facilities offering physical activity classes for older adults can develop a comprehensive risk management plan by referring to the ACSM's publication.

The five ACSM standards that apply to working with older adults are as follows:

1. Be able to respond in a timely manner to any emergency event, and post a written emergency response plan that is known to all personnel and that includes periodic emergency response drills for all staff. (More on this topic is provided later in the chapter.)

2. Administer a preactivity screening to each participant to ensure safe programs. Chapter 5 provides detailed information on this topic.

3. Require instructors to demonstrate professional competence, including a current CPR card and certification in first aid.

4. Post instructions on equipment use, and post warnings of any relevant risks.

5. Follow all relevant laws, regulations, and published standards.

Facilities can also minimize equipment-related injuries and subsequent liability by installing equipment in accordance with the manufacturers' or sellers' instructions, inspecting equipment prior to installation, providing initial and ongoing user instruction and supervision, establishing a regular schedule for the inspection and maintenance of equipment, and having a set of procedures in place for the prompt removal of defective and potentially dangerous equipment (Eickhoff-Shemek et al., 2009).

Injury and Medical Emergency Prevention

A comprehensive risk management plan should also address injury and medical emergency procedures. Chapter 17 discussed safety precautions and strategies for adapting exercises for older adults with chronic medical problems. The following additional 10 strategies are provided to help you design a safe and effective exercise environment that minimizes clients' risk of injury or medical emergency:

- Conduct a preexercise health screening and assessment of all participants (see chapters 5 and 6). Preexercise and health screenings help determine which clients (1) would find your

class suitable to their needs and goals, *or* (2) would be better served attending a different class, *or* (3) should be referred back to their physicians for additional testing to determine whether it is safe to exercise and at what level.

- If you are considering accepting clients who are at a moderate to high risk for an adverse event while exercising (e.g., cardiac arrest), it is imperative that you conduct a preactivity cardiovascular screening (American College of Sports Medicine, 2012; Springer, Eickhoff-Shemek, & Zuberbuehler, 2009) prior to enrollment, and monitor and record blood pressure and heart rate (using a heart rate monitor or the CR10 Rating of Perceived Exertion scale) before exercise and, if necessary, several times during the exercise session.

- People with diabetes should bring their own portable glucometers to the fitness center and measure blood glucose before and after each exercise session. Orange juice and other high-carbohydrate snacks should be available for those participants who become hypoglycemic (glucose level below 60 milligrams per deciliter).

- An infectious waste container for blood specimens should be available for clients who must check their blood glucose levels. Blood specimens should be obtained in a clean setting, away from equipment and high-volume traffic areas. Floors where blood specimens are taken should be washed daily with bleach and water.

- Make every effort to prevent clients from experiencing prolonged or unusual fatigue or delayed-onset muscle soreness. Although this is a common side effect of participation in any new exercise program, soreness and fatigue can prevent older adults from completing their normal activities of daily living.

- Be observant of warning signs of heart distress (e.g., chest pain, irregular pulse, difficulty breathing, and dizziness). If any of these symptoms occur, exercise should be stopped immediately and the client's doctor notified.

- To protect clients from heat-related medical problems, monitor the temperature in the exercise area. If there is no thermostat, have one installed.

- Class participants should wear properly fitted athletic shoes with sturdy arch support and soles that provide ample cushioning (although thickly cushioned shoes are contraindicated for older adults with balance problems and sensation loss in the feet). For outdoor exercise, clients should be encouraged to wear protective sunscreen, sunglasses, and hats or visors.

- Encourage participants to wear multiple layers of lightweight clothing that can be removed as body temperature rises during exercise and then replaced as the body cools.

- Participants should be taught how to rate their own perceived exertion, use equipment safely, and understand the warning signs for when to stop exercising. These warning signs, listed in the consent form in chapter 5, should be reviewed with all participants, but especially those who have a diagnosis of coronary heart disease. Once the participant understands these warning signs and can repeat them back to the instructor, both parties should sign the form. This ensures that the client has a basic understanding of how to watch for these warning signs.

Creating a Safe Environment

Physical activity instructors who teach groups of older adults are especially challenged to provide safe environments when their participants have a variety of medical problems. It can be even more difficult to provide a safe and effective exercise environment for clients who are visually or hearing impaired. Clients with visual impairments must exercise in a safe environment that protects them from falls and related injuries.

Following are safety guidelines for establishing a safe instructional environment for older adults with visual and hearing problems:

- Two major obstacles for sight-challenged participants are glare and dim lighting. With proper lighting, mirrored walls may help participants see the instructor's movement demonstrations. In large classes, teaching from a raised platform can also help participants more easily follow the workout.

- Participants with visual or hearing impairments should never be in the back row. Positioning participants with visual problems toward the front of the class maximizes their view of the instructor's movements. Also, review clients' health histories to determine the exact nature of their visual impairments for a better understanding of what they can and cannot see.

- People who are visually impaired often do not see objects in their path and can easily trip over equipment that is not stored properly. Make sure that all equipment is stored after use and that no obstacles are left along travel routes.

- Use specific directional signs around the facility, and mark the routes to different areas with bright colors to make them easier to follow.

- Speak slowly and clearly, and try to make verbal instructions easy to understand.

- Any written materials that you distribute should be typed in large print for individuals who have difficulty reading standard-size print or recorded on audiotape for individuals who are blind.

Hearing impairments are common among older adults. It is imperative that all clients understand the proper way to exercise, signs and symptoms of overexertion, and any other instructions necessary for a safe and effective environment. Here is a list of things you can do to provide a safer environment for older adults with hearing problems:

- Use visual cues when giving instructions (e.g., pictures of the exercises, demonstrations).

- Project your voice, but without a simultaneous rise in pitch.

- Be sure to face the client so that he or she has a clear view of your face. Some clients with limited hearing may be able to read lips or interpret facial expressions and thus be able to understand your spoken directions.

- Find out if the person has better hearing in one ear and speak to the client on the side with better hearing. Background noises can be very distracting. If a person is having difficulty understanding something you are trying to explain, it may be a good idea to move to a quiet area where there is no background noise.

- Speak slowly (but not too slowly) and clearly. Enunciate your words, but do not exaggerate your lip movements; some clients may read lips so you should form words naturally. Speaking too fast or slurring words can also make it difficult for an older adult with hearing loss to understand you. It may be necessary to repeat instructions. Do not shout at the client. Shouting distorts the sound and makes it even more difficult to understand instructions.

- For participants who use hearing aids, excessive volume results in an unpleasant cacophony of competing sounds. In fact, loud music hinders most participants' abilities to follow verbal instructions. To determine the optimal music volume, ask for feedback from your clients while simultaneously observing their performance. Some participants may prefer instrumental tunes so the instructor's voice does not have to compete with music lyrics.

Responding to an Emergency Situation

An essential part of a risk management plan is establishing and maintaining policies and response procedures for handling emergencies. In your capacity as a physical activity instructor, the standard of care as a reasonably prudent instructor may include the following:

- Having a current certification in CPR
- Knowing how to administer basic first aid
- Obtaining a complete health history from your client so that you know what types of health problems may be present
- Consulting with the client's physician if you have questions about the safety of a program you have designed
- Knowing the signs and symptoms of a particular health problem
- Knowing the response needed for a particular problem (e.g., if your client has diabetes, what to do if he or she feels faint)
- Knowing the location of the nearest telephone for contacting emergency personnel

Following are some policies and procedures to respond to an emergency situation.

- Having a written emergency plan is essential. Figure 18.1 provides an example of an emergency plan. If you work for a facility that does not have emergency procedures in place, it places you at risk for being liable.

- You should have immediate access to each client's permanent file, which includes his or her medical history and whom to contact in case of an emergency.

- Identify the telephone closest to the exercise area and near the phone post a clear sign with the first responders' emergency contact number and directions to the facility. Post similar signs at various areas in the facility so people can use their mobile phones to calls. An example is provided in figure 18.2.

- After an emergency or injury, be sure to complete an accident form similar to the one provided in figure 18.3. Completing such a form documents what procedures were taken during the incident or injury and helps to protect you in a liability case.

- Many health and fitness facilities now routinely use **automated emergency defibrillators (AEDs)**. In fact, according to Abbott (2012), where there has been an event in which a participant dies, the primary litigation against fitness facilities results from the facility not having an **emergency response plan (ERP)** and no available AED. In facilities where older adults exercise, an AED is strongly recommended, even if a heart attack is a rare occurrence. An AED works by delivering a controlled electric shock to the heart, forcing all of the heart muscles to contract at once and,

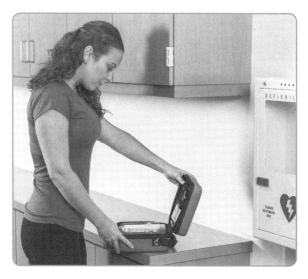

It is important to regularly check the batteries on your Automated Emergency Defibrillator (AED) to make sure it is ready for use in case of an emergency.

In the event of an emergency when no medical personnel are present, these guidelines should be followed:

1. A staff person trained in CPR should identify himself or herself. This helps to reassure the victim and bystanders. If the victim is conscious, legally you must ask permission to assist the victim. (The law assumes that an unconscious person would give consent.) A senior staff person should stay with the individual at all times. The staff person should attempt to reassure the victim and protect him or her from personal bodily harm. The senior staff person should assume control of the situation and issue further orders as needed.

2. A second staff member should call 9-1-1 (or, outside the United States, your local first responders' emergency number). Please review specific emergency procedures and directions posted near the phones.

3. The victim should be monitored at all times:
   a. Check heart rate, noting the regularity and strength of each heart beat.
   b. Monitor and record blood pressure.
   c. Observe skin color and breathing pattern.
   d. Maintain an open airway.
   e. Establish unresponsiveness and initiate CPR when appropriate.
   f. Before the individual is transported (if unconscious), give the emergency medical technicians (EMTs) as much information as possible regarding the individual:
      • Name
      • Age
      • Medical considerations
      • Home phone number
      • Emergency phone numbers
      • Physician
   g. Ask EMTs the hospital to which the member will be transported.

4. Once the individual is transported, the senior staff person in charge should do the following:
   a. Notify the director and request that the participant's emergency contacts be notified.
   b. Assume responsibility for the individual's personal belongings and valuables. Please remember that it is important to respect the individual's privacy. Be as brief as possible when disclosing information pertinent to the event.
   c. Immediately fill out an accident report, and file one copy in the member's folder and one copy with the center's director.

FIGURE 18.1 Emergency plan.

From Centers for Disease Control and Prevention, *Promoting Active Lifestyles Among Older Adults. National Center for Chronic Disease Prevention and Health Promotion. Nutrition and Physical activity.* (2002). http://www.cdc.gov/nccdphp/dnpa/physical/lifestyles.htm

---

Emergency Procedures and Directions

- Dial 9-1-1.
- The 9-1-1 dispatcher will need to know
    1. **WHERE** the emergency is
    2. **WHAT** the emergency is and **HOW MANY** people are involved
    3. **PHONE NUMBER** from which you are calling
    4. What is currently being done

IMPORTANT: Stay on the phone. Do not hang up until dispatcher instructs you to do so. Send someone out to flag down the emergency medical technicians and direct them to the scene.

Directions to the Fitness Center

- Go south on State College Road.
- Turn left into the campus on Gym Drive.
- Go through the first stop sign.
- The Kinesiology and Health Science building is on the right side of the street.
- Someone will meet you next to the back entrance of the building to guide you to the scene.

FIGURE 18.2   Emergency procedures and directions.

©Debra J. Rose, Center for Successful Aging, California State University, Fullerton.

hopefully, jolting it back into a regular rhythm. Current AEDs are very user friendly and verbally guide users through the process of applying the patches and delivering the electric shock appropriately. Additional training in the use of AEDs is also readily available.

Ethical Guidelines for the Physical Activity Instructor

Failure to adhere to the ethical guidelines associated with your profession probably will not result in legal action. However, ethics deal with very important issues, such as the quality of your relationship with your client, your level of professionalism, and how you represent the profession of physical activity instruction of older adults. Ethical behavior involves keeping the best interests of your clients in mind, being truthful and fair, and being guided by profes-

sional integrity in your decisions. The IDEA Health and Fitness Association has published excellent codes of ethics for both personal fitness trainers and group fitness instructors (see appendixes B and C).

In addition to the IDEA codes of ethics, the following suggestions are provided to assist you with maintaining the highest professional ethics:

- Do not guarantee results. Let your clients know that each individual responds differently to an exercise or nutrition program.
- Discuss fees with your clients before you begin working with them. More important, have a written agreement setting forth services to be performed and fees to be paid. You should have a separate agreement with each client and both of you should date and sign the agreement. Then give the client one copy and keep the original in each client's permanent file.
- Charge fees uniformly. Do not charge one client one fee and another client a different fee unless there is a logical basis for doing so. Keep payment records.

Date of injury _____ Time _____ a.m./p.m.

               Date/Month/Year   Hour:Minutes

Name of injured person _____ Sex _____ Age _____

Address _____ _____

           Street   City   State   ZIP code   Area code and phone number

Check suspected cause of injury or illness

__ Fall   __ Overexposure   __ Hyperflexion   __ Other: _____

__ Blunt trauma   __ Overexertion   __ Hyperextension

Nature of injury/illness in detail (Did it happen before, during, or after exercise? How?)

_____

_____

Check site of injury/illness

__ None	__ Back (lower)	__ Fingers/thumb	__ Leg	__ Stomach
__ Abdomen	__ Chest/ribs	__ Foot	__ Mouth	__ Teeth
__ Ankle	__ Ear	__ Hand	__ Neck/throat	__ Toes
__ Arm	__ Elbow	__ Head	__ Nose	__ Wrist
__ Back (upper)	__ Face	__ Knee	__ Shoulder/	
__ Other: _____			collarbone	

Check sign or symptom

__ Abrasion	__ Dislocation	__ Loss of function	__ Pain
__ Contusion	__ Fracture	__ Lung involvement	__ Shock
__ Cut	__ Heart involvement	__ Nausea/vomiting	__ Sprain/strain
__ Discoloration	__ Internal injury	__ Numbness	__ Swelling
__ Other: _____			

What was done for the injured person? _____

_____

By whom? _____

Was the injured person sent to a hospital? __ Yes __ No To a physician? __ Yes __ No

To whom was the injured person released? __ Self __ Relative __ Other:_____

Signature of person filling out form _____ Date _____

Witness signature _____ Date _____

Witness address_____

Witness phone number _____

FIGURE 18.3   Accident report form.

- Be punctual. One of the hallmarks of a professional is being on time to all personal training sessions and group classes. Always assume your clients' time is valuable; it is to them, even if they are retired. Being punctual is a sign of respect. If you are going to be late, call to let them know or to see if the session can be rescheduled.

- Provide full measure. If you are paid for a one-hour training session, be sure you provide an hour's worth of time.

- Provide advance notice of sessions or classes from which you will be absent. Part of your written agreement may ask clients to give 24 hours' notice if they are going to have to cancel a session.

- Do what you say you will do in a timely fashion. If you offer to do something for the client, do it in a timely fashion. Otherwise, don't offer.

- Maintain confidentiality. It is important to establish a relationship of trust with a client that encourages the client to freely discuss the exercise program and related questions. To gain a client's confidence and to keep it, do not talk about one client with another. Client communications should be confidential. If you want to discuss a client with his or her medical professional, first obtain the client's written permission and keep it in his or her file.

- Establish good relationships with your clients. Develop a caring attitude and genuine interest in the goals of your clients, their progress, and their concerns. In other words, *listen to your* *clients*. This is particularly important with older adults, because listening is how you can learn about challenges that may have to be addressed in an exercise program. Keep in mind that people are less likely to sue someone they like.

Summary

A number of health and fitness organizations and associations publish standards and guidelines for health and fitness facilities and for physical activity instructors. The best way to provide a safe physical activity environment for older adults and avoid legal problems is to know the standard of care to which you are held: the degree of care a reasonable and prudent physical activity instructor would exercise under the same or similar circumstances.

This chapter summarized components of a risk management plan, including health and fitness facility standards and guidelines, steps to prevent injuries and medical emergencies, and plans to respond to emergency situations. It also provided information regarding professional ethics for personal trainers and group instructors. In the future, more specific standards and guidelines for physical activity instructors of older adults will be published and recognized by the leading associations in the industry. You should stay abreast of these developments by being involved as a member in your professional organization and by regularly attending conferences and training workshops to update your knowledge and hone your skills as a physical activity instructor.

Key Terms

allegations

assumption of risk

automated emergency defibrillator (AED)

breached

causation

comparative negligence

damages

defendant

defenses

duty

emergency response plan (ERP)

guidelines

negligence

plaintiff

risk management plan (RMP)

standard of care

standards

Recommended Readings

American College of Sports Medicine. (2012). *ACSM's health/fitness facility standards and guidelines* (4th ed.). Champaign, IL: Human Kinetics.

Eickhoff-Shemek, J., Herbert, D., & Connaughton, D. (2009). *Risk management for health/ fitness professionals*. Philadelphia, PA: Lippincott Williams and Wilkins.

Study Questions

1. In legal terms, the party accused of having caused an injury resulting from fitness training is referred to as the

   a. plaintiff

   b. defendant

   c. defense team

   d. plaintiff team

2. The *standard of care* to which you are held is that of

   a. a reasonably prudent physical activity instructor of older adults

   b. an expert physical activity instructor of older adults

   c. a degreed physical activity instructor of older adults

   d. a certified physical activity instructor of older adults

3. You can reduce your risk of liability as an instructor of physical activity of older adults if you

   a. tolerate sexual harassment

   b. keep medical and emergency information on each client posted up on the wall for easy access

   c. have a written emergency response plan readily available

   d. don't let on to your clients that you made a mistake

4. When working with older adults with hearing problems you should *not*

   a. use visual cues

   b. project your voice and raise the pitch

   c. face your clients when talking

   d. project your voice, but don't raise the pitch

5. Which of the following will help you design a safe and effective exercise environment that minimizes clients' risk of injury or medical emergency?

   a. ask your clients with diabetes to bring their own portable glucometers to the fitness class

   b. monitor the room temperature during exercise

   c. observe for warning signs of heart distress

   d. all of the above

Application Activities

1. An 80-year-old woman contacts you about starting an exercise program. She says her health is good, although she appears to be about 50 pounds (23 kg) overweight. She says her doctor has approved an exercise program. Set up a file for this potential client, and list all the paperwork you feel you should have before designing and starting a program for her.

2. An 85-year-old man you have been training for several weeks in his home seems to be flirting with you. He takes every opportunity to touch your arm or shoulder, stands too close, wears workout clothes that are inappropriate, and tells suggestive jokes. You have tried to discuss your discomfort with his behavior tactfully with him but to no avail. Write a letter to this client setting forth the problem and proposing a solution that will work for you.

3. You teach group exercise classes to older adults at a facility that does not have an emergency response plan (ERP). Develop your own ERP.

Appendix A

International Curriculum Guidelines for Preparing Physical Activity Instructors of Older Adults

Executive Summary

Nancy A. Ecclestone, Canada

C. Jessie Jones, United States

The recognized value of physical activity in preserving functional capacity and reducing physical frailty in later years, combined with the support of the medical community, has resulted in numerous senior fitness and physical activity classes springing up in various facilities (e.g., senior centers, hospitals, recreation departments, health and fitness clubs, churches, YMCAs, community centers, retirement communities, long-term care facilities) throughout the world. Because of the lack of licensure or endorsement of training guidelines for preparing physical activity instructors of older adults, facility directors can hire whom they want, regardless of the instructors' educational backgrounds. People receiving little or no specialized training can advertise themselves as senior fitness instructors. Most older adults lack the knowledge and experience to determine whether the physical activity program in which they are participating is safe and effective. Experts in the field have argued that because of the range of medical conditions and functional abilities of the 65-and-older population, physical activity instructors of older adults require more knowledge, skills, and experience than instructors of younger adults. Unfortunately, because of the lack of endorsed curriculum training guidelines to prepare physical activity instructors of older adults, some training programs have not required instructors to attain essential knowledge and skills for instructing older adults in a safe and effective way.

Historical Background

Historically, the development of the *International Curriculum Guidelines for Preparing Physical Activity Instructors of Older Adults* began at the 1996 World International Congress on Physical Activity, Aging and Sport held in Heidelberg, Germany. Delegates from several countries met and developed a draft document; however, the guidelines were never published. Subsequently, Canada developed national guidelines in 2003 (appendix A) under the leadership of the Canadian Centre for Activity and Aging and with the support of Health Canada. In the United States, representatives from six national organizations developed and published national standards in 1998 (appendix B).

In 2003, the two separate documents from the United States (national standards) and Canada (national guidelines) were condensed into one document and titled the *International Curriculum Guidelines for Preparing Physical Activity Instructors of Older Adults*. Then, a coalition of members from 13 countries and a committee from the United States (appendix C) agreed to review and make recommendations for this document. These international guidelines were then presented at the 6th World Congress on Aging and Physical Activity held in London, Ontario, Canada (August 3 to 7, 2004) by the cochairs of this initiative, Nancy Ecclestone (Canada) and C. Jessie Jones (United States).

The *International Curriculum Guidelines for Preparing Physical Activity Instructors of Older Adults* is a consensus document that outlines each of the major content areas that experts recommend should be included in any entry-level training program with the goal of preparing physical activity instructors to work with older adults. The principles and perspectives of the World Health Organization (WHO) Active Ageing Policy Framework are reflected in this document. Organizations and coalitions currently endorsing the guidelines are listed in appendix D.

These guidelines can be applied to older adults across the continuum from healthy, independent older adults in community settings to functionally dependent older adults in long-term care. Advanced training would be necessary for instructors interested in working with older adults with severe disabilities or cognitive impairment in rehabilitation settings or managing and directing facilities, especially ones providing insurance reimbursement and those that serve a more frail older adult population.

Because of the complexity of the fitness industry and the differences in state and national requirements throughout the world, we believe that it is the responsibility of individual associations and organizations to develop the details of each major content area within each curriculum module, to develop appropriate areas of emphasis, and to develop performance standards that indicate the level of achievement expected of their students. Because of the varied functional ability levels of older adults, it is important to be aware of the target population (community-dwelling, able older adults versus homebound or institutionalized frail older adults) and to develop the content to meet the specific needs of that population.

Purposes and Delimitations

The purpose of the *International Curriculum Guidelines for Preparing Physical Activity Instructors of Older Adults* is to (1) ensure safe, effective, and accessible physical activity and fitness programs for older adults; (2) develop competent physical activity instructors of older adults; (3) provide more consistency among instructor training programs preparing physical activity instructors of older adults; (4) inform administrators, physical activity instructors, and others about the minimum training guidelines recommended by the profession when recruiting physical activity instructors of older adults; (5) clarify the definition and role of a physical activity instructor for older adults; and (6) establish the level of expertise required to help protect instructors and other facility staff from litigation (lawsuits). *These curriculum guidelines are not being developed to promote one certification or licensing body of physical activity instructors of older adults, but rather to provide curriculum guidelines to encourage more consistency among instructor training programs throughout the world.*

These guidelines do not include recommendations for (1) qualifications and experience of trainers and course tutors, (2) methods of curriculum delivery, (3) assessment requirements for students, or (4) requirements of the training providers.

Definitions of Terms

The following terms are commonly used when discussing training modules.

instructor—A physical activity instructor is broadly defined as a professional who teaches, educates, and trains people to do physical activities.

physical activity—An encompassing term to mean any body movement produced by a skeletal muscle that results in energy expenditure.

exercise—A subset of physical activity. It is planned and repetitive body movement, which improves or maintains one or more components of physical fitness (e.g., cardiovascular endurance, muscular strength, balance, flexibility).

Training Module 1: Overview of Aging and Physical Activity

Recommended areas of study include general background information about the aging process and the benefits of an active lifestyle.

Suggested Topics

1. Demographic considerations (e.g., ethnicity, culture, gender) as they relate to individual participation in physical activity programs

2. Various definitions of aging (including pathological, usual, and successful aging)

3. The difference between the terms chronological, biological, and functional aging

4. The benefits of physical activity as it relates to the multiple dimensions of wellness (e.g., intellectual, emotional, physical, vocational, social, spiritual) and the prevention of chronic

medical conditions, health promotion, and quality of life throughout the lifespan

5. Current research and epidemiology related to health and physical activity

Training Module 2: Psychological, Sociocultural, and Physiological Aspects of Physical Activity and Older Adults

Recommended areas of study include psychological, sociocultural, and physiological aspects of physical activity in order to develop safe and effective physical activity and exercise programs for older adults.

Suggested Topics

1. Exercise science: Basic anatomy, physiology, neurology, motor learning and control, and exercise psychology

2. Myths, stereotypes, and barriers associated with aging and physical activity participation in later life

3. Predictors of successful aging (e.g., biological, psychological, and sociological theories of aging, environmental factors, and lifestyle choices)

4. The relationship between physical activity and psychosocial well-being

5. Age-associated physiological and biomechanical changes in multiple body systems (e.g., cardiovascular and respiratory systems, musculoskeletal system, and central nervous system) and how these changes affect functional mobility and independence

Training Module 3: Screening, Assessment, and Goal Setting

Recommended areas of study include information on selection, administration, and interpretation of preexercise health and activity screening and fit-

ness and mobility assessments appropriate for older adults. This information will provide the basis for exercise program design and appropriate referrals to other health professionals.

Suggested Topics

1. Guidelines and procedures for the selection, administration, and interpretation of screening tools to determine the health, physical activity, and disability status of older adult participants

2. Health, activity, and other lifestyle appraisals, including identification risk factors for falls and cardiovascular complications

3. How and when to make appropriate referrals to, or seek advice from, physicians and other qualified allied health and fitness professionals

4. Physiological and functional fitness assessments (e.g., heart rate, blood pressure, body mass index, and field tests for strength, flexibility, submaximal endurance, and functional mobility such as balance, agility, gait, coordination, and power)

5. Psychological (e.g., self-efficacy, depression) and sociological (e.g., social support) assessments

6. For homebound or institutionalized older adults, assessments of functional abilities (e.g., mobility, grooming, dressing, toileting) with input from caregivers

It is further recommended that training programs include information on establishing, with client input, realistic and measurable short-term, medium-term, and long-term goals.

Suggested Topics

1. Factors influencing physical activity participation among older adults, including barriers, motivators, regular involvement in physical activity, and behavior modification

2. Developing, monitoring, and modifying short-term and long-term activity goals based on results from screening and assessments and input from the participants and caregivers if appropriate

3. Importance of encouraging lifetime leisure physical activities (e.g., dancing, gardening, hiking, tennis, swimming) in addition to structured exercise programs

Training Module 4: Program Design and Management

Recommended areas of study include information about using results from screening, assessment, and client goals to make appropriate decisions regarding individual and group physical activity and exercise program design and management.

Suggested Topics

1. Interpretation of prescreening and assessment data, and consideration of client goals, for effective program development

2. Exercise variables (e.g., mode, frequency, duration, intensity) and principles (i.e., overload, functional relevance, challenge, accommodation) for program design in both individual and group settings

3. Exercise training components and methods, including warm-up and cool-down, flexibility, resistance, aerobic endurance, balance and mobility, mind–body exercise, and aquatics for program design in both individual and group settings

4. Applied movement analysis for proper selection and implementation of specific exercises

5. Training formats and session designs for various functional abilities and individual and group exercise sequencing for exercise programming

6. Economic considerations and consequent options for equipment (e.g., quality for cost, safety, and age-friendliness)

7. Importance of making healthy lifestyle choices (e.g., proper nutrition, stress management, and smoking cessation)

8. An organizational system for participant recruitment, tracking exercise compliance, and maintaining other client information

9. Methods for client reassessment and program evaluation

Training Module 5: Program Design for Older Adults With Stable Medical Conditions

Recommended areas of study include information on common medical conditions of older adults, signs and symptoms associated with medication-related negative interactions during activity and how to adapt exercise for clients with varying fitness levels, and stable medical conditions to help prevent injury and other emergency situations.

Suggested Topics

1. Age-related medical conditions (e.g., cardiovascular disease, stroke, hypertension, respiratory disorders, obesity, arthritis, osteoporosis, back pain, diabetes, balance and motor control deficits, visual and hearing disorders, dementia, and urinary incontinence)

2. How to adapt group and individual exercise programs to accommodate for age-related medical conditions and for people who have experienced falls, operations, and illness

3. How to adapt group and individual exercise programs to accommodate for prosthetics (e.g., artificial hips, knees, legs)

4. How to design programs for preventive health (e.g., exercises to reduce risk of falling, control diabetes, heart disease)

5. Recognizing signs and symptoms associated with medication-related negative interactions during physical activity (e.g., postural hypotension, arrhythmias, fatigue, weakness, dizziness, balance and coordination problems, altered depth perception, depression, confusion, dehydration, and urinary incontinence) and refer back to health professional

Training Module 6: Teaching Skills

Recommended areas of study include information about motor learning principles that guide the selection and delivery of effective individualized and group exercises and physical activities and the construction of safe and effective practice environments.

Suggested Topics

1. Application of motor learning principles for proper client instruction, verbal cues, feedback, and reinforcement

2. Structure of the learning environment to facilitate optimal learning of motor skills

3. Development of safe, friendly, and fun exercise and physical activity environments (e.g., appropriate use of humor, special equipment, creative movements, music, novelty, and props)

4. Issues facing older adults that may affect motivation (e.g., depression, social isolation, learned helplessness, low self-efficacy)

5. Development of lesson plans and elements of instruction

6. Methods for self-evaluation of teaching effectiveness

7. Monitoring and adjustment of exercise variables (e.g., frequency, intensity, duration, mode)

Training Module 7: Leadership, Communication, and Marketing Skills

Recommended areas of study include information on incorporating effective motivational, communication, and leadership skills related to teaching individual and group exercise classes as well as professional leadership skills, and how to create effective marketing tools for program and self.

Suggested Topics

1. Principles of individual and group dynamics in structured exercise settings

2. Translation of technical terminology into client-friendly language

3. Incorporating leadership skills into personal training and group physical activity classes

to enhance teaching effectiveness and client satisfaction

4. Application of positive interpersonal interaction behaviors to work with a heterogeneous older adult population (e.g., gender, ethnicity, education level) in both group and individual exercise settings

5. Listening skills and reception to participants' feedback

6. Development of social support strategies (e.g., buddy system, telephone support)

7. Development of effective, age-friendly marketing strategies and tools of program and self, and methods of delivering the "right" message

Training Module 8: Client Safety and First Aid

Recommended areas of study include information on developing a risk-management plan to promote a safe exercise environment and respond to emergency situations.

Suggested Topics

1. Signs that indicate need for immediate exercise cessation or immediate medical consultation

2. Appropriate response to emergency situations such as would be covered in standard first-aid and CPR classes (e.g., cardiac arrest; airway obstruction; emergencies requiring rescue breathing; heat- and cold-related injuries; musculoskeletal injuries including strains, sprains, and fractures; diabetic emergencies; bleeding; falls; seizures; and shock)

3. Establishment of an emergency action plan

4. Identification of a safe and age-friendly exercise environment (e.g., working condition of equipment, accessibility, ventilation, lighting, floor surfaces, proper footwear, access to water and washroom facilities) and precautions for environmental extremes (e.g., high or low temperatures and excessive humidity)

Training Module 9: Ethics and Professional Conduct

Recommended areas of study include information on legal, ethical, and professional conduct.

Suggested Topics

1. Legal issues related to delivering physical activity programs to older adults, including legal concepts and terminology

2. Issues related to lawsuits, including scope of practice, industry standards, and negligence and types of applicable insurance coverage

3. Ethical standards and personal conduct and scope of practice for physical activity instructors of older adults

4. Accessing resources for the enhancement of professional skills (e.g., position stands, ethical practices, professional practice guidelines consistent with the standards of care)

5. Methods of continuing education to enhance one's professional skills

Appendix A Canadian Guidelines

Canadian Guidelines for Leaders of Physical Activity Programs for Older Adults in Long-Term Care, Home Care and the Community (2003) can be found on the Web site of the Canadian Centre for Activity and Aging at www.uwo.ca/actage.

These guidelines were produced as a result of the release, in the International Year of Older Persons (1999), of the following:

- *Canada's Physical Activity Guide to Healthy Active Living* (endorsed by more than 56 organizations)

- *Blueprint for Action for Active Living and Older Adults: Moving Through the Years* (contributors: La Fondation en adaptation motrice [FAM], Active Living Coalition for Older Adults [ALCOA], Canadian Centre for Activity and Aging [CCAA], and Health Canada)

- Recommendations from the *Roundtable of Leaders in Physical Activity and Aging* (1998)

and the *ALCOA National Forum—Older Adults and Active Living* (1999).* Both events were hosted by the Canadian Centre for Activity and Aging.

Several delegates representing a cross-section of health-related perspectives were instrumental in contributing to the development of the Canadian Guidelines. These contributions were solicited on the basis of their expertise and not necessarily their affiliations. Delegates (66) to the forums ([1]Long-Term Care Forum, [2]Home Care and Community Forum) that contributed to the Canadian guidelines included the following:

Newfoundland

Elsie McMillan, St. John's Nursing Home Board, St. John's[1]

Janet O'Dea, Memorial University of Newfoundland, Health Sciences Centre, St. John's[1]

Fran Cook, Memorial University Recreation Complex, St. John's[2]

Moira Hennessey, Department of Health and Community Services, St. John's[2]

Patricia Nugent, Health and Community Services, St. John's Region, St. John's[2]

Prince Edward Island

Marilyn Kennedy, Acute and Continuing Care, Department of Health and Social Services, Charlottetown[1]

Pat Malone, Senior Services Liaison—Acute and Continuing Care, Department of Health and Social Services, Charlottetown[1]

Lona Penny, Dr. John Gillis Memorial Lodge, Belfast[1]

Sharon Claybourne, Island Fitness Council, Charlottetown[2]

Nova Scotia

Denise Dreimanis, Nova Scotia Fitness & Lifestyle Leaders Association, ALCOA Speakers Bureau Dartmouth[1]

Debra Leigh, Continuing Care Association of Nova Scotia, Halifax[1]

Lygia Figueirado, Continuing Care, Government of Nova Scotia, Halifax[2]

Andrea Leonard, Home Support Association of Nova Scotia, Halifax[2]

New Brunswick

Flora Dell, Active Living Coalition for Older Adults (ALCOA), Fredericton[1]

Vicky Knight, Fredericton[1]

Ron Davis, Camden Park Terrace, Moncton[2]

Québec

Phillipe Markon, Ste-Famille, Ile d'Orleans[1]

Jaques Renaud, Association des Etablissments Prives Conventionnes, Montreal[1]

Clermont Simard, DEP-PEPS, Université Laval, Sainte-Foy[2]

Ontario

Jane Boudreau-Bailey, Chelsey Park Nursing Home, London[1]

Liz Cyarto, Canadian Centre for Activity and Aging, London[1,2]

Nancy Ecclestone, Canadian Centre for Activity and Aging, London[1,2]

Clara Fitzgerald, Canadian Centre for Activity and Aging, London[1,2]

Janice Hutton, Canadian Association of Fitness Professionals, Markham[1]

Marita Kloseck, Division of Geriatric Medicine, Parkwood Hospital, London[1]

Jody Kyle, YMCA St. Catherines, St. Catherines[1]

Darien Lazowski, Canadian Centre for Activity and Aging, London[1]

Stephanie Luxton, Canadian Centre for Activity and Aging, London[1,2]

Karen Macdonald, Canadian Red Cross Link to Health Program, Mississauga[1]

Sandra Mallett, Allendale Long Term Care, Milton[1]

Colleen Sonnenberg, Ministry of Health and Long-Term Care, Toronto[1]

Sue Veitch, Kingston[1]

Gabriel Blouin, Institute for Positive Health for Seniors, ALCOA, Ottawa[2]

Lynne Briggs, Advocacy Committee, Older Adult Centres Association of Ontario, Evergreen Seniors Centre, Guelph[2]

Carol Butler, PSW Program, Fanshawe College, London[2]

Trish Fitzpatrick, Client Services and Program Development, CCAC Oxford County, Woodstock[2]

Hania Goforth, Recreation Services, Lifestyle Retirement Communities, Mississauga[2]

John Griffin, George Brown College, Toronto[2]

Joan Hunter, Link to Health, Canadian Red Cross, Toronto[2]

Janice Hutton, Canadian Association of Fitness Professionals, Markham[2]

Jane Miller, Ontario Fitness Council, Toronto[2]

Don Paterson, University of Western Ontario, Canadian Centre for Activity and Aging, London[1,2]

Sheila Schuehlein, VON Canada, Kitchener[2]

Nancy Stelpstra, Ontario Fitness Council, Guelph[2]

Bert Taylor, University of Western Ontario, London[1]

Bruce Taylor, Health Canada, Ottawa[2]

Sue Thorning, Ontario Community Support Association, Toronto[2]

Manitoba

Cindy Greenlay-Brown, West St. Paul[1]

Jim Hamilton, Manitoba Seniors Directorate, Winnipeg[1,2]

Hope Mattus, Health Accountability Policy and Planning, Seniors and Persons With Disabilities,

Manitoba Health, Winnipeg[1,2]

Russell Thorne, Manitoba Fitness Council, University of Manitoba, Winnipeg[2]

Saskatchewan

Angela Nunweiler, Community Care Branch, Saskatchewan Health, Regina[1]

Bob Lidington, Saskatoon Home Support Services, Ltd, Saskatoon[2]

Alberta

Jennifer Dechaine, Alberta Centre for Active Living, Edmonton[1]

Timothy Fairbank, Capital Health Authority ADL/CRP, Edmonton[2]

Debbie Lee, Calgary Regional Health Authority, Calgary[2]

Debbie Ponich, Alberta Fitness Leadership Certification Association, Provincial Fitness Unit[2]

Faculty of Physical Education & Recreation, University of Alberta, Edmonton[2]

British Columbia

Carol Hansen, Kwantlan University College, Surrey[1, 2]

Linda Mae Ross, Continuing Care Renewal Regional Programs, Victoria[1]

Catherine Rutter, McIntosh Lodge, Chilliwack[1]

Barbara Harwood, NLTI Project Advisory Committee, Speakers Bureau ALCOA, North Saanich[2]

Cheryl Hedgecock, British Columbia Parks and Recreation, Richmond[2]

Yukon

Willy Shippey, Yukon Health and Social Services, Thompson Centre, Whitehorse[1,2]

Northwest Territory

Marjorie Sandercock, Yellowknife[1]

Nunavut

Jason Collins, Recreation and Leadership Division, Government of Nunavut, Igloolik[2]

Federal

Health Canada

Appendix B U.S. Standards

The *National Standards for Preparing Senior Fitness Instructors* were published by Jones, C.J. & Clark, J. (1998). National standards for preparing senior fitness instructors. *Journal of Aging and Physical Activity, 6*, 207-221.

Coalition Members

Chair: C. Jessie Jones, Council on Aging and Adult Development, American Association for Active Lifestyles and Fitness

Members

Janie Clark, American Senior Fitness Association

Richard Cotton, American Council on Exercise

Laura Gladwin, Aerobics and Fitness Association of America

Gwen Hyatt, Desert Southwest Fitness, Inc.

Lee Morgan, Cooper Institute of Aerobic Research

Kay Van Norman, Council on Aging and Adult Development, American Association for Active Lifestyles and Fitness

Appendix C International Recommendations

A coalition of members from 13 countries and a committee from the United States made recommendations for the *International Curriculum Guidelines for Preparing Physical Activity Instructors of Older Adults.*

International Coalition

Cochairs

Nancy Ecclestone, Canada, and C. Jessie Jones, United States

Members

Susie Dinan	England
Dorothy Dobson	Scotland
Ellen Freiberger	Germany
Linda Halliday	South Africa
Carol Hansen	Canada
Eino Heikkinen	Finland
Keith Hill	Australia
Marijke Hopman-Rock	The Netherlands
Gareth Jones	Canada
Alexandre Kalache	WHO
Stephanie Luxton	Canada
Michele Porter	Canada
Suely Santos	Brazil
Federico Schena	Italy
Cody Sipe	United States
Kiyoji Tanaka	Japan
Janice Tay	Singapore
Bruce Taylor	Canada
Catrine Tudor-Locke	United States

United States Coalition

Chair

C. Jessie Jones	American College of Sports Medicine (ACSM)

Members

Kazuko Aoyagi	World Instructor Training Schools (WITS)
Ken Baldwin	A.H. Ismail Center for Health, Exercise & Nutrition, Purdue University
Grant Clark American	Senior Fitness Association
Janie Clark American	Senior Fitness Association
Wojtek Chodzko-Zajko	National Blueprint on Active Aging
Laura Gladwin	American Fitness and Aerobic Association
Carol Kennedy	Indiana University
Steve Keteyian	ACSM
Rainer Martens	Human Kinetics
Julie McNeney	International Council on Active Aging
Colin Milner	International Council on Active Aging
Tammy Peterson	American Academy of Health and Fitness
Jerry Purvis	American Kinesiotherapy Association
Roberta Rikli	Center for Successful Aging, Cal State University, Fullerton
Debra Rose	Center for Successful Aging, Cal State University, Fullerton
Christine Schnitzer	Healthy Strides, Kisco Senior Living Facilities
Cody Sipe	A.H. Ismail Center for Health, Exercise & Nutrition, Purdue University
Christian Thompson	Council on Adult Development and Aging (CAAD), American Association for Active Lifestyles and Fitness (AAALF)
Mary Visser	CAAD, AAALF
Judy Wright	Human Kinetics

Appendix D Supporting Organizations and Coalitions

Organizations and coalitions supporting the *International Curriculum Guidelines for Preparing Physical Activity Instructors of Older Adults* as of this printing include the following:

- American Association for Active Lifestyles and Fitness, Council on Adult Development and Aging
- American Kinesiotherapy Association
- American Fitness and Aerobic Association
- American Senior Fitness Association
- Desert Southwest Fitness, Inc.
- International Council on Active Aging
- National Blueprint: Increasing Physical Activity Among Adults Age 50 and Older
- World Instructor Training Schools

Organizations and coalitions endorsing the *International Curriculum Guidelines for Preparing Physical Activity Instructors of Older Adults* as of this printing include the following:

- Active Living Coalition for Older Adults
- Canadian Centre for Activity and Aging
- Canadian Society for Exercise Physiology

Reprinted from International Society for Aging and Physical Activity, 2004.

Appendix B

IDEA Code of Ethics For Personal Trainers

As a member of IDEA Health & Fitness Association, I will be guided by the best interests of the client and will practice within the scope of my education and knowledge. I will maintain the education and experience necessary to appropriately train clients; will behave in a positive and constructive manner; and will use truth, fairness and integrity to guide all my professional decisions and relationships.

Ethical Practice Guidelines for Personal Fitness Trainers

1. **Always be guided by the best interests of the client.**
   a. Remember that a personal trainer's primary responsibility is to the client's safety, health and welfare; never compromise this responsibility for your own self-interest, personal advantage or monetary gain.
   b. Recommend products or services only if they will benefit the client's health and well-being, not because they will benefit you financially or occupationally.
   c. If recommending products or services will result in financial gain for you or your employer, be aware that disclosure to the client may be appropriate.
   d. Base the number of training sessions on the client's needs, not your financial requirements.

2. **Maintain appropriate professional boundaries.**
   a. Never exploit—sexually, economically or otherwise—a professional relationship with a supervisor, an employee, a colleague or a client.
   b. Respect the client's right to privacy. A client's conversations, behavior, results and—if appropriate—identity should be kept confidential.
   c. Use physical touching appropriately during training sessions, as a means of correcting alignment and/or focusing a client's concentration on the targeted area. Immediately discontinue the use of touch at a client's request or if the client displays signs of discomfort.
   d. Focus on the business relationship, not the client's personal life, except as appropriate.
   e. When you are unable to maintain appropriate professional boundaries or to work within the legitimate agenda of the training relationship, whether because of your own attitudes and behaviors or those of the client, either terminate the relationship or refer the client to an appropriate professional, such as another trainer, a medical doctor or a mental health specialist.
   f. Avoid sexually oriented banter and inappropriate physical contact.

(continued)

(continued)

3. **Maintain the education and experience necessary to appropriately train clients.**

   a. Continuously strive to keep abreast of the new developments, concepts and practices essential to providing the highest-quality services to clients.

   b. Recognize your limitations in services and techniques, and engage only in activities that fall within the boundaries of your professional credentials and competencies. Refer clients to other professionals for issues that fall beyond the boundaries of a personal fitness trainer's profession or your current competencies.

   c. For health screening, fitness assessment, prudent progression and exercise technique, follow the standards outlined by professionals in the fields of medicine and health and fitness.

4. **Use truth, fairness, and integrity to guide all professional decisions and relationships.**

   a. In all professional and business relationships, clearly demonstrate and support honesty, integrity and trustworthiness.

   b. Accurately represent your qualifications.

   c. In advertising materials, be truthful and fair. When describing personal training services, be guided by the primary obligation of helping the client develop informed judgments, opinions and choices. Avoid ambiguity, sensationalism, exaggeration and superficiality.

   d. Make your contract language clear and understandable.

   e. Administer consistent pricing and procedural policies.

   f. Never solicit business from another trainer's client. When interacting with clients of other trainers, be open and honest so those clients cannot interpret the interaction as solicitation of their business.

   g. If you work for a business that finds clients and assigns them to you, recognize that the clients belong to that business.

5. **Show respect for clients and fellow professionals.**

   a. Act with integrity in your relationships with colleagues, facility owners and other health professionals to help ensure that each client benefits optimally from all professionals.

   b. Never discriminate based on race, creed, color, gender, age, sexual orientation, physical handicap or nationality.

   c. When disagreements or conflicts occur, focus on behavior, factual evidence and nonderogatory forms of communication, not on judgmental statements, hearsay, the placing of blame or other destructive responses.

   d. Present fitness information completely and accurately in order to help the client make informed decisions.

6. **Uphold a professional image through conduct and appearance.**

   a. Avoid smoking, substance abuse and unhealthy eating habits.

   b. Speak and dress in a manner that increases the client's comfort level.

Appendix C

IDEA Code of Ethics For Group Fitness Instructors

As a member of IDEA Health & Fitness Association, I will be guided by the best interests of the client and will practice within the scope of my education and knowledge. I will maintain the education and experience necessary to appropriately teach classes; will behave in a positive and constructive manner; and will use truth, fairness and integrity to guide all my professional decisions and relationships.

Ethical Practice Guidelines for Group Fitness Instructors

1. **Always be guided by the best interests of the group, while acknowledging individuals.**
   a. Remember that a group fitness instructor's primary obligation is to the group as a whole, taking class level and class description into account.
   b. Strive to provide options and realistic goals that take individual variations into account.
   c. Offer modifications for all levels of fitness and experience (i.e., demonstrate easy and more challenging options).
   d. Recommend products or services only if they will benefit a client's health and well-being, not because they will benefit you or your employer financially or occupationally.

2. **Provide a safe exercise environment.**
   a. Prioritize all movement choices by (1) safety, (2) effectiveness and (3) creativity. Do not allow creativity to compromise safety.
   b. Use good judgment in exercise selection. Assess all class moves according to risk versus reward, making sure rewards and benefits always outweigh risks.
   c. Adhere to safe guidelines for music speed in all classes.
   d. Follow guidelines for maximum music volume. IDEA recommends that "music intensity during group exercise classes should measure no more than 90 decibels (dB). Since the instructor's voice needs to be about 10 dB louder than the music in order to be heard, the instructor's voice should measure no more than 100 dB."
   e. Consider whether exercises that can be properly monitored in a one-to-one setting are appropriate in a group environment.

3. **Obtain the education and training necessary to lead group exercise.**
   a. Obtain the education and training necessary to lead group exercise.
   b. Continuously strive to keep abreast of the latest research and exercise techniques essential to providing effective and safe classes.
   c. Maintain certifications and continuing education.

(continued)

(continued)

    d. Obtain specific training for teaching specialty classes or instructing special populations. Teach a class such as kickboxing or yoga only after mastering the skill and understanding the important aspects of the class. Instruct a special population, like older adults or perinatal women, only after studying the specific needs of the group.

    e. Work within the scope of your knowledge and skill. When necessary, refer participants to professionals with appropriate training and expertise beyond your realm of knowledge.

4. **Use truth, fairness, and integrity to guide all professional decisions and relationships.**

    a. In all professional relationships, clearly demonstrate and support honesty, integrity and trustworthiness.

    b. Speak in a positive manner about fellow instructors, other staff, participants and competitive facilities and organizations or say nothing at all.

    c. When disagreements or conflicts occur, focus on behavior, factual evidence and nonderogatory forms of communication, not on judgmental statements, hearsay, the placing of blame or other destructive responses.

    d. Accurately represent your certifications, training and education.

    e. Do not discriminate based on race, creed, color, gender, age, sexual orientation, physical handicap or nationality.

5. **Maintain appropriate professional boundaries.**

    a. Never exploit—sexually, economically or otherwise—a professional relationship with a supervisor, an employee, a colleague or a client.

    b. Use physical touching appropriately during classes, as a means of correcting alignment and/or focusing a client's concentration on the targeted area. Immediately discontinue the use of touch at a client's request or if the client displays signs of discomfort.

    c. Avoid sexually oriented banter and inappropriate physical contact.

6. **Uphold a professional image through conduct and appearance.**

    a. Model behavior that values physical ability, function and health over appearance.

    b. Demonstrate healthy behaviors and attitudes about bodies (including your own). Avoid smoking, substance abuse and unhealthy exercise and eating habits.

    c. Encourage healthful eating for yourself and others.

    d. Dress in a manner that allows you to perform your job while increasing the comfort level of class participants. Be more conservative in dress, decorum and speech when the class standard is unclear.

    e. Establish a mood in class that encourages and supports individual effort and all levels of expertise.

Study Questions
Answer Key

Chapter 1
1. d.
2. c.
3. b.
4. c.
5. a.
6. b.

Chapter 2
1. b.
2. a.
3. b.
4. d.
5. d.

Chapter 3
1. d.
2. d.
3. b.
4. c.
5. d.
6. a.
7. d.

Chapter 4
1. d.
2. a.
3. b.
4. d.
5. a.
6. b.
7. c.

Chapter 5
1. c.
2. d.
3. a.
4. b.
5. b.
6. a.
7. c.

Chapter 6
1. a.
2. d.
3. a.
4. b.

Chapter 7
1. d.
2. d.
3. d.
4. c.
5. a.
6. b.
7. a.
8. b.

Chapter 8
1. a.
2. b.
3. c.
4. d.
5. d.
6. a.

Chapter 9
1. b.
2. a.
3. c.
4. d.

Chapter 10
1. c.
2. d.
3. b.
4. a.
5. d.
6. d.
7. d.

Chapter 11
1. b.
2. b.
3. c.
4. c.
5. d.
6. a.
7. c.
8. c.
9. c.
10. d.

Chapter 12
1. a.
2. b.
3. c.

4. d.
5. d.
6. d.
7. a.
8. b.

Chapter 13
1. c.
2. c.
3. a.
4. a.
5. c.
6. b.
7. c.

Chapter 14
1. d.
2. d.
3. a.
4. d.
5. b.
6. d.
7. d.
8. d.

Chapter 15
1. c.
2. d.
3. d.
4. b.
5. a.

6. c.
7. b.
8. b.
9. b.
10. a.

Chapter 16
1. d.
2. c.
3. a.
4. c.
5. a.
6. d.
7. d.
8. b.

Chapter 17
1. d.
2. b.
3. a.
4. c.
5. b.
6. d.

Chapter 18
1. b.
2. a.
3. c.
4. d.
5. d.

References

Preface

Ecclestone, N.A., & Jones, C.J. (2004). International curriculum guidelines for preparing physical activity instructors of older adults. *Journal of Aging and Physical Activity, 12,* 467-479.

He, W., Goodkind, D., & Kowal, P. (2016). *An aging world: 2015.* International population reports, P95/16-1. Washington, DC: U.S. Census Bureau, U.S. Government Publishing Office.

Jones, C.J., & Clark, J. (1998). National standards for preparing senior fitness instructors. *Journal of Aging and Physical Activity, 6,* 207-221.

Chapter 1

Campbell, A.J., Robertson, M.C., Gardner, M.M., Norton, R.N., Tilyard, M.W., & Buchner, D.M. (1997). Randomised controlled trial of a general practice programme of home based exercise to prevent falls in elderly women. *British Medical Journal, 315,* 1065-1069.

Carlson, S.A., Fulton, J.E., Pratt, M., Yang, Z., & Adams, E.K. (2015). Inadequate physical activity and health care expenditures in the United States. *Progress in Cardiovascular Disease, 57,* 315-323. doi:10.1016/j.pcad.2014.08.002

de Jong, L.D., Peters, A., Hooper, J., Chalmers, N., Henderson, C., Laventure, R.M. E., & Skelton, D.A. (2016). The functional fitness MOT test battery for older adults: Protocol for a mixed-method feasibility study. *Journal of Medical Internet Research Protocols, 20,* e108.

Department of Health. (2009). Falls and fractures: Exercise training to prevent falls. In Prevention Package for Older People. Department of Health, London, UK. Retrieved from http://webarchive. nationalarchives.gov.uk/+/http://www.dh.gov. uk/en/Publicationsandstatistics/Publications/ DH_103146.

Ecclestone, N.A., & Jones, C.J. (2004). International curriculum guidelines for preparing physical activity instructors of older adults. *Journal of Aging and Physical Activity, 6,* 207-221.

Fries, J.F., & Crapo, L.M. (1981). *Vitality and aging.* San Francisco: Freeman.

Gawler, S., Skelton, D.A., Dinan-Young, S., Masud, T., . . . Iliffe, S. (2016) Reducing falls among older people in general practice: The ProAct65+ exercise intervention trial. *Archives of Gerontology & Geriatrics, 67,* 46-54.

Hawley-Hague, H., Horne, M., Campbell, M.C., Demack, S., Skelton, D.A., & Todd C.J. (2014). Multiple layers of influence on older adults' attendance and adherence to community exercise classes. *Gerontologist, 54,* 599-610.

Hawley-Hague, H., Horne, M., Skelton, D.A., & Todd, C. (2016). Older adults' uptake and adherence to exercise classes: Instructors' perspectives. *Journal of Aging & Physical Activity, 24,* 119-128.

He, W., Goodkind, D., & Kowal, P. (2016). *An aging world: 2015.* International population reports, P95/16-1. Washington, DC: U.S. Census Bureau, U.S. Government Publishing Office.

Hoffman, S.J., & Knudson, D.V. (Eds.). (2017). *Introduction to kinesiology* (5th ed.). Champaign, IL: Human Kinetics.

Iliffe, S., Kendrick, D., Morris, R., Masud, T., Gage, H., Skelton, D.A., . . . Belcher, C. (2014). Multi-centre cluster randomised trial comparing a community group exercise programme with home based exercise with usual care for people aged 65 and over in primary care. *Health Technology Assessment, 18,* 49. Retrieved from www.journalslibrary.nihr. ac.uk/hta/hta18490#/s1

International Council on Active Aging (2017a). Trends and environments for active aging. ICAA Active-Aging Industry Development Survey 2017. Retrieved from www.icaa.cc/listing. php?type=industry_research

International Council on Active Aging (2017b). ICAA/ ProMatura Wellness Benchmarks, The National Wellness Benchmark Report 2016. Retrieved from www.icaa.cc/listing.php?type=industry_research

Jones, C.J., & Rikli, R.E. (1994). The revolution in aging: Implications for curriculum development and professional preparation in physical education. *Journal of Aging and Physical Activity, 2,* 261-272.

Jones, C.J. & Rose, D.J. (2005). *Physical activity instruction of older adults.* Champaign, IL: Human Kinetics.

Katz, S., Branch, L.G., Branson, M.H., Papsidero, J.A., Beck, J.C., & Greer, D.S. (1983). Active life expectancy. *New England Journal of Medicine, 309,* 1218-1224.

Kerse, N., Elley, C.R., Robinson, E., & Arroll, B. (2005). Is physical activity counseling effective for older people? A cluster randomized, controlled trial in primary care. *Journal of the American Geriatric Society, 53,* 1951-1956.

King, A.C., Rejeski, W.J., & Buchner, D.M. (1998). Physical activity interventions targeting older adults. A critical review and recommendations. *American Journal of Preventive Medicine, 15,* 316-33.

Laventure, B., & Aherne, C. (2009, September/October) Living well with dementia: A framework for programs. *Journal on Active Aging,* 24-33.

Laventure, B., & Aherne, C. (2010, September/October) Living well with dementia: Guidance for exercise instructors & wellness leaders. *Journal on Active Aging,* 62-68.

Laventure, B. & Skelton, D. (2016). Evaluating the impact of the use of the functional fitness MOT tool by active aging professionals. *Journal of Aging & Physical Activity, 24,* S24-S25.

Laventure, R.M.E., Dinan, S.M., & Skelton, D.A. (2008). Someone like me: Increasing participation in physical activity among seniors with senior peer health motivators. *Journal of Aging & Physical Activity, 16,* S76-S77.

Laventure, R.M.E., Hetherington, S., Street, R., & Penington, A. (2016). Changing hearts and minds: Strategies to improve exercise perceptions and behaviours. *Journal of Aging & Physical Activity, 24,* S5.

Mead, G.E., Greig, C.A., Cunningham, I., Lewis, S.J., Dinan, S., Saunders, D.H., . . . Young, A. (2007). Stroke: A randomized trial of exercise or relaxation. *Journal of the American Geriatric Society, 55,* 892-899.

National Health Interview Survey, 2015. Retrieved from www.cdc.gov/nchs/nhis/shs/tables.htm

National Institute for Health and Clinical Excellence (NICE) (2007). *Behaviour change at population, community and individual levels.* NICE public health guidance 6. National Institute for Health and Clinical Excellence, London. Retrieved from www.nice.org.uk/Guidance/ph6

Nelson, M.E., Rejeski, W.J., Blair, S.N., Duncan, P.W., . . . Castaneda-Sceppa, C. (2007). Physical activity and public health in older adults: Recommendation from the American College of Sports Medicine and the American Heart Association. *Medicine & Science in Sports & Exercise, 39,* 1435-1445.

Noordman, J., Verhaak, P., & van Dulmen, S. (2010). Discussing patient's lifestyle choices in the consulting room: Analysis of GP-patient consultations between 1975 and 2008. *BMC Family Practice, 11,* 87.

PAGAC (Physical Activity Guidelines Advisory Committee). (2018). *2018 Physical activity guidelines advisory committee scientific report.* Washington, DC: U.S. Department of Health and Human Services.

Public Health England (2018). *Return on investment of falls prevention programmes in older people in the community.* Public Health England, London, UK. Retrieved from https://www.gov.uk/government/publications/falls-prevention-cost-effective-commissioning.

Rikli, R.E. & Jones, C.J. (1999). Functional fitness normative scores for community-residing older adults aged 60-94. *Journal of Aging and Physical Activity, 7,* 162-181.

Rikli, R.E. & Jones, C.J. (2013). *Senior fitness test manual* (2nd ed.). Champaign, IL: Human Kinetics.

Rowe, J.W., & Kahn, R.L. (1987). Human aging: Usual and successful. *Science, 237,* 143-149.

Royal College of Physicians. (2012). *Older people's experiences of therapeutic exercise as part of a falls prevention service.* RCP London, UK. Retrieved from www.rcplondon.ac.uk/projects/outputs/older-peoples-experience-therapeutic-exercise-part-falls-prevention-service

Skelton, D.A. (2004). The Postural Stability Instructor: Qualification in the UK for Effective Falls Prevention Exercise. *Journal of Aging & Physical Activity, 12,* 375-376.

Skelton, D.A., Dinan, S.M., Campbell, M.G., & Rutherford, O.M. (2005). Tailored Group Exercise (Falls Management Exercise–FaME) reduces falls in community-dwelling older frequent fallers (an RCT). *Age Ageing, 34,* 636-639.

Skelton, D.A., Dinan, S.M., & Laventure, R.E.M. (2004). Later Life Training: Exercise and physical activity training for working with older people in the UK. *Journal of Aging & Physical Activity, 12,* 274-275.

Skelton, D.A., & Gawler, S. (2008). Otago home based exercise for older people. *Sport & Exercise, 19,* 18-20.

Skelton, D.A., & Townley, B. (2008). Take a seat: Chair based exercise for older people. *SportEx, 18,* 9-11.

Skelton, D.A., Townley, R., & Gawler, S. (2015). Otago strength and balance exercise programme to prevent falls. *E-REPS Journal, 40,* 19-24.

Spirduso, W.W., Francis, K.L., & MacRae, P.G. (2005). *Physical dimensions of aging* (2nd ed.). Champaign, IL: Human Kinetics.

Taylor, A.W., & Johnson, M.J. (2008). *Physiology of exercise and healthy aging.* Champaign, IL: Human Kinetics.

U.S. Census Bureau (2015). *International Data Base.* Retrieved from www.census.gov/population/international/data/ib/informationGateway.php

U.S. Department of Health and Human Services (2008). *2008 Physical activity guidelines for Americans.* Retrieved from https://health.gov/paguidelines/pdf/paguide.pdf

Watson, R. R. (2017). *Physical activity and the aging brain.* San Diego, CA: Academic Press.

Yardley, L., Beyer, N., Hauer, K., McKee, K., Ballinger, C., & Todd, C. (2007). Recommendations for promoting the engagement of older people in preventative healthcare. *Quality & Safety in Health Care, 16,* 230-234.

Chapter 2

Angevaren, M., Aufdemkampe, G., Verhaar, H.J., Aleman, A., & Vanhees, L. (2008). Physical activity and enhanced fitness to improve cognitive function in older people without known cognitive impairment. Cochrane Database Systematic Review, 3, CD005381. doi:10.1002/14651858.CD005381.pub3

Atchley, R.C. (1971). *Retirement and leisure participation: Continuity or crisis? The Gerontologist, 11,* 13-17.

Atchley, R.C. (1999). *Continuity and adaptation in aging: Creating positive experiences.* Baltimore, MD: Johns Hopkins University Press.

Baker, J., Meisner, B.A., Logan, A.J., Kungl, A., & Weir, P. (2009). Physical activity and successful aging in Canadian older adults. *Journal of Aging & Physical Activity, 17,* 223-235.

Baltes, M.M., & Baltes, P.B. (1980). Plasticity and variability in psychological aging: Methodological and theoretical issues. In G.E. Gurski (Ed.), *Determining the effects of aging on the central nervous system* (pp. 41-66). Berlin, Germany: Schering.

Baltes, M.M., & Baltes, P.B. (1990). Psychological perspectives on successful aging: The model of selective optimization with compensation. In M.M Baltes & P.B. Baltes (Eds.), *Successful aging: Perspectives from the behavioral sciences (pp. 1-34).* Cambridge, UK: Cambridge University Press.

Baltes, P.B., & Mayer, K.U. (1999). *The Berlin Aging Study: Aging from 70 to 100.* New York, NY: Cambridge University Press.

Brawley, L.R, Flora, P.K., Locke, S.R., & Gierc, M.S.H. (2016). Social influence in promoting change among older adults: Group-mediated cognitive behavioral interventions. *Kinesiology Review, 5,* 39-49. doi:10.1123/kr.2015-0051

Centers for Disease Control and Prevention (2007). *Healthy aging for older adults.* Retrieved August 10, 2007, from www.cdc.gov/aging

Centers for Disease Control and Prevention (2013). *The state of aging and health in America 2013.* Atlanta, GA: Centers for Disease Control and Prevention, US Department of Health and Human Services.

Charles, S.& Carstensen, L.L. (2010). Social and emotional aging. *Annual Reviews of Psychology, 61,* 383-409. doi:10.1146/annurev.psych.093008.100448

Colcombe, S., & Kramer, A.F. (2003). Fitness effects on the cognitive function of older adults: A meta-analytic study. *Psychological Science, 14,* 125-130.

Depp, C.A., & Jeste, D.V. (2006). Definitions and predictors of successful aging: A comprehensive review of larger quantitative studies. *American Journal of Geriatric Psychology,14,* 6-20.

Diggs, J. (2008a). The cross-linkage theory of aging. In S. Loue & M. Sajatovic (Eds.), *Encyclopedia of Aging and Public Health* (pp. 250-252). Boston, MA: Springer Science.

Diggs, J. (2008b). Activity theory of aging. In S. Loue & M. Sajatovic. (Eds.), *Encyclopedia of Aging and Public Health* (pp. 79-81). Boston, MA: Springer Science.

Erikson, E., Erikson, J., & Kivnick. (1986). *Vital involvement in old age.* New York, NY: Norton.

Faber, M.J., Bosscher, R.J., Chin A Paw, M.J., & van Wieringen, P.C. (2006). Effects of exercise programs on falls and mobility in frail and pre-frail older adults: A multicenter randomized controlled trial. *Archives of Physical Medicine & Rehabilitation, 87,* 885-896.

Ferri, C., & James, I. (2009). Successful aging: Definitions and subjective assessment according to older adults. *Clinical Gerontology, 32,* 379-388.

Freund, A. M., & Baltes, P. B. (2007). Toward a theory of successful aging: Selection, optimization, and compensation. In R. Fernández-Ballesteros (Ed.), *Geropsychology. European perspectives for an aging world* (pp. 239-254). Göttingen, Germany: Hogrefe.

Frost, S.S., Goins, R.T., Hunter, R.H., Hooker, S.P., Bryant, L.L., Kruger, J., . . . Pluto, D. (2010). Effects of the built environment on physical activity of adults living in rural settings: A review of the literature. *American Journal of Health Promotion, 24,* 267-283. doi:10.4278/ajhp.08040532

Harman, D. (1956). Aging: A theory based on free radical and radiation chemistry. *Journal of Gerontology, 11,* 298-300.

Havighurst, R.J. (1961). Successful aging. *Gerontologist, 1,* 8-13.

Hayflick, L. (1961). The limited in vitro lifetime of human diploid cell strains. *Experimental Cell Research, 37,* 614-636.

Haywood, K.M. & Getchell, N. (2014). *Lifespan motor development* (6th ed.). Champaign, IL: Human Kinetics.

Hillman, C.H., Belopolsky, A.V., Snook, E.M., Kramer, A.F., & McAuley, E. (2004). Physical activity and executive control: Implications for increased cognitive health during older adulthood. *Research Quarterly for Exercise & Sport, 75,* 176-185.

Jopp, D., & Smith, J. (2006). Resources and life-management strategies as determinants of successful aging: On the protective effect of selection, optimization, and compensation. *Psychology and Aging, 21,* 253-265

Liffiton, J.A., Horton, S., Baker, J., & Weir, P.L. (2012). Successful aging: How does physical activity influence engagement in life? *European Review of Aging and Physical Activity, 9,* 98. doi:10.1007/s11556-012-0098-0

Marcus, B.H., Williams, D.M., Dubbert, P.M., Sallis, J.F., King, A.C., Yancey, A.K., . . . Claytor, R.P. (2006). Physical activity intervention studies: What we know and what we need to know: A scientific statement from the American Heart Association Council on Nutrition, Physical Activity, and Metabolism (subcommittee on physical activity); Council on Cardiovascular Disease in the Young; and the Interdisciplinary Working Group on Quality of Care and Outcomes Research. *Circulation, 114,* 2739-2752.

Maslow, A. (1943). A theory of human motivation. *Psychological Review, 50,* 370-396.

Maslow, A., & Lowery, R. (Eds.). (1998). *Toward a psychology of being* (3rd ed.). New York, NY: Wiley.

McLaughlin, S.J., Connell, C.M, Heeringa, S.G., Li, L.W., & Roberts, J.S. (2009). Successful aging in the United States: prevalence estimates from a national sample of older adults. *Journals of Gerontology: Psychological Science Sociological Science , 65B,* 216-226.

Medvedev, Z.A. (1981). Age changes and the rejuvenation processes related to reproduction. *Mechanisms of Ageing and Development, 17,* 331-349.

Meisner, B.A., Dogra, S., Logan, J.A., Baker, J., & Weir, P.L. (2010). Do or decline?: Comparing the effects of physical inactivity on biopsychosocial components of successful aging. *Journal of Health Psychology, 15,* 688-696.

Nelson, M.E., Rejeski, W.J., Blair, S.N., Duncan, P.W., Judge, J.O., King, A.C., . . . Castaneda-Sceppa, C. (2007). Physical activity and public health in older adults: Recommendation from the American College of Sports Medicine and the American Heart Association. *Medicine & Science in Sports & Exercise, 39,* 1435-1445.

Palmore, E.B. (1979). Predictors of successful aging. *Gerontologist, 19,* 427-431.

Passarino, G., De Rango, F., & Montesanto, A. (2016). Human longevity: Genetics or lifestyle? It takes two to tango. *Immunity & Ageing, 13,* 12. doi:10.1186/s12979-016-0066-z

Paterson, D. H., & Warburton, D.E.R. (2010). Physical activity and functional limitations in older adults: A systematic review related to Canada's Physical Activity Guidelines. *International Journal of Behavioral Nutrition and Physical Activity, 7,* 38. doi:10.1186/1479-5868-7-38

Peiffer, R., Darby, L.A., Fullenkamp, A., & Morgan, A.L. (2015). Effects of acute aerobic exercise on executive function in older women. *Journal of Sports Science Medicine, 14,* 574-583.

Phelan, E.A., Anderson, L.A., Lacroix, A.Z., & Larson, E.B. (2004). Older adults' views of "successful aging": How do they compare with researchers' definitions? *Journal of the American Geriatric Society, 52,* 211-216.

Pope, A.M., & Tarlov, A.R. (1999). *Disability in America: Toward a national agenda for prevention.* Washington, DC: National Academies Press.

Pruchno, R.A., Wilson-Genderson, M., & Cartwright, F. (2010). A two-factor model of successful aging. *Journal of Gerontology: Biological Sciences, 65B,* 671-679.

Reichstadt, J., Sengupta, G., Depp, C.A., Palinkas, L.A., & Jeste, D.V. (2010). Older adults' perspectives on successful aging: Qualitative Interviews. *American Journal of Geriatric Psychiatry, 18,* 567-575.

Rejeski, W.J., Brawley, L.R., & Haskell, W.L. (Eds.). (2003). Physical activity: Preventing physical disablement in older adults (Special issue). *American Journal of Preventive Medicine, 25,* (3Sii).

Rowe, J.W., & Kahn, R.L. (1987). Human aging: Usual and successful. *Science, 237,* 143-149.

Rowe, J.W., & Kahn, R.L. (1998). *Successful aging.* New York, NY: Pantheon Books.

Spirduso, W., Francis, K., & MacRae, P. (2005). *Physical dimensions of aging* (2nd ed.). Champaign, IL: Human Kinetics.

Strawbridge, W.J., Wallhagen, M.I., & Cohen, R.D. (2002). Successful aging and well-being: Self rated compared with Rowe and Kahn. *Gerontologist, 42,* 727-733.

Tay, L., & Diener, E. (2011). Needs and subjective well-being around the world. *Journal of Personality and Social Psychology, 101*(2), 354-365. doi:10.1037/a0023779

Umberson, D. & Montez, J.K. (2010). Social relationships and health: A flashpoint for health policy. *Journal of Health and Social Behavior, 51 (suppl),* S54-S66. doi:10.1177/0022146510383501

Warburton, D.E.R., Nicol, C.W., & Bredin, S.S. (2006). Health benefits of physical activity: The evidence. *Canadian Medical Association Journal, 174,* 801-809.

World Health Organization (1996). *The Heidelberg Guidelines for Promoting Physical Activity among Older Persons,* D.o.H.P. WHO Ageing and Health Programme, Education, and Communication. Geneva, Switzerland.

Young, J., Angevaren, M., Rusted, J., & Tabet, N. (2015). Aerobic exercise to improve cognitive function in older people without known cognitive impairment. *Cochrane Database Systematic Review, 4,* CD005381. doi:10.1002/14651858. CD005381.pub4

Chapter 3

AARP (2006). *Physical activity survey, 2006.* Washington, DC: AARP.

Acree, L.S., Longfors, J., Fjeldstad, A.S., Fjeldstad, C., Schank, B., Nickel, K.J., . . . Gardner, A.W. (2006). Physical activity is related to quality of life in older adults. *Health and Quality of Life Outcomes, 4,* 37. doi:10.1186/1477-7525-4-37

American College of Sports Medicine (ACSM). (2009). ACSM position stand on exercise and physical activity for older adults. *Medicine & Science in Sports & Exercise, 41,* 1510-1530.

Anderson-Hanley, C., Arciero, P.J., Brickman, A.M., Nimon, J.P., Okuma, N., Westen, S.C., . . . Zimmerman, E.A. (2012). Exergaming and older adult cognition: A cluster randomized clinical trial. *American Journal of PreventiveMedicine, 42*(2), 109-119.

Angus, J., & Reeve, P. (2006). Ageism: A threat to "aging well" in the 21st century. *Journal of Applied Gerontology, 25*(2), 137-152. doi:10.1177/0733464805285745

Aparicio-Ting, F. E., Farris, M., Courneya, K., Schiller, A., & Friedenreich, C. M. (2015). Predictors of physical activity at 12 month follow-up after a supervised exercise intervention in post-menopausal women. *International Journal of Behavioral Nutrition and Physical Activity, 12*: 55. doi:10.1186/s12966-015-0219-z

Armstrong, S., (2001). National blueprint: Increasing physical activity among adults age 50 and older [Special supplement]. *Journal of Aging and Physical Activity, 9.*

Bandura, A. (1997). *Self-efficacy. The exercise of control.* New York, NY: Freeman.

Bandura, A. (2005). The primacy of self-regulation in health promotion. *Applied Psychology, 54*(2), 245-254.

Barbour, K.A., & Blumenthal, J.A. (2005). Exercise training and depression in older adults. *Neurobiology of Aging, 26*(1, Supplement), 119-123. doi:10.1016/j. neurobiolaging.2005.09.007

Baumeister, R.F. and Leary, M.R. (1995). The need to belong: Desire for interpersonal attachments as a fundamental human motivation. *Psychological Bulletin, 117,* 497-529.

Beauchamp, M.R., Carron, A.V., McCutcheon, S., & Harper, O. (2007). Older adults' preferences for exercising alone versus in groups: Considering contextual congruence. *Annals of Behavioral Medicine, 33,* 200-206.

Benedetti, T.R.B., Schwingel, A., & Torres, T.D.L. (2011). Physical activity acting as a resource for social support among older adults in Brazil. *Journal of Human Sport and Exercise, 6,* 452-461. doi:10.4100/jhse.2011.62.26

Black, S.V., Cooper, R., Martin, K.R., Brage, S., Kuh, D., & Stafford, M. (2015) Physical Activity and Mental Well-being in a Cohort Aged 60–64 Years. *American Journal of Preventive Medicine, 49,* 172-180.

Bowling, A. (2007). Aspirations for older age in the 21st century: What is successful aging? *International Journal of Aging and Human Development, 64,* 263-297.

Bowling, A. & Iliffe, S. (2011) Psychological approach to successful aging predicts future quality of life in older adults. *Health and Quality of Life Outcomes, 9,* 13.

Brookmeyer, R., Evans, D.A., Hebert, L., Langa, K.M., Heeringa, S.G., Plassman, B.L., & Kukull, W.A. (2011). National estimates of the prevalence of Alzheimer's disease in the United States. *Alzheimer's & Dementia: The Journal of the Alzheimer's Association, 7*(1), 61-73.

Burton, N.W., Kahn, A., & Brown, W.J., (2012). How, where, and with whom? Physical activity context preferences of three adult groups at risk of inactivity. *British Journal of Sports Medicine, 46,* 1125-1131.

Butler, R.N., & Lewis, M.I. (1982). *Aging and mental health* (3rd ed.). St. Louis, MO: Mosby.

Cairney, J., Faught, B.E., Hay, J., Wade, T.J., & Corna, L. (2005). Physical activity and depressive symptoms in older adults. *Journal of Aging and Physical Activity, 2,* 98-114.

Chodzko-Zajko, W.J. (1995). The roots of ageism in contemporary society: An historical and scientific perspective. *Gerontologist, 35,* 105.

Chodzko-Zajko, W.J., Proctor, D.N., Singh, M.A.F., Minson, C.T., Nigg, C.R., Salem, G.J., & Skinner, J.S. (2009). American College of Sports Medicine position stand. Exercise and physical activity for older adults. *Medicine & Science in Sports & Exercise,* 1510-1530. doi:10.1249/MSS.0b013e3181a0c95c

Coelho, F.G.d.M, Gobbie, S., Andreatto, C.A.A., Corazza, D.I., Pedroso, R.V., & Santos-Galduroz, R.F. (2013). Physical exercise modulates peripheral levels of brain-derived neurotrophic factor (BDNF): A systematic review of experimental studies in the elderly. *Archives of Gerontology and Geriatrics, 56,* 10-15. doi:10.1016/j.archger.2012.06.003

Cohen-Mansfield, J., Marx, M.S., Biddison, J.R., & Guralnik, J.M. (2004). Socio-environmental exercise preferences among older adults. *Preventive Medicine, 38,* 804-11.

Colcombe, S., & Kramer, A.F. (2003). Fitness effects on the cognitive function of older adults: A meta-analytic study. *Psychological Science, 14,* 125-130.

Crombie, I.K., Irvine, L., Williams, B., McGinnis, A.R., Slane, P.W., Alder, E.M., & McMurdo, M.E.T. (2004). Why older people do not participate in leisure time physical activity: A survey of activity levels, beliefs and deterrents. *Age and Ageing, 33,* 287-292. doi:10.1093/ageing/afh089

Depp, C.A., & Jeste, D.V. (2009). Definitions and predictors of successful aging: A comprehensive review of larger quantitative studies. *Focus, VII,* 137-150.

Elavsky, S., McAuley, E., Motl, R.W., Konopack, J.F., Marquez, D.X., Hu, L., . . . Diener, E. (2005). Physical activity enhances long-term quality of life in older adults: Efficacy, esteem, and affective influences. *Annals of Behavioral Medicine, 30,* 138-145.

Erickson, K.I., Voss, M.W., Prakash, R.S., Basak, C., Szabo, A., Chaddock, L., . . . Kramer, A.F. (2011). Exercise training increases size of hippocampus and improves memory. *Proceedings of the National Academy of Sciences, 108*(7), 3017-3022. doi:10.1073/pnas.1015950108

Fox, K.R., Stathi, A., McKenna, J., & Davis, M.G., (2007). Physical activity and mental well-being in older people participating in the Better Ageing Project. *European Journal of Applied Physiology, 100,* 591-602.

Garber, C.E., Blissmer, B., Deschenes, M.R., Franklin, B.A., Lamonte, M.J., Lee, I.M., . . . American College of Sports Medicine (2011). American College of Sports Medicine position stand. Quantity and quality of exercise for developing and maintaining cardiorespiratory, musculoskeletal and neuromotor fitness in apparently healthy adults: Guidance for prescribing exercise. *Medicine & Science in Sports & Exercise, 43,* 1334-1359. doi:10.1249/MSS.0b013e318213fefb

Gellert, P., Ziegelmann, J.P., Warner, L.M., & Schwarzer, R. (2011). Physical activity intervention in older adults: Does a participating partner make a difference? *European Journal of Ageing, 8*(3), 211-219. doi:10.1007/s10433-011-0193-5

Gillison, F.B., Skevington, S.M., Sato, A., Standage, M., & Evangelidou, S. (2009). The effects of exercise interventions on quality of life in clinical and healthy populations: A meta-analysis. *Social Science & Medicine, 68,* 1700-1710.

Haselwandter, E.M., Corcoran, M.P., Folta, S.C., Hyatt, R., Fenton, M., & Nelson, M.E. (2015). The built environment, physical activity, and aging in the United States: A state of the science review. *Journal of Aging and Physical Activity, 23,* 323-329. doi:10.1123/japa.2013-0151

Hausdorff, J.M., Levy, B., & Wei, J.Y. (1999). The power of ageism on physical function of older persons: Reversibility of age-related gait changes. *Journal of the American Geriatrics Society, 47,* 1346-9.

Higgins, T.J., Middleton, K.R., Winner, L., & Janelle, C.M. (2014). Physical activity interventions differentially affect exercise task and barrier self-efficacy: A meta-analysis. *Health Psychology, 33,* 891-903. doi:10.1037/a0033864

Horton, S., Baker, J., Cote, J., & Deakin, J.M. (2008). Understanding seniors' perceptions and stereotypes of aging. *Educational Gerontology, 34*(11), 997-1017. doi:10.1080/03601270802042198

House, J.S., Umberson, D., & Landis, K.R. (1988). Structures and processes of social support. *Annual Reviews of Sociology, 14,* 293-318.

Kamal, A. (2011). Exergaming: New Age Gaming for Health, Rehabilitation and Education. In N. Meghanathan, B. Kaushik, & D. Nagamalai (Eds.), *Advanced Computing* (Vol. 133, pp. 421-430): New York, NY: Springer Berlin Heidelberg.

King, A. & King, D. (2010). Physical activity for an aging population. *Public Health Reviews, 32,* 401-426.

King A.C., Marcus, B., Ahn, D., Dunn, A.L., Rejeski, W.J., Sallis, J.F., & Coday M. (2006). Identifying subgroups that succeed or fail with three levels of physical activity intervention: the Activity Counseling Trial. *Health Psychology. 25,* 336-47.

Kirk-Sanchez, N.J., & McGough, E.L (2014). Physical exercise and cognitive performance in the elderly: Current perspective. *Clinical Interventions in Aging, 9,* 51-62.

Klusmann, V., Evers, A., Schwarzer, R., & Heuser, I. (2012). Views on aging and emotional benefits of physical activity: Effects of an exercise intervention in older women. *Psychology of Sport and Exercise, 13,* 236-242.

Koeneman, M., Verheijden, M., Chinapaw, M., & Hopman-Rock, M. (2011). Determinants of physical activity and exercise in healthy older adults: A systematic review. *International Journal of Behavioral Nutrition and Physical Activity, 8*(1), 142.

Komulainen, P., Kivipelto, M., Lakka, T.A., Savonen, K., Hassinen, M., Kiviniemi, V., . . . Rauramaa, R. (2010). Exercise, fitness and cognition—A randomised controlled trial in older individuals: The DR's EXTRA study. *European Geriatric Medicine, 1*(5), 266-272. doi:10.1016/j.eurger.2010.08.001

Kramer, A.F., & Erickson, K.I. (2007). Effects of physical activity on cognition, well-being, and brain: Human interventions. *Alzheimer's & Dementia: The Journal of the Alzheimer's Association, 3*(2), S45-S51.

Lee, C., & Russell, A., (2003). Effects of physical activity on emotional well-being among older Australian women. Cross-sectional and longitudinal analyses. *Journal of Psychosomatic Research, 54,* 155-160.

Levy, B.R. (1996). Improving memory in old age through implicit self-stereotyping. *Journal of Personality and Social Psychology, 71,* 1092-1107. doi:10.1037/0022-3514.71.6.1092

Levy, B.R. (2009). Stereotype embodiment: A psychosocial approach to aging. *Current Directions in Psychological Science, 18,* 332-336. doi:10.1111/j.1467-8721.2009.01662.x

Levy, B.R., & Myers, L.M. (2004). Preventive health behaviors influenced by self-perceptions of aging. *Preventive Medicine, 39*(3), 625-629. doi:10.1016/j.ypmed.2004.02.029

Levy, B.R., Slade, M.D., & Kasl, S.V. (2002). Longitudinal benefit of positive self-perceptions of aging on functional health. *The Journals of Gerontology Series B: Psychological Sciences and Social Sciences, 57*(5), P409-P417. doi:10.1093/geronb/57.5.P409

Levy, B.R., Slade, M.D., Kunkel, S.R., & Kasl, S.V. (2002). Longevity increased by positive self-perceptions of aging. *Journal of Personality and Social Psychology, 83*(2), 261-270. doi:10.1037/0022-3514.83.2.261

Lindland, E., Fond, M., Haydon, A., & Kendall-Taylor, N. (2015). *Gauging aging: Mapping gaps between expert and public understandings of aging in America.* Washington, DC: FrameWorks Institute.

Liu-Ambrose, T., Nagamatsu, L.S., Voss, M.W., Khan, K.M., & Handy, T.C. (2012). Resistance training and functional plasticity of the aging brain: A 12-month randomized controlled trial. *Neurobiology of Aging, 33*(8), 1690-1698.

Mathews, A.E., Laditka, S.B., Laditka, J.N., Wilcox, S., Corwin, S.J., Liu, R., . . . Logsdon, R.G. (2010). Older adults' perceived physical activity enablers and barriers: A multicultural perspective. *Journal of Aging and Physical Activity, 18*(2), 119-140.

McAuley, E., Doerksen, S.E., Morris, K.S., Motl, R.W., Hu, L., Wojcicki, T.R., . . . Rosengren, K.R. (2008). Pathways from physical activity to quality of life in older women. *Annals of Behavioral Medicine, 36,* 13-20. doi:10.1007/s12160-008-9036-9

McAuley, E., Elavsky, S., Motl, R.W., Konopack, J.F., Hu, L., & Marquez, D.X. (2005). Physical activity, self-efficacy, and self-esteem: Longitudinal relationships in older adults. *The Journals of Gerontology Series B: Psychological Sciences and Social Sciences, 60*(5), P268-P275. doi:10.1093/geronb/60.5.P268

McAuley, E., & Katula, J. (1998). Physical activity interventions in the elderly: Influence on physical health and psychological function. In R. Schulz, M.P. Lawton, & G. Maddox (Eds.), *Annual review of gerontology and geriatrics* (Vol. 18, pp. 115-154). New York, NY: Springer.

McAuley, E., Konopack, J.F., Motl, R.W., Morris, K.S., Doerksen, S.E., & Rosengren, K.R. (2006). Physical activity and quality of life in older adults: Influence of health status and self-efficacy. *Annals of Behavioral Medicine, 31,* 99-103.

McAuley, E., Kramer, A.F., & Colcombe, S.J., (2004). Cardiovascular fitness and neurocognitive function in older adults: A brief review. *Brain, Behavior, and Immunity, 18,* 214-220.

Moore, J.B., Mitchell, N.G., Beets, M.W., & Bartholomew, J.B., (2012). Physical self-esteem in older adults: A test of the indirect effect of physical activity. *Sport, Exercise and Performance Psychology, 1,* 231-241.

Motl, R.W., Konopack, J.F., McAuley, E., Elavsky, S., Jerome, G.J., & Marquez, D.X. (2005). Depressive symptoms among older adults: Long-term Reduction after a physical activity intervention. *Journal of Behavioral Medicine, 28*(4), 385-394. doi:10.1007/s10865-005-9005-5

Murphy, M., Nevill, A., Neville, C., Biddle, S., & Hardman, A. (2002). Accumulating brisk walking for fitness, cardiovascular risk and psychological health. *Medicine & Science in Sports & Exercise, 34,* 1468-1474. doi:10.1249/01.MSS.0000027686.50344.77

Nathan, A., Wood, L., & Giles-Corti, B. (2014). Perceptions of the built environment and associations with walking among retirement village residents. *Environment and Behavior, 46,* 46-69. doi:10.1177/0013916512450173

Nelson, M.E., Rejeski, W.J., Blair, S.N., Duncan, P.W., Judge, J.O., King, A.C., . . . Castaneda-Sceppa, C. (2007). Physical activity and public health in older adults: Recommendation from the American College of Sports Medicine and the American Heart Association. *Medicine & Science in Sports & Exercise, 39*(8), 1435-1445.

Netz, Y., & Raviv, S. (2004). Age differences in motivational orientation toward physical Activity: An application of social–cognitive theory. *The Journal of Psychology, 138*(1), 35-48.

Netz, Y., Wu, M.-J., Becker, B.J., & Tenenbaum, G. (2005). Physical activity and psychological well-being in advanced age: A meta-analysis of intervention studies. *Psychology and Aging, 20*(2), 272-284. doi:10.1037/0882-7974.20.2.272

Opdenacker, J., Delecluse, C., & Boen, F. (2009). The longitudinal effects of a lifestyle physical activity intervention and a structured exercise intervention on physical self-perceptions and self-esteem in older adults. *Journal of Sport & Exercise Psychology, 31,* 743-760.

Orsega-Smith, E.M., Payne, L.L., Mowen, A.J., Ching-Hua, H., & Godbey, G.C. (2007). The role of social support and self-efficacy in shaping the leisure time physical activity of older adults. *Journal of Leisure Research, 39,* 705-727.

Ory, M., Kinney Hoffman, M., Hawkins, M., Sanner, B., & Mockenhaupt, R. (2003). Challenging aging stereotypes: Strategies for creating a more active society. *American Journal of Preventive Medicine, 25,* 164-171.

PAGAC (Physical Activity Guidelines Advisory Committee). (2018). *2018 Physical activity guidelines advisory committee scientific report.* Washington, DC: U.S. Department of Health and Human Services.

Palmore, E. (2004). Research note: Ageism in Canada and the United States. *Journal of Cross-Cultural Gerontology, 19*(1), 41-46. doi:10.1023/B:JCCG.0000015098.62691.ab

Park, C.-H., Chodzko-Zajko, W., Ory, M.G., Gleason-Senior, J., Bazzarre, T.L., & Mockenhaupt, R. (2010). The impact of a national strategy to increase physical activity among older adults on national organizations. *Journal of Aging and Physical Activity, 18*(4), 425-438.

Powell, K.E., Paluch, A.E., & Blair, S.N. (2011). Physical activity for health: What kind? How much? How intense? On top of what? *Annual Review of Public Health, 32,* 349-365. doi:10.1146/annurev-publhealth-031210-101151

Rennemark, M., Lindwall, M., Halling, A., & Berglund, J. (2009). Relationships between physical activity and perceived qualities of life in old age. Results of the SNAC study. *Aging & Mental Health, 13,* 1-9.

Rosenberg, M., Schooler, C., Schoenbach, C., & Rosenberg, F. (1995). Global self-esteem and specific self-esteem: Different concepts, different outcomes. *American Sociological Review, 60*(1), 141-156. doi:10.2307/2096350

Schutzer, K.A., & Graves, B.S. (2004). Barriers and motivations to exercise in older adults. *Preventive Medicine, 39,* 1056-1061.

Singh, N.A., Stavrinos, T.M., Scarbek, Y., Galambos, G., Liber, C., & Fiatarone Singh, M.A. (2005). A randomized controlled trial of high versus low intensity weight training versus general practitioner care for clinical depression in older adults. *The Journals of Gerontology Series A: Biological Sciences and Medical Sciences, 60*(6), 768-776. doi:10.1093/gerona/60.6.768

Smith, P.J., Blumenthal, J.A., Hoffman, B.M., Cooper, H., Strauman, T.A., Welsh-Bohmer, K., . . . Sherwood, A. (2010). Aerobic exercise and neurocognitive performance: A meta-analytic review of randomized controlled trials. *Psychosomatic Medicine, 72,* 239-252. doi:10.1097/PSY.0b013e3181d14633

Snowden, M., Steinman, L., Mochan, K., Grodstein, F., Prohaska, T. R., Thurman, D.J., . . . Anderson, L.A. (2011). Effect of exercise on cognitive performance in community-dwelling older adults: Review of intervention trials and recommendations for public health practice and research. *Journal of the American Geriatrics Society, 59*(4), 704-716. doi:10.1111/j.1532-5415.2011.03323.x

Sonstroem, R.J., Harlow, L.L., & Josephs, L. (1994). Exercise and self-esteem: Validity of model expansion and exercise associations. *Journal of Sport & Exercise Psychology, 16,* 29-42.

Sonstroem, R.J., & Morgan, W.P., (1989). Exercise and self-esteem: Rationale and model. *Medicine & Science in Sports & Exercise, 21,* 329-337.

Spence, J.E., McGannon, K.R., & Poon, P. (2005). The effect of exercise on global self-esteem: A quantitative review. *Journal of Sport & Exercise Psychology, 27,* 311-334.

Strachan, S.M., Brawley, L.R., Spink, K., & Glazebrook, K. (2010). Older adults' physically-active identity: Relationships between social cognitions, physical activity and satisfaction with life. *Psychology of Sport and Exercise, 11*(2), 114-121. doi:10.1016/j.psychsport.2009.09.002

Steinmo, S., Hagger-Johnson, G., & Shahab, L. (2014). Bidirectional association between mental health and physical activity in older adults: Whitehall II prospective cohort study. *Preventive Medicine, 66,* 74-79.

Thomas, P.A. (2010). Is it better to give or to receive? Social support and the well-being of older adults. *Journal of Gerontology, 65B,* 351-357.

Thornton, J.E. (2002). Myths of aging or ageist stereotypes. *Educational Gerontology, 28*(4), 301-312. doi:10.1080/036012702753590415

Tilvis, R.S., Routasalo, P., Karppinen, H., Strandberg, T.E., Kautiainen, H., & Pitkala, K.H., (2012). Social isolation, social activity and loneliness as survival indicators in old age; A nationwide survey with a 7-year follow-up. *European Geriatric Medicine, 3,* 18-22.

Troiano, R P., Berrigan, D., Dodd, K.W., Masse, L.C., Tilert, T., & McDowell, M. (2008). Physical activity in the United States measured by accelerometer. *Medicine & Science in Sports & Exercise, 40,* 181-188.

U.S. Department of Health and Human Services (2008). *2008 Physical activity guidelines for Americans.* Retrieved from https://health.gov/paguidelines/pdf/paguide.pdf

U.S. Surgeon General. (1996). *Physical activity and health.* Washington, DC: U.S. Department of Health and Human Services.

Vance, D. E., Wadley, V. G., Ball, K. K., Roenker, D. L., & Rizzo, M. (2005). The effects of physical activity and sedentary behavior on cognitive health in older adults. *Journal of Aging and Physical Activity, 13,* 294–313.

Warburton, D., Nicol, C.W., & Bredin, S. (2006). Health benefits of physical activity: The evidence. *Canadian Medical Association Journal, 174,* 801-809.

Warner, L.M., Schuz, B., Wolff, J.K., Parschau, L., Wurm, S. & Schwarzer, R. (2014). Sources of self-efficacy for physical activity. *Health Psychology, 33,* 1298-1308. doi:10.1037/hea0000085

Warner, L.M., Ziegelmann, J.P., Schuz, B., Wrum, S., & Schwarzer, R. (2011). Synergistic effect of social support and self-efficacy on physical exercise in older adults.. *Journal of Aging and Physical Activity, 19*(3), 249-261.

White, S.M., Wojcicki, T.R., & McAuley, E. (2009). Physical activity and quality of life in community dwelling older adults. *Health and Quality of Life Outcomes, 7,* 10.

White, S.M., Wojcicki, T.R., & McAuley, E (2012). Social cognitive influences on physical activity behavior in middle-aged and older adults. *Journals of Gerontology, 67B,* 18-26.

Wilcox, S., King, A.C., Brassington, G.S., & Ahn, D.K. (1999). Physical Activity Preferences of Middle-Aged and Older Adults: A Community Analysis. *Journal of Aging and Physical Activity, 7,* 386-399.

Wilcox, S., Dowda, M., Leviton, L.C., Bartlett-Prescott, J., Bazzarre, T., Campbell-Voytal, K., . . . Wegley, S. (2008). Active for life. Final results from the translation of two physical activity programs. *American Journal of Preventive Medicine, 35,* 340-351.

Wilson, K.S., & Spink, K.S. (2006). Exploring older adults' social influences for physical activity. *Activities, Adaptation & Aging, 30,* 47-60. doi:10.1300/J016v30n03_03

Wilson, K.S., & Spink, K.S. (2009). Social influence and physical activity in older females: Does activity preference matter? *Psychology of Sport and Exercise, 10,* 481-488. doi:10.1016/j.psychsport.2009.01.002

World Health Organization. (1998). *Growing older—Staying well: Aging and physical activity in everyday life.* Geneva, Switzerland: World Health Organization.

World Health Organization. (2018). *Global action plan on physical activity 2018-2030: More active people for a healthier world.*

Wurm, S., Tesch-Römer, C., & Tomasik, M.J. (2007). Longitudinal findings on aging-related cognitions, control beliefs, and health in later life. *The Journals of Gerontology Series B: Psychological Sciences and Social Sciences, 62*(3), P156-P164.

Wurm, S., Tomasik, M.J., & Tesch-Römer, C. (2010). On the importance of a positive view on aging for physical exercise among middle-aged and older adults: Cross-sectional and longitudinal findings. *Psychology & Health, 25*(1), 25-42.

Chapter 4

Aagaard, P., Suetta, C., Caserotti, P., Magnusson, S.P., & Kjær, M. (2010). Role of the nervous system in sarcopenia and muscle atrophy with aging: Strength training as a countermeasure. *Scandinavian Journal of Medicine & Science in Sports, 20*, 49-64.

Ahlskog, J.E., Geda, Y.E., Graff-Radford, N.R., & Petersen, R C. (2011). Physical exercise as a preventive or disease-modifying treatment of dementia and brain aging. *Mayo Clinic Proceedings, 86*, 876-884.

American College of Sports Medicine (2017). *ACSM's Guidelines for Exercise Testing and Prescription* (10th ed.). Philadelphia, PA: Lippincott Williams & Wilkins.

Bassey, E.J., Fiatarone, M.A., O'Neill, E.F., Kelly, M., Evans, W. J., & Lipsitz, L. A. (1992). Leg extensor power and functional performance in very old men and women. *Clinical Science, 82,* 321-327.

Betik, A.C., & Hepple, R.T. (2008). Determinants of $\dot{V}O_2$max decline with aging: An integrated perspective. *Applied Physiology, Nutrition, and Metabolism, 33,* 130-140.

Billman, G.E. (2002). Aerobic exercise conditioning: a nonpharmacological antiarrhythmic intervention. *Journal of Applied Physiology, 92,* 446-454. doi:10.1152/japplphysiol.00874.2001

Brunner, F., Schmid, A., Sheikhzadeh, A., Nordin, M., Yoon, J., & Frankel, V. (2007). Effects of aging on type II muscle fibers: A systematic review of the literature. *Journal of Aging and Physical Activity, 15*(3), 336-348.

Chodzko-Zajko, W.J., Proctor, D.N., Fiatarone Singh, M.A., Minson, C.T., Nigg, C.R., Salem, G.J., & Skinner, J.S. (2009). American College of Sports Medicine Position Stand. Exercise and physical activity for older adults. *Medicine & Science in Sports & Exercise, 41,* 1510-1530. doi: 10.1249/MSS.0b013e3181a0c95c

Colcombe, S., & Kramer, A.F. (2003). Fitness effects on the cognitive function of older adults: A meta-analytic study. *Psychological Science, 14*(2), 125-130.

Cruz-Jentoft, A.J., Landi, F., Topinková, E., & Michel, J.P. (2010). Understanding sarcopenia as a geriatric syndrome. *Current Opinions in Clinical Nutritional Metabolism Care, 1,* 1-7. doi:10.1097/MCO.0b013e328333c1c1

Cunningham, D.A., Paterson, D.H., Koval, J.J., & St. Croix, C.M. (1997). A model of oxygen transport capacity changes for independently living older men and women. *Canadian Journal of Applied Physiology, 22*(5), 439-453.

Eagan, M.S., & Sedlock, D.A. (2001). Kyphosis in active and sedentary postmenopausal women. *Medicine & Science in Sports & Exercise, 33*(5), 688-695.

Erickson, K.I., & Kramer, A.F. (2009). Aerobic exercise effects on cognitive and neural plasticity in older adults. *British Journal of Sports Medicine, 43*(1), 22-24.

Fagard, R.H. (2001). Exercise characteristics and the blood pressure response to dynamic physical training. *Medicine & Science in Sports & Exercise, 3*(6; Supp.), S484-S492.

Farage, M.A., Miller, K.W., Ayaji, F., & Hutchins, D. (2012). Design principles to accommodate older adults. *Global Journal of Health Science, 4,* 2-25. doi: 10.5539/gjhs.v4n2p2

Fiatarone, M.A., O'Neill, E.F., Ryan, N.D., Clements, K.M., Solares, G.R., Nelson, M.E., . . . Evans, W.J. (1994). Exercise training and nutritional supplementation for physical frailty in very elderly people. *New England Journal of Medicine, 330,* 1769-1775.

Fitzgerald, M. D., Tanaka, H., Tran, Z. V., & Seals, D. R. (1997). Age-related declines in maximal aerobic capacity in regularly exercising vs. sedentary women: A meta-analysis. *Journal of Applied Physiology, 83,* 160-165.

Flegal, K.E., and Reuter-Lorenz, P.A. (2010). Commentary aging and brain fitness. *European Journal of Neuroscience, 31*, 165–166.

Frontera, W.R., Meredith, C.N., O'Reilly, K.P., Knuttgen, H.G., & Evans, W.J. (1988). Strength conditioning in older men: Skeletal muscle hypertrophy and improved function. *Journal of Applied Physiology, 64*(3), 1038-1044.

Gomez-Cabello, A., Ara, I., González-Agüero, A., Casajus, J.A., & Vicente-Rodriguez, G. (2012). Effects of training on bone mass in older adults. *Sports Medicine, 42*(4), 301-325.

Hedman, A.M., van Haren, N.E., Schnack, H.G., Kahn, R.S., Pol, H., & Hilleke, E. (2012). Human brain changes across the life span: A review of 56 longitudinal magnetic resonance imaging studies. *Human Brain Mapping, 33*(8), 1987-2002.

Hepple, R.T. (2000). Skeletal muscle: Microcirculatory adaptation to metabolic demand. *Medicine & Science in Sports & Exercise, 32*(1), 117-123.

Holloszy, J.O. (2001). Cellular adaptations to endurance exercise: Master athletes. *International*

Journal of Sport Nutrition and Exercise Metabolism, 11, 186-188.

Huang, G., Gibson, C.A., Tran, Z.V., & Osness, W.H. (2005). Controlled endurance exercise training and V̇O₂max changes in older adults: A meta-analysis. *Preventive Cardiology, 8*(4), 217-225.

Huggett, D.L., Connelly, D.M., & Overend, T.J. (2005). Maximal aerobic capacity testing of older adults: A critical review. *The Journals of Gerontology: Series A, 60*, 57-66. doi:10.1093/gerona/60.1.57

Katzel, L.I., Sorkin, J.D., & Fleg, J.L. (2001). A comparison of longitudinal changes in aerobic fitness in older endurance athletes and sedentary men. *Journal of the American Geriatrics Society, 49*(12), 1657-1664.

Kukuljan, S., Nowson, C.A., Bass, S.L., Sanders, K., Nicholson, G.C., Seibel, M.J., . . . Daly, R.M. (2009). Effects of a multi-component exercise program and calcium–vitamin-D3-fortified milk on bone mineral density in older men: A randomised controlled trial. *Osteoporosis International, 20*(7), 1241-1251.

Liu-Ambrose, T., Nagamatsu, L.S., Voss, M.W., Khan, K.M., & Handy, T.C. (2012). Resistance training and functional plasticity of the aging brain: A 12-month randomized controlled trial. *Neurobiology of Aging, 33*(8), 1690-1698.

MacRae, P.G., Feltner, M.E., & Reinsch, S.A. (1994). One-year exercise program for older women: Effects on falls, injuries, and physical performance. *Journal of Aging and Physical Activity, 2*, 127-142.

Marcus, R. (2001). Role of exercise in preventing and treating osteoporosis. *Rheumatic Disease Clinics of North America, 27*(1), 131-141.

Marques, E.A., Mota, J., Machado, L., Sousa, F., Coelho, M., Moreira, P., & Carvalho, J. (2011). Multicomponent training program with weight-bearing exercises elicits favorable bone density, muscle strength, and balance adaptations in older women. *Calcified Tissue International, 88*(2), 117-129.

Martini, F.H., Tallitsch, R.B., & Nath, J.L. (2017). *Human anatomy* (9th ed.). New York, NY: Pearson Publishing.

Martins, R.A., Veríssimo, M.T.,Coelho e Silva, M.J., Cumming, S.P., & Teixeira, A.M. (2010). Effects of aerobic and strength-based training on metabolic health indicators in older adults. *Lipids in Health and Disease, 9*(1), 1.

Metcalfe, L., Lohman, T., Going, S., Houtkooper, L., Ferriera, D., Flint-Wagner, H., . . . Cussler, E. (2001). Postmenopausal women and exercise for prevention of osteoporosis: The Bone, Estrogen, Strength Training (BEST) Study. *ACSM's Health & Fitness Journal, 5*(3), 6-14.

National Center for Injury Prevention and Control (2015). Preventing falls: A guide to implementing effective community-based fall prevention programs (2nd ed.). Atlanta, GA: Centers for Disease Control and Prevention.

Nelson, M.E., Rejeski, W.J., Blair, S.N., Duncan, P.W., Judge, J.O., King, A.C., . . . Castaneda-Sceppa, C. (2007). Physical activity and public health in older adults: Recommendation from the American College of Sports Medicine and the American Heart Association. *Circulation, 116*(9), 1094.

Nieman, D.C. (2010). *Exercise testing and prescription: A health related approach* (7th ed.). Columbus, OH: McGraw-Hill Education.

Paterson, D.H., Cunningham, D.A., Koval, J.J., & St. Croix, C.M. (1999). *Medicine & Science in Sports & Exercise, 31*, 1813-20. PMID:10613433

Perini, R., Fisher, N., Veicsteinas, A., & Pendergast, D.R. (2002). Aerobic training and cardiovascular responses at rest and during exercise in older men and women. *Medicine & Science in Sports & Exercise, 34*(4), 700-708.

Persinger, R., Foster, C., Gibson, M., Fater, D.C., & Porcari, J.P. (2004). Consistency of the talk test for exercise prescription. *Medicine & Science in Sports & Exercise, 36*(9), 1632-1636.

Peters, R. (2006). Ageing and the brain. *Postgraduate Medical Journal, 82*, 84-88. doi:10.1136/pgnj.2005.036665

Peterson, M. D., & Gordon, P. M. (2011). Resistance exercise for the aging adult: clinical implications and prescription guidelines. *The American Journal of Medicine, 124*(3), 194-198.

Peterson, M.D., Rhea, M.R., Sen, A., & Gordon, P.M. (2010). Resistance exercise for muscular strength in older adults: A meta-analysis. *Ageing Research Reviews, 9*(3), 226-237.

Reid, K.F., & Fielding, R.A. (2012). Skeletal muscle power: A critical determinant of physical functioning in older adults. *Exercise and Sport Sciences Reviews, 40*(1), 4.

Reid, K.F., Doros, G., Clark, D.J., Patten, C., Carabello, R.J., Cloutier, G.J., . . .Fielding, 2012. Muscle power failure in mobility-limited older adults: preserved single fiber function despite lower whole muscle size, quality and rate of neuromuscular activation. *European Journal of Applied Physiology, 112*, 2289-2301. doi: 10.1007/s00421-011-2200-0.

Rosenberg, I.H. (2011). Sarcopenia: Origins and clinical relevance. *Clinics in Geriatric Medicine, 27*(3), 337-339.

Salthouse, T. (2012). Consequences of age-related cognitive declines. *Annual Review of Psychology, 63,* 201.

Sayer, S.P. (2007). High-speed power training: a novel approach to resistance training in older men and women. A brief review and pilot study. *Journal of Strength and Conditioning Research, 21,* 518-26. PMID: 17530980.

Sayer, S.P., & Gibson, K. (2010). A comparison of high-speed power training and traditional slow-speed resistance training in older men and women. *Journal of Strength and Conditioning Research, 24,* 3369-80.

Sayer, A.A., Syddall, H., Martin, H., Patel, H., Baylis, D., & Cooper, C. (2008). The developmental origins of sarcopenia. *The Journal of Nutrition Health and Aging, 12*(7), 427-432.

Scheuermann, B.W., Bell, C., Paterson, D.H., Barstow, T.J., & Kowalchuk, J.M. (2002). Oxygen uptake kinetics for moderate exercise are speeded in older humans by prior heavy exercise. *Journal of Applied Physiology, 92*(2), 609-616.

Seals, D.R., Monahan, K.D., Bell, C., Tanaka, H., & Jones, P.P. (2001). The aging cardiovascular system: Changes in autonomic function at rest and in response to exercise. *International Journal of Sport Nutrition and Exercise Metabolism, 11,* 189-195.

Shephard, R.J. (1997). *Aging, physical activity, and health.* Champaign, IL: Human Kinetics.

Short, K.., & Nair, K.S. (2001). Muscle protein metabolism and the sarcopenia of aging. *International Journal of Sport Nutrition and Exercise Metabolism, 11,* 119-127.

Spirduso, W.W. (1975). Reaction and movement time as a function of age and physical activity level. *Journal of Gerontology, 30*(4), 435-440.

Spirduso, W.W., & Clifford, P. (1978). Replication of age and physical activity effects on reaction and movement time. *Journal of Gerontology, 33*(1), 26-30.

Spirduso, W. W., Francis, K. L., & MacRae, P. G. (2005). *Physical dimensions of aging.* Champaign, IL: Human Kinetics.

Sprung, J., Gajic, O., & Warner, D.O. (2006). Review article: Age related alterations in respiratory function—anesthetic considerations. *Canadian Journal of Anesthesia, 53*(12), 1244-1257.

U.S. Department of Health and Human Services (2015). Surgeon General's Report on Bone Health and Osteoporosis. What It Means To You. Available at: https://www.bones.nih.gov/sites/bones/files/SGRBoneHealthEnglish2015_022516_0.pdf

Tanaka, H., Monahan, K.D., & Seals, D.R. (2001). Age-predicted maximal heart rate revisited. *Journal of the American College of Cardiology, 37*(1), 153-156.

Tanaka, H., & Seals, D.R. (2008). Endurance exercise performance in Masters athletes: Age-associated changes and underlying physiological mechanisms. *The Journal of Physiology, 586*(1), 55-63.

Taylor, B.J., & Johnson, B.D. (2010). The pulmonary circulation and exercise responses in the elderly. In *Seminars in respiratory and critical care medicine* (Vol. 31, No. 5, pp. 528-538). New York, NY: Thieme Medical Publishers.

Tschopp, M., Sattelmayer, M.K., & Hilfiker, R. (2011). Is power training or conventional resistance training better for function in elderly persons? A meta-analysis. *Age and Ageing, 40*(5), 549-556.

U.S. Department of Health and Human Services (2004). Bone health and osteoporosis. A Report of the Surgeon General. Rockville, MD: U.S. Department of Health and Human Services.

Vandervoort, A.A. (2009). Potential benefits of warm-up for neuromuscular performance of older athletes. *Exercise and Sport Sciences Reviews, 37*(2), 60-65.

Voelcker-Rehage, C., & Niemann, C. (2013). Structural and functional brain changes related to different types of physical activity across the life span. *Neuroscience & Biobehavioral Reviews, 37*(9), 2268-2295.

Volkers, K.M., de Kieviet, J.F., Wittingen, H.P., & Scherder, E.J.A. (2012). Lower limb muscle strength (LLMS): Why sedentary life should never start? A review. *Archives of Gerontology and Geriatrics, 54*(3), 399-414.

Voss, M.W., Nagamatsu, L.S., Liu-Ambrose, T., & Kramer, A.F. (2011). Exercise, brain, and cognition across the life span. *Journal of Applied Physiology, 111*(5), 1505-1513.

Wiebe, C.G., Gledhill, N., Jamnik, V.K., & Ferguson, S.(1999). Exercise cardiac function in young through elderly endurance trained women. *Medicine & Science in Sports & Exercise, 31*(5), 684-691.

Wilson, T.M., & Tanaka, H. (2000). Meta-analysis of the age-associated decline in maximal aerobic capacity in men: Relation to training status. *American Journal of Physiology: Heart and Circulatory Physiology, 278*(3), H829-H834.

Zehnacker, C.H., & Bemis-Dougherty, A. (2007). Effect of weighted exercises on bone mineral density in postmenopausal women: A systematic review. *Journal of Geriatric Physical Therapy, 30*(2), 79-88.

Chapter 5

American College of Sports Medicine. (2017). *ACSM's guidelines for exercise testing and prescription* (10th ed.). Philadelphia, PA: Lippincott Williams & Wilkins.

Expert Panel on the Identification, Evaluation, and Treatment of Overweight and Obesity in Adults. (1998). Executive summary of the clinical guidelines on the identification, evaluation, and treatment of overweight and obesity in adults. *Archives of Internal Medicine, 158,* 1855-1867.

Flint, A.J., Rexrode, K.M., Hu, F.B., Glynn, R.J., Caspard, H., Manson, J.E., . . . Rimm, E.B. (2010). Body mass index, waist circumference, and risk of coronary heart disease: A prospective study among men and women. *Obesity Research & Clinical Practice, 4,* e171-e181. doi:10.1016/j.orcp.2010.01.001

Jamnik, V.J., Warburton, D.E.R., Makarski, J., McKenzie, D.C., Shephard, R.J., Stone, J., & Gledhill, N. (2011). Enhancing the effectiveness of clearance for physical activity participation; Background and overall process. *Applied Physiology, Nutrition, & Metabolism, 36,* S3-S13.

Rikli, R.E., & Jones, C.J. (1998). The reliability and validity of a 6-minute walk test as a measure of physical endurance in older adults. *Journal of Aging and Physical Activity, 6,* 363-375.

Rikli, R.E., & Jones, C.J. (2013). *Senior fitness test manual* (2nd ed.). Champaign, IL: Human Kinetics.

Soares-Miranda, L., Siscovick, D.S., Psaty, B.M., Longstreth, W.T., & Mozaffarian, D. (2016). Physical activity and risk of coronary heart disease and stroke in older adults: The cardiovascular health study. *Circulation, 133,* 147-155. doi:10.1161/CIRCULATIONAHA.115.018323

Tennant, R., Hiller, L., Fishwick, R., Platt, S., Joseph, S., Weich, S. . . . Stewart-Brown, S. (2007). The Warwick-Edinburgh mental well-being scale (WEMWBS): development and UK validation. *Health and Quality of Life Outcomes, 5,* 63.

Thompson, P.D., Franklin, B.A., Balady, G.J., Blair, S.N., Corrado, D., Estes, N.A.M., III, . . . Costa, F., in collaboration with the American College of Sports Medicine (2007). Exercise and acute cardiovascular events: Placing the risks into per-spective. A scientific statement from the American Heart Association Council on Nutrition, Physical Activity, and Metabolism and the Council on Clinical Cardiology. *Circulation, 115,* 2358-2368.

Warburton, D.E.R., Gledhill, N., Jamnik, V.K., Bredin, S.S.D., McKenzie, D.C., Stone, J., . . . Shephard, R.J. (2011). Evidence-based risk assessment and recommendations for physical activity clearance: Consensus document. *Applied Physiology, Nutrition, & Metabolism, 36,* S266-S298.

World Health Organization (2008). *Waist circumference and waist-hip ratio: Report of a WHO expert consultation.* Geneva, Switzerland: World Health Organization.

Chapter 6

Berg, K., Wood-Dauphinee, S.L., & Williams, J.T. (1992). Measuring balance in the elderly: Validation of an instrument. *Canadian Journal of Public Health, 83,* S9-S11.

Berg, K.O., Wood-Dauphinee, S.L., Williams, J.I., & Gayton, D. (1989). Measuring balance in the elderly: Preliminary development of an instrument. *Physiotherapy Canada, 41,* 304-311.

Cesari, M. (2011). Role of gait speed in the assessment of older patients. *Journal of the American Medical Association, 305,* 93-94.

Giuliani, C. A., Gruber-Baldini, A. L., Park, N. S., Schrodt, L.A., Rokoske, F., Sloane, P.D., & Zimmerman, S. (2008). Physical performance characteristics of assisted living residents and risk for adverse health outcomes. *The Gerontologist, 48,* 203-212. doi:10.1093/geront/48.2.203

Guralnik, J.M., Ferrucci, L., Pieper, C., Leveille, S.G., Markides, K.S., Ostir, G.V., . . . Wallace, R.B. (2000). Lower extremity function and subsequent disability: Consistency across studies, predictive models, and value of gait speed alone compared with the short physical performance battery. *Journal of Gerontology: Medical Sciences, 55,* M221-M231.

Guralnik, J. M., Simonsick, E. M., Ferrucci, L., Glynn, R.J., Berkman, L.F., Blazer, D.G., . . . Wallace, R.B. (1994). A short physical performance battery assessing lower extremity function: Association with self-reported disability and prediction of mortality and nursing home admission. *Journal of Gerontology, Medical Sciences, 49,* M85-M94.

Hernandez, D., & Rose, D.J. (2008). Predicting which older adults will or will not fall using the Fullerton Advanced Balance Scale. *Archives of Physical Medicine & Rehabilitation, 89,* 2309-2315.

Rikli, R.E. & Jones, C.J. (1999a), "Development and validation of a functional fitness test for community-residing older adults," *Journal of Aging and Physical Activity 7*, 129-161.

Rikli, R.E., & Jones, C.J. (1999b). Functional fitness normative scores for community-residing older adults, ages 60-94. *Journal of Aging and Physical Activity, 7,* 162-181.

Rikli, R.E., & Jones, C.J. (2013a). Development and validation of criterion-referenced clinically relevant fitness standards for maintaining physical independence in later years. *The Gerontologist, 2,* 255-267. doi:10.1093/geront/gns071.

Rikli, R.E., & Jones, C.J. (2013b). *Senior fitness test manual* (2nd ed.). Champaign, IL: Human Kinetics.

Rose, D.J. (2010) *FallProof!: A comprehensive balance and mobility training program* (2nd ed.). Champaign, IL: Human Kinetics.

Rose, D.J., Lucchese, N., & Wiersma, L.D. (2006). Development of a multidimensional balance scale for use with functionally independent older adults. *Archives of Physical Medicine & Rehabilitation, 87,* 1478-1485.

Seeman, T. E., Charpentier, P. A., Berkman, L. F., Tinetti, M.E., Guralnik, J.M., Albert, M. (1994). Predicting changes in physical performance in a high-functioning elderly cohort: MacArthur Studies of Successful Aging. *Journal of Gerontology, 49,* M97-M108.

Studenski, S., Perera, S., Patel, K., Rosano, C., Faulkner, K., Inzitari, M., . . . Guralnik, J. (2011). Gait speed and survival in older adults. *Journal of the American Medical Association, 305,* 50-58.

VanSwearingen, J.M., & Brach, J.S. (2001). Making geriatric assessment work: Selecting useful measures. *Physical Therapy, 81,* 1233-1252.

World Health Organization (2002). *Active ageing: A policy framework.* Geneva, Switzerland: Author.

Chapter 7

Ajzen, I. (1991). The theory of planned behavior. *Organizational Behavior and Human Decision Processes, 50,* 179-211.

Ajzen, I. (2011). The theory of planned behavior: Reactions and reflections. *Psychology and Health, 26,* 1113-1127.

Ajzen, I., & Fishbein, M. (1980). *Understanding attitudes and predicting social behavior.* Englewood Cliffs, NJ: Prentice-Hall.

Ashworth, N.L., Chad, K.E., Harrison, E.L., Reeder, B.A., & Marshall, S.C. (2005). Home versus center based physical activity programs in older adults. *Cochrane Database of Systematic Reviews, 1.* doi:10.1002/14651858.CD004017.pub2

Bandura, A. (1977). Self-efficacy: Toward a unifying theory of behavioral change. *Psychological Review, 84,* 191-215.

Bandura, A. (1982). Self-efficacy mechanism in human agency. *American Psychologist, 37,* 122-147.

Bandura, A. (1986a). *Social foundations of thought and action: A social cognitive theory.* Englewood Cliffs, NJ: Prentice-Hall.

Bandura, A. (1986b). The explanatory and predictive scope of self-efficacy theory. *Journal of Social and Clinical Psychology, 4,* 359-373.

Bandura, A. (1997). *Self-efficacy: The exercise of control.* New York, NY: W.H. Freeman Company.

Baranowski, T., Perry, C.L., & Parcel, G.S. (2002). How individuals, environments, and health behavior interact. Social cognitive theory. In K. Glanz, B.K. Rimer, & F.M. Lewis (Eds.), *Health behavior and health education: Theory, research, and practice* (3rd ed., pp. 165-184). San Francisco, CA: Jossey-Bass.

Beauchamp, M.R., Carron, A.V., McCutcheon, S., & Harper, O. (2007). Older adults' preferences for exercising alone versus in groups: Considering contextual congruence. *Annals of Behavioral Medicine, 33,* 200-206. doi:10.1080/08836610701310037

Brittain, E.L., Jones, C.J., & Rikli, R.E. (2002). Barriers to physical activity in older adults as a function of age, gender, and activity level [Abstract]. *Medicine & Science in Sports & Exercise, 33,* S75.

Brown, D.S., Finkelstein, E.A., Brown, D.R., Buchner, D.M., & Johnson, F.R. (2009). Estimating older adults' preferences for walking programs via conjoint analysis. *American Journal of Preventive Medicine, 36,* 201-207, e204.

Buman, M.P., Giacobbi, P.R., Jr., Dzierzewski, J.M., Aiken Morgan, A., McCrae, C.S., Roberts, B.L., & Marsiske, M. (2011). Peer volunteers improve long-term maintenance of physical activity with older adults: A randomized controlled trial. *Journal of Physical Activity and Health, 8 Suppl 2,* S257-266.

Burke, L.E., Wang, J., & Sevick, M.A. (2011). Self-monitoring in weight loss: A systematic review of the literature. *Journal of the American Dietetic Association, 111,* 92-102.

Castro, C.M., Pruitt, L.A., Buman, M.P., & King, A.C. (2011). Physical activity program delivery by professionals versus volunteers: The Team randomized trial. *Health Psychology, 30,* 285-294.

Centers for Disease Control and Prevention. (2007). U.S. Physical Activity Statistics. Retrieved

October 18, 2012, from http://apps.nccd.cdc.gov/PASurveillance/DemoComparev.asp

Conroy, M.B., Yang, K., Elci, O.U., Gabriel, K.P., Styn, M.A., Wang, J., . . . Burke, L. E. (2011). Physical activity self-monitoring and weight loss: 6-month results of the Smart Trial. *Medicine & Science in Sports & Exercise, 43*, 1568-1574.

Cress, M. E., Buchner, D. M., Prohaska, T., Rimmer, J., Brown, M., Macera, C., . . . Chodzko-Zajko, W. (2005). Best practices for physical activity programs and behavior ounseling in older adult populations. *Journal of Aging and Physical Activity, 13*, 61-74.

Dunlop, W.L., & Beauchamp, M.R. (2013). Birds of a feather stay active together: A case study of an all-male older adult exercise program. *Journal of Aging and Physical Activity, 21*, 222-232. doi:10.1123/japa.21.2.222

Ettinger, W.H., Jr., Burns, R., Messier, S.P., Applegate, W., Rejeski, W.J., Morgan, T., . . . Craven, T. (1997). A randomized trial comparing aerobic exercise and resistance exercise with a health education program in older adults with knee osteoarthritis. The Fitness Arthritis and Seniors Trial (Fast). *Journal of the American Medical Association, 277*, 25-31.

Fishbein, M., & Ajzen, I. (1975). *Belief, attitude, intention and behavior*. Don Mills, NY: Addison Wesley.

Gardiner, P.A., Eakin, E.G., Healy, G.N., & Owen, N. (2011). Feasibility of reducing older adults' sedentary time. *American Journal of Preventive Medicine, 41*, 174-177.

Gerber, J.B., Bloom, P.A., & Ross, J.S. (2010). The physical activity contract tailored to promote physical activity in a geriatric outpatient setting: A pilot study. *Journal of the American Geriatrics Society, 58*, 604-606.

Goldstein, A.P., & Higginbotham, H.N. (1991). Relationship enhancement methods. In F.H. Kanfer & A.P. Goldstein (Eds.), *Helping people change. A textbook of methods* (4th ed., pp. 20-69). New York, NY: Pergamon Press.

Haber, D., & Rhodes, D. (2004). Health contract with sedentary older adults. *Gerontologist, 44*, 827-835.

Heneman, K., Block-Joy, A., Zidenberg-Cherr, S., Donohue, S., Garcia, L., Martin, A., . . . Steinberg, F.M. (2005). A "contract for change" increases produce consumption in low-income women: A pilot study. *Journal of the American Dietetic Association, 105*, 1793-1796.

Hughes, S.L., Seymour, R.B., Campbell, R.T., Huber, G., Pollak, N., Sharma, L., & Desai, P. (2006). Long-term impact of Fit and Strong! on older adults with osteoarthritis. *Gerontologist, 46*, 801-814.

Jette, A.M., Lachman, M., Giorgetti, M.M., Assmann, S.F., Harris, B.A., Levenson, C., . . . Krebs, D. (1999). Exercise—It's never too late: The Strong-for-Life Program. *American Journal of Public Health, 89*, 66-72.

Justine, M., Azizan, H., Hassan, V., Salleh, Z., & Manaf, H. (2013). Barriers to participation in physical activity and exercise among middle-aged and elderly individuals. *Singapore Medical Journal, 54*, 581-6.

King, A.C., Friedman, R., Marcus, B., Castro, C., Napolitano, M., Ahn, D., & Baker, L. (2007). Ongoing physical activity advice by humans versus computers: The Community Health Advice by Telephone (Chat) Trial. *Health Psychology, 26*, 718-727.

King, A.C., Haskell, W.L., Taylor, C.B., Kraemer, H.C., & DeBusk, R.F. (1991). Group- vs home-based exercise training in healthy older men and women. A community-based clinical trial. *Journal of the American Medical Association, 266*, 1535-1542.

King, A.C., Pruitt, L.A., Phillips, W., Oka, R., Rodenburg, A., & Haskell, W.L. (2000). Comparative effects of two physical activity programs on measured and perceived physical functioning and other health-related quality of life outcomes in older adults. *Journal of Gerontology, 55*, M74-M83.

King, A.C., Sallis, J.F., Frank, L.D., Saelens, B.E., Cain, K., Conway, T.L., . . . Kerr, J. (2011). Aging in neighborhoods differing in walkability and income: Associations with physical activity and obesity in older adults. *Social Science and Medicine, 73*, 1525-1533.

Kolt, G.S., Schofield, G.M., Kerse, N., Garrett, N., Ashton, T., & Patel, A. (2012). Healthy Steps Trial: Pedometer-based advice and physical activity for low-active older adults. *Annals of Family Medicine, 10*, 206-212.

Kolt, G.S., Schofield, G.M., Kerse, N., Garrett, N., & Oliver, M. (2007). Effect of telephone counseling on physical activity for low-active older people in primary care: A randomized, controlled trial. *Journal of the American Geriatrics Society, 55*, 986-992.

Layne, J.E., Sampson, S.E., Mallio, C.J., Hibberd, P.L., Griffith, J.L., Das, S.K., . . . Castaneda-Sceppa, C. (2008). Successful dissemination of a community-based strength training program for older adults by peer and professional leaders: The People Exercising program. *Journal of the American Geriatrics Society, 56*, 2323-2329.

Lewis, M., Peiris, C.L., & Shields, N. (2017). Long-term home and community-based exercise programs improve function in community-dwelling older people with cognitive impairment: a systematic review. *Journal of Physiotherapy, 63,* 23-29. doi: 10.1016/j.jphys.2016.11.005.

Marcus, B.H, & Forsyth, L.H. (2003). *Motivating people to be physically active.* Champaign, IL: Human Kinetics.

Marlatt, G.A., & Gorden, J.R. (1985). *Relapse prevention: Maintenance strategies in the treatment of addictive behaviors.* New York, NY: Guilford Press.

Martinson, B.C., Sherwood, N.E., Crain, A.L., Hayes, M.G., King, A.C., Pronk, N.P., & O'Connor, P.J. (2010). Maintaining physical activity among older adults: 24-month outcomes of the Keep Active Minnesota randomized controlled trial. *Preventive Medicine, 51,* 37-44.

Marzano. R.J. (2007) *The art & science of teaching: A comprehensive framework for effective instruction.* Alexandria, VA: Association for Supervision & Curriculum Development.

Matthews, C.E., Chen, K.Y., Freedson, P.S., Buchowski, M.S., Beech, B.M., Pate, R.R., & Troiano, R.P. (2008). Amount of time spent in sedentary behaviors in the United States, 2003-2004. *American Journal of Epidemiology, 167,* 875-881. doi:10.1093/aje/kwm390

Opdenacker, J., Boen, F., Coorevits, N., & Delecluse, C. (2008). Effectiveness of a lifestyle intervention and a structured exercise intervention in older adults. *Preventive Medicine, 46,* 518-524.

Opdenacker, J., Delecluse, C., & Boen, F. (2011). A 2-year follow-up of a lifestyle physical activity versus a structured exercise intervention in older adults. *Journal of the American Geriatrics Society, 59,* 1602-1611.

Pahor, M., Blair, S.N., Espeland, M., Fielding, R., Gill, T.M., Guralnik, J.M., . . . Studenski, S. (2006). Effects of a physical activity intervention on measures of physical performance: Results of the Lifestyle Interventions and Independence for Elders pilot (Life-P) study. *Journal of Gerontology, 61,* M1157-1165.

PAGAC (Physical Activity Guidelines Advisory Committee). (2018). *2018 Physical activity guidelines advisory committee scientific report.* Washington, DC: U.S. Department of Health and Human Services.

Picorelli, A.M.A., Pereira, L.S.M., Pereira, D.S., Felicio, D., & Sherrington, C. (2014). Adherence to exercise programs for older people is influenced by program characteristics and personal factors: A systematic review. *Journal of Physiotherapy, 60,* 151-156.

Prochaska, J.O., DiClemente, C.C., & Norcross, J.C. (1992). In search of how people change. Applications to addictive behaviors. *American Psychologist, 47,* 1102-1114.

Prochaska, J.O., & Marcus, B.H. (1994). The Transtheoretical Model: Applications to exercise. In R.K. Dishman (Ed.), *Advances in exercise adherence* (pp. 161-180). Champaign, IL: Human Kinetics.

Proper, K.I., Singh, A.S., van Mechelen, W., & Chinapaw, M.J. (2011). Sedentary behaviors and health outcomes among adults: A systematic review of prospective studies. *American Journal of Preventive Medicine, 40,* 174-182.

Rejeski, W.J., Brawley, L.R., Ambrosius, W.T., Brubaker, P.H., Focht, B.C., Foy, C.G., & Fox, L.D. (2003). Older adults with chronic disease: Benefits of group-mediated counseling in the promotion of physically active lifestyles. *Health Psychology, 22,* 414-423.

Sallis, J.F., & Owen, N. (1999). *Physical activity and behavioral medicine.* Thousand Oaks, CA: Sage.

Stewart, A.L., Mills, K.M., Sepsis, P.G., King, A.C., McLellan, B.Y., Roitz, K., & Ritter, P.L. (1997). Evaluation of Champs, a physical activity promotion program for older adults. *Annals of Behavioral Medicine, 19,* 353-361.

Stewart, A.L., Verboncoeur, C.J., McLellan, B.Y., Gillis, D.E., Rush, S., Mills, K.M., . . . Bortz, W. M., 2nd. (2001). Physical activity outcomes of Champs II: A physical activity promotion program for older adults. *Journal of Gerontology, 56,* M465-M470.

Troiano, R.P., Berrigan, D., Dodd, K.W., Masse, L.C., Tilert, T., & McDowell, M. (2008). Physical activity in the United States measured by accelerometer. *Medicine &d Science in Sports & Exercise, 40,* 181-188.

Trost, S.G., Owen, N., Bauman, A.E., Sallis, J.F., & Brown, W. (2002). Correlates of adults' participation in physical activity: Review and update. *Medicine & Science in Sports & Exercise, 34,* 1996-2001.

Van Cauwenberg, J., De Bourdeaudhuij, I., De Meester, F., Van Dyck, D., Salmon, J., Clarys, P., & Deforche, B. (2011). Relationship between the physical environment and physical activity in older adults: A systematic review. *Health and Place, 17,* 458-469.

van Stralen, M.M., de Vries, H., Mudde, A.N., Bolman, C., & Lechner, L. (2011). The Long-term efficacy of two computer-tailored physical activity interventions for older adults: Main effects and mediators. *Health Psychology, 30,* 442-452.

West, D.S., Bursac, Z., Cornell, C.E., Felix, H.C., Fausett, J.K., Krukowski, R.A., . . . Beck, C. (2011). Lay health educators translate a weight-loss intervention in senior centers: A randomized controlled trial. *American Journal of Preventive Medicine, 41,* 385-391.

Wilcox, S., Dowda, M., Leviton, L.C., Bartlett-Prescott, J., Bazzarre, T., Campbell-Voytal, K., . . . Wegley, S. (2008). Active for life. Final results from the translation of two physical activity programs. *American Journal of Preventive Medicine, 35,* 340-351.

Wilcox, S., Tudor-Locke, C.E., & Ainsworth, B.E. (2002). Physical activity patterns, assessment, and motivation in older adults. In R.J. Shephard (Ed.), *Gender, physical activity, and aging* (pp. 13-39). Boca Raton, FL: CRC Press.

Chapter 8

American College of Sports Medicine (2018). *ACSM's resources for the personal trainer* (5th ed.). Philadelphia, PA: Wolters Kluwer.

Centers for Disease Control and Prevention (2013). *The state of aging and health in America 2013.* Atlanta, GA: Centers for Disease Control and Prevention, U.S. Department of Health and Human Services.

Chodzko-Zajko, W., Proctor, D.N., Fiatarone Singh, M.A., Minson, C.T., Nigg, C.R., Salem, G.J., & Skinner. J.S. (2009). Exercise and physical activity for older adults. *Medicine & Science in Sports & Exercise, 41,* 1510-1530. doi:10.1249/MSS.0b013e3181a0c95c

Daniels, R., van Rossum, E., de Witte, L., Kempen, G.I., & van den Heuvel, W. (2008). Interventions to prevent disability in frail community-dwelling elderly: A systematic review. *BMC Health Services Research, 8,* 278. doi:10.1186/1472-6963-8-278

de Souto Barreto, P. (2013). *Bulletin of the World Health Organization, 91,* 390-390A. doi:10.4271/BLT.13.120790

Dumurgier J., Elbaz, A., Ducimetiere, P., Tavernier B., Alperovitch, A., & Tzourio, C. (2009). Slow walking speed and cardiovascular death in well functioning older adults: Prospective cohort study. *British Medical Journal, 339,* b4460. doi:10.1136/bmj.b4460

Garber, C.E., Blissmer, B., Deschenes, M.R., Franklin, B.A., Lamonte, M.J., Lee, I.M., . . . Swain, D.P. (2011). Quantity and quality of exercise for developing and maintaining cardiorespiratory, musculoskeletal, and neuromotor fitness in apparently healthy adults: Guidance for prescribing exercise. *Medicine & Science in Sports & Exercise, 43,* 1334-1359. doi:10.1249/MSS.0b013c318213fefb

Gillis, D.E. & Stewart, A.L. (2005). A new approach to designing exercise programs for older adults. In C.J. Jones, & D.J. Rose (Eds), *Physical activity instruction of older adults.* Champaign, IL: Human Kinetics.

Harris, C.D., Watson, K.B., Carlson, S.A., Fulton, J.E., Dorn, J.M., & Elam-Evans, L. (2013). Adult participation in aerobic and muscle strengthening physical activities: United States, 2011. *Morbidity and Mortality Weekly Report, 62,* 17, 326-330. Retrieved from www.cdc.gov/mmwr/preview/mmwrhtml/mm6217a2.htm

Jindai, K., Nielson, C.M., Vorderstrasse, B.A., & Quinones, A.R. (2016). Multimorbidity and functional limitations among adults 65 or older, NHANES 2005-2012. *Preventing Chronic Disease, 13,* 160174. doi:10.5888/pcd13.160174

Loprinzi, P.D., Lee, H., & Cardinal, B.J. (2015). Evidence to support including lifestyle light-intensity recommendations in physical activity guidelines for older adults. *American Journal of Health Promotion, 29,* 277-284. doi:10.4278/ajhp.130709-QUAN-354

Nagi, S.Z. (1976). An epidemiology of disability among adults in the United States. *Milbank Memorial Fund Quarterly, 54,* 439-467.

Nagi, S.Z. (1991). Disability concepts revisited: Implications for prevention. In A.M. Pope & A.R. Tarlov (Eds.), *Disability in America: Toward a national agenda for prevention* (pp. 309-327). Washington DC: National Institutes of Health.

National Center for Health Statistics. National Health and Nutrition Examination Survey 1999-2016 Survey Content Brochure. Available at: https://www.cdc.gov/nchs/data/nhanes/survey content 99 16.pdf.

PAGAC (Physical Activity Guidelines Advisory Committee). (2018). *2018 Physical activity guidelines advisory committee scientific report.* Washington, DC: U.S. Department of Health and Human Services.

Pahor M., Blair, S.N., et al. LIFE Study Investigators (2006). Effects of a physical activity intervention on measures of physical performance: Results of the lifestyle interventions and independence for elders pilot (LIFE-P) study. *Journals of Gerontology A: Biological Sciences, Medical Sciences, 61,* 1157-1165.

Rikli, R.E., & Jones, C.J. (2013). *Senior fitness test manual* (2nd ed.). Champaign, IL: Human Kinetics.

Rose, D.J. (2010). *FallProof! A comprehensive balance and mobility training program.* Champaign, IL: Human Kinetics.

Seeman, T.E., Merkin, S.S., Crimmins, E.M., & Karlamangla, A.S. (2010). Disability trends among older Americans: National health and nutrition examination surveys, 1988-1994 and 1999-2004. *American Journal of Public Health, 100,* 100-107. doi:10.2105/AJPH.2008.157388

Shephard, R.J. (1993). Exercise and aging: Extending independence in older adults. *Geriatrics, 48,* 61-64.

Tucker, J.M., Welk, G.J., & Beyler, N.K. (2011). Adults: Compliance with the physical activity guidelines for Americans. *American Journal of Preventive Medicine, 40,* 454-461. doi:10.1016/j.amepre.2010.12.016

U.S. Department of Health and Human Services (2008). *2008 Physical activity guidelines for Americans.* Retrieved from https://health.gov/paguidelines/pdf/paguide.pdf

Verbrugge, L.M., & Jette, A.M. (1994). The disablement process. *Social Science and Medicine, 38,* 1-14.

Vita, A.J., Terry, R.B., Hubert, H.B., & Fries, J.F. (1998). Aging, health risks, and cumulative disability. *New England Journal of Medicine, 338,* 1035-1041.

World Health Organization (2011). World Health Statistics. Geneva, Switzerland: WHO Press.

Chapter 9

Bherer, I., Erickson, K.I., & Liu-Ambrose, T. (2013). A review of the effects of physical activity and exercise on cognitive and brain functions in older adults. *Journal of Aging Research, 657508.* doi:10.1155/2013/657508

Bridle, C., Spanjers, K., Patel, S., Atherton, N.M., & Lamb, S. (2012). Effect of exercise on depression severity in older people: Systematic review and meta-analysis of randomized controlled trials. *The British Journal of Psychiatry, 201,* 180-185. doi:10.1192/bjp.bp.111.095174

Centers for Disease Control and Prevention, U.S. Department of Health and Human Services (2013). *National Vital Statistics, 61,* 4.

Dunn, H.L. (1961). *High level wellness.* Arlington, VA: Beatty Press.

Edelman, P., & Montague, J.M. (2006). Whole-person wellness outcomes in senior living communities: The resident whole-person wellness survey. *Seniors Housing & Care Journal, 14,* 1-21.

Edelman, P., & Montague, J.M. (2008). Whole-person wellness: First national survey identifies changing expectations for LTC. *Long-Term Living, 57,* 4, 20-25.

Fry, C.L. (2012). Paper 3: *Measuring up success.* Retrieved from https://healthyandsuccessfulaging.wordpress.com/2012/11/12/paper-3-measuring-up-success/

Global Wellness Institute (2016). *History of wellness.* Retrieved from www.globalwellnessinstitute.org/history-of-wellness

Guure, C.B., Ibrahim, N.A., Adam, M.B., & Said, S.M. (2017). Impact of physical activity on cognitive decline, dementia, and its subtypes: Meta-analysis of prospective studies. *BioMed Research International.* doi:10.1155/2017/9016924

International Council on Active Aging (2015). *ICAA Active-Aging Industry Development Survey 2015: Trends in wellness programs and development.* Retrieved from www.icaa.cc/business/research.htm

Kahana, E., & Kahana, B. (2012). Paper 5: Interventions to promote successful aging. Retrieved from https://healthyandsuccessfulaging.wordpress.com/2012/11/12/paper-5-interventions-to-promote-successful-aging/.

Konopack, J.F., & McAuley, E. (2012). Efficacy-mediated effects of spirituality and physical activity on quality of life: A path analysis. *Health Quest Life Outcomes.* doi:10.1186/1477-7525-10-57

Kramer, A.F., Hahn, S., Cohen, N.J., Banich, M.T., McAuley, E., Harrison, C.R., . . . Colcombe, A. (1999). Ageing, fitness and neurocognitive function. *Nature, 400,* 418-419.

Levy, B.R., Slade, M.D., Kunkel, S.R., & Kasl, K.V. (2002). Longevity increased by positive self-perceptions of aging. *Journal of Personality & Social Psychology, 83,* 261-270.

McMahon, S., & Fleury, J. (2012). Wellness in older adults: A concept analysis. *Nursing Forum, 47,* 30-51.

Merriam-Webster (2016). [Definition of *wellness*] Retrieved from www.merriam-webster.com/dictionary/wellness&gt

Miller, J.W. (2005). Wellness: The history and development of a concept. *Spektrum Freiziet, 27,* 84-106.

Montague, J.M., & Frank, B.H. (2007, July/August). Creating whole-person wellness. *Assisted Living Consult, 1-5.*

National Wellness Institute (2016). Retrieved from www.nationalwellness.org/?page=AboutWellness

Poon, L.W., Gueldner, S.H., & Sprouse, B.M. (2003). *Successful aging and adaptation with chronic diseases.* New York, NY: Springer.

Rose, D.J. (2013). Aging successfully: Predictors and pathways. In J.M. Rippe (Ed.), *Lifestyle medicine* (2nd ed., pp. 1247-1267). Boca Raton, FL: CRC Press.

Rose, D.J., (2016). The future of aging research: Should the focus be on not growing old or growing old better? *Kinesiology Review, 5,* 65-74.

Rowe, J.W., & Kahn, R.L. (1998). *Successful aging.* New York, NY: Pantheon Books.

Sarkisian, C.A., Prohaska, T.R., Wong, M., Hirsch, S., & Mangione, C.M. (2005). The relationship between expectations for aging and physical activity among older adults. *Journal of General Internal Medicine, 20,* 911-915. doi:10.1111/j.1525-1497.2005.0204.x

Strawbridge, W.J., & Wallhagen, M.I. (2003) *What can be learned about successful aging from those experiencing it?* New York, NY: Springer.

Strout, K.A., &Howard, E.P., (2012). The six dimensions of wellness and cognition in aging adults. *Journal of Holistic Nursing, 30,* 195-204.

UnitedHealth Group. (2013). *Doing good is good for you: 2013 Health and Volunteering Study.* Retrieved from www.unitedhealthgroup.com/SocialResponsibility/Volunteering.aspx

United States Census. (2014). Retrieved from www.census.gov/population/projections/data/national/2014.html

Vaillant, G. (2002). *Aging Well: Surprising guideposts to a happier life from the landmark Harvard study of adult development.* Boston, MA: Little Brown.

Vaillant, G. (2014). Aging well: Thoughts from a 75-year-old study. *AgingToday.* Retrieved from http://asaging.org/blog/aging-well-thoughts-75-year-old-study

Web MD. (2016). *What is wellness?* Retrieved from www.webmdhealthservices.com

White House Conference on Aging Policy Brief (2015). Retrieved from www.whitehouseconferenceonaging.gov/blog/policy/file.axd?file=/Healthy%20Aging%20Policy%20Brief/Healthy%20Aging%20Issue%20Brief.pdf

World Health Organization (1946). *Preamble to the constitution of the World Health Organization as adopted by the international health conference, New York.* Retrieved from www.who.int/library/collections/historical/en/index3.html

Chapter 10

American College of Sports Medicine (2012). *ACSM's health/fitness facility standards and guidelines* (4th ed). Champaign, IL: Human Kinetics.

Bandura, A. (1997). *Self-efficacy: The exercise of control.* New York, NY: Freeman.

Bean, J.F., Vora, A., & Frontera, W.R. (2013). Benefits of exercise for community dwelling older adults. *Archives of Physical Medicine and Rehabilitation, 85,* S31-S42.

Borg, G. (1998). *Borg's perceived exertion and pain scales.* Champaign, IL: Human Kinetics.

Chodzko-Zajko, W.J., Proctor, D.N., Fiatarone, M.A., Minson, C.T., Nigg, C.R., Salem, G.J., & Skinner, J.S. (2009). Exercise and physical activity for older adults. *Medicine & Science in Sports & Exercise, 41,* 1510-1530. doi:10.1249/MSS.0b013e3181a0c95c

Ferrini, A., & Ferrini, R. (2012). *Health in the later years* (5th ed.) St. Louis, MO: McGraw-Hill.

Hogan, C.L., Mata, J., & Carstensen, L.L. (2013). Exercise holds immediate benefits for affect and cognition in younger and older adults. *Psychology of Aging, 28,* 587-594. doi:10.1037/a0032634

Inoue, S., Yorifuji, T.K., Sugiyama, M., Ohta, T., Ishikawa-Takata, K., & Doi, H. (2013). Does habitual physical activity prevent insomnia? A cross-sectional and longitudinal study of elderly Japanese. *Journal of Physical Activity and Aging, 2,* 119-139.

Kluge, M.A., & Savis, J.C. (November/December, 2000). Using chronobiology to enhance exercise quality in older adults. *American College of Sports Medicine Health & Fitness Journal, 4,* 20-25.

Kluge, M.A., & Savis, J.C. (2001). Charting a course: A guide for activity professionals who lead exercise programs for older adults. *Activities, Adaptation, and Aging, 25,* 73-93.

Melone, L. (2014). *A new way to stretch.* Retrieved from www.arthritistoday.org/what-you-cando/staying-active/fitness-benefits/stretching-benefits.php

Nieman, D.C. (1999). *Exercise testing and prescription: A health-related approach.* Mountain View, CA: Mayfield.

Page, P. (2012). Current concepts in muscle stretching for exercise and rehabilitation. *The International Journal of Sports Physical Therapy, 7,* 109-119.

Reid, D.A., & McNair, P.J. (2011). Effects of a six-week lower limb stretching programme on range of motion, peak passive torque and stiffness in people with and without osteoarthritis of the knee. *New Zealand Journal of Physiotherapy, 39,* 5-12.

Speer, K.P. (2005). *Injury prevention and rehabilitation for active older adults.* Champaign, IL: Human Kinetics.

Ullman, G. (2012). Dialog on JAPA's mission: Mind-body exercises are "physical activity." *Journal of Aging and Physical Activity, 20,* 399-401.

Van Norman, K. (2005). Principles of the warm-up and cool-down. In C.J. Jones & D.J. Rose (Eds.), *Physical activity instruction of older adults* (pp. 142-153). Champaign, IL: Human Kinetics.

Vandervoort, A.A. (2009). Potential benefits of warm-up for neuromuscular performance of older athletes. *Exercise and Sport Sciences Reviews, 37,* 60-65. doi:10.1097/JES.0b013e31819c2f5c

Wise, J.B., & Trunnell, E.P. (2001). The influence of sources of self-efficacy upon efficacy strength. *Journal of Sport and Exercise Psychology, 23,* 268-280.

Chapter 11

Ashwell, K., Foulcher, T., & Baker, M. (2014). *The student's anatomy of stretching manual.* Hauppage, NY: Barron's.

Batista, L.H., Vilar, A.C., De Almeida Ferreira, J.J., Rebelatto, J.R., & Salvini, T.F. (2009). Active stretching improves flexibility, joint torque, and functional mobility in older women. *American Journal of Physical Medicine and Rehabilitation, 88,* 815-822.

Bell, R., & Hoshizaki, T. (1981). Relationships of age and sex with joint range of motion of seventeen joint actions in humans. *Canadian Journal of Applied Sport Sciences, 6,* 202-206.

Brooks, S.V., & Faulkner, J.A. (1996). The magnitude of the initial injury induced by stretches of maximally activated muscle fibres of mice and rats increases in old age. *Journal of Physiology, 497,* 573-580.

Brown, M., Sinacore, D.R., Ehsani, A.A., Binder, E.F., & Holloszy, J.O. (2000). Low-intensity exercise as a modifier of physical frailty in older adults. *Archives of Physical Medicine and Rehabilitation, 81,* 960-965.

Buckwalter, J.A., Woo, S.L., Goldberg, V.M., Hadley, E.C., Booth, F., Oegema, T.R., & Eyre, D.R. (1993). Soft tissue aging and musculoskeletal function. *Journal of Bone and Joint Surgery, 75,* 1533-1548.

Cetta, G., Tenni, R., Zanaboni, G., & Maroudas, A. (1982). Biochemical and morphological modifications in rabbit Achilles tendon during maturation and ageing. *Biomechanics Journal, 204,* 61-67.

Christiansen, C.L. (2008). The effects of hip and ankle stretching on gait function of older people. *Archives of Physical Medicine and Rehabilitation, 89,* 1421-1428.

Cristopoliski, F., Barela, J.A., Leite, N., Fowler, E., and Rodacki, A.L.F. (2009). Stretching exercise program improves gait in the elderly. *Gerontology, 55,* 614-620.

Eddinger, T.J., Cassens, R.G., & Moss, R.L. (1986). Mechanical and histochemical characterization of skeletal muscles from senescent rats. *American Journal of Physiology, 251,* C421-C430.

Einkauf, D.K., Gohdes, M.L., Jensen, G.M., & Jewell, M.J. (1987). Changes in spinal mobility with increasing age in women. *Physical Therapy, 67,* 370-375.

Gajdosik, R.L., Vander Linden, D.W., McNair, P.J., Williams, A.K. & Riggin, T.J. (2005). Effects of an eight-week stretching program on the passive-elastic properties and function of the calf muscles of older women. *Clinical Biomechanics, 20,* 973-983.

Golding, L.A., & Lindsay, A. (1989). Flexibility and age. *Perspective, 15,* 28-30.

Hall, D.A. (1976). *The aging of connective tissue.* New York, NY: Academic Press.

Holland, G.J., Tanaka, K., Shigematsu, R., & Nakagaichi, M. (2002). Flexibility and physical functions of older adults: A review. *Journal of Aging and Physical Activity, 10,* 169-206.

James, B., & Parker, A.W. (1989). Active and passive mobility of lower limb joints in elderly men and women. *American Journal of Physical Medicine and Rehabilitation, 68,* 162-167.

Keogh, J.W.L., Kilding, A., Pidgeon, P., Ashley, L., & Gillis, D. (2009). Physical benefits of dancing for healthy older adults: A review. *Journal of Aging and Physical Activity, 17,* 1-23.

King, A.C., Pruitt, L.A., Phillips, W., Oka, R., Rodenburg, A., & Haskell, W.L. (2000). Comparative effects of two physical activity programs on measured and perceived physical functioning and other health-related quality of life outcomes in older adults." *Journals of Gerontology Series A, 55,* M74-M83.

Klein, D.A., Stone, W.J., Phillips, W.T., Gangi, J., & Hartman, S. (2002). PNF training and physical function in assisted living older adults. *Journal of Aging and Physical Activity, 10,* 476-488.

Lindsay, D.M., Horton, J.F., & Vandervoort, A.A. (2000). A review of injury characteristics, aging factors and prevention programmes for the older golfer. *Sports Medicine, 30,* 89-103.

Lung, M.W., Hartsell, H.D., & Vandervoort, A.A. (1996). Effects of aging on joint stiffness: Implications for exercise. *Physiotherapy Canada, 48,* 96-106.

McHugh, M.P., Connolly, D.A., Eston, R.G., Kremenic, I.J., Nicholas, S.J., & Gleim, G.W. (1999). The role of passive muscle stiffness in symptoms of exercise-induced muscle damage. *American Journal of Sports Medicine, 27,* 594-599.

Moskowitz, R.W. (1989). Clinical and laboratory findings in osteoarthritis. In D.J. McCarty (Ed.),

Arthritis and allied conditions (pp. 1605-1630). Philadelphia, PA: Lea & Febiger.

Nigg, B.M., Fisher, V., Allinger, T.L., Ronsky, J.R., & Engsberg, J.R. (1992). Range of motion of the foot as a function of age. *Foot and Ankle, 13,* 336-343.

Noonan, T.J., & Garrett, W.E., Jr. (1999). Muscle strain injury: Diagnosis and treatment. *Journal of American Orthopaedic Surgery, 7,* 262-269.

Ploutz-Snyder, L.L., Giamis, E.L., Formikell, M., & Rosenbaum, A.E. (2001). Resistance training reduces susceptibility to eccentric exercise-induced muscle dysfunction in older women. *Journal of Gerontology: Biological Sciences, 56,* B384-B390.

Rosenberg, I.H. (2011). Sarcopenia: Origins and clinical relevance. *Clinics in Geriatric Medicine, 27,* 337-339.

Stanziano, D.C., Roos, B.A. Perry, A.C., Lai, S., & Signorile, J.F. (2009). The effects of an active-assisted stretching program on functional performance in elderly persons: A pilot study. *Clinical Interventions in Aging, 4,* 115-120.

Stathokostas, L., McDonald, M.W., Little, R.M.D., & Paterson, D.H. (2013). Flexibility of older adults aged between 55-86 years and the influence on physical activity. *Journal of Aging Research.* doi:10.1155/2013/743843

Svenningsen, S., Terjesen, T., Auflem, M., & Berg, V. (1989). Hip motion related to age and sex. *Acta Orthopaedica Scandinavica, 60,* 97-100.

Tainaka, K., Takizawa, T., Katamoto, S., & Aoki, J, (2009). Six-year prospective study of physical fitness and incidence of disability among community-dwelling Japanese elderly women. *Geriatrics and Gerontology International, 9,* 21-28.

Taylor-Piliae, R.E., Haskell, W.L., Stotts, N.A., & Froelicher, E.S. (2006). Improvement in balance, strength, and flexibility after 12 weeks of tai chi exercise in ethnic Chinese adults with cardiovascular disease risk factors. *Alternative Therapies in Health and Medicine, 12,* 50-58.

U.S. Department of Health and Human Services (2008). *2008 Physical activity guidelines for Americans.* Retrieved from https://health.gov/paguidelines/pdf/paguide.pdf

Vandervoort, A.A., Chesworth, B.M., Cunningham, D.A., Paterson, D.H., Rechnitzer, P.A., & Koval, J. (1992). Age and sex effects on mobility of the human ankle. *Journal of Gerontology, 47(1),* M17-21.

Walker, J.M., Sue, D., Miles-Elkousy, N., Ford, G., & Trevelyan, H. (1984). Active mobility of the extremities in older subjects. *Physical Therapy, 64,* 919-923.

Chapter 12

Baechle, T.R., & Earle, R.W. (2016). *Essentials of strength training and conditioning* (4th ed.). Champaign, IL: Human Kinetics.

Barnett, C., Carey, M., Proietto, J., Cerin, E., Febbraio, M.A., & Jenkins, D. (2004). Muscle metabolism during sprint exercise in man: Influence of sprint training. *Journal of Science and Medicine in Sport, 7,* 314-322.

Bassey, E.J., Fiatarone, M.A., O'Neill, E.F., Kelly, M., Evans, W.J., & Lipsitz, L.A. (1992). Leg extensor power and functional performance in very old men and women. *Clinical Science (London), 82,* 321-327.

Beebe, J.A., Hines, R.W., McDaniel, L.T., & Shelden, B.L. (2013). An isokinetic training program for reducing falls in a community-dwelling older adult: A case report. *Journal of Geriatric Physical Therapy, 36,* 146-53. doi:10.1519/JPT.0b013e31826e73d5

Bendall, M.J., Bassey, E.J., & Pearson, M.B. (1989). Factors affecting walking speed of elderly people. *Age and Ageing, 18,* 327-332.

Charette, S.L., McEvoy, L., Pyka, G., Snow-Harter, C., Guido, D., Wiswell, R.A., & Marcus, R. (1991). Muscle hypertrophy response to resistance training in older women. *Journal of Applied Physiology, 70,* 1912-1916.

Clark, B.C., & Manini, T.M. (2012). What is dynapenia? *Nutrition, 28,* 495-503.

Clyman, B. (2001). Exercise in the treatment of osteoarthritis. *Current Rheumatology Reports, 3,* 520-523.

Cruz-Jentoft, A.J., Baeyens, J.P., Bauer, J.M., Boirie, Y., Cederholm, T., Landi, F.,...Zamboni, M.(2010). Sarcopenia: European consensus on definition and diagnosis. Report of the European Working Group on Sarcopenia in Older People. *Age & Ageing, 39,* 412-423.

Cuoco, A., Callahan, D.M., Sayers, S., Frontera, W.R., Bean, J., & Fielding, R.A. (2004). Impact of muscle power and force on gait speed in disabled older men and women. *Journals of Gerontology A: Biological Sciences, Medical Sciences, 59,* 1200-1206.

Ebbeling, C.B., & Clarkson, P.M. (1989). Exercise-induced muscle damage and adaptation. *Sports Medicine, 7,* 207-234.

Evans, W.J. (1996). Reversing sarcopenia: How weight training can build strength and vitality. *Geriatrics, 51,* 46-47, 51-53.

Faigenbaum, A.D., Skrinar, G.S., Cesare, W.F., Kraemer, W.J., & Thomas, H.E. (1990).

Physiologic and symptomatic responses of cardiac patients to resistance exercise. *Archives of Physical Medicine and Rehabilitation, 71*, 395-398.

Feigenbaum, M.S., & Pollock, M.L. (1999). Prescription of resistance training for health and disease. *Medicine and Science in Sports and Exercise, 31*, 38-45.

Fiatarone, M.A., Marks, E.C., Ryan, N.D., Meredith, C.N., Lipsitz, L.A., & Evans, W.J. (1990). High-intensity strength training in nonagenarians. *Journal of the American Medical Association, 263*, 3029-3034.

Fleck, S.J., & Kraemer, W.J. (2004). *Designing resistance training programs* (3rd ed.). Champaign, IL: Human Kinetics.

Foldvari M., Clark, M., Laviolette, L.C., Bernstein, M.A, Kaliton, D., Castaneda, C., . . . Singh, M.A. (2000). Association of muscle power with functional status in community-dwelling elderly women. *Journals of Gerontology A: Biological Science, Medical Science, 55*, M192-M199.

Frontera, W.R., Meredith, C.N., O'Reilly, K.P., Knuttgen, H.G., & Evans, W.J. (1998). Strength conditioning in older men: Skeletal muscle hypertrophy and improved function. *Journal of Applied Physiology, 64*, 1038-1044.

Gersten, J.W. (1991). Effect of exercise on muscle function decline with aging. *Western Journal of Medicine, 154*, 579-582.

Haff, G.G. & Triplett, N.T. (2016). *Essentials of strength training and conditioning* (4th ed.). Champaign, IL: Human Kinetics.

Häkkinen, K., Newton, R.U., Gordon, S.E., McCormick, M., Volek, J.S., Nindl, B.C.,….Kramer, W.J. (1998). Changes in muscle morphology, electromyographic activity, and force production characteristics during progressive strength training in young and older men. *Journal of Gerontology: Biological Sciences, 53*, B415-B423.

Hather, B.M., Tesch, P.A., Buchanan, P., & Dudley, G.A. (1991). Influence of eccentric actions on skeletal muscle adaptations to resistance training. *Acta Physiologica Scandinavica, 143*, 177-185.

Hedayatpour, N. & Falla, D. (2015). Physiological and neural adaptations to eccentric exercise: Mechanisms and considerations for training. *Biomed Research International.* doi:10.1155/2015/193741

Heitkamp, H.C., Horstmann, T., Mayer, F., Weller, J., & Dickhuth, H.H. (2001). Gain in muscular strength and muscular balance after balance training. *International Journal of Sports Medicine, 22*, 285-290. doi:10.1055/s-2001-13819

Hunter, G.R., & Treuth, M.S. (1995). Relative training intensity and increases in older women. *Journal of Strength and Conditioning Research, 9*, 188-191.

Hurley, B.F., & Roth, S.M. (2000). Strength training in the elderly: Effects on risk factors for age-related diseases. *Sports Medicine, 30*, 249-268.

Kelley, G.A., & Kelley, K.S. (2000). Progressive resistance exercise and resting blood pressure: A meta-analysis of randomized controlled trials. *Hypertension, 35*, 838-843.

Knutzen, K.M., Brilla, L.R., & Caine, D. (1999). Validity of 1RM prediction equations for older adults. *Journal of Strength and Conditioning Research, 13*, 242-246. doi:10.1519/00124278-199908000-00011

Komi, P.V., Kaneko, M., & Aura, O. (1987). EMG activity of the leg extensor muscles with special reference to mechanical efficiency in concentric and eccentric exercise. *International Journal of Sports Medicine, 8*(Suppl. 1), 22-29.

Kosek, D.J., Kim, J-S., Petrella, J.K., Cross, J.M., & Bamman, M.M. (2006). Efficacy of 3 days/wk resistance training on myofiber hypertrophy and myogenic mechanisms in young vs. older adults. *Journal of Applied Physiology, 101*, 531–544. doi:10.1152/japplphysiol.01474.2005

Kraemer, W.J., Adams, K., Cafarelli, E., Dudley, G.A., Dooly, C., Feigenbaum, M.S., ….Triplett-McBride, T. (2002). American College of Sports Medicine position stand: Progression models in resistance training for healthy adults. *Medicine & Science in Sports & Exercise, 34*, 364-380.

Kraemer, W.J., & Ratamess, N.A. (2000). Physiology of resistance training: Current issues. *Orthopaedic Physical Therapy Clinics of North America: Exercise Technologies, 9*, 467-513.

Kraemer, W. J., & Ratamess, N.A. (2004). Fundamentals of resistance training: Progression and exercise prescription. *Medicine & Science in Sports & Exercise, 36*, 674-688.

Kraemer, W.J., Ratamess, N.A., & French, D.N. (2002). Resistance training for health and performance. *Current Sports Medicine Reports, 1*, 165-171.

Liu, C.-J., & Latham, N. (2011). Can progressive resistance strength training reduce physical disability in older adults? A meta-analysis study. *Disability and Rehabilitation, 33*, 87-97.

Liu, C.-J., Shiroy, D.M., Jones, L.Y., & Clark, D.O. (2014). Systematic review of functional training on muscle strength, physical functioning, and activities of daily living in older adults. *European*

Review of Aging and Physical Activity, 11, 144. doi:10.1007/s11556-014-0144-1

Linossier, M.T., Dormois, D., Perier, C., Frey, J., Geyssant, A., & Denis, C. (1997). Enzyme adaptations of human skeletal muscle during bicycle short-sprint training and detraining. *Acta Physiologica Scandinavica, 161,* 439-445.

Metter, E.J., Conwitt, R., Tobin, J., & Fozard, J.L. (1997). Age-associated loss of power and strength in the upper extremities in women and men. *Journal of Gerontology: Biological Sciences, 52A,* B267-B276.

Pescatello, L.S. (2015). Updating ACSM's recommendations for exercise preparticipation health screening. *Medicine & Science in Sports & Exercise, 47,* 2473-2479.

Pollock, M.L., Franklin, B.A., Balady, G.J., Chaitman, B.L., Fleg, J.L., Fletcher, B., ...Bazarre, T. (2000). Resistance exercise in individuals with and without cardiovascular disease: Benefits, rationale, safety, and prescription. *Circulation, 101,* 828-833.

Ratamess, N.A., Alvar, B.A., Evetoch, T.K., Housh, T.J., Kibler, W.B., & Kraemer, W.J. (2009). ACSM position stand: Progression models in resistance training for healthy adults. *Medicine & Science in Sports & Exercise, 41,* 687-708.

Rhea, M.R., Alvar, B.A., Burkett, L.N., & Ball, S.D. (2003). A meta-analysis to determine the dose response for strength development. *Medicine & Science in Sports & Exercise, 35,* 456-464.

Rikli, R.E., & Jones, C.J. (2013). *Senior fitness test manual* (2nd ed). Champaign, IL: Human Kinetics.

Rogers, M.A., & Evans, W.J. (1993). Changes in skeletal muscle with aging: Effects of exercise training. *Exercise and Sport Sciences Reviews, 21,* 65-102.

Rogers, M.W., & Mille, M.L. (2003). Lateral stability and falls in older people. *Exercise & Sport Science Reviews, 31,* 182-187.

Shaw, C.E., McCully, K.K., & Posner, J.D. (1995). Injuries during the one repetition maximum assessment in the elderly. *Journal of Cardiopulmonary Rehabilitation, 15,* 283-287.

Signorile, J.F. (2011). *Bending the aging curve: The complete exercise guide for older adults.* Champaign, IL: Human Kinetics.

Signorile, J.F., Carmel, M.P., Czaja, S.J., Asfour, S.S., Morgan, R.O., Khalil, T.M., . . . Roos, B.A. (2002). Differential increases in average isokinetic power by specific muscle groups of older women due to variations in training and testing. *Journals of Gerontology A: Biological Sciences, Medical Sciences, 57,* M683-M690.

Signorile, J.F., Carmel, M.P., Lai, S., & Roos, B.A. (2005). Early plateaus of power and torque gains during high- and low-speed training in older women. *Journal of Applied Physiology, 98,* 1213-1220.

Simão, R., Spineti, J., de Salles, B.F., Oliveira, L.F., Matta, T., Miranda, F., . . . Costa, P.B. (2010). Influence of exercise order on maximum strength and muscle thickness in untrained men. *Journal of Sports Science & Medicine, 1,* 1-7.

Sipila, S., Elorinne, M., Alen, M., Suominen, H., & Kovanen, V. (1997). Effects of strength and endurance training on muscle fibre characteristics in elderly women. *Clinical Physiology, 17,* 459-474.

Tomlin, D.L. (2001). The relationship between aerobic fitness and recovery from high intensity intermittent exercise. *Sports Medicine (Auckland). 31,* 1-11.

Whipple, R.K., Wolfson, M.D., & Amerman, P.M. (1987). The relationship of knee and ankle weakness to falls in nursing home residents: An isokinetic study. *Journal of the American Geriatric Society, 35,* 13-20.

Willardson, J.M. (2007). The application of training to failure in periodized multiple-set resistance exercise programs. *Journal of Strength and Conditioning Research, 21,* 628-631.

Willoughby, D.S. (2014) Resistance training and the older adult. American College of Sports Medicine Current Comment. Retrieved from http://acsm.org/docs/current-comments/resistancetrainingandtheoa.pdf

Chapter 13

Akushevich, I., Kravchenko, J., Ukraintseva, S., & Arbeev, K.A.I. (2013). Time trends of incidence of age-associated diseases in the U.S. elderly population: Medicare-based analysis. *Age & Ageing 42*(4): 494-500.

Alves, E.S., Souza, H.S., Rosa, J.P., Lira, F.S., Pimentel, G.D., Santos, R.V., . . . de Mello, M.T. (2012). Chronic exercise promotes alterations in the neuroendocrine profile of elderly people. *Hormone & Metabolic Research, 44*(13), 975-979.

American College of Sports Medicine. (2009). ACSM position stand on exercise and physical activity for older adults. *Medicine & Science in Sports & Exercise, 41*(7), 1510-1530.

American College of Sports Medicine. (2017). *ACSM's guidelines for exercise testing and prescription* (10th ed.). Philadelphia, PA: Lippincott Williams & Wilkins.

Arnett, S.W., Laity, J.H., Agrawal, S.K., Cress, M,E. (2008). Aerobic reserve and physical functional performance in older adults. *Age & Ageing, 37*(4), 384-389.

Batacan, R.B. Jr., Duncan, M.J., Dalbo, V.J., Tucker, P.S., & Fenning, A.S. (2017). Effects of high-intensity interval training on cardiometabolic health: a systematic review and meta-analysis of intervention studies. *British Journal of Sports Medicine,* 51(6), 494-503.

Bell, J.M., & Bassey, E.J. (1996). Post exercise heart rates and pulse palpation as a means of determining exercising intensity in an aerobic dance class. *British Journal of Sports Medicine, 30,* 48-52.

Bocalini, D.S., Serra, A.J., Murad, N., & Levy, R.F. Water- versus land-based exercise effects on physical fitness in older women. *Geriatrics & Gerontology International, 8,* 265-271.

Bompa, T.O., & Buzzichelli, C. (2018). *Periodization: Theory and Methodology of Training.* (6th ed.). Champaign, IL: Human Kinetics.

Borg, G.A. (1982). Psychophysical bases of perceived exertion. *Medicine & Science in Sports & Exercise, 14,* 377-381.

Borg, G., & Hassmen, P. (1999). Physical activity and perceived exertion: Basic knowledge with applications for the elderly. *Advances in Rehabilitation, 1,* 17-34.

Brooks, D.S. (1997). *Program design for personal trainers.* Champaign, IL: Human Kinetics.

Brovold, T., Skelton, D.A., & Bergland, A. (2013). Older patients recently discharged from hospital: The effect of aerobic interval exercise on health-related quality of life, physical fitness and physical activity. *Journal of the American Geriatrics Society, 61*(9), 1580-1585.

Brown, D.R., Wang, Y., Ward, A., Ebbeling, C.B., Fortlage, L., Puleo, E., . . . Rippe, J.M. (1995). Chronic psychological effects of exercise and exercise plus cognitive strategies. *Medicine & Science in Sports & Exercise, 27,* 765-775.

Cho, C., Han, C., Sung, M., Lee, C., Kim, M., Ogawa, Y., & Kohzuki, M. (2017). Six-month lower limb aerobic exercise improves physical function in young-old, old-old, and oldest-old adults. *Tohuku Journal of Experimental Medicine, 242,* 251-257.

Colcombe, S.J., Erickson, K.I., Scalf, P.E., Kim, J.S., Prakash, R., McAuley, E., . . . Kramer, A.F. (2006). Aerobic exercise training increases brain volume in aging humans. *Journals of Gerontology: Series A Biological Sciences, Medical Sciences, 61*(11), 1166-1170.

Dinan, S. (2002). Exercise for vulnerable patients. In A. Young & M. Harries (Eds.), *Physical activity for patients: An exercising prescription* (53-70). London: Royal College of Physicians.

Dinan, S., Lenihan, P., Tenn, T., Iliffe, S. (2006). Is the promotion of physical activity in vulnerable older people feasible and effective in general practice? *British Journal of General Practice, 56,* 791-793.

Dinan, S., & Skelton, D.A. (2008). *Exercise for the prevention of falls and injuries in frailer older people: A manual for the postural stability instructor* (4th ed.). London, UK: Later Life Training.

Donath, L., Zahner, L., Cordes, M., Hanssen, H., Schmidt-Trucksäss, A., & Faude, O. (2013) Recommendations for aerobic endurance training based on subjective ratings of perceived exertion in healthy seniors. *Journal of Aging and Physical Activity, 21,* 100-111.

Erickson, K.I., Prakash, R.S., Voss, M.W., Chaddock, L., Hu, L., Morris, K.S., . . . Kramer, A.F. (2009). Aerobic fitness is associated with hippocampal volume in elderly humans. *Hippocampus, 19*(10), 1030-1039.

Fiatarone Singh, M.A. (2002). The exercise prescription. In M.A. Fiatarone Singh (Ed.), *Exercise, nutrition, and the older woman: Wellness for women over fifty.* Boca Raton, FL: CRC Press.

Fiatarone Singh, M.A. (2011). *Exercise, nutrition and the older adult: Wellness for optimal aging,* (2nd ed.). Boca Raton, FL: CRC Press.

Fitzsimons, C.F., Greig, C.A., Saunders, D.H., Lewis, S.H., Shenkin, S.D., Lavery, C., Young, A. (2005). Responses to walking-speed instructions: Implications for health promotion for older adults. *Journal of Aging and Physical Activity, 13*(2), 172-183.

Globas, C., Becker, C., Cerny, J., Lam, J.M., Lindemann, U., Forrester, L.W., . . . Luft, A.R. (2012). Chronic stroke survivors benefit from high-intensity aerobic treadmill exercise: A randomized control trial. *Neurorehabilitation & Neural Repair, 26*(1), 85-95.

Hassmen, P., & Koivula, N. (1997). Mood, physical working capacity and cognitive performance in the elderly as related to physical activity. *Aging (Milano), 9,* 136-142.

Heyward, V.H. & Gibson, A. (2014). *Advanced fitness assessment and exercise prescription* (7th ed.). Champaign, IL: Human Kinetics.

Hill, R.D., Storandt, M., & Malley, M. (1993). The impact of long-term exercise training on psychological function in older adults. *Journal of Gerontology, 48,* 12-17.

Ilarraza, H., Myers, J., Kottman, W., Rickli, H., & Dubach, P. (2004). An evaluation of training responses using self-regulation in a residential rehabilitation program. *Journal of Cardiopulmonary Rehabilitation, 24,* 27-33.

King, A.C., Rejeski, J., & Buchner, D.M. (1998). Physical activity interventions targeting older adults—A critical review and recommendations. *American Journal of Preventative Medicine, 15,* 316-333.

Kobayashi, H. (2013). Effect of measurement duration on accuracy of pulse-counting. *Ergonomics, 56,* 1940-1944. doi:10.1080/00140139.2013.840743

Kohrt, W.M., Spina, R.J., Holloszy, J.O., & Ehsani, A.A. (1998). Prescribing exercise intensity for older women. *Journal of the American Geriatrics Society, 46,* 129-133.

Lavie, C.J., & Milani, R.V. (1995). Effects of cardiac rehabilitation programs on exercise capacity, coronary risk factors, behavioral characteristics, and quality of life in a large elderly cohort. *American Journal of Cardiology, 76,* 177-179.

Lovell, D.I., Cuneo, R., & Gass, G.C. (2010). Can aerobic training improve muscle strength and power in older men? *Journal of Aging & Physical Activity, 18*(1), 14-26.

Malbut, K.E., Dinan, S., & Young, A. (2002). Aerobic training in the "oldest old" – the effects of 24 weeks of training. *Age and Ageing, 31,* 255-260.

Malbut-Shennan, K.E., Greig, C., & Young, A. (2000). Aerobic exercise. In A. Young (Ed.), section on "muscle," (Eds.) J.G. Evans, T.F. Williams, B.L. Beattie, J.P. Michel, and G.K. Wilcock, 968-972. *Oxford textbook of geriatric medicine* (2nd ed.). Oxford: Oxford University Press.

Masuki, S., Morikawa, M., & Nose, H. (2017). Interval Walking Training Can Increase Physical Fitness in Middle-Aged and Older People. *Exercise & Sport Science Review,* 45(3), 154-162.

Ministry of Health, New Zealand. (2013) *Guidelines on physical activity for older people (aged 65 years and over).* Wellington, New Zealand: Author.

Nelson, M.E., Rejeski, W.J., Blair, S.N., Duncan, P.W., Judge, J.O., King, A.C., . . . Castaneda-Sceppa, C. (2007). Physical activity and public health in older adults: Recommendation from the American College of Sports Medicine and the American Heart Association. *Medicine & Science in Sports & Exercise, 39*(8), 1435-1445.

Nemoto, K., Gen-no, H., Masuki, S., Okazaki, K., & Nose, H. (2007). Effects of high-intensity interval walking training on physical fitness and blood pressure in middle-aged and older people. *Mayo Clinic Proceedings, 82*(7), 803-811.

PAGAC. (Physical Activity Guidelines Advisory Committee). (2018). *2018 Physical activity guidelines advisory committee scientific report.* Washington, DC: U.S. Department of Health and Human Services.

Puggaard, L., Larsen, J., Stovring, H., & Jeune, B. (2000). Maximal oxygen uptake, muscle strength and walking speed in 85-year-old women: Effects of increased physical activity. *Aging, Clinical and Experimental Research, 12,* 180-189.

Scharff-Olsen, M., Williford, H.N., & Smith, F.H. (1992). The heart rate $\dot{V}O_2$ relationship of aerobic dance: A comparison of target heart rate methods. *Journal of Sports Medicine and Physical Fitness 32,* 372-377.

Shephard, R.J. (1990). The scientific basis of exercise prescribing for the very old. *Journal of the American Geriatrics Society, 38,* 62-70.

Shephard, R.J. (1991). Exercise prescription for the healthy aged: Testing and programs. *Clinical Journal of Sports Medicine, 1,* 88-99.

Shephard, R.J. (2009). Maximal oxygen intake and independence in old age. *British Journal of Sports Medicine, 43,* 342-346.

Sherrington, C., Whitney, J.C., Lord, S.R., Herbert, R.D., Cumming, R.G. & Close, J.C. (2008). Effective exercise for the prevention of falls: A systematic review and meta-analysis. *Journal of the American Geriatrics Society, 56,* 2234-2243.

Skelton, D.A., & Beyer, N. (2003). Exercise and injury prevention in older people. *Scandinavian Journal of Medicine & Science in Sports, 13,* 77-85.

Skelton, D.A., & Dinan, S.M. (1999). Exercise for falls management: Rationale for an exercise programme to reduce postural instability. *Physiotherapy: Theory and Practice, 15,* 105-120.

Skelton, D.A., & Dinan, S.M. (2008). Ageing and older people. In J.P. Buckley (Ed.), *Exercise physiology in special populations. Advances in sport and exercise science* (pp. 161-223). Edinburgh, UK: Elsevier Books.

Skelton, D.A., Young, A., Greig, C.A., & Malbut, K.E. (1995). Effects of resistance training on strength, power and selected functional abilities of women aged 75 and over. *Journal of the American Geriatrics Society, 43,* 1081-1087.

Tanaka, H., Monahan, K.D., & Seals, D.R. (2001). Age-predicted maximal heart rate revisited. *Journal of the American College of Cardiology, 37,* 153-156.

Taylor, A.H., Cable, N.T., Faulkner, G., Hillsdon, M., Narici, M.,Van Der Bij, A.K. (2004). Physical activity and older adults: A review of health benefits and the effectiveness of interventions. *Journal of Sports Sciences, 22*(8), 703-725.

U.K. Department of Health. (2011). *Start active, stay active. A report on physical activity for health from the four home countries' Chief Medical Officers.* London, UK: Department of Health.

U.S. Department of Health and Human Services. (2008). *Physical activity guidelines for Americans: A report of the Surgeon General.* Atlanta, GA: Centers for Disease Control and Prevention, National Center for Chronic Prevention and Health Promotion, and the President's Council on Physical Fitness and Sports.

Warburton E.R., Whitney C., Shannon, N., & Bredin,S.D. (2006) Health benefits of physical activity: The evidence. *Canadian Medical Association Journal, 174*(6), 801-809.

Whitehurst, M. (2012). High-intensity interval training: An alternative for older adults. *American Journal of Lifestyle Medicine,6,* 382-386. doi:10.1177/1559827612450262

Wilcox, S., Dowda, M., Griffin, S.F., Rheaume. C., Ory, M.G., Leviton, L., . . . Mockenhaupt, R. (2006). Results of the First year of Active for Life: Translation of 2 evidence-based physical activity programs for older adults into community settings. *American Journal of Public Health, 96,* 1201-1209.

Williams, P., & Lord, S.R. (1995). Predictors of adherence to a structured exercise program for older women. *Psychology and Aging, 10,* 617-624.

Yessis, M. (1987). *The secret of Soviet sports fitness and training.* London, UK: Arbour House.

Young, A. (2001). An exercise prescription for a healthier old age. In A. Young & M. Harries (Eds.), *Physical activity for patients: An exercise prescription.* London, UK: Royal College of Physicians.

Young, A., & Dinan, S. (2005). Active in later life. *British Medical Journal, 330,* 189-191.

Yu, F., Leon, A.S, Bliss, D., Dysken, M., Savik, K., Wyman, J.F. (2011). Aerobic training for older men with Alzheimer's disease: Individual examples of progression. *Research in Gerontological Nursing, 4*(4), 243-250.

Chapter 14

Alexander, N.B. (1994). Postural control in older adults. *Journal of the American Geriatrics Society, 42,* 93-108.

Arshad, Q., & Seemungal, B.M. (2016). Age-related vestibular loss: Current understanding and future research directions. *Frontiers in Neurology, 7,* 231. doi:10.3389/fneur.2016.00231

Centers for Disease Control and Prevention (CDC, 2016). Falls are leading cause of injury and death in older Americans. Retrieved from www.cdc.gov/media/releases/2016/p0922-older-adult-falls.html

Dijkstra, B.W., Horak, F.B., Kamsma, Y.P., & Peterson, D.S. (2015). Older adults can improve compensatory stepping with repeated postural perturbations. *Frontiers in Aging Neuroscience, 7,* 201.

Hu, M., & Woollacott, M.H. (1994). Multisensory training of standing balance in older adults: I. Postural stability and one-leg stance balance. *Journal of Gerontology, 49,* M52-M61.

Kanekar, N., & Aruin, A.S. (2014). The effect of aging on anticipatory postural control. *Experimental Brain Research, 232,* 1127-1136. doi:10.1007/s00221-014-3822-3

Li, L., Simonsick, E.M., Ferucci, L., & Lin, F.R. (2013). Hearing loss and gait speed among older adults in the United States. *Gait & Posture, 38,* 25-29. doi:10.1016/j.gaitpost.2012.10.006

Lin, F.R. & Ferucci, L. (2012). Hearing loss and falls among older adults in the United States. *Archives of Internal Medicine, 172,* 369-371. doi:10.1001/archinternmed.2011.728

Maki, B.E., & McIlroy, W.E. (2006). Control of rapid limb movements for balance recovery: Age-related changes and implications for fall prevention. *Age and Ageing, 35*(Supp. 2), ii12-ii18.

McCrum, C., Gerards, M.H.G., Karamanidis, K., Zijlstra, W., & Meijer, K. (2017). A systematic review of gait perturbation paradigms for improving reactive stepping responses and falls risk among healthy older adults. *European Review of Aging & Physical Activity. 14,* 3. doi:10.1186/s11556-017-0173-7

Melzer, I., Liebermann, D.G., Krasovsky, T., & Oddsson, L.I.E. (2010). Cognitive load affects lower limb force–time relations during voluntary rapid stepping in healthy old and young adults. *Journals of Gerontology A: Biological Science & Medical Science, 4,* 400-406. doi:10.1093/gerona/glp185

Mille, M.L., Johnson, M.E., Martinez, K.M., and Rogers, M.W. (2005). Age-dependent differences in lateral balance recovery through protective stepping. *Clinical Biomechanics, 20,* 607-616. doi:10.1016/j.clinbiomech.2005.03.004

Mille, M.L., Johnson-Hilliard, M., Martinez, K.M., Zhang, Y., Edwards, B.J., & Rogers, M.W. (2013).

One step, two steps, three steps more. Directional vulnerability to falls in community-dwelling older people. *Journals of Gerontology A: Biological Science & Medical Science, 68,* 1540-1548. doi:10.1093/gerona/glt062

O'Connor, K.W., Loughlin, P.J., Redfern, M.S., & Sparto, P.J. (2008). Postural adaptations to repeated optic flow stimulation in older adults. *Gait & Posture, 28,* 385-391. doi:10.1016/j.gaitpost.2008.01.010

Panel on Prevention of Falls in Older Persons, American Geriatrics Society, and British Geriatrics Society (2011). Summary of the updated American Geriatrics Society/British Geriatrics Society clinical practice guideline for prevention of falls in older persons. *Journal of the American Geriatric Society, 59,* 148-157.

Perry, S.D. (2006). Evaluation of age-related plantar-surface insensitivity in older adults using vibratory and touch sensation tests. *Neuroscience Letters, 392,* 62-67.

Ribeiro, F., & Oliveira, J. (2007). Aging effects on joint proprioception: The role of physical activity in proprioception preservation. *European Review of Aging and Physical Activity, 4,* 26. doi:10.1007/s11556-007-0026-x

Rose, D.J. (2010). *FallProof! A comprehensive balance and mobility training program (2nd ed.).* Champaign, IL: Human Kinetics.

Shaffer, S.W., & Harrison, A.L. (2007). Aging of the somatosensory system: A translational perspective. *Physical Therapy, 87,* 193-207.

Shumway-Cook, A., & Woollacott, M.H. (2017). *Motor control: Translating research into clinical practice* (5th ed.). Philadelphia: Lippincott Williams & Wilkins.

Spirduso, W., MacRae, P., & Francis, K. (2005). *Physical dimensions of aging (2nd ed.).* Champaign, IL: Human Kinetics.

Stockel, T., Wunsch, K., & Hughes, C.M.L. (2017). Age-related decline in anticipatory motor planning and its relation to cognitive and motor proficiency. *Frontiers in Aging Neuroscience, 9,* 283. doi:10.3389/fnagi.2017.00283

Thelen, D.G., Wojcik, L.A., Schultz, A.B., Ashton-Miller, J.A., & Alexander, N.B. (1997). Age differences in using a rapid step to regain balance during a forward fall. *Journal of Gerontology: Medical Sciences, 52A,* M8-M13.

Chapter 15

Ashford, D., Bennett, S.J., & Davids, K. (2006). Observational modeling effects for movement dynamics and movement outcome measures across differing task constraints: A meta-analysis. *Journal of Motor Behavior, 38,* 185-205.

Behrman, A.L., Vander Linden, D.W., & Cauraugh, J.H. (1992). Relative frequency knowledge of results: Older adults learning a force-time modulation task. *Journal of Human Movement Studies, 23,* 233-250.

Chiviacowsky, S., & Wulf, G. (2007). Feedback after good trials enhances learning. *Research Quarterly for Exercise and Sport, 78,* 40-47.

Chiviacowsky, S., Wulf, G., Wally, R., & Borges, T. (2009). Knowledge of results after good trials enhances learning in older adults. *Research Quarterly for Exercise and Sport, 80,* 663-668.

Gentile, A.M. (1972). A working model of skill acquisition with application to teaching [Monograph]. *Quest, 17,* 3-23.

Gentile, A.M. (2000). Skill acquisition: Action, movement, and neuromotor processes. In J.H. Carr & R.B. Shephard (Eds.), *Movement science: Foundations for physical therapy* (2nd ed., pp. 111-187). Rockville, MD: Aspen.

Guadagnoli, M.A. & Lee, T.D. (2004). Challenge point: A framework for conceptualizing the effects of various practice conditions in motor learning. *Journal of Motor Behavior, 36,* 212-224.

Knudson, D.V. (2013). *Qualitative analysis of human movement* (3rd ed.). Champaign, IL: Human Kinetics.

Knudson, D.V., & Morrison, C.S. (2002). *Qualitative analysis of human movement* (2nd ed.). Champaign, IL: Human Kinetics.

Landin, D. (1994). The role of verbal cues in skill learning. *Quest, 46,* 299-313.

Magill, R.A., & Anderson, D. (2014). *Motor learning: Concepts and applications* (7th ed.), New York, NY: McGraw-Hill.

McCullagh, P., Law, B., & Ste-Marie, D. (2012). Modeling and performance. In S.M. Murphy (Ed.), *The Oxford handbook of sport and performance psychology* (pp. 250-272). New York, NY: Oxford University Press.

McCullagh, P., & Weiss, M.R. (2001). Modeling: Considerations for motor skill performance and psychological responses. In R.N. Singer, H.A. Hausenblas, & C.M. Janelle (Eds.), *Handbook of sport psychology* (2nd ed., pp. 205-238). New York, NY: Wiley.

Rodrigue, K.M., Kennedy, K.M., & Raz, N. (2005). Aging and longitudinal change in perceptual-motor skill acquisition in healthy adults. *Journals* of Gerontology B: Psychological Science and Social Sciences, 60, 174-181.

Rose, D.J., & Christina, R.W. (2006). A multilevel approach to the study of motor control and learning (2nd ed.). San Francisco, CA: Benjamin-Cummings.

Schmidt, R.A., & Lee, T.D. (2014). Motor learning and performance (5th ed.). Champaign, IL: Human Kinetics.

Spirduso, W.W., Francis, K.L., & MacRae, P.G. (2005). Physical dimensions of aging (2nd ed.). Champaign, IL: Human Kinetics.

Townley, R, & Dinan, S. (2003). The chair-based exercise programme for frailer, older adults and disabled adults: "Sit tall, stand strong" knowledge base manual (2nd ed.). London, UK: Later Life Training.

Voelcker-Rehage, C. (2008). Motor skill learning in older adults: A review of studies on age-related differences. European Review of Aging and Physical Activity, 5, 5-16. doi:10.1007/s11556-008-0030-9

Wishart, L.R., & Lee, T.D. (1997). Effects of aging and reduced relative frequency of knowledge of results on learning a motor skill. Perceptual and Motor Skills, 84, 1107-1122.

Woods D.L., Wyma J., Yund, E.W., Herron T.J., & Reed, B. (2015a). Factors influencing the latency of simple reaction time. Frontiers in Human Neuroscience, 9, 131. doi:10.3389/fnhum.2015.00131

Woods, D.L., Wyma, J.M., Yund, E.W., Herron, T.J., & Reed, B. (2015b). Age-related slowing of response selection and production in a visual choice reaction time task. Frontiers in Human Neuroscience, 9, 193. doi:10.3389/fnhum.2015.00193

Chapter 16

Akushevich, I., Kravchenko, J., Ukraintseva, S., & Arbeev, K.A.I. (2013). Time trends of incidence of age-associated diseases in the U.S. elderly population: Medicare-based analysis. Age and Ageing 42, 494-500.

American College of Sports Medicine. (2009). ACSM position stand on exercise and physical activity for older adults. Medicine & Science in Sports & Exercise, 41, 1510-1530.

Arnold, E.C., & Underman Boggs, K. (2016) Interpersonal relationships: Professional communication skills for nurses (7th ed.). Amsterdam, The Netherlands: Elsevier.

British Heart Foundation, National Centre for Physical Activity & Health, Glasgow Caledonian University, and Later Life Training (2014). Functional fitness MOT training for professionals. Retrieved from www.bhfactive.org.uk/older-adults-training-and-events-item/370/index.html

Buchner, D.M., & Coleman, E.A. (1994) Exercise considerations for older adults. Physical Medicine and Rehabilitation Clinics of North America, 5, 5-9.

Chemers, M.M., Watson, C.B., & May, S.T. (2000). Dispositional affect and leadership effectiveness: A comparison of self-esteem, optimism and efficacy. Personality & Social Psychology Bulletin, 26, 3, 267-277.

Chodzko-Zajko, W.J., Resnick, B. (2004) Beyond screening: The need for new preactivity counseling protocols to assist older adults' transition from sedentary living to physically active lifestyles. Journal on Active Aging, 3, 26-30.

Costello, E., Kafchinski, M., Vrazel, J., & Sullivan, P. (2011). Motivators, barriers, and beliefs regarding physical activity in an older adult population, Journal of Geriatric Physical Therapy. 34,138-147. doi:10.1519/JPT.0b013e31820e0e71

Craig, A., Dinan, S., Smith, A., Taylor, A., & Webborn, N. (2001). NHS exercise referral systems: A national quality assurance framework. London, UK: Department of Health, HMSO, Stationary Office.

De Groot, G.C.L., & Fagerstrom, L. (2011). Older adults' motivating factors and barriers to exercise to prevent falls. Scandinavian Journal of Occupational Therapy, 18, 153-160. doi:10.3109/11038128.2010.487113

Dennis, J., Wicebloom-Paul, S., Townley, B., Dinan-Young, S. (2013). Design and delivery of exercise and fitness training after stroke. In: G.E. Mead, G.E. & F. van Wijck, F. (Eds), Exercise and fitness training after a stroke. A handbook for practice. (pp. 169-212). Edinburgh, UK: Elsevier Publications, UK.

Department of Health. (2011). Start active, stay active. A report on physical activity for health from the four home counties' Chief Medical Officers. London, UK: Department of Health.

Digman, J.M. (1990). Personality structure: Emergence of the five-factor model. Annual Review of Psychology, 41, 417-440.

Dinan, S., Buckley , J., Lister, C., Gittus, B., & Webborn, N. (2001-2009). National occupational standards (NOS) for instructing physical activity and exercise; NOS for physical activity and exercise instructors of older adults (D441), 2001, 2006, 2009; Specialist physical activity and health instructors of exercise for the prevention of falls *in frailer older people* (D551), 2000, 2009. Skills Active UK. Retrieved from www.skillsactive.com/training/standards/level-3/Instructing-Physical-Activity-and-Exercise

Dinan, S., Lenihan, P., Tenn, T., & Iliffe, S. (2006). Is the promotion of physical activity in vulnerable older people feasible and effective in general practice? *British Journal of General Practice, 56,* 791-793.

Dinan, S., & Skelton, D.A. (2008). *Exercise for the prevention of falls and injuries in frailer older people: A manual for the postural stability instructor* (4th ed.). London, UK: Later Life Training.

Dinan, S., & Skelton, D.A. (2013). Sit to stand exercise. In S. Gawler (Ed.), *Chair-based exercise program for frailer older adults and adults with disabilities : A manual for the Chair Based Exercise Leader* (4th ed.). London, UK: Later Life Training.

Ecclestone, N.A., & Jones, C.J. (2004). International curriculum guidelines for preparing physical activity instructors of older adults. *Journal of Aging and Physical Activity 12,* 5-21.

Estabrooks, P.A., Munroe, K.J., Fox, E.H., Gyurcsik, N.C., Hill, J.L., Lyon, R., . . . Shannon, V.R. (2004). Leadership in physical activity groups for older adults: A qualitative analysis. *Journal of Aging and Physical Activity, 12,* 232-245.

Fox, K.R., Stathi, A., McKenna, J., & Davis, M.G. (2007). Physical activity and mental well-being in older people participating in the Better Ageing Project. *European Journal of Applied Physiology, 100,* 591-602.

Hawley, H. (2011). *The role of the exercise instructor in older adults' uptake and adherence to exercise classes.* PhD thesis, University of Manchester.

Hawley, H., Skelton, D.A., Campbell, M., & Todd, C. (2012) Are attitudes of exercise instructors who work with older adults influenced by their training and personal characteristics? *Journal of Aging and Physical Activity, 20,* 47-63.

Hawley-Hague, H., Horne, M., Campbell, M., Demack, S., Skelton, D.A., & Todd, C. (2014). Multiple levels of influence on older adults' attendance and adherence to community exercise classes. *The Gerontologist, 54,* 599-610. doi:10.1093/geront/gnt075

Hawley-Hague, H., Horne, M., Skelton, D.A., & Todd, C. (2015). Older adults' uptake and adherence to exercise classes: Instructors' perspectives. *Journal of Aging and Physical Activity, 24,* 119-128.

Hawley-Hague, H., Horne, M., Skelton, D.A., & Todd, C. (2016). Review of how we should define (and measure) adherence in studies examining older adults' participation in exercise classes. *British Medical Journal Open, 6*(6), e011560. doi:10.1136/bmjopen-2016-011560

Hawley-Hague, H., Laventure, R., & Skelton, D.A. (2018) The role of the instructor in exercise and physical activity programmes for older people. In Samuel R. Nyman et al. (Eds.), *The Palgrave Handbook of Ageing and Physical Activity Promotion,* 337-358.

Horne, M., Skelton, D., Speed, S., & Todd, C. (2010) The influence of primary care health professionals in encouraging exercise and physical activity uptake amongst White and South Asian older adults: Experiences of young older adults. *Patient Education and Counselling, 78,* 97-103.

Jones, C.J., & Rose, D.J. (Eds.). (2005). *Physical activity instruction of older adults.* Champaign, IL: Human Kinetics.

Karageorghis, C.I., Terry, P.C., Lane, A.M., Bishop, D.T., & Priest, D.L. (2012). The BASES expert statement on use of music in exercise. *Journal of Sports Science, 30,* 953-956. doi:10.1080/02640414.2012.676665

Kennedy-Armbruster, C., & Yoke, M.M. (2014). *Methods of group exercise instruction* (3rd ed.). Champaign, IL: Human Kinetics.

King, A.C., Haskell, W.L., Taylor, C.B., Kraemer, H.C., & Debusk, R.F. (1991). Group- vs. home-based exercise training in healthy older men and women: A community-based clinical trial. *Journal of the American Medical Association, 266,* 1535-1542.

King, A.C., Rejeski, J., & Buchner, D.M. (1998). Physical activity interventions targeting older adults: A critical review and recommendations. *American Journal of Preventative Medicine, 15,* 316-333.

King, A.C., Taylor, C.B., & Haskell, W.L. (1993). Effects of differing intensities and formats of 12 months of exercise training on psychological outcomes in older adults. *Health Psychology 12,* 292-300.

Lachman, M.E. (2006). Perceived control over aging-related declines: Adaptive beliefs and behaviors. *Current Directions in Psychological Science, 15,* 282-286.

Laventure, R.M.E., Dinan, S.M., & Skelton, D.A. (2008) Someone Like Me: Increasing participation in physical activity among seniors with senior peer health motivators. *Journal of Aging and Physical Activity, 16*(Suppl.), S76-S77.

Loughead, T.M., & Carron, A.V. (2004). The mediating role of cohesion in the leader behaviour-satisfaction relationship. *Psychology of Sport and Exercise, 5,* 355-371. doi:10.1016/S1469-0292(03)00033-5

Marzano, R.J. (2007) *The art and science of teaching: A comprehensive framework for effective instruction*. Alexandria, VA: Association for Supervision & Curriculum Development.

Marzano, R.J. (2009). *Designing and teaching learning goals and objectives: Classroom strategies that work*. Bloomington, IN: Marzano Research Laboratory

Maxwell, J. (1993). *The winning attitude. Nashville, TN: Thomas Nelson.*

Ministry of Health. (2013) *Guidelines on physical activity for older people (aged 65 years and over)*. Wellington, New Zealand: Ministry of Health.

Nelson, M.E., Rejeski, W.J., Blair, S.N., Duncan, P.W., Judge, J.O., King, A.C., . . . Castaneda-Sceppa, C. (2007). Physical activity and public health in older adults: Recommendation from the American College of Sports Medicine and the American Heart Association. *Medicine & Science in Sports & Exercise, 39,* 1435-1445.

Newson, R., & Kemps, E. (2007) Factors that promote and prevent exercise engagement in older adults. *Journal of Aging and Health, 19,* 470-481.

Norris, C.M. (2011) *Managing sports injuries: A guide for students and clinicians*. London, UK: Churchill Livingstone.

Rikli, R.E., & Jones, C.J. (2013a). *Senior fitness test manual* (2nd ed.). Champaign, IL: Human Kinetics.

Rikli, R.E., & Jones, C.J. (2013b). Development and validation of criterion-referenced clinically relevant fitness standards for maintaining physical independence in later years. *The Gerontologist, 53,* 255-267.

Rose, D.J. (2010) *FallProof! A comprehensive balance and mobility training program*. (2nd ed.). Champaign, IL: Human Kinetics.

Schutzer, K.A., & Graves, B.S. (2004). Barriers and motivations to exercise in older adults. *Preventive Medicine, 39*(5), 1056-1061.

Scott, F., Young, A., Dinan -Young, S., Harding, M., Lewis, S., , . . Fisken, S. (2008). *Expert survey on physical activity programmes and physical activity promotion strategies for older people*. European Network on Physical Activity & Ageing (EUNAAPA). Work Package 5. Cross National Report. Retrieved from http://www.eunaapa.org/media/cross-national_report_expert_survey_on_pa_programmes_and_promotion_strategies_2008_.pdf Seguin, R.A., Economos, C.D., Palombo, R., Hyatt, R., Kuder, J., & Nelson, M.E.

(2010). Strength training and older women: A cross-sectional study examining factors related to exercise adherence. *Journal of Aging and Physical Activity, 2,* 201-218.

Sjösten, N.M., Salonoja, M., Piirtola, M, Vahlberg, T.J, Isoaho, R, Hyttinen, H.K, . . . Kivelä, S.L. (2007). A multifactorial fall prevention programme in the community-dwelling aged: Predictors of adherence. *European Journal of Public Health. 17,* 464-470.

Skelton, D.A., & Dinan, S.M. (2008). Ageing and older people. In J.P. Buckley (Ed.), *Exercise physiology in special populations: Advances in sport and exercise science* (pp.161-223). Edinburgh: Elsevier.

Skelton, D.A, Dinan, S, Campbell, M.G, & Rutherford, O.M. (2005) Tailored group exercise (Falls Management Exercise) reduces falls in community dwelling older frequent fallers (an RCT). *Age and Ageing 34,* 636-639.

Stathi, A., McKenna, J., & Fox, K.R. (2010). Processes associated with participation and adherence to a 12-month exercise program for adults aged 70 and older. *Journal of Health Psychology, 15,* 838-47. doi:10.1177/1359105309357090.

Stigglebout, M., Hopman-Rock, M., Crone, M., Lecher, L., Van Mechelen, W. (2006) Predicting older adults' maintenance in exercise participation using an integrated social psychological model. *Health Education Research. 21,* 1-14.

Taylor, A.H., Cable, N.T., Faulkner, G., Hillsdon, M., Narici, M., & Van Der Bij, A.K. (2004). Physical activity and older adults: A review of health benefits and the effectiveness of interventions. *Journal of Sports Sciences, 22*(8), 703-725.

Townley, R., & Dinan-Young, S. (2013) The functional model. In S.Gawler (Ed.), *The Otago Strength and Balance Exercise Programme for Older Adults: A manual for the older adult Otago exercise leader* (2nd ed.). London, UK: Later Life Training.

U.S. Department of Health and Human Services. (2008). *Physical activity guidelines for Americans: A report of the Surgeon General. Atlanta, GA:* Centers for Disease Control and Prevention, National Center for Chronic Prevention and Health Promotion, and the President's Council on Physical Fitness and Sports.

Winters, A. (2005). Perceptions of body posture and emotion: A question of methodology. *The New School Psychology Bulletin, 3*(2), 35-45.

Yardley, L., Bishop, F., Beyer, N., Hauer, K., Kempen, G.I., Piot-Ziegler, C., . . . Holt, A.R. (2006) Older people's views of falls: Prevention interventions in six European countries. *The Gerontologist, 46,* 650-660.

Young, A. (2001).An exercise prescription for a healthier old age. In A. Young & M. Harries (Eds.), *Physical activity for patients: An exercise prescription*. London, UK: Royal College of Physicians.

Young, A., & Dinan, S. (2005). Active in later life. *British Medical Journal, 330,* 189-191.

Chapter 17

American Heart Association. (2018). *Understanding Blood Pressure Readings*. Retrieved from: http://www.heart.org/HEARTORG/Conditions/HighBloodPressure/KnowYourNumbers/Understanding-Blood-Pressure-Readings_UCM_301764_Article.jsp

Becker, B.E. (2009). Aquatic therapy: Scientific foundations and clinical rehabilitation applications. *Physical Medicine & Rehabilitation,1,* 859-872. doi:10.1016/j.pmrj.2009.05.017

Bennell, K.L., Dobson, F., & Hinman, R.S. (2014). Exercise in osteoarthritis: Moving from prescription to adherence. *Best Practice & Research: Clinical Rheumatology, 28,* 93-117. doi:10.1016/j.berh.2014.01.009

Blakey, J.D., Woolnough, K., Fellows, J., Walker, S., Thomas, M., & Pavord, I.D. (2013). Assessing the risk of attack in the management of asthma: A review and proposal for revision of the current control-centred paradigm. *Primary Care Respiratory Journal, 22,* 344-352. doi:10.4104/pcrj.2013.00063

Cadore, E.L., Pinto, R.S., Bottaro, M., & Izquierdo, M. (2014). Strength and endurance training prescription in healthy and frail elderly. *Aging and Disease, 5,* 183-195. doi:10.14336/ad.2014.0500183

Carnethon, M.R., Rasmussen-Torvik, L.J., & Palaniappan, L. (2014). The obesity paradox in diabetes. *Current Cardiology Reports, 16,* 446. doi:10.1007/s11886-013-0446-3

Carson, K.V., Chandratilleke, M.G., Picot, J., Brinn, M.P., Esterman, A.J., & Smith, B.J. (2013). Physical training for asthma. *Cochrane Database System Review, 9,* CD001116. doi:10.1002/14651858. CD001116.pub4

Caspersen, C.J., Thomas, G.D., Boseman, L.A., Beckles, G.L., & Albright, A.L. (2012). Aging, diabetes, and the public health system in the United States. *American Journal of Public Health, 102,* 1482-1497. doi:10.2105/ajph.2011.300616

Centers for Disease Control and Prevention. (2013). *Asthma facts: CDC's National Asthma Control Program*. Atlanta, GA: U.S. Department of Health and Human Services, Centers for Disease Control and Prevention.

Clark, C., & Cochrane, L. (2009). *Asthma* (3rd ed.). Champaign, IL: Human Kinetics.

Colberg, S.R., Albright, A.L., Blissmer, B.J., Braun, B., Chasan-Taber, L., Fernhall, B., . . . Sigal, R.J. (2010). American College of Sports Medicine and the American Diabetes Association joint position statement. Exercise and type 2 diabetes. *Medicine & Science in Sports & Exercise, 42,* 2282-2303. doi:10.1249/MSS.0b013e3181eeb61c

Cooper, C. (2009). *Chronic obstructive pulmonary disease* (3rd ed.). Champaign, IL: Human Kinetics.

Dawson-Hughes, B., Looker, A.C., Tosteson, A.N., Johansson, H., Kanis, J.A., & Melton, L.J., 3rd. (2012). The potential impact of the National Osteoporosis Foundation guidance on treatment eligibility in the USA: An update in NHANES 2005-2008. *Osteoporosis International, 23*(3), 811-820. doi:10.1007/s00198-011-1694-y

De Schutter, A., Lavie, C.J., & Milani, R.V. (2014). The impact of obesity on risk factors and prevalence and prognosis of coronary heart disease: The obesity paradox. *Progress in Cardiovascular Diseases, 56,* 401-408. doi:10.1016/j.pcad.2013.08.003

Dorsey, E.R., George, B.P., Leff, B., & Willis, A.W. (2013). The coming crisis: Obtaining care for the growing burden of neurodegenerative conditions. *Neurology, 80*(21), 1989-1996. doi:10.1212/WNL.0b013e318293e2ce

Ebersbach, G., Moreau, C., Gandor, F., Defebvre, L., & Devos, D. (2013). Clinical syndromes: Parkinsonian gait. *Movement Disorders, 28,* 1552-1559. doi:10.1002/mds.25675

Ehsani, A.A. (2001). Exercise in patients with hypertension. *American Journal of Geriatric Cardiology, 10,* 253-259, 273.

Eves, N.D., & Davidson, W.J. (2011). Evidence-based risk assessment and recommendations for physical activity clearance: Respiratory disease. *Applied Physiology, Nutrition, and Metabolism, 36*(Suppl. 1), S80-S100. doi:10.1139/h11-057

Fielding, R.A., Guralnik, J.M., King, A.C., Pahor, M., McDermott, M.M., Tudor-Locke, C., . . . Rejeski, W.J. (2017). Dose of physical activity, physical functioning and disability risk in mobility-limited older adults: Results from the LIFE study randomized trial. *PLOS ONE, 12:* e0182155. doi:10.1371/journal.pone.0182155

Gibofsky, A. (2012). Overview of epidemiology, pathophysiology, and diagnosis of rheumatoid arthritis. *American Journal of Managed Care, 18*(13 Suppl), S295-S302.

Gill, T.M. (2014). Disentangling the disabling process: Insights from the precipitating events project. *Gerontologist, 54*(4), 533-549. doi:10.1093/geront/gnu067

Gillespie, L.D., Robertson, M.C., Gillespie, W.J., Sherrington, C., Gates, S., Clemson, L.M., & Lamb, S.E. (2012). Interventions for preventing falls in older people living in the community. *Cochrane Database System Review, 9*, CD007146. doi:10.1002/14651858.CD007146.pub3

Go, A.S., Mozaffarian, D., Roger, V.L., Benjamin, E.J., Berry, J.D., Borden, W.B., . . . Turner, M.B. (2013). Executive summary: Heart disease and stroke statistics—2013 update. A report from the American Heart Association. *Circulation, 127*, 143-152. doi:10.1161/CIR.0b013e318282ab8f

Gooneratne, N.S., Patel, N.P., & Corcoran, A. (2010). Chronic obstructive pulmonary disease diagnosis and management in older adults. *Journal of the American Geriatric Society, 58*, 1153-1162.

Gordon, N. (2009). *Hypertension* (3rd ed.). Champaign, IL: Human Kinetics.

Gordon, N.F., Gulanick, M., Costa, F., Fletcher, G., Franklin, B.A., Roth, E.J., & Shephard, T. (2004). Physical activity and exercise recommendations for stroke survivors: An American Heart Association Scientific Statement From the Council on Clinical Cardiology, Subcommittee on Exercise, Cardiac Rehabilitation, and Prevention; the Council on Cardiovascular Nursing; the Council on Nutrition, Physical Activity, and Metabolism; and the Stroke Council. *Circulation, 109*, 2031-2041. doi:10.1161/01.cir.0000126280.65777.a4

Hamm, L.F., Wenger, N.K., Arena, R., Forman, D.E., Lavie, C.J., Miller, T.D., & Thomas, R.J. (2013). Cardiac rehabilitation and cardiovascular disability: Role in assessment and improving functional capacity. A position statement from the American Association of Cardiovascular and Pulmonary Rehabilitation. *Journal of Cardiopulmory Rehabilitation and Prevention, 33*, 1-11. doi:10.1097/HCR.0b013e31827aad9e

Hornsby, W., & Albright, A.L. (2009). *Diabetes* (3rd ed.). Champaign, IL: Human Kinetics.

Howe, T. E., Shea, B., Dawson, L. J., Downie, F., Murray, A., Ross, C., . . . Creed, G. (2011). Exercise for preventing and treating osteoporosis in postmenopausal women. *Cochrane Database System Review, 7*, CD000333. doi:10.1002/14651858.CD000333.pub2

Interiano, B., & Guntupalli, K.K. (1996). Clinical aspects of asthma. *Current Opinions in Pulmonary Medicine, 2*, 60-65.

Iversen, M.D., Brawerman, M., & Iversen, C.N. (2012). Recommendations and the state of the evidence for physical activity interventions for adults with rheumatoid arthritis: 2007 to present. *International Journal of Clinical Rheumatology, 7*, 489-503. doi:10.2217/ijr.12.53

Johnson, V.L., & Hunter, D.J. (2014). The epidemiology of osteoarthritis. *Best Practice and Research: Clinical Rheumatology, 28*, 5-15. doi:10.1016/j.berh.2014.01.004

Kalyani, R.R., & Egan, J.M. (2013). Diabetes and altered glucose metabolism with aging. *Endocrinology and Metabolism Clinics of North America, 42*, 333-347. doi:10.1016/j.ecl.2013.02.010

King, M.J., & Hanania, N.A. (2010). Asthma in the elderly: Current knowledge and future directions. *Current Opinion in Pulmonary Medicine, 16*, 55-59. doi:10.1097/MCP.0b013e328333acb0

Kirkland, J.L. (2013). Translating advances from the basic biology of aging into clinical application. *Exp Gerontol, 48*(1), 1-5. doi:10.1016/j.exger.2012.11.014

Knittle, K., De Gucht, V., & Maes, S. (2012). Lifestyle- and behaviour-change interventions in musculoskeletal conditions. *Best Practice and Research: Clinical Rheumatology, 26*, 293-304. doi:10.1016/j.berh.2012.05.002

Kwakkel, G., & Kollen, B. J. (2013). Predicting activities after stroke: What is clinically relevant? *International Journal of Stroke, 8*, 25-32. doi:10.1111/j.1747-4949.2012.00967.x

Liu, C.J., & Latham, N.K. (2009). Progressive resistance strength training for improving physical function in older adults. *Cochrane Database System Review, 3*, CD002759. doi:10.1002/14651858.CD002759.pub2

Maniu, C., Flipse, T., Patton, N., & Fletcher, G. (2010). Physical activity and the cardiovascular system. In M. Crawford (Ed.), *Cardiology* (Vol. 3). Philadelphia, PA: Mosby/Elsevier.

McFadden, E.R., Jr. & Gilbert, I.A. (1992). Asthma. *New England Journal of Medicine, 327*, 1928-1937.

Minino, A.M. (2013). Death in the United States, 2011. *NCHS Data Brief, 115*, 1-8.

Modi, A., Sajjan, S., & Gandhi, S. (2014). Challenges in implementing and maintaining osteoporosis therapy. *International Journal of Women's Health, 6*, 759-769. doi:10.2147/ijwh.s53489

Nelson, M.E., Rejeski, W.J., Blair, S.N., Duncan, P.W., Judge, J.O., King, A.C., . . . Castaneda-Sceppa,

C. (2007). Physical activity and public health in older adults: Recommendation from the American College of Sports Medicine and the American Heart Association. *Circulation, 116,* 1094-1105. doi:10.1161/circulationaha.107.185650

Nicola, T., & Rimmer, J. (2010). *Stroke.* Philadelphia: Wolters Kluwer Health/Lippincott Williams & Wilkins Health.

O'Donnell, D.E., Laveneziana, P., Webb, K., & Neder, J.A. (2014). Chronic obstructive pulmonary disease: Clinical integrative physiology. *Clinics in Chest Medicine, 35,* 51-69. doi:10.1016/j.ccm.2013.09.008.

Pahor, M., Guralnik, J.M., Ambrosius, W.T., Blair, S., Bonds, D.E., Church, T.S., . . . Williamson, J.D. (2014). Effect of structured physical activity on prevention of major mobility disability in older adults: The LIFE study randomized clinical trial. *Journal of the American Medical Association, 311,* 2387-2396. doi:10.1001/jama.2014.5616

Reitz, C., & Mayeux, R. (2014). Alzheimer disease: Epidemiology, diagnostic criteria, risk factors and biomarkers. *Biochemical Pharmacology, 88,* 640-651. doi:10.1016/j.bcp.2013.12.024

Robinson, T., Brodie, F., & Manios, E. (2010). *Complications of hypertension: Stroke.* Philadelphia, PA: Mosby/Elsevier.

Rosenstock, J. (2001). Management of type 2 diabetes mellitus in the elderly: Special considerations. *Drugs and Aging, 18,* 31-44.

Smith, S., Wang, C., & Bloomfield, S. (2009). *Osteoporosis* (3rd ed.). Champaign, IL: Human Kinetics.

Stevens, M., Reininga, I.H., Bulstra, S.K., Wagenmakers, R., & van den Akker-Scheek, I. (2012). Physical activity participation among patients after total hip and knee arthroplasty. *Clinics in Geriatric Medicine, 28,* 509-520. doi:10.1016/j.cger.2012.05.003

Stolker, J., & Rich, M. (2010). *Aging and geriatric heart disease.* Philadelphia, PA: Mosby/Elsevier.

Tseng, C. L., Soroka, O., Maney, M., Aron, D. C., & Pogach, L. M. (2014). Assessing potential glycemic overtreatment in persons at hypoglycemic risk. *Journal of the American Medical Association*

Internal Medicine, 174, 259-268. doi:10.1001/jamainternmed.2013.12963

van der Kolk, N.M., & King, L.A. (2013). Effects of exercise on mobility in people with Parkinson's disease. *Movement Disorders, 28,* 1587-1596. doi:10.1002/mds.25658

Xie, J., Wu, E.Q., Zheng, Z.-J., Sullivan, P.W., Zhan, L., & Labarthe, D.R. (2008). Patient-reported health status in coronary heart disease in the United States: Age, sex, racial, and ethnic differences. *Circulation, 118,* 491-497. doi:10.1161/circulationaha.107.752006

Chapter 18

Abbott, A. (2012). Emergency response plan. *ACSM's Health & Fitness Journal, 16,* 33-36. doi:10.1249/FIT.0b013e318264cc4b

American College of Sports Medicine (2012). *ACSM's health/fitness facility standards and guidelines* (4th ed.). Champaign, IL: Human Kinetics.

Eickhoff-Shemek, J.M., Herbert, D.L., & Connaughton, D.P. (2009). *Risk management for health/fitness professionals: Legal issues and strategies.* Philadelphia, PA: Wolters Kluwer/Lippincott Williams & Wilkins.

National Strength and Conditioning Association. (2017). *NSCA strength and conditioning professional standards and guidelines.* Available at: https://www.nsca.com/uploadedFiles/NSCA/Resources/PDF/Education/Tools_and_Resources/NSCA_strength_and_conditioning_professional_standards_and_guidelines.pdf

Riebe, D., Franklin, B.A., Thompson, P.D., Garber C.E., Whitfield, G.P., Magal, M., & Pescatello, L.S. (2015). Updating ACSM's recommendations for exercise preparticipation health screening. *Medicine & Science in Sports & and Exercise, 47,* 2473-2479. doi:10.1249/MSS.0000000000000664.

Springer, J.B., Eickhoff-Shemek, J.M., & Zuberbuehler, E.J. (2009). An investigation of pre- activity cardiovascular screening procedures in health/fitness facilities-Part II: Rationale for low adherence with national standards. *Preventive Cardiology, Fall,* 176-183.

Index

Note: The italicized *f* and *t* following page numbers refer to figures and tables, respectively.

About the Editor

Debra Rose, PhD, is a professor in the division of kinesiology and health science and director of the Center for Successful Aging at California State University at Fullerton. She also serves as codirector of the Fall Prevention Center of Excellence at the University of Southern California. Her primary research focus is on the enhancement of mobility, postural control, and the prevention of falls in later years.

Rose is nationally and internationally recognized for her work in assessment and programming for fall risk reduction. Her research in fall risk reduction in the elderly has been published in numerous peer-reviewed publications, including the Journal of the American Geriatric Society, Archives of Physical Medicine and Rehabilitation, Neurology Report, and the Journal of Aging and Physical Activity—where she also served as an editor in chief. She was an expert contributor to the Global Report on Falls Prevention in Older Age published by the World Health Organization in 2007.

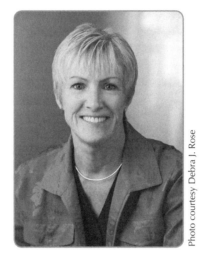

Photo courtesy Debra J. Rose

Rose is the creator of the innovative fall risk reduction program, FallProof, which was recognized by the Health Promotion Institute of the National Council on Aging (NCOA) in 2006 as a "Best Practice" program in health promotion. This program is currently being implemented in numerous community-based settings and retirement communities throughout the United States.

Rose was also the recipient of the 2013 Herbert A. DeVries Award for Distinguished Research on Aging from the Council on Aging and Adult Development, American Association for Physical Activity and Recreation. She is a fellow and past president of the National Academy of Kinesiology and former executive board member of the North American Society for the Psychology of Sport and Physical Activity.

Contributors

Judy Aprile, MS
California State University, Fullerton

Susie Dinan-Young, MS
Royal Free and University College London Medical School, United Kingdom

Helen Hawley-Hague, PhD
University of Manchester, United Kingdom

C. Jessie Jones, PhD
California State University, Fullerton

Abby C. King, PhD, FACSM
Stanford University, Palo Alto, California

Mary Ann Kluge, PhD
University of Colorado, Colorado Springs, Colorado

Priscilla MacRae, PhD
Pepperdine University, California

Janis Montague, MS
President, Whole Person Wellness International

Matthew Peterson, PhD
Wright State University, Ohio

Roberta Rikli, PhD, FACSM, FNAK
California State University, Fullerton

Joseph Signorile, PhD, FACSM
University of Miami, Coral Gables, Florida

Dawn Skelton, PhD
Glasgow Caledonian University, Scotland

Sara Wilcox, PhD, FNAK
University of South Carolina, Columbia

Kathleen Wilson, PhD
California State University, Fullerton

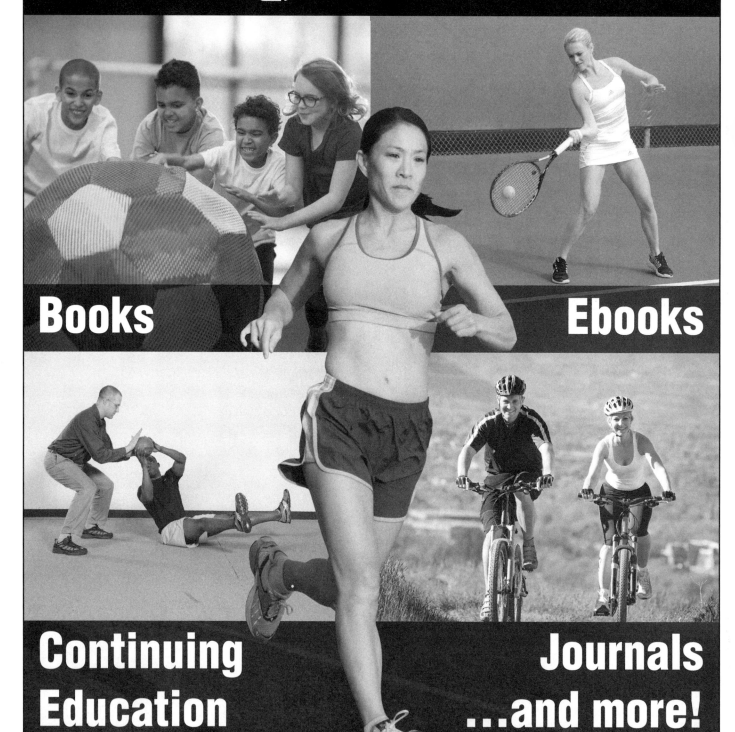